AF327942

A Practical Approach to Pediatric Infections

For Churchill Livingstone

Publisher: Lucy Gardner
Copy editor: Graham Wild
Indexer: Laurence Errington
Project Controller: Anita Sekhri

A Practical Approach to Pediatric Infections

David Isaacs
MB BChir MD MRCP FRACP
Head, Department of Immunology and Infectious Diseases,
Royal Alexandra Hospital for Children, Westmead, Sydney, Australia
Clinical Associate Professor, University of Sydney

E. Richard Moxon
MA MB BChir FRCP
Action Research Professor Paediatrics
University of Oxford, John Radcliffe Hospital, Oxford UK

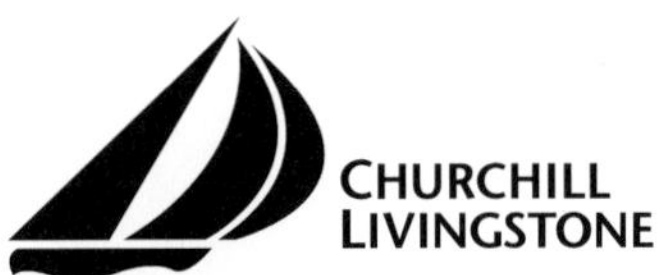

NEW YORK EDINBURGH LONDON MADRID MELBOURNE SAN FRANCISCO AND TOKYO 1996

CHURCHILL LIVINGSTONE
Medical Division of Pearson Professional Limited

Distributed in the United States of America by Churchill Livingstone Inc.,
650 Avenue of the Americas, New York, N.Y. 10011, and by associated
companies, branches and representatives throughout the world.

© Pearson Professional Limited 1996

All rights reserved. No part of this publication may be reproduced,
stored in a retrieval system, or transmitted in any form or by any means,
electronic, mechanical, photocopying, recording or otherwise, without
either the prior permission of the publishers (Churchill Livingstone,
Robert Stevenson House, 1-3 Baxterís Place, Leith Walk, Edinburgh, EH1
3AF), or a licence permitting restricted copying in the United Kingdom
issued by the Copyright Licensing Agency Ltd, 90 Tottenham Court
Road, London, W1P 9HE.

First Published 1996

ISBN 0443 051429

British Library Cataloguing in Publication Data
A catalogue record for this book is available from the British Library.

Library of Congress Cataloging in Publication Data
A catalog record for this book is available from the library of Congress.

Medical Knowledge is constantly changing. As new information
becomes available, changes in treatment, procedures, equipment and the
use of drugs become necessary. The editors/authors/contributors and
the publishers have, as far as it is possible, taken sure that the information
given in this text is accurate and up to date. However, readers are
strongly advised to confirm that the information, especially with regard
to drug usage, complies with the latest legislation and standards of
practice.

The
publisher's
policy is to use
**paper manufactured
from sustainable forest**

Printed in Hong Kong
SP/01

Contents

Contributors

I. Andrews MB BS FRACP
Department of Neurology, The Prince of Wales Children's Hospital, Randwick, NSW, Australia

F. Bell MB MRCP
Lecturer in Paediatric Infectious Diseases, Sheffield Children's Hospital, Sheffield, UK

M. Bellemore MB BS FRACS
Consultant Orthopaedic Surgeon, Royal Alexandra Hospital for Children, Westmead, Australia

R. Booy MB BS FRACP
Lecturer, Paediatric Infectious Diseases, St Mary's Hospital, London, UK

D. Brewster BA MD FRACP MPH
Associate Professor of Paediatrics, College of Medicine, University of Malawi, Malawi and Professor of Paediatrics, Royal Darwin Hospital, Darwin, NT, Australia

M. A. Burgess MD FRACP
Head, Australian Centre for Immunisation Research, Royal Alexandra Hospital for Children, Westmead and Clinical Associate Professor, University of Sydney, Australia

D. Candy MD FRCP
Professor of Child Health, Kings College School of Medicine and Dentistry, London, UK

A. Cameron BDS (Hons) MDSc FRACDS
Specialist and Senior Clinical Lecturer Consultant, Division of Paediatric Dentistry, Royal Alexandra Hospital for Children, Westmead, Australia

J. Craig MB FRACP NHMRC
Fellow in Paediatric Nephrology, Royal Alexandra Hospital for Children, Westmead, Sydney, Australia

E. G. Davies MB FRCP
Consultant Immunologist and Senior Lecturer in Child Health, St. George's Hospital Medical School, London, UK

S. Dobson MD MRCP (UK) FRCPC
Assistant Professor, Division of Pediatric Infectious Diseases, British Columbia Children's Hospital, Vancouver, British Columbia, Canada

C. Donaldson MBBS FRACS FRACO
Fellow in Ophthalmology, Hospital for Sick Children, Toronto, Canada

G. M. Eagles MB FRCPA
Head, Department of Microbiology, Royal Alexandra Hospital for Children, Westmead, Australia

M. J. Ferson MB BS MPH FRACP FAF PHM
Director, Public Health Unit, Eastern Sydney Area Health Service, NSW, Australia

A. Finn MD MRCP
Consultant in Infectious Diseases, Sheffield Children's Hospital, Sheffield, UK

J. M. Forrest MD
Research Fellow, Australian Centre for Immunisation Research, Royal Alexandra Hospital for Children, Westmead, Australia

P. Grattan-Smith MB FRACP
Consultant Neurologist, Royal Alexandra Hospital for Children, Westmead, Australia

P. R. Gully MD FRCP
Department of Pediatrics, University of Ottawa, Children's Hospital of Eastern Ontario, Canada

W. Hanekom MD
Department of Pediatrics, Northwestern University Medical School, USA

M. A. Herbert MB MRCP
Fellow in Paediatrics, Oxford Vaccine Group, John Radcliffe Hospital, Oxford, UK

P. H. Hewson MD FRACP
Senior Lecturer, Department of Paediatrics, University of Melbourne, Australia

D. Isaacs MD MRCP FRACP
Head, Department of Immunology and Infectious Diseases, Royal Alexandra Hospital for Children, Westmead, Sydney, Australia

A. Kakakios MB BS FRACP
Staff Specialist in Paediatric Immunology and Allergy, Royal Alexandra
Hospital for Children, Westmead, Australia

C. R. Kennedy MD FRCP
Consultant in Paediatric Neurology, Southampton General Hospital,
Southampton, UK

H. Kilham MB BS FRACP
Head, Subdivision of General Medicine, Physician, Respiratory
Department, Royal Alexandra Hospital for Children, Westmead, Australia

N. Klein BSc MB BS MRCP PhD
Consultant and Senior Lecturer in Infectious Diseases, Hospital for Sick
Children, London, UK

J. Knight MB FRACP
Renal Physician and Head of Research and Development, Royal
Alexandra Hospital for Children, Westmead, Australia

J. S. Kroll MA FRCP
Professor of Paediatrics and Molecular Infectious Diseases, St Mary's
Hospital Medical School, Imperial College of Science, Technology and
Medicine, London, UK

M. Levin PhD FRCP
Professor of Paediatrics, St Marys Hospital Medical School, London

N. E. Macdonald BSc MSc MD FRCP(C)
Professor of Pediatrics and Microbiology, University of Ottawa,
Children's Hospital of Eastern Ontario, Canada

P. Malleson MB BS MRCP (UK) FRCPC
Associate Professor, Department of Pediatrics, University of British
Columbia, Vancouver, Canada

F. Martin MBBS FRACS FRACO
Head, Department of Ophthalmology, Royal Alexandra Hospital for
Children, Westmead, Sydney, Australia

E. D. McIntosh MB BS MPH FAFPHM FRACP
Royal Alexandra Hospital for Children, Westmead, Sydney, Australia

P. McIntyre MB PhD FRACP FAFPHM
Senior Staff Specialist, Paediatric Infectious Diseases, Royal Alexandra
Hospital for Children, Westmead, Sydney, Australia

C. Mellis MB BS MPH FRACP
Consultant Chest Physician, Royal Alexandra Hospital for Children, Westmead and Clinical Associate Professor, University of Sydney, Australia

J. Mertsola MD Dr Sc M
Assistant Professor, Department of Paediatrics, Turku University Hospital, Turku, Finland

E. R. Moxon MA MB BChir FRCP
Action Research Professor, Paediatrician, University of Oxford, John Radcliffe Hospital, Oxford, UK

S. Nadel MB MRCP
Research Fellow, Department of Paediatric Infectious Diseases, St. Mary's Hospital Medical School, London, UK

C. R. J. C. Newton MD MRCP
Lecturer in Department of Paediatrics, University of Oxford, Oxford UK

R. A. Ouvrier MD FRACP
Head, Department of Neurology, Royal Alexandra Hospital for Children, Westmead and Clinical Associate Professor, University of Sydney, Australia

E. Pichichero MD
Professor of Pediatrics and Medicine, University of Rochester Medical Center, Rochester, New York, USA

A. Putto-Laurilla MD
Division of Infectious Diseases, Department of Paediatrics, Turku University Hospital, Turku, Finland

M. Rogers MB BS FACD
Head, Department of Dermatology, Royal Alexandra Hospital for Children, Westmead, Sydney, Australia

P. Roy MB BS BSc (Med) FRACP
Head, Department of Nephrology, Royal Alexandra Hospital for Children, Westmead, Sydney, Australia

O. Ruuskanen MD
Chief, Division of Infectious Diseases, Department of Paediatrics, Turku University Hospital, Turku, Finland

S. T. Shulman MD
Professor of Pediatrics and Associate Dean for Faculty Affairs, Northwestern University Medical School, USA

J. Smith MBBS FRACS FRACO
Staff Specialist in Ophthalmology, Royal Alexandra Hospital for Children, Westmead, Australia

M. C. Steinhoff MD
Division of Anesthesiology and Critical Care Medicine, John Hopkins, Baltimore, Maryland, USA

M. Tarlow MB FRCP
Senior Lecturer in Paediatrics, Birmingham, Heartlands Hospital, UK

A. Thomson MD FRCP
Consultant Paediatrician in Respiratory Diseases, John Radcliffe Hospital, Oxford, UK

G. Tudor Williams MB MRCP
Senior Lecturer, Paediatric Infectious Diseases, St. Mary's Hospital Medical School, London, UK

E. R. Wald MD
Professor of Pediatrics, University of Pittsburgh School of Medicine, Pittsburgh, Pennsylvania, USA

D. W. Webb MD MRCP
Consultant Paediatric Neurologist, Royal Belfast Children's Hospital, Belfast, Northern Ireland

R. Widmer MDSc FRACDS
Head of Paediatric Dentistry, Westmead Hospital and Royal Alexandra Hospital for Children, Sydney and Adjunct Associate Professor, University of Sydney

Foreword

Diagnosis, management and prevention of infectious diseases comprise greater than 60% of a pediatrician's practice. In an era of extensive international travel and rapid communication the physician is faced with a bewildering array of exotic infectious disease issues, some in the form of advice for prophylaxis during trips abroad and others involving treatment of infections that have heretofore been considered textbook curiosities. Additionally, some organisms have regained their virulence in causing life-threatening disease (i.e. group A streptococci) and new agents such as *Borrelia burgdorferi* and *Bartonella henselae* have been identified as the cause of Lyme disease and cat scratch infection, respectively.

The physician is fortunate to have a large number of antimicrobial agents available for therapy of most infections of infants and children. This turns out, however, to be a mixed blessing. Despite an extensive armamentarium from which to select treatments, these agents are excessively used, often inappropriately and for prolonged periods in a vain attempt to prevent superinfection. This worldwide pattern of abuse has resulted in emergence of resistant organisms, especially Gram positive coccal pathogens that can be difficult or impossible to treat.

These medical dilemmas are not rare events and soon will face every physician on a regular basis. The struggle to keep abreast of these changing events is challenging, especially in an era of multiple new texts, journals, newsletters, meetings and mednet. Thus, it is refreshing to encounter a textbook designed especially for the harried physician and busy student, resident and fellow.

This text by Professors Isaacs and Moxon provides practical, current information about most pediatric infectious diseases. The format is user-friendly and specific questions about diagnosis and management of infections are easy to locate and to assimilate quickly. The authors, internationally recognized experts in the field, have included many interesting chapters not regularly found in textbooks on infectious diseases. For example, in the chapter on "Oral and Facial Infections", the authors provide useful information on management of odontogenic infections, recurrent gingival disease and ulceration and chronic apthous disease. There is a section on "Cough" (Chapter 12) which organizes the causes of cough by frequency and age of occurrence as well as by pattern and nature of the cough. There is an interesting chapter devoted to "Viral-induced Asthma" or wheezy bronchitis that describes briefly the epidemiology, pathogenesis and management of children who wheeze. There is a marvelous chapter on "The Child with Paralysis or Weakness" in which a table outlines the clinical findings that assist the physician in localizing the putative site in the central nervous system. There are sections on "Daycare" and on "Recurrent Infections" and a unique chapter on "Infections in Travellers". The latter is a handy review of recommended immunizations and supplies that every traveller should have, depending on the destination, as well as a reference for common infections that might be encountered and how they can be avoided or treated.

For the 59 chapters in their text Professors Issacs and Moxon selected authors who had extensive clinical experience that could be imparted in a simple and practical way. The book will certainly remain in a handy place on my shelf for convenient reference.

George H. McCraken
Professor of Pediatrics
Dallas, Texas, USA

Preface

Children do not present to a doctor with a disease, such as bacterial meningitis, but with symptoms and signs, such as fever, vomiting and neck stiffness. It is for the doctor to interpret the significance of constellations of symptoms, perform a physical examination, order appropriate tests and initiate appropriate therapy. The doctor does this using scientific information and training, but also on the basis of clinical experience. This is the art of medicine. The art of medicine is difficult to teach, but is the essence of good clinical practice.

The aim of this book is for experts in paediatric infectious diseases, from three continents, North America, Australia and Europe, to present an approach to their specialist area, which concentrates on practical aspects of diagnosis and management, based on personal experience. Paediatric infectious diseases is a rapidly emerging sub-speciality and an extremely exciting one. We hope this book conveys something of the art of paediatric infectious diseases.

Acknowledgements

We should like to thank the many colleagues who have been instrumental in helping us to develop our philosophy of medicine, and in particular, paediatric infectious diseases.

Special thanks to Dr Henry Kilham for his illustrations, to Pixie Maloney for medical photography, and to our secretaries, Francine Sanhard and Dorian Watson for their organisation.

Finally, thanks to our long-suffering wives, Carmel and Marianne.

David Isaacs and E. Richard Moxon

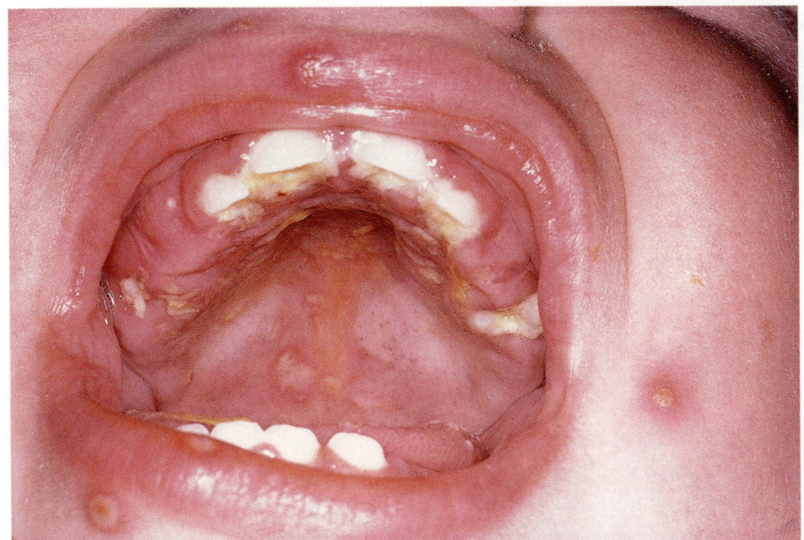

Fig. 1A.6.4 Herpetic gingivostomatitis. (see p. 57).

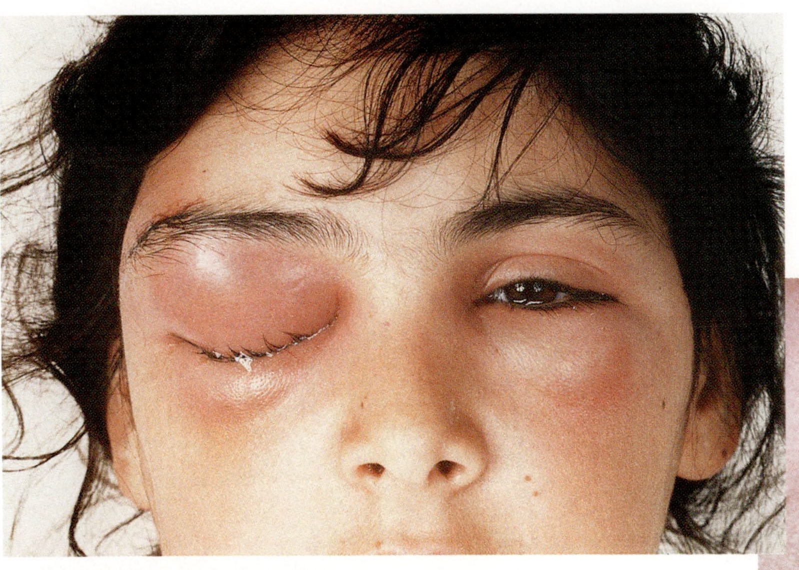

Fig. 1A.6.8 Periorbital cellulitis due to *Haemophilus influenzae* type b. (see p. 63 and p. 362).

Fig. 1A.7.2 White exudate from parotoid duct (see p. 71).

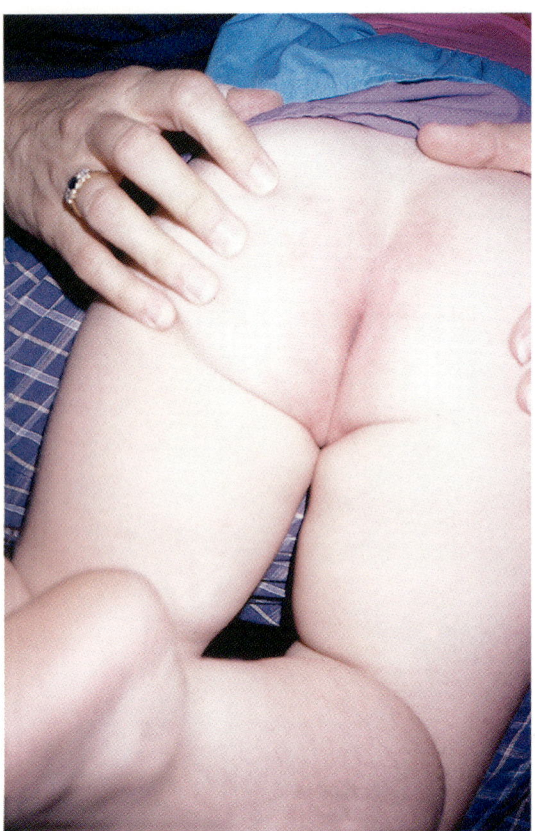

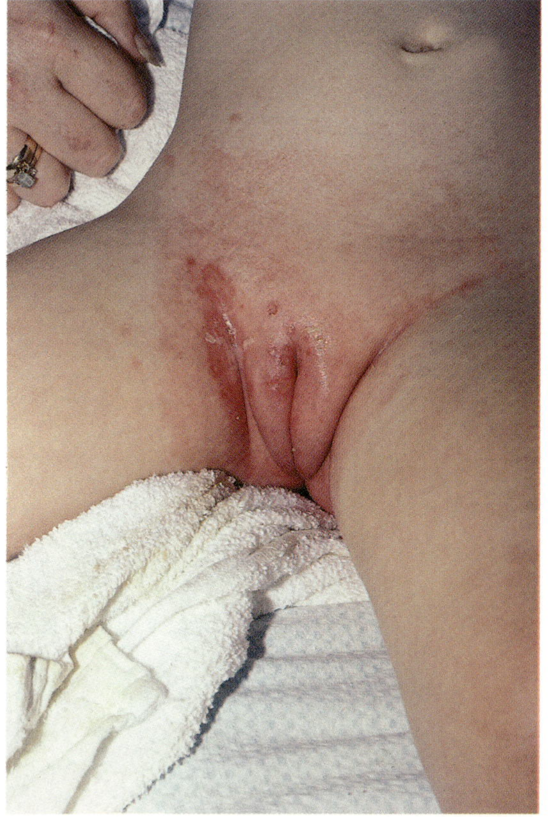

Fig. 5.1.1 Group A streptococcal vulvovaginitis. (see p. 248).

Fig. 5.1.2 Primary herpes simplex virus vulvovaginitis. Note ulcerated lesions. (see p. 249).

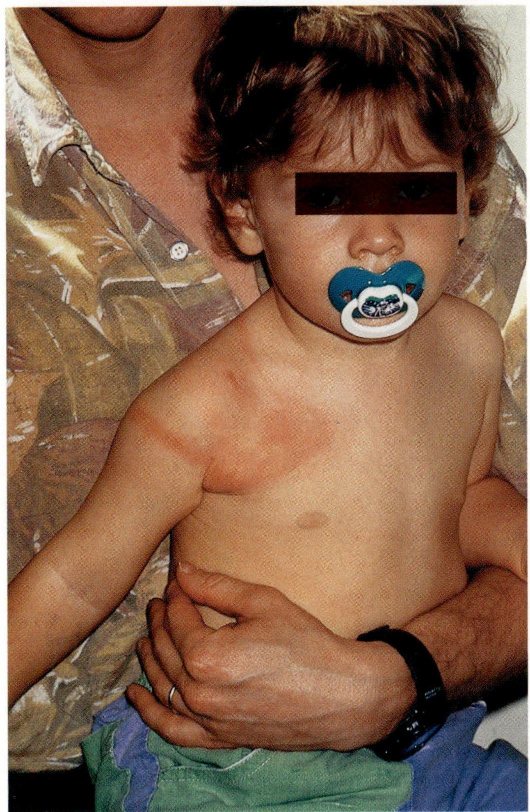

Fig. 8.1.1 Lyme disease. Erythema migrans with central clearing. (see p. 348).

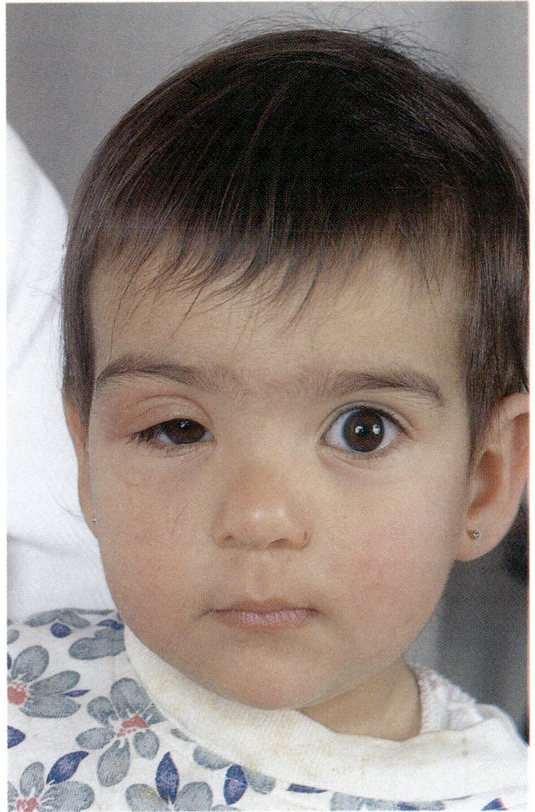

Fig. 9.1.1 Preseptal cellulitis. (see p. 360).

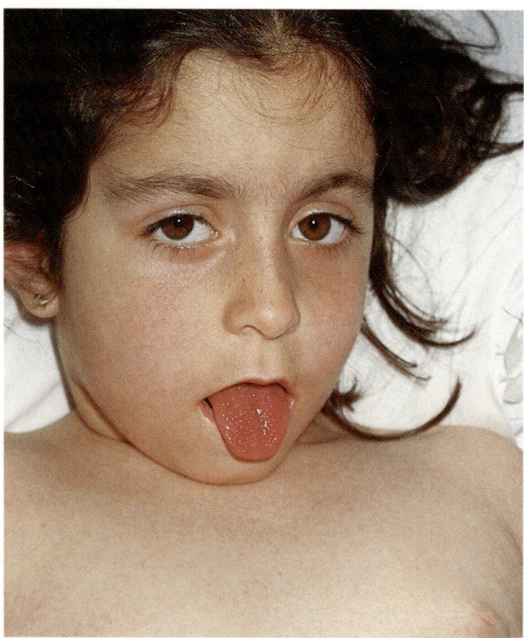

Fig. 10.1.1 This child presented with fever, sore throat and rash. A throat swab grew group A streptococcus. The rash of 'scarlatina' does not show all the features of classical scarlet fever. Note the 'strawberry tongue'. (see p. 372).

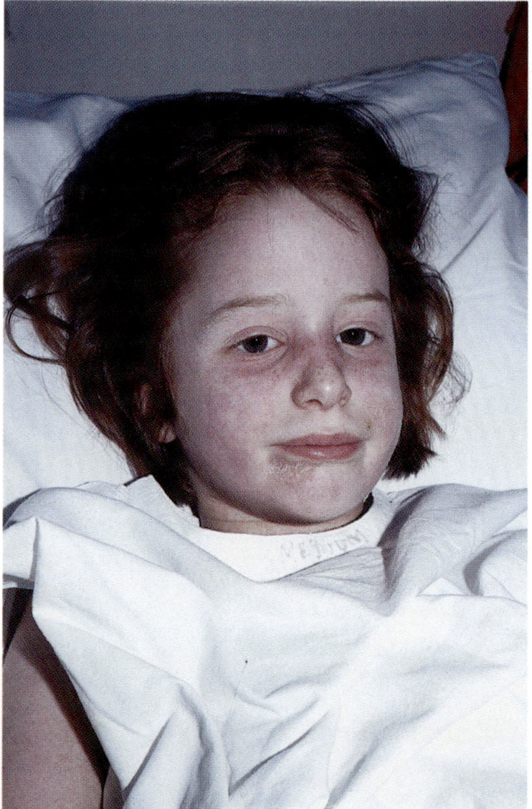

Fig. 10.1.2 Scarlet fever. Diffuse erythroderma with circumoral pallor. (see p. 373).

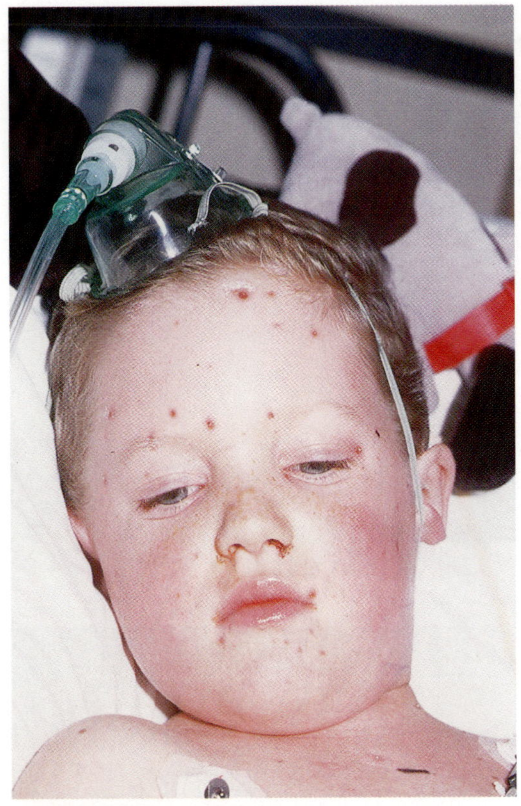

Fig. 10.1.3 Scarlet fever complicating chickenpox. Chickenpox lesions on forehead and rash with circumoral pallor. (see p. 374).

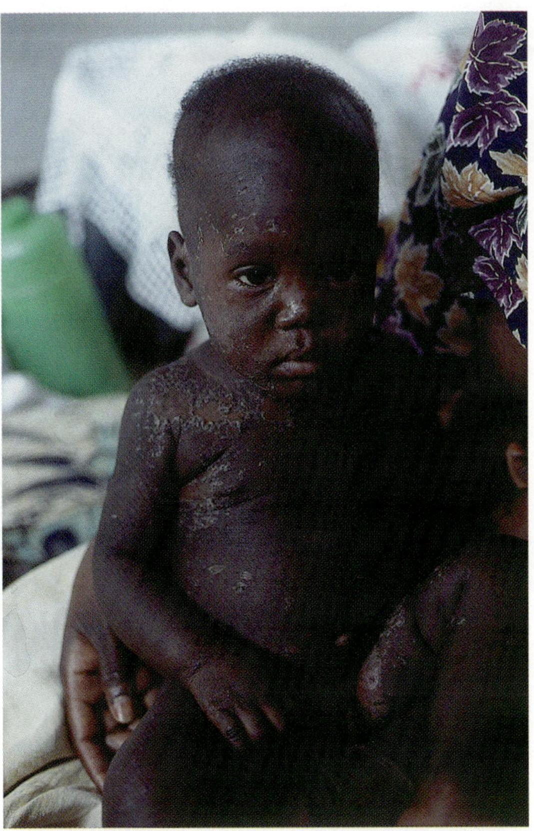

Fig. 10.1.4 (b) Measles in a black child: desquamating rash. (see p. 376)

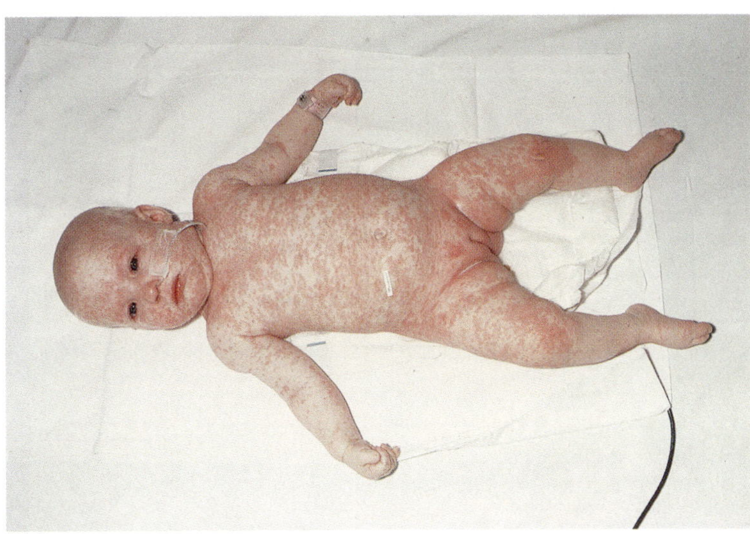

Fig. 10.1.4 (a) Maculopapular rash, confluent in places, of measles. (see p. 376)

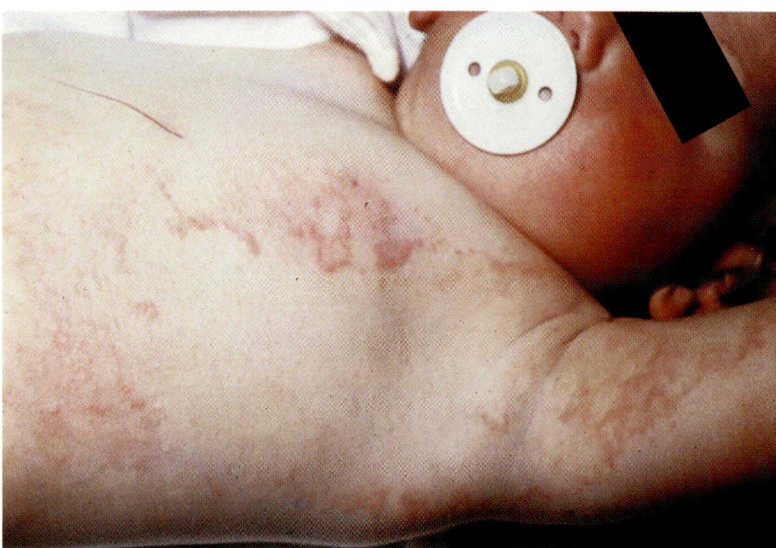

Fig. 10.1.5 Fifth disease. Slapped cheek appearance and lacy rash on trunk. (see p. 379).

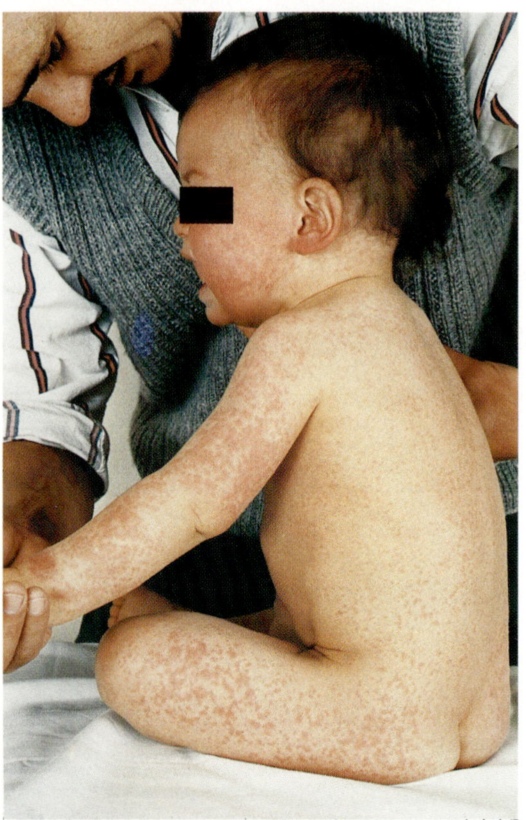

Fig. 10.1.6 Roseola infantum exanthem subitum or sixth disease. Morbilliform rash. (see p. 380).

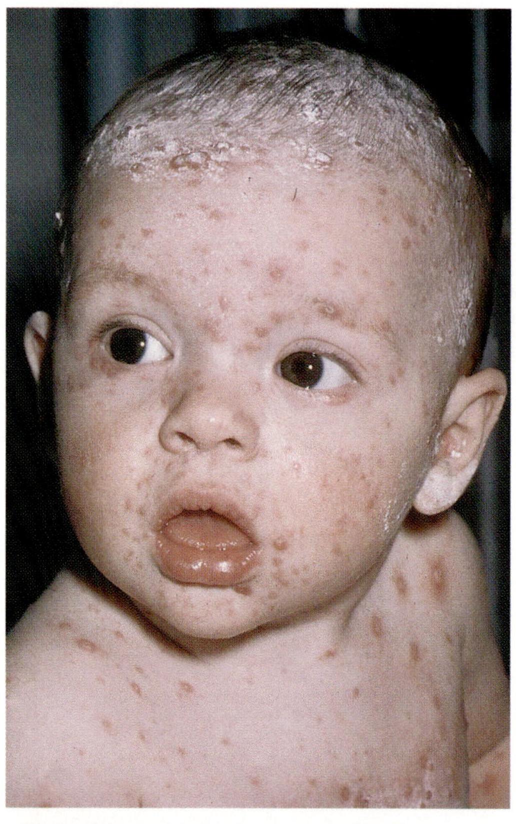

Fig. 10.1.7 Chickenpox. Vesicular lesions at different stages of development. White scalp due to calamine lotion to reduce itching. (see p. 382).

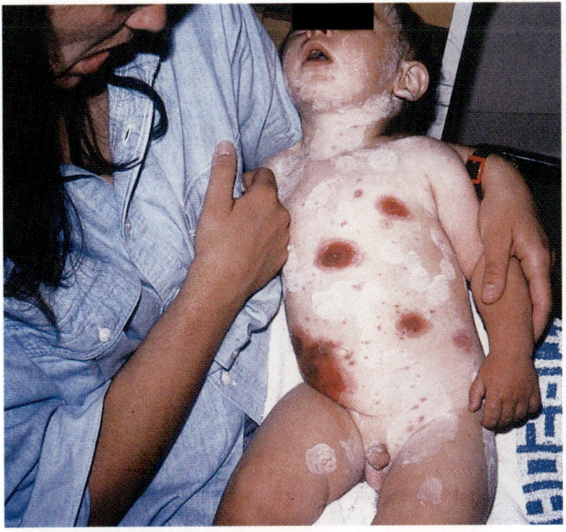

Fig. 10.1.8 Bullous varicella. Alarming appearance caused by staphylococcal superinfection of chickenpox. (see p. 383).

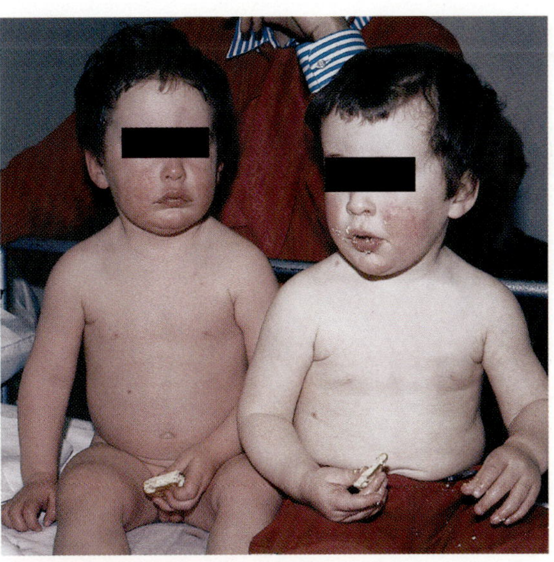

Fig. 10.1.9 Varicella and ampicillin. Ampicillin can cause a diffuse rash, here seen in one of twins with chickenpox, in VZV as well as EBV infections. (see p. 383).

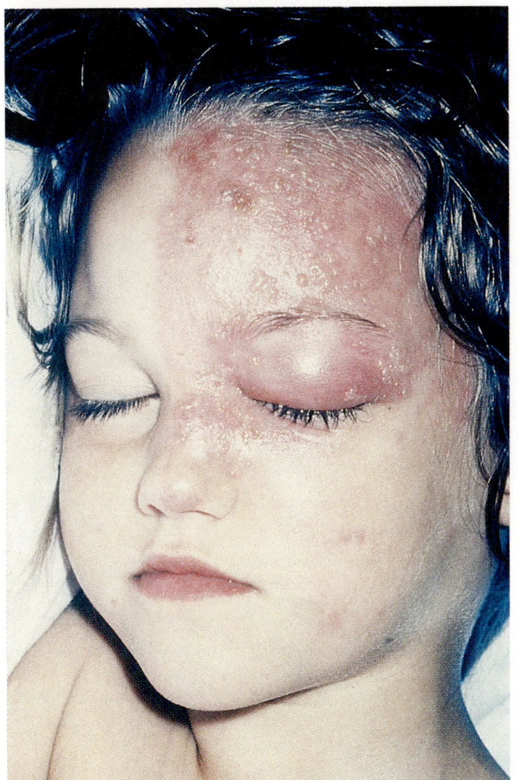

Fig. 10.1.10 Ophthalmic zoster: Herpes zoster of the ophthalmic division of the trigeminal nerve. (see p. 384).

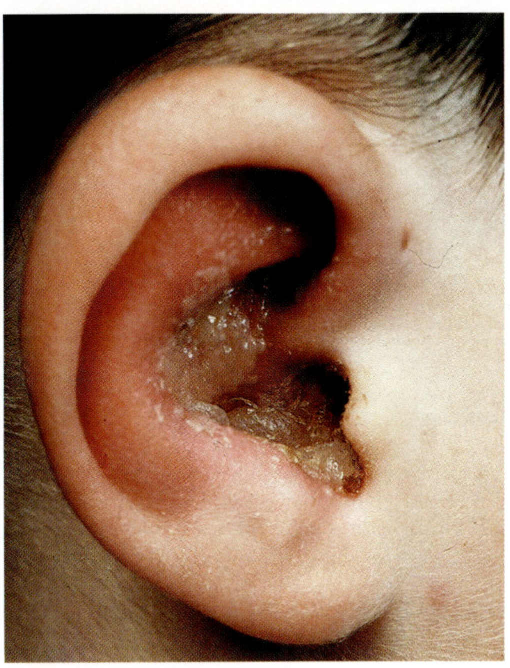

Fig. 10.1.11 Ramsay-Hunt syndrome: herpes zoster of the geniculate ganglion causing eruption on the pinna. (see p. 385).

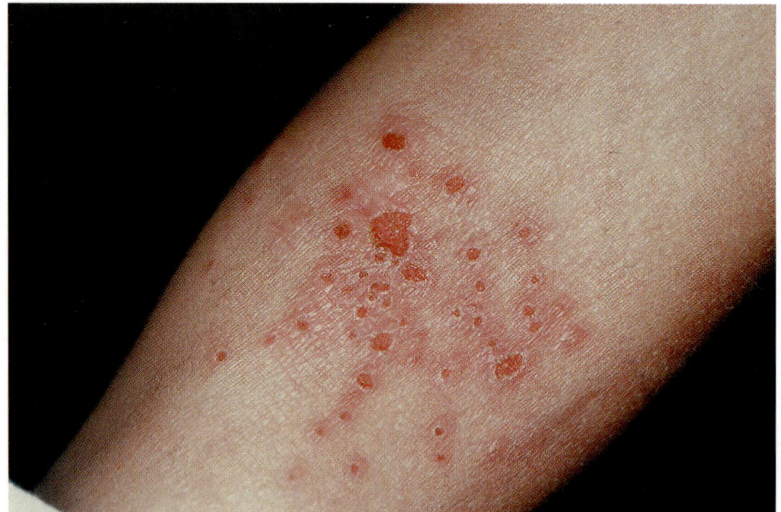

Fig. 10.2.1 Papular acro-located syndrome (PALS). (see p. 388).

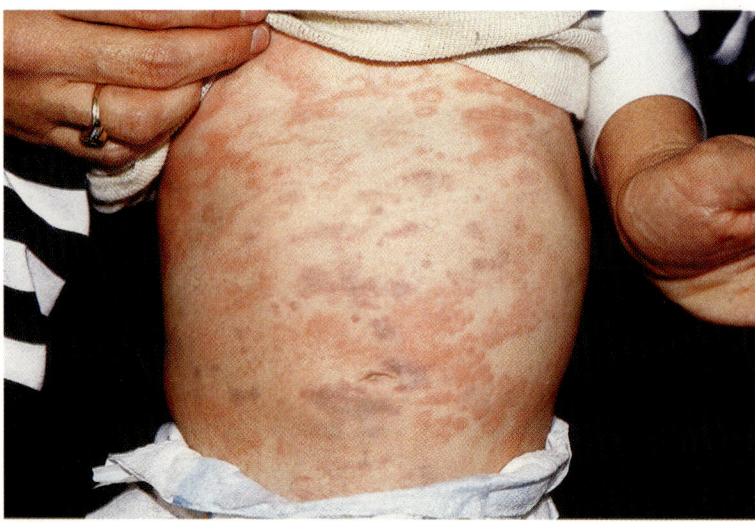

Fig. 10.2.2 Purple urticaria. Urticarial rash with purpura in some lesions; common and benign. (see p. 388).

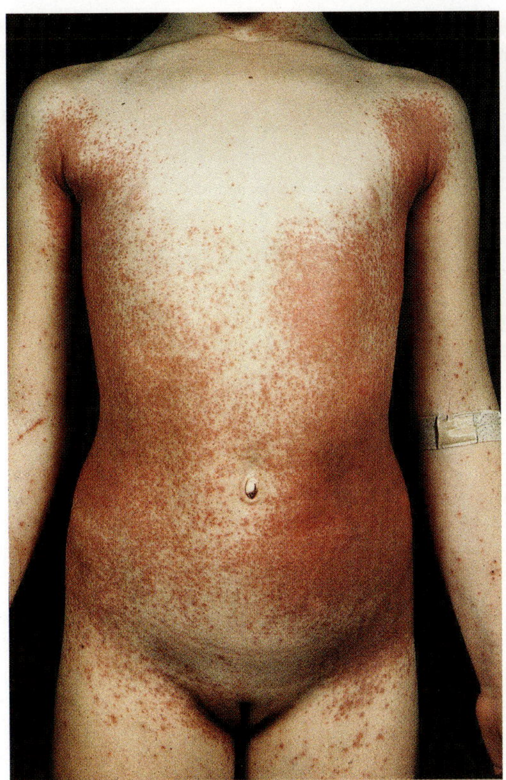

Fig. 10.2.6 Enterovirus exanthem. Dramatic rash, purpuric in places. (see p. 390).

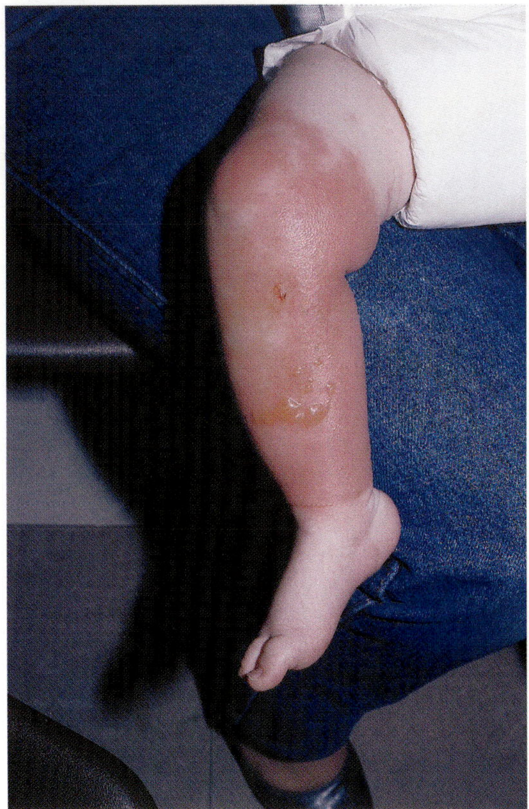

Fig. 10.3.3 Erysipelas. Group A streptococcal cellulitis with sharp leading edge. (see p. 395).

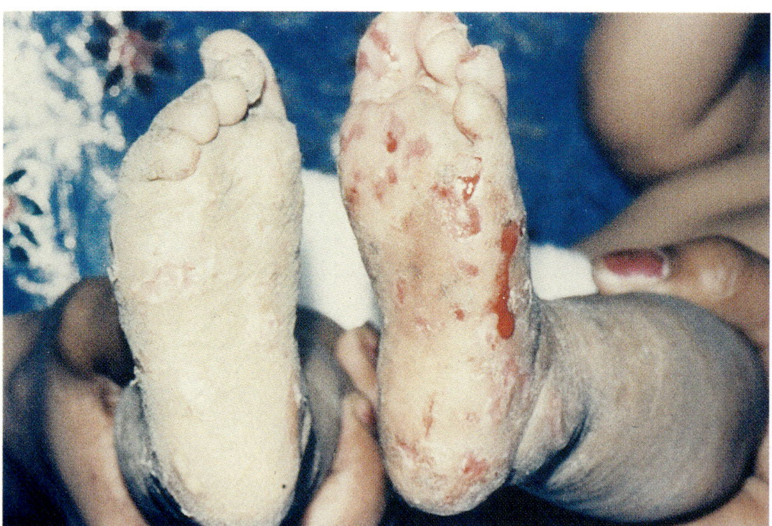

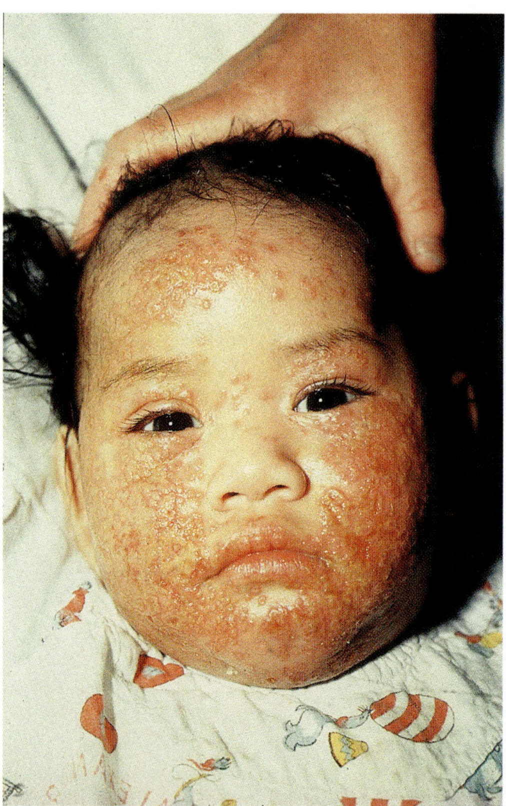

Fig. 10.3.15   Eczema herpeticum (Kaposi's varicelliform eruption). Vesicular and umbilicated lesions. Note sparing of nose. (see p. 405).

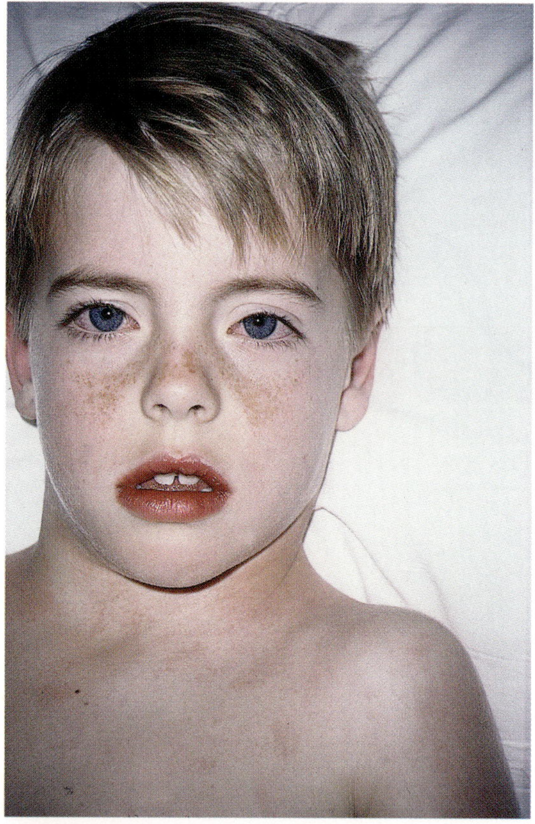

Fig. 11.2.1   Child with Kawasaki disease. Note red, cracked lips ("lipstick sign") and bilateral conjunctivitis (see p. 418).

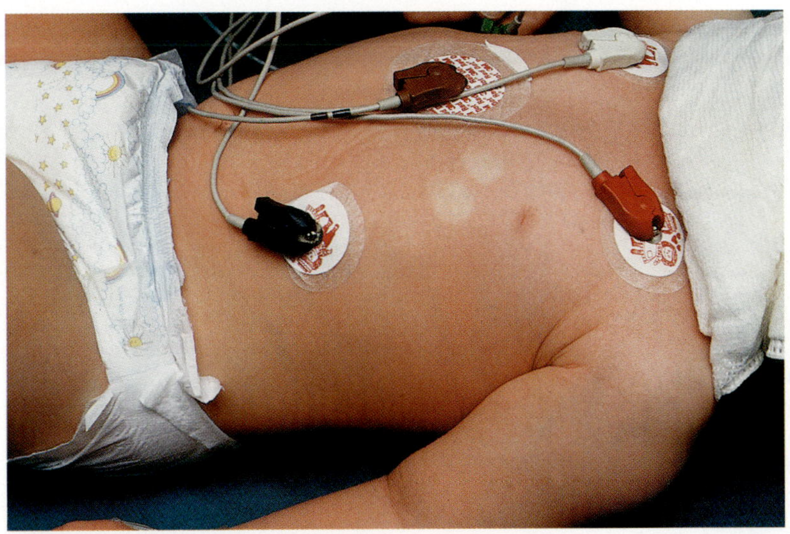

Fig. 11.3.4 Toxic shock syndrome. Intense erythema with prolonged blanching on fingertip pressure. (see p. 439).

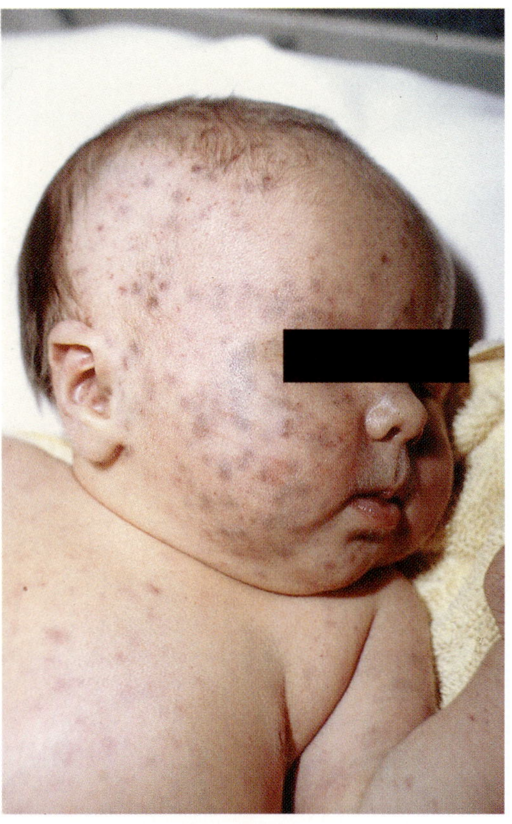

Fig. 12.1.1 Rash of congenital infection. Appearance is due to areas of extramedullary erythropoiesis in skin, sometimes referred to as blueberry muffin. Suggestive of rubella or toxoplasmosis. (see p. 454).

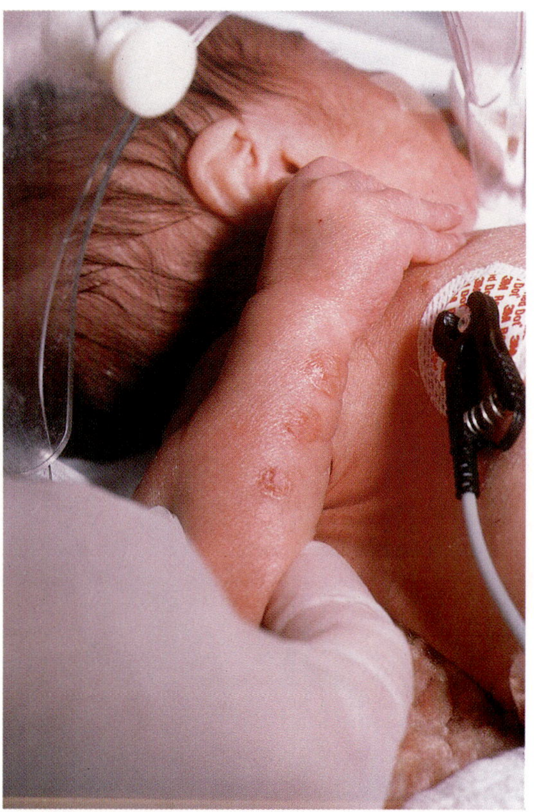

Fig. 12.1.11 Congenital syphilis. Baby born with blistering lesions, which turn brown as they heal. (see p. 467).

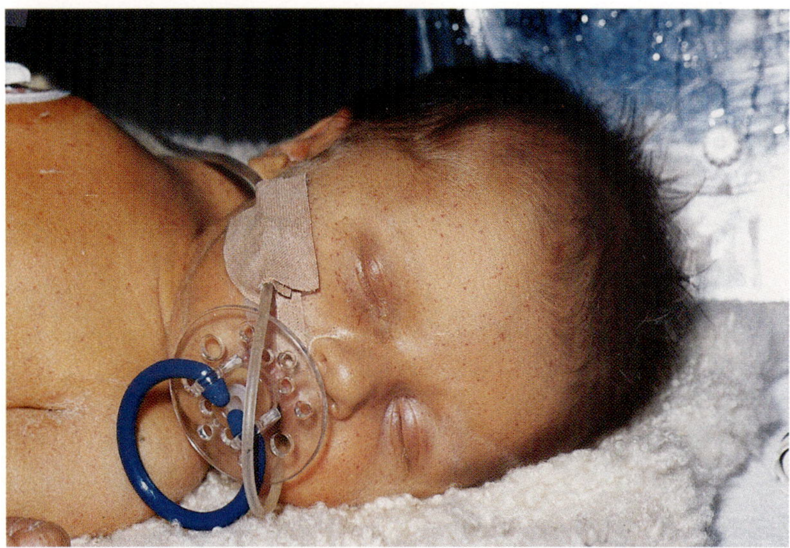

Fig. 12.1.2 Congenital CMV infection, age 2 days. Jaundice and fine petechial rash. (see p. 455)

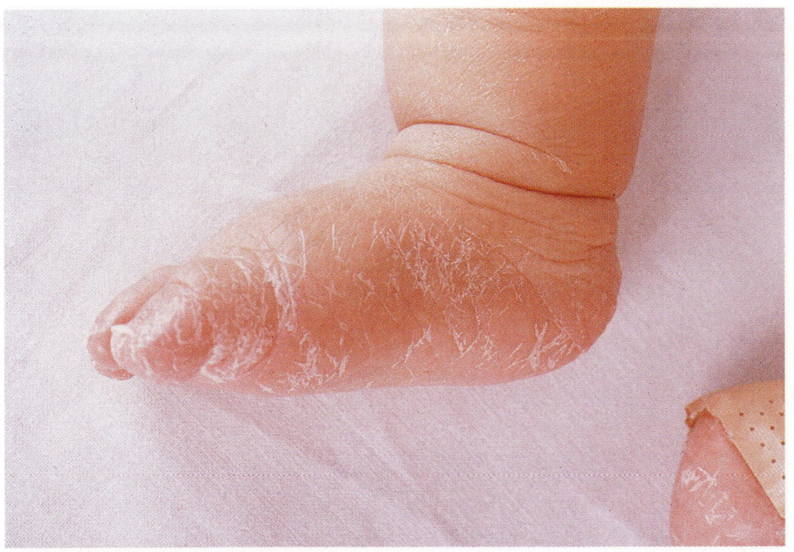

Fig. 12.1.12 Congenital syphilis. Late presentation (age 4 months) with anaemia, oedema, hepatosplenomegaly and this appearance of red, dry feet. (see p. 468).

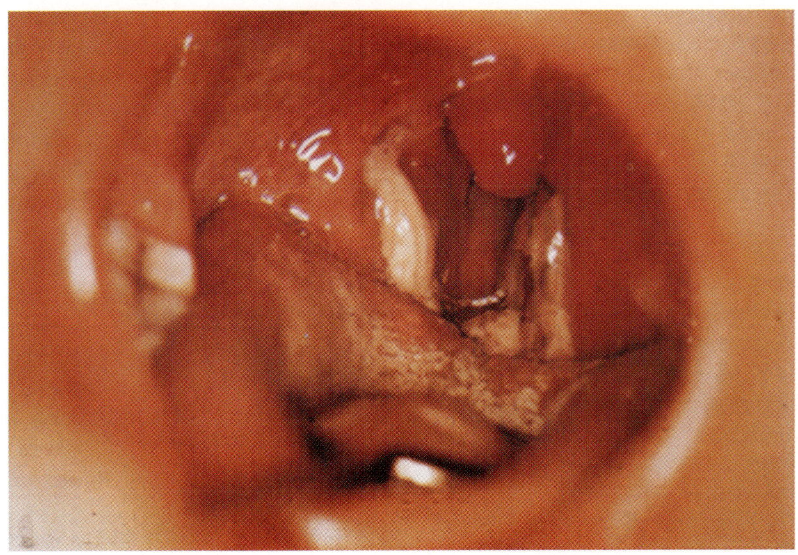

Fig. 18.1.1 Diphtheria. Adherent grey membrane. (see p. 550).

UPPER RESPIRATORY TRACT INFECTIONS

1A.1 Infections of the upper respiratory tract

INTRODUCTION

Infections of the upper respiratory tract are of major importance for a number of reasons. Firstly they are extremely common, causing substantial paediatric morbidity in terms of minor illness, visits to doctors, days of school lost, parental work-days lost, and general family disruption. Secondly, infection may spread to involve the lower respiratory tract, and lower respiratory tract infections, as will be discussed in Chapter 1B, are one of the leading causes of child mortality in the world. Thirdly, upper respiratory infections may predispose to a number of infectious and para-infectious conditions: they are a common antecedent of bacterial meningitis, acute rheumatic fever, Henoch–Schönlein purpura and sudden infant death syndrome, among many other conditions. Finally, the same viruses that cause upper respiratory infections in one child or adult may cause severe disease in another child due to younger age and no prior exposure (such as respiratory syncytial virus (RSV), bronchiolitis and parainfluenza virus infection) or due to an altered response to the virus (e.g. most respiratory viruses can precipitate wheezing in predisposed children).

CLINICAL FEATURES

Donald Court,[1] in his important paper defining categories of acute respiratory infections, described an 'upper respiratory infection syndrome', in which affected children are very frequently febrile with some or all of red pharynx, red tonsils with or without exudate, red ear drums, cough and nasal discharge. To this description can be added cervical lymphadenopathy. Children with such infections are usually described as having upper respiratory tract infections or URTIs. If one symptom or sign predominates, then this conventionally becomes the diagnosis, e.g. intense redness of the pharynx is called pharyngitis; or marked redness of the ear drum is acute otitis media.

AETIOLOGY

Upper respiratory tract infections are caused by viruses.[2] Experimental studies using adult volunteers have shown that filtered nasal secretions from children with URTIs will transmit infection. It has been consistently shown that oral antibiotics do not shorten the duration of upper respiratory infections, nor do they prevent their complications.[3] Despite this, antibiotics are frequently prescribed for children with URTIs, both in developed and developing countries.

Even though there is strong clinical, experimental and circumstantial evidence that URTIs are caused exclusively by viruses, the rate of virus isolation in tissue cultures of nasal secretions from children with URTIs is only 30–40% in the most careful studies. There are a number of reasons. The virus isolation rate is highly dependent on the techniques employed. Optimum specimens are respiratory secretions containing cells; nasopharyngeal secretions obtained by suction at the back of the nasal cavity are better than nose or throat swabs alone.[2] If throat swabs are the specimen used, then moderately vigorous swabbing of the pharynx is necessary to dislodge cells, since these are the site of viral replication. Once the specimens are obtained, they should ideally be inoculated direct into tissue culture. If, as is usually the case, the specimens need transporting, this should be done by placing the secretions in viral transport medium and on melting ice if for short periods of time, or frozen on dry ice for long periods. However, the process of freezing can itself reduce the viability of some viruses. Viruses may grow poorly or not at all in conventional tissue culture.

Rhinoviruses grow best on Ohio Hela cells, while coronaviruses will usually grow only in tracheal organ cultures, and are best detected by antigen detection using enzyme-linked immunosorbent assay (ELISA) tests. When the problem of ideal specimen collection is combined with the fastidiousness of growth of some respiratory viruses in tissue culture, and the fact that we have not yet identified all viruses responsible for URTIs, it becomes clear why virus isolation rates might be only 30–40% from children with definite viral infection. In one study,[4] vigorous attempts were made to isolate viruses from nasal washings taken from 38 adults with naturally acquired colds. Viruses were cultured from 25 (66%). Secretions from the remaining 13 adults were inoculated into volunteers, causing colds in 5, even though no virus could be detected. Respiratory viruses implicated in causing URTIs and their approximate relative frequency are shown in Table 1A.1.1.

EPIDEMIOLOGY

Upper respiratory infections are a normal part of childhood, like tears and tantrums. Children are relatively protected in the first 6 months of life, by transplacentally acquired IgG antibody, and respiratory infections then are uncommon. The peak incidence of respiratory infections is between 6 months and 5 years of age, and the most critical determinant of the incidence is exposure. In Table 1A.1.2, it can be seen that the peak incidence was between 1 and 4 years of age in studies of preschool children at home, but when children were studied in a day care centre, often being placed there from 6 weeks of age, the peak incidence was in the first year of life.[5-7] Dingle[6] showed that preschool children attending day care

Table 1A.1.1 Relative frequency of virus isolation in acute respiratory infections of childhood

Infection	Adeno	Entero	Corona	Influenza	Para influenza	Rhino viruses	RSV	EBV	Herpes simplex	CMV	Reoviruses	Measles
Common cold	+	++	+++	+	+	++++	+				+	
URTI	+	++	+++	+	+	++++	+					
Sinusitis	+			+	+	+						
Pharyngitis	++++	++	++	++	++	+	+	+++	++	+	+	++
Otitis media	++	+	+	+	+	+++	++		+	++		++
Croup	++	+	+	+++	++++	+	++		+			+
Bronchiolitis		+		+	++	+	++++					
Bronchitis	+	+	++	++	+++	++++	++++					++
Pneumonia	++	+	+	+	++	+++	++++		+	+		++

Table 1A.1.2 Mean number of upper respiratory infections per child per year observed in different studies

Study	Location of child	Age (years)				
		0–1	1–2	2–3	3–4	4–5
North Carolina[5]	Day care	9.6	8.6	8.1	7.2	7.6
Cleveland[6]	Home	6.9	8.3	8.5	8.6	8.1
Seattle[7]	Home	4.4	4.9	4.8	4.8	4.8

or kindergarten had as many as 12 infections per year, while preschool children at home had more infections if they had an older sibling at school (Figs 1A.1.1 and 1A.1.2). This theme of older siblings bringing home infections, despite having no or minimal symptoms themselves, is repeated in many studies, although isolation of viruses from the nasopharynx of asymptomatic children is very unusual. It is interesting to speculate that school children might be bringing home infected respiratory secretions on their hands, but this has not been studied. Although

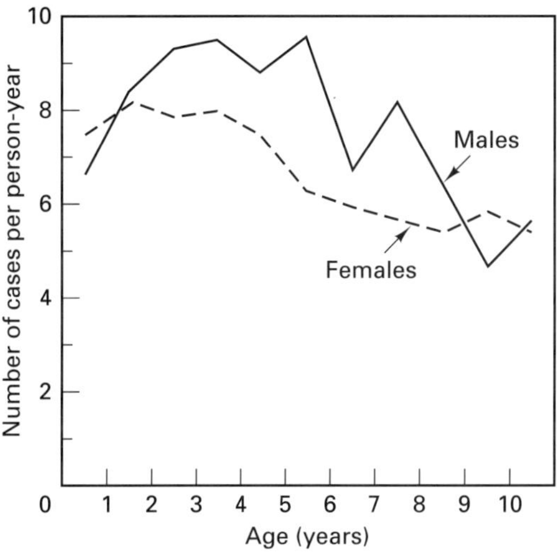

Fig. 1A.1.1 Incidence of common respiratory disease among children by age and sex. (From Dingle et al.[6])

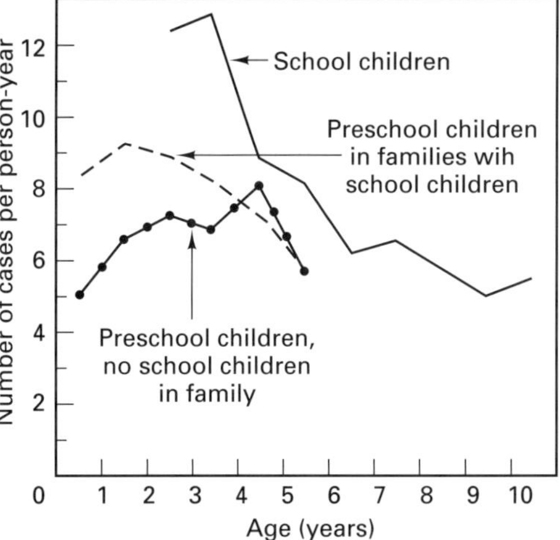

Fig. 1A.1.2 Incidence of common respiratory disease by school status. (From Dingle et al.[6])

the peak incidence of respiratory infections is preschool, there is a secondary but lesser peak at school entry, presumably due to exposure to new organisms. Boys generally experience somewhat more infections than girls (Fig. 1A.1.1).

Other factors which have been shown to result in an increase in the observed incidence of respiratory infections are passive exposure to tobacco smoke, and an urban as opposed to a rural environment, implying that air pollution makes children more susceptible to infection, exacerbates symptoms of respiratory virus infection, or causes respiratory symptoms that mimic infection. Breast-feeding is protective against respiratory virus infections. Boyce et al[8] found that children who had experienced recent stressful life events had longer respiratory illnesses, although no more frequent, than children without such stress. In contrast, Cohen et al[9] found a linear correlation between a score of stress and susceptibility to respiratory virus infection in adult volunteers, although no tendency to increased severity. The most stressed were twice as likely to catch an experimental cold as the least stressed.

Children in day care not only have more respiratory infections than those at home, but the infections last longer.[10] On average, infections last about 7–9 days, but more than 13% of children aged 2–3 years in day care had infections lasting over 15 days. Respiratory infections are commoner in winter in temperate climates and in the rainy season in the tropics.

Clearly, when children are having six to eight infections per year lasting 7–9 days, it can seem, particularly in winter, that they are always ill. For the parents of children in day care, whose children are excluded while symptomatic, this perception is reinforced by having to find alternative means of caring for the child.

PATHOPHYSIOLOGY

The pathophysiology of upper respiratory infections has been studied mainly in adult volunteers inoculated experimentally with respiratory viruses. Virus replicates in the nasal and pharyngeal epithelium, causing symptoms after 2–3 days, coinciding with maximum viral shedding. Submucosal oedema and shedding of ciliated cells may occur, with maximal epithelial damage at 5 days, and regeneration over the next 10 days. Often there is relatively little damage to the nasal epithelium, and it is thought that the host response contributes significantly to the symptoms of upper respiratory infections. Concentrations of kinins, particularly bradykinin, increase markedly in nasal secretions during colds, while interferons, produced in respiratory secretions in response to virus infections, can cause influenza-like symptoms such as fever, headache, myalgia and malaise, and local symptoms of nasal stuffiness and sore throat.[11]

Almost all adults with colds have transient evidence of sinus involvement with mucosal changes and fluid in the sinuses which resolves within 2–3 weeks.[12]

IMMUNITY

There are three aspects of immunity which should be considered. The first is *innate immunity* to infection: why should one child and not another be infected during a class outbreak? This is a complex question, and may depend as much on the quantity of virus and the site of inoculation as anything else, although passively acquired antibody is clearly important in infancy. For some viruses, such as herpes simplex virus (HSV), natural killer cell activity has been shown to be important in innate resistance.

The second question is one of *recovery* from viral upper respiratory infection. Antibody is of little importance in this process, since boys with congenital agammaglobulinaemia recover normally from viral infections. Recovery depends on the interplay of a number of host factors, of which T lymphocyte function ('cell-mediated immunity') and interferon are probably the most important, but natural killer cell activity and even neutrophil activity are also important in some infections.

The third question is that of *resistance* to reinfection with respiratory viruses, and here antibody becomes more important, though not for all viruses. In general, upper respiratory viral infections are localized to the upper respiratory tract, and infected children do not become viraemic. It is perhaps not surprising that the presence of secretory IgA antibody specific to a strain of respiratory virus usually correlates better with protection against reinfection with that virus than the presence of specific serum IgG. However, for some respiratory virus infections, such as RSV and parainfluenza virus infections, reinfections can occur despite the presence of specific serum and secretory antibody.

SPREAD

During the Second World War, the importance of respiratory infections in reducing the efficiency of workers, and the belief that respiratory droplets were the major vehicle of spread, were encapsulated in posters urging people to use handkerchiefs (Fig. 1A.1.3). 'Coughs and sneezes spread diseases' was the slogan of the time.

Subsequent research has shown that droplet spread is certainly important, but that at least some respiratory viruses may be spread as often or even more often

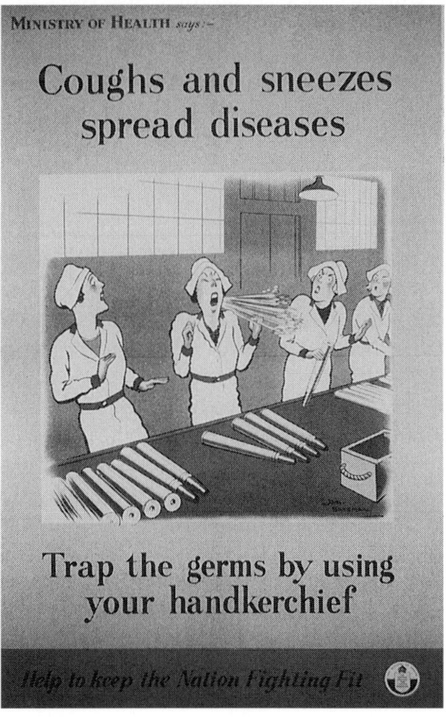

Fig. 1A.1.3 Ministry of Health poster from the Second World War: trying to prevent colds in the munitions factory.

on hands or intermediate objects (fomites). Soon after the war, the droplet theory was lent great weight by experiments at the Common Cold Research Unit in Salisbury, UK. In one experiment, volunteers with natural upper respiratory infections were separated from children by a large blanket across the room which did not reach the ceiling; the children became infected when a fan was placed behind the volunteers, blowing droplets over the blanket. The 'artificial sneeze' was even more elegant: a bellows was used to puff a suspension of a coxsackievirus into a wardrobe, then volunteers poked their heads into the wardrobe and became infected.

However, other possible modes of spread were emerging. Bynoe and colleagues showed that rhinovirus inoculated onto the nasal epithelium or the conjunctiva, but not the external nares or pharynx, caused colds in volunteers.[13] This suggested the possibility of spread of virus on hands or by droplet. Dick and coworkers then undertook an ingenious series of experiments involving cardplayers with and without rhinovirus colds. In the first experiments, uninfected players who used virucidal wipes on their cards were protected from catching colds from infected players, while those without wipes got colds. Not content that this showed whether the virus was rubbed into the nose or eyes, or was airborne from the cards, Dick's card-players were fitted with splints to prevent them reaching their eyes or nose, and still got colds. So droplet spread still seemed important.[13]

Nevertheless, spread on hands, sometimes via fomites, at least in hospital, appears to be more important than droplet spread for RSV (see Chapter 1B.1 on Bronchiolitis). Kissing is an extremely low-risk activity, at least in terms of transmitting rhinoviruses.[13] Close proximity appears to be important in encouraging spread: an 85% transmission rate of a rhinovirus was found when men were crowded together in a small hut in the Arctic.[13]

One thing is clear: although respiratory viral infections are more common in winter, catching a cold has nothing to do with being cold. At Salisbury, volunteers who were stood out in a hockey field or immersed in cold water until they had dropped their rectal temperature by 1°C were no more susceptible to rhinovirus infections than the lucky controls who were not thus exposed.

DIAGNOSIS

The diagnosis of an URTI is a clinical one, based on the constellation of symptoms and signs described by Donald Court, and outlined in the 'Clinical features' section of this chapter (p. 3).

It is arguable whether it is necessary to attempt to demonstrate the virus responsible, other than as part of a research project or when there are unusual complications. If it is elected to do so, then nasopharyngeal secretions, aspirated using a mucus extractor or catheter, are the best specimen, with a higher yield than nose or throat swabs.[2]

Although inoculation of respiratory secretions into tissue cultures has been the traditional mainstay of diagnosis, some laboratories are making increasing use of antigen detection techniques and even of molecular techniques. The problem with these is that they are almost *too* specific, being best when only one virus such as measles or RSV is suspected; yet URTIs can be caused by an enormous range of viruses (see Table 1A.1.1). To be comprehensive, each specimen of nasopharyngeal secretions would need to be tested against the range of viruses using multiple separate antigen detection methods. Molecular techniques for detecting viral nucleic acid are extraordinarily sensitive, but have the same problem as antigen detection methods in being too specific, are expensive, and almost exclusively a research tool.

Serology for diagnosing respiratory viral infections is generally disappointing. This is because of the wide range of possible infecting viruses, the difficulty in getting acute and convalescent sera from children, and the poor serological response to infection of young children. However, for coronaviruses, which are particularly difficult to grow, serological studies, and more recently ELISA tests to detect antigen and PCR for nucleic acid, have been valuable in research studies.

TREATMENT

Viral upper respiratory infections are associated with a range of bacterial infections, such as bacterial pneumonia and bacterial meningitis, and the evidence suggests that this association is more than a chance one. Thus, children with bacterial meningitis are more likely to have had a recent URTI than age-matched controls. This implies that URTIs predispose to bacterial meningitis, either by a local effect on the nasal mucosa allowing bacteria to infect and/or invade the nasal epithelium, or by exerting a degree of immunosuppression. However, the vast majority of URTIs are self-limiting and uncomplicated. Large studies have consistently shown that antibiotic treatment of URTIs does not alter the natural history, nor prevent complications.[3] Furthermore, it is dubious whether oral antibiotics would ever prevent bacterial meningitis. The practice, particularly common in some developing countries, of prescribing antibiotics for simple URTIs should be strongly discouraged as likely to cause side-effects to the patient and to induce antibiotic resistance.

Antihistamines and decongestants do not reduce symptoms and may cause unwarranted side-effects.[14] Even the use of paracetamol (acetaminophen) to control fever is controversial, and aspirin actually increases viral shedding.

SUMMARY

Upper respiratory tract infections are extremely common in preschool children, who experience around six to eight episodes per year. This is because of the wide range of potential infecting viruses and multiple serotypes of many respiratory viruses. A child's incidence of URTIs is determined primarily by exposure, with child care centre or kindergarten attendance, school-aged siblings, urban environment and passive smoking as particular risk factors, while breast-feeding is relatively protective. Spread is by droplets and/or direct inoculation from hands. Although URTIs are of importance because of their high incidence, and because of their association with bacterial infections and non-infectious complications, in large studies such complications are not prevented by antibiotic treatment. Antibiotics, antihistamines and decongestants should not be used in children with uncomplicated URTIs.

REFERENCES

See end of Chapter 1A.2 (p. 15) for references to this Part.

1A.2 Nose: rhinitis

INTRODUCTION

Acute, chronic and recurrent rhinitis can occur at any age, but are particularly common problems in childhood. Acute rhinitis is predominantly caused by respiratory viruses ('the common cold'), but there are important alternative diagnoses (Table 1A.2.1). The distinction between chronic and recurrent rhinitis is not always clear cut, as recurrent episodes of rhinitis may merge into each other to resemble chronic rhinitis. Rhinitis may be considered also in descriptive terms as being either a clear or a mucopurulent nasal discharge.

The significance of upper respiratory tract infections has been considered in the previous chapter, and the common cold is of major social and economic importance. Allergic rhinitis can be extremely disabling, and is a diagnosis that is easily overlooked. Sinusitis is another under-diagnosed condition of childhood.

ACUTE RHINITIS

The vast majority of episodes of acute rhinitis are due to common colds, this being the diagnosis in the majority of the six to eight upper respiratory infections suffered each year by preschool children. However, allergy, sinusitis and other important infections may all cause acute rhinitis (see Table 1A.2.1).

Common cold

Preschool children have around three to eight common colds per year, according to various studies. Court[1] defines the common cold as an illness in which the

Table 1A.2.1 Causes of rhinitis in children

Acute rhinitis	Viral infections	Common cold
		Upper respiratory tract infection
	Bacterial infections	Acute sinusitis
		Congenital syphilis
		Pertussis
		Nasal diphtheria
	Allergy	Allergic rhinitis (seasonal)
Chronic or recurrent rhinitis	Recurrent viral infections	
	Chronic sinusitis	
	Allergic rhinitis (perennial)	
	Immune deficiency	Antibody
		Ciliary dyskinesia
	Foreign body	
	Choanal atresia	
	Nasopharyngeal tumours	

principal symptom is excessive mucoid or purulent nasal discharge, and in which more than half the affected children have a red pharynx, a cough and are febrile.

During a cold, the nasal discharge is initially clear and watery. After 2–3 days, the discharge becomes thick and mucopurulent, due to the presence of desquamated cells and polymorphs. This is part of the natural history of a cold, is not due to bacterial superinfection, and is not an indication for antibiotics, which do not alter the clinical course.[14]

The pathogenesis of rhinitis in the common cold probably owes more to inflammatory mediators such as bradykinin and related kinins, than it does to transudation or exudation of proteins due to direct viral damage.[11]

The epidemiology, diagnosis and management of colds is essentially similar to that of upper respiratory tract infections (URTIs), and has been considered in the previous chapter. It should be stressed additionally that vitamin C, which has been widely advocated for treatment, has not been shown to have any benefit in large clinical trials. Although in modest doses vitamin C is almost certainly harmless, high doses are potentially hazardous due to its antioxidant effect.[15]

Acute sinusitis

This will be discussed in detail in Ch. 1A.5. Most respiratory viral infections last 5–7 days. Even though sinus changes occur in most adults with colds, the sinus changes resolve without antibiotics within 2–3 weeks.[12] Nasal discharge not resolving after 10 days, particularly when accompanied by cough, painless periorbital swelling and bad breath, with or without fever, may be due to sinusitis.[16] Frontal headache or tenderness over the sinuses is highly suggestive of acute sinusitis.

Congenital syphilis

Congenital syphilis is an important cause of nasal discharge in the neonatal period or first 3 months of infancy, although rare in countries which employ universal antenatal screening for syphilis. Nasal discharge is not present at birth, usually beginning in the second week of life or later, as a watery discharge. This subsequently becomes thick and mucopurulent, and crusts around the nose, obstructing respiration and causing the characteristic 'snuffles'. It may be associated with a soundless cry, due to laryngeal involvement. Other signs of congenital syphilis, anaemia, oedema, rash, red soles of the feet, lymphadenopathy, hepatosplenomegaly and pseudoparalysis of a limb should be sought, though may not be present. There may be mucous patches (condylomata lata) in the mouth. The diagnosis of congenital syphilis can be made by serology or by dark-field microscopy of the nasal discharge.

Pertussis

The early, 'catarrhal' phase of whooping cough or pertussis is characterized by a mucopurulent nasal discharge, which usually lasts for a week before the paroxysmal stage of coughing supervenes. If there is a history of contact with whooping cough, the use of erythromycin should be considered, as it is only effective in limiting the severity and duration of the illness when given in the catarrhal phase of whooping cough. A full blood count may be helpful in revealing the characteristic lymphocytosis.

Nasal diphtheria

Although usually tonsillopharyngeal, diphtheria may sometimes be nasal. The child is initially systemically well and develops a thin watery nasal discharge, usually unilateral. This becomes serosanguinous and then mucopurulent with a foul-smelling, bloody discharge and excoriation of the upper lip. Inspection of the nares often reveals a white membrane. Absorption of toxin is slow, and systemic symptoms only develop gradually. Nasal diphtheria only occurs in unimmunized children, and is more common in infants. The diagnosis of nasal diphtheria should be considered in an unimmunized child with a unilateral bloody nasal discharge, although in developed countries foreign body will be a far more likely diagnosis in this clinical situation.

Allergic rhinitis (seasonal)

Seasonal allergic rhinitis (hay fever) is most common in spring, when the pollen count is high, and rhinitis is accompanied by sneezing, itchy nose and red, watery eyes. It is generally diagnosed in school-aged children, although is not uncommon in preschool children and even in infancy. An atopic personal or family history and the extreme itchiness of the nose are possible indicators of allergic rhinitis.

Streptococcosis

Ellen Wald[17] describes an indolent illness occurring in children under 3 years of age, associated with group A streptococcal infection and characterized by low-grade fever, purulent nasal discharge and cervical lymphadenopathy, and lasting weeks to months, which she calls 'streptococcosis'. She contrasts this to acute streptococcal infection in school-aged children with acute sore throat and high fever. Todd and colleagues[14] found that 8% of 142 children with purulent naso-pharyngitis had group A streptococcus in nasal swabs, but that antibiotic therapy with cephalexin did not alter the nature or duration of the nasal discharge.

Management of acute rhinitis

Most episodes of acute rhinitis are due to colds, and the main problem is with over-treatment with antibiotics, antihistamines and decongestants. Other causes of acute rhinitis described above may be suggested by history or examination, but are relatively rare, particularly in industrialized countries with high rates of childhood immunization. Most proprietary cold remedies are not without side-effects, which may be severe. Antihistamines can cause drowsiness or hallucinations, and when combined with decongestants can cause major dystonic reactions and CNS depression. Yet controlled trials have shown no benefit.[18] Vitamin C has been shown to be ineffective and although harmless in moderate doses is potentially harmful in high dose due to its antioxidant effects. Aspirin increases the duration of viral shedding in adults with colds. As Sir William Osler stated, 'there is just one way to treat a cold, and that is with contempt'.

CHRONIC RHINITIS

Chronic mucopurulent nasal discharge is sometimes known as catarrh, and John Fry has written a book on *The catarrhal child*. It is not always apparent whether such discharge is persistent, i.e. chronic, or in fact recurrent, with short intervening periods of remission. Chronic nasal discharge is more common in children in non-industrialized countries and in native children living in poverty in industrialized countries. The most likely explanation is chronic or recurrent nasal infection with bacteria and viruses, due to close exposure to these organisms, rather than genetic or even anatomical reasons which have sometimes been proposed.

Recurrent viral infections

It seems likely that a number of children with supposedly constant mucopurulent nasal discharge are in fact having repeated infections with different respiratory viruses. This was found to be the case during an intensive study of preschool children.[2] The discharge might only dry up for one or two days between infections, but a new respiratory virus could be cultured when the nasal discharge recurred.

Chronic sinusitis

If a child has chronic mucopurulent nasal discharge which persists for 30 days, particularly if associated with a cough which is present in the day and night, then chronic sinusitis should be considered. Supportive signs and symptoms are bad breath and painless periorbital swelling in the morning. Facial pain and frontal headache or tenderness are uncommon, but their presence strongly suggests chronic sinusitis (see Chapter 1A.5 on Sinusitis).

Allergic rhinitis (perennial)

Perennial allergic rhinitis is more common than seasonal rhinitis in young children. Chronic nasal discharge is usually less prominent than nasal stuffiness, extreme nasal itch and blocked nose. The child, even infant, continually rubs their nose on the back of their hand (the 'allergic salute') or a parent's shoulder, until a lateral crease develops across the nose (the 'allergic crease'). The child may have dark rings under the eyes: 'allergic shiners'. The nasal mucosa is red and inflamed, and polyps may be present. The diagnosis is mainly clinical, but nasal smears can be stained, and the presence of eosinophils and/or mast cells strongly supports allergic rhinitis.[19] Treatment is with topical steroids and/or cromoglycate, but can be difficult to administer to young children.

Immune deficiency

Some forms of immune deficiency predispose to upper and lower respiratory infections, including sinusitis, and may cause chronic nasal discharge, although this is usually part of a broader clinical picture.

Children with low immunoglobulin levels, or those with normal immunoglobulin levels, but dysfunctional immunoglobulins, most commonly have recurrent ear infections and recurrent lower respiratory tract infections as their predominant infections. Those with IgG subclass deficiency, particularly deficiency of IgG_2, may present with chronic ear infections and/or chronic bronchitis. In all these groups of immune deficient children, chronic nasal discharge is more likely to be an additional symptom rather than the sole one.

In immotile cilia syndrome, the symptoms of neonatal respiratory distress, purulent nasal discharge due to chronic sinusitis, purulent ear discharge, and chronic productive cough due to bronchiectasis, result from abnormal ciliary clearance. Half the affected children have dextrocardia (Kartagener's syndrome).

Foreign body

Persistent unilateral nasal discharge is likely to be due to foreign body, unilateral choanal atresia or tumour (see below). Nasal foreign bodies are most likely in children aged 9–24 months with the ability to put an object up their nose and not enough experience to avoid doing so. However, siblings may push objects up the noses of young babies, and older children sometimes experiment. The discharge is characteristically foul-smelling and somewhat, or even heavily, blood-stained.

Choanal atresia

Complete bilateral choanal atresia causes neonatal respiratory distress which is relieved when the baby cries. However, there may be partial choanal atresia (perhaps better called choanal stenosis), or unilateral choanal atresia, which will cause chronic bilateral or unilateral mucopurulent discharge. Affected children usually present in early infancy. If choanal atresia is suspected, an attempt should be made to pass a small feeding tube.

Tumours

Nasopharyngeal tumours can be benign or malignant, and cause nasal blockage with mucopurulent or bloody discharge. Diagnosis is made by CT scan and a tissue diagnosis obtained by endoscopy and biopsy.

REFERENCES

1 Court S D M. The definition of acute respiratory illnesses in children. Postgrad Med J 1973; 49: 771–776.
2 Isaacs D, Clarke J R, Tyrrell D A J, Valman H B. Selective involvement of the lower respiratory tract by respiratory viruses in children with recurrent respiratory tract infections. Br Med J 1982; 284: 1746–1748.
3 Sutrisna B, Frerichs R R, Reingold A L. Randomised, controlled trial of effectiveness of ampicillin in mild acute respiratory infections in Indonesian children. Lancet 1991; 338: 471–474.
4 Larson H E, Reed S E, Tyrrell D A J. Isolation of rhinoviruses and coronaviruses from 38 colds in adults. J Med Virol 1980; 5: 221–229.
5 Loda F A, Glezen W P, Clyde W A. Respiratory diseases in group day care. Pediatrics 1972; 49: 428–437.
6 Dingle J H, Badger G F, Jordan W S. Illness in the home. Cleveland, OH: Western Reserve University Press, 1964.
7 Fox J P, Elveback L R, Spigland I, Frothingham T E, Stevens D A, Huger A. The virus watch program: a continuing surveillance of viral infections in metropolitan New York families. I. Overall plan, methods of collecting and handling information and a summary report of specimens collected and illnesses observed. Am J Epidemiol 1966; 88: 389–412.
8 Boyce W T, Jensen E W, Cassel J C et al. Influence of life events and family routines on childhood respiratory tract illness. Pediatrics 1977; 60: 609–615.
9 Cohen S, Tyrrell D A J, Smith A P. Psychological stress and susceptibility to the common cold. N Engl J Med 1991; 325: 606–612.
10 Wald E R, Guerra N, Byers C. Upper respiratory tract infections in young children: duration of and frequency of complications. Pediatrics 1991; 87: 129–133.
11 Isaacs D. Cold comfort for the catarrhal child. Arch Dis Child 1990; 65: 1295–1296.
12 Gwaltney J M, Phillips C D, Miller R D, Riker A K. Computed tomographic study of the common cold. N Engl J Med 1994; 330: 25–30.
13 Isaacs D. Respiratory virus infections. In: Weatherall D J, Ledingham J G G, Warrell D A, eds. Oxford textbook of medicine, 3rd ed. Oxford: Oxford University Press, 1995.
14 Todd J K, Todd N, Damato J, Todd W A. Bacteriology and treatment of purulent nasopharyngitis: a double-blind, placebo-controlled evaluation. Pediatr Infect Dis 1984; 3: 226–232.
15 Barness L A. Safety considerations with high ascorbic acid dosage. Ann NY Acad Sci 1975; 258: 523–528.
16 Wald E R. Sinusitis in children. N Engl J Med 1992; 326: 319–323.
17 Wald E R. Purulent nasal discharge. Pediatr Infect Dis J 1991; 10: 329–333.
18 Hutton N, Wilson M H, Mellits E et al. Effectiveness of an antihistamine–decongestant combination for young children with the common cold: a randomised controlled clinical trial. J Pediatr 1991; 118: 125–130.
19 Kemp A, Bryan L. Perennial rhinitis: a common childhood complaint. Med J Aust 1984; 141: 640–643.

A. Putto-Laurila   O. Ruuskanen

1A.3 Throat: tonsillopharyngitis, retropharyngeal abscess

ACUTE TONSILLOPHARYNGITIS

INTRODUCTION

Acute tonsillopharyngitis is an inflammatory disease of the throat with definite erythema with or without tonsillar exudate, ulceration or vesicles. Its great frequency in children and adolescents makes it a common clinical problem in a paediatric outpatient practice.

AETIOLOGY

For practical purposes, tonsillopharyngitis can be classified as streptococcal or non-streptococcal (Fig. 1A.3.1). The proportions of the different aetiological pathogens detected vary according to the season of the year, epidemiological

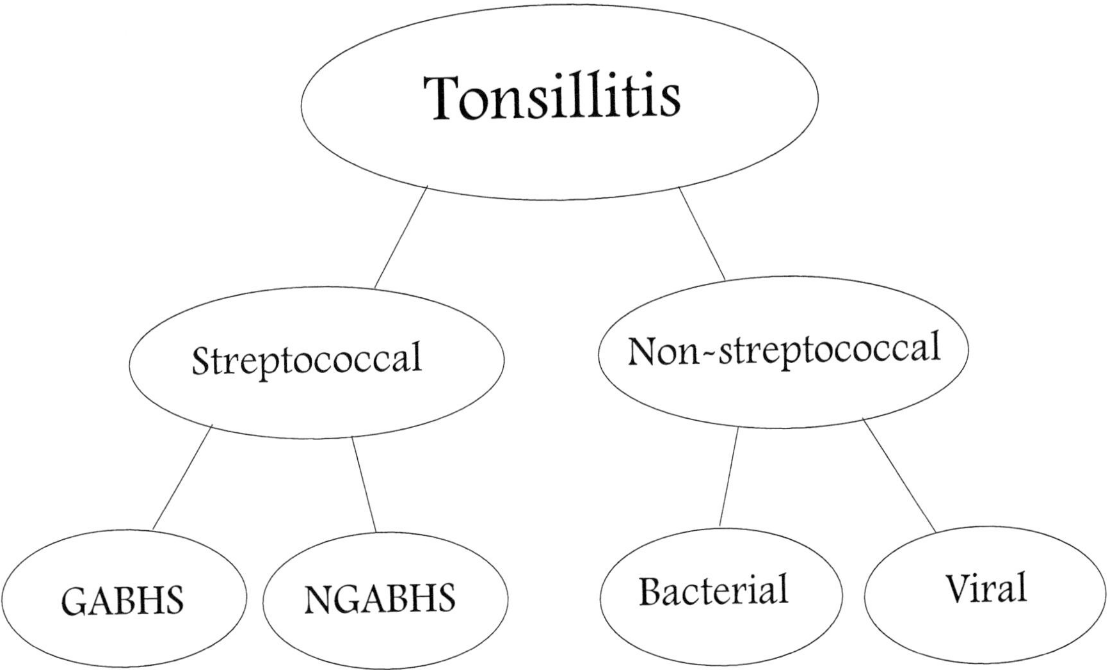

Fig. 1A.3.1   Classification of tonsillitis.

Table 1A.3.1   Aetiology of acute tonsillopharyngitis

	Evans & Dick[1] 1964	Glezen et al[2] 1967	Douglas et al[3] 1984	Putto[4] 1987	Huovinen et al[5] 1989
Number of patients:	308	715	178	110	106
Age of patients (years):	Adults	Adults, children	1–10	< 18	Adults
	%	%	%	%	%
GAS	26	37	47	12	5
Non-GAS	NS	NS	5	21	18
Mycoplasma pneumoniae	9	3	NS	5	9
Chlamydia pneumoniae	NS	NS	NS	NS	8
Adenovirus	2	6	7	19	3
EBV	NS	NS	NS	9	2
Parainfluenza viruses	3	3	1	7	2
Influenza viruses	4	0	1	3	7
Enteroviruses	4	1	14	4	1
No pathogen	36	50	28	35	31

GAS, group A streptococci; NS, not studied.

conditions, the age of population studied and the microbiological methods used. Grouping of the results presented in Table 1A.3.1 shows that 20–40% of throat infections are caused by β-haemolytic streptococci and at least 20–40% by viruses. In one-third of the patients no possible aetiological agent can be found.

Group A β-haemolytic streptococcus (GABHS) is the most frequent and important aetiological agent of tonsillopharyngitis, because of its potential capacity to cause post-infectious complications like rheumatic fever. Non-group-A β-haemolytic streptococci (NGABHS) also can cause symptomatic throat infections.[6–8] Although they are common in patients with pharyngitis, and although outbreaks caused by these organisms have been described, their role in sporadic cases remains obscure. They are not usually associated with post-infectious complications, thus making them of less importance to the clinician. Many small children are carriers of NGABHS.[9] Also a quarter of symptomless contacts of the GABHS tonsillitis patients can carry bacteria in their throats.

Mycoplasma pneumoniae may be responsible for about 5% of tonsillopharyngitis in children, occurring most frequently in older children.[2,4] On the other hand positive cultures for *M. pneumoniae* have been found equally often from controls as from patients with pharyngitis.[10] The role of *M. pneumoniae* should be emphasized because the recommended treatment is erythromycin. Acute antibodies to *Chlamydia pneumoniae* have been found in 8% of adults with pharyngitis.[5] The role of chlamydia species in childhood tonsillopharyngitis is unresolved. *Arcanobacterium haemolyticum* has been detected in tonsillopharyngitis, clinically indistinguishable from streptococcal pharyngitis.[11] Also *Neisseria gonorrhoeae, N. meningitidis, Haemophilus influenzae* and anaerobes are known to cause tonsillitis. Although rare, *Corynebacterium diphtheriae* should be remembered as a possible aetiological agent of exudative tonsillopharyngitis in the non- or under-immunized and exposed person.

Adenoviruses are the most common cause of non-streptococcal tonsillitis in children.[12] They are the viral group most likely to cause isolated exudative tonsillitis, in which the symptoms resemble those of streptococcal tonsillitis.[13] Epstein–Barr virus (EBV) can induce exudative tonsillitis also in small children.[14] Other viruses, e.g. respiratory syncytial virus, parainfluenza viruses, influenza viruses, rhinoviruses and coronaviruses, are more likely to cause upper or lower respiratory syndromes involving the pharynx rather than isolated tonsillopharyngitis. Enteroviruses and herpes simplex virus can cause ulcerative pharyngotonsillitis.[15] The proportion of other viruses causing tonsillopharyngitis is the same as that of adenovirus alone. However, it is probable that most patients in whom no aetiological agent can be found have viral infections.

EPIDEMIOLOGY

Group A streptococci are spread by respiratory secretions and droplets. The transmission of GABHS is facilitated by close contact and crowding. The period of maximal infectivity is in the acute phase of the illness, with most secondary cases occurring within 2 weeks after acquisition. The incubation period of streptococcal pharyngitis is 12 h to 5 days. Untreated patients often become asymptomatic in 3–4 days and upon return to normal activities may become an occult source for spread to others.

Up to 20% of children carry GABHS in the throat. The role of carriers in the spread of infection is controversial. They appear less likely to transmit the organism than acutely infected patients and are at significantly reduced risk of developing rheumatic fever.[16]

In temperate climates streptococcal infection is present throughout the year. The peak months of infection are January to May, although in many areas streptococcal pharyngitis is seen in autumn after school has commenced.

CLINICAL FEATURES

For therapeutic reasons it is important to differentiate between viral and streptococcal infection. Furthermore it is important to differentiate GABHS from other β-haemolytic streptococci, which are not so important when thinking of the risk of postinfectious complications. Contrary to the popular belief of clinicians, findings in the throat are insufficient for a definite differentiation between a viral and a bacterial infection. In particular, the clinical features of adenoviral tonsillitis may mimic those of streptococcal tonsillitis.[13]

The colour or extent of the exudates do not help in distinguishing bacterial from viral tonsillitis. Enlarged and tender cervical lymph nodes and pain on swallowing are found to be the most specific clinical symptoms in streptococcal tonsillitis (Table 1A.3.2).[17] Also headache, high fever and gastrointestinal symptoms in children are more commonly connected to streptococcal than to viral infections.

Coughing, hoarseness and rhinorrhoea favour viral rather than streptococcal aetiology. In adenoviral tonsillitis, 30–50% of children have cough and rhinitis.[13] Otitis media is often recorded in children with adenoviral tonsillitis. High and long-lasting fever is typical for adenoviral infection.[18] More than half of children

Table 1A.3.2   Classic features of streptococcal pharyngitis

Age 5–15 years
Sudden onset
Sore throat (pain on swallowing)
Fever
Headache
Nausea, vomiting, abdominal pain
No nasal discharge or cough
Patchy discrete exudate
Marked inflammation of throat and tonsils
Palatal petechiae
Tender, enlarged anterior cervical nodes

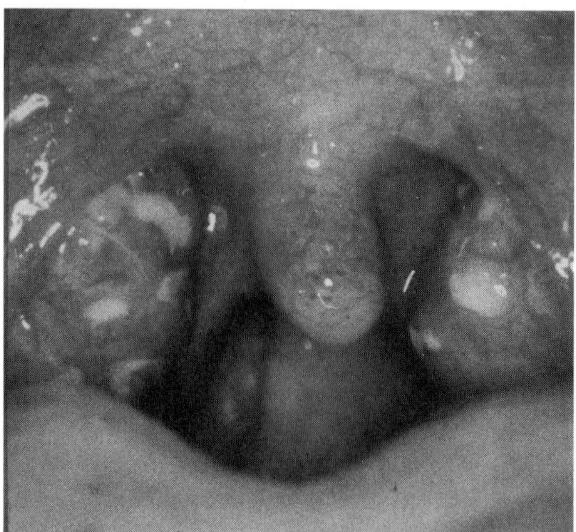

Fig. 1A.3.2 Exudative tonsillitis: could be due to group A streptococcal infection or viral (adenovirus, herpes simplex virus or EBV).

with adenoviral tonsillitis have fever ⩾ 40°C, and more than one-third have fever lasting for 5 days or more. The longest duration of fever is caused by EBV. Almost half of the children with this virus have fever lasting for 5 days or longer.[4,14]

The appearance of the tonsils is not diagnostic (Fig. 1A.3.2). The best predictor of the aetiological agent is the age of the child. In children younger than 3 years of age, streptococcal tonsillitis is uncommon.[2,4,19] In this age group the most important aetiological agent of non-streptococcal tonsillitis is adenovirus. GABHS is most common in school-aged children and in adolescence.[2] Groups C and G streptococcal infections tend to occur during the teenage and early adult years. Half the children aged 6 years or less have viral aetiology, but only one-third of children older than 6 years. In this age group the most important viral agent is Epstein–Barr virus.

DIAGNOSIS

Clinical diagnosis

The presumptive clinical diagnosis of streptococcal pharyngitis can be based on probability using epidemiological factors and observations from the clinical examination. The probability of streptococcal pharyngitis is increased when the patient has symptoms and findings presented in Table 1A.3.2. Also exposure to a person with known streptococcal pharyngitis or scarlatina rash increases the risk of streptococcal infection.

Bacterial diagnosis

Throat culture onto sheep blood agar plate is the most satisfactory method of confirming streptococcal infection.[20] All groups of β-haemolytic streptococci should be studied, as all can induce the illness. The preliminary culture result is available within 24–48 h. It has clearly been pointed out that it is useful economically as well as considering the treatment of the patient to culture the throat and wait for the result.[21] Nevertheless, many physicians will place patients with tonsillopharyngitis on antibiotics while awaiting the results of the throat culture and, in one survey, as many as as 40% of the physicians admitted to continuing antibiotics even after the throat culture had been reported as negative.[22]

Throat culture is also important to determine the sensitivity of antimicrobial drugs.

There are many rapid group A streptococcal antigen detection tests available nowadays. The advantage of the rapid tests is the speed of obtaining a result, generally within 10–20 min. The consequences of having rapidly available results in the office are important. The patient is often very interested in obtaining a rapid diagnosis so that treatment can begin and the child can be returned to day care or school somewhat sooner. There is also psychological benefit from recognizing streptococci on the day of the visit. The available tests are very specific but sensitivity varies.[20] The sensitivity of the tests decreases especially when the number of colonies on the throat culture is small: false negative test results usually occur in cultures with fewer than 10 colonies. Less than 10% of symptomatic patients will have so few colonies. On the other hand, one-third of patients with sore throat and a small number of colonies on the culture plate will have a significant serological response, so the negative test result can miss a real infection. One explanation for the weak growth of bacteria can be a poor sample.

GABHS antigen detection test and throat culture should be used wisely together. The common opinion is that negative rapid test results should be confirmed by throat culture, at least from children older than 3 years of age.[23] Treatment is started if necessary after the result of throat culture. Even if treatment is delayed for several days, it does not predispose the child to acute rheumatic fever. It has even been suggested that those with early treatment have more recurrences because the formation of type-specific antibodies will be prevented.[24] A negative rapid test result of a child under the age of 3 years has to be confirmed only when there is a strong clinical suspicion of streptococcal infection (e.g. there is a GABHS-positive person in the family or in day care).

If the child has been fully immunized against diphtheria, there is little to gain from seeking other bacteria than streptococci from the throat culture. They do not cause postinfectious complications, they occur infrequently and the effect of antimicrobial treatment is largely unknown or minimal. Streptococcal serology does not help in the diagnosis of acute tonsillitis. The greatest benefit of serology can be achieved in the aetiological diagnosis of a patient with non-suppurative complications.

Viral diagnosis

A nasopharyngeal mucus specimen for rapid viral diagnosis from children with exudative tonsillitis with no GABHS can be useful.[25] The specimen should be tested at least for adenoviral antigen, if available. Although the viral diagnosis as such does not have value in treatment it makes it possible to name the aetiological agent in the acute phase of the disease. This will decrease parents' concern about the child's disease and especially from fever, which in adenoviral infection can be high and long-lasting. With known aetiology it is also easier for the doctor to advise parents about the infection, its prognosis and spread in the family.

The rapid slide test for heterophile antibodies or measurement of IgM antibodies are useful tests for EBV tonsillopharyngitis in children older than 4 years of age. In younger children, measurement of IgM antibodies to EBV capsid antigen is recommended,[26] as the slide test is often negative despite EBV infection. Coinfection with GABHS may occur in 5–30% of EBV infections.

Other viral serology or virus isolation in the diagnosis of tonsillitis is indicated only in special cases.

Non-specific laboratory methods

Routine haematological tests are not helpful in differentiating between viral and streptococcal tonsillopharyngitis. Increased values of white blood cell count, erythrocyte sedimentation rate and C-reactive protein are found so often in adenoviral and EBV tonsillitis that the differences between values recorded in streptococcal tonsillitis are marginal and not helpful.[27] The presence of lymphocytosis or characteristic atypical lymphocytes may aid in the diagnosis of infectious mononucleosis.

TREATMENT

There is no specific treatment for viral tonsillopharyngitis. Some relief can be achieved with anti-inflammatory drugs, especially in highly febrile children.

The antimicrobial therapy of tonsillopharyngitis should be based on the detection of β-haemolytic streptococci in the throat. Children with NGABHS tonsillopharyngitis can be treated by the regimens used for group A infections.

The optimal treatment of streptococcal tonsillopharyngitis includes four goals: clinical recovery is hastened, the patient becomes non-infectious for contacts, suppurative complications are avoided and rheumatic fever is prevented. The recent resurgence of rheumatic fever and the appearance of severe streptococcal infections remind us of the importance of treating GABHS infections properly.

The drug of choice in the treatment of streptococcal tonsillopharyngitis is peroral penicillin (Table 1A.3.3).[28] The dose is 50 000–100 000 units/kg per day divided in two doses. Twice daily oral penicillin has the same effect as three times daily, with better compliance.[29] Erythromycin, first-generation cephalosporins or clindamycin may be used for patients with penicillin allergy. The new macrolides, clarithromycin and azithromycin, have a susceptibility pattern similar to that of erythromycin but cause less gastrointestinal distress. Cephalosporins have been compared favourably with penicillin. They have been shown to be as effective as, or probably even more effective than, penicillin in the treatment of GABHS tonsillopharyngitis.[30] There is also evidence that a single daily dose of cefadroxil is as effective as penicillin V given more frequently.[31] The possibility of erythromycin-resistant group A streptococci, which have been identified in Finland, Sweden, Germany and Japan, should be remembered.[32]

Tetracyclines, sulphonamides and trimethoprim/sulphamethoxazole are in-

Table 1A.3.3   Treatment of GABHS tonsillopharyngitis

Antimicrobial treatment	Comments
Drug of first choice	
Penicillin V	No penicillin-resistant streptococci described, inexpensive, safe
Other possibilities	
Cephalexin, cefadroxil	
Erythromycin	Resistant strains possible
Clindamycin	
Ineffective antimicrobials	
Tetracyclines	Resistant strains common
Trimethoprim/sulphamethoxazole	GAS always resistant
Fluoroquinolones	No effect confirmed
Ampicillin/amoxycillin	Rash reaction with EBV
Cefaclor/cefuroxime	No benefits compared with first-generation cephalosporins, side-effects more common, expensive
Recurrent or complicated infections	
Cephalexin, cefadroxil	Consult an ENT specialist when considering tonsillectomy (e.g. more than four
Clindamycin	to six episodes of tonsillitis per year, peritonsillar abscess, obstruction because of
Dicloxacillin	hypertrophy)

effective antimicrobials in the treatment of streptococcal tonsillopharyngitis. Amoxycillin is not recommended for the treatment of throat infections because of the rash reaction in infectious mononucleosis. The duration of penicillin V treatment should be 10 days.[33] A 4- to 7-day course of cephalosporin treatment may be as effective as penicillin V for 10 days. A 5-day course of therapy with azithromycin is sufficient.[30,34]

The potential advantage of immediate treatment is more prompt clinical improvement. The maximal benefit can be achieved when the treatment is started during the first 24 h. However, the early treatment may be associated with more relapses and recurrences than delayed treatment.[24] All children treated with penicillin will be afebrile after 24–48 h.[4] However, throat culture will be negative only in a small proportion of children after 12 h of treatment. This makes it possible to take the throat culture even after the first dose of antibiotics.[35]

If the patient is not asymptomatic after 2 days of therapy with penicillin, there is possibly a coinfection with virus, and it is of no benefit to change the antimicrobial therapy. Although there will be relapses in 10–20% after penicillin treatment, the primary efficacy of penicillin has continued to be good in GABHS infections. Patients who remain asymptomatic after stopping treatment need no bacteriological follow-up. Children can be sent back to day care or school after completing a full 24 h of antibiotics, if they otherwise feel well enough.[35]

RECURRENT TONSILLOPHARYNGITIS

Recurrent tonsillopharyngitis is a common infectious problem in paediatric and adolescent patients. Many reasons have been proposed for recurrent infections (Table 1A.3.4). The frequency or clinical significance of any single reason is obscure, but several factors may interact simultaneously and are probably not independent of each other.[36]

In recurrent infections the diagnosis should be based on the result of throat culture. Assessment of the complete pharyngeal flora may be useful as a guide to appropriate therapy. The rapid antigen detection test will not give adequate information in these cases. If the recurrences are always caused by GABHS, two-thirds of these recurrences are relapses caused by the same bacteria.[37] A change of antimicrobial therapy will sometimes stop the recurrences (Table 1A.3.3). Treatment with erythromycin, a penicillinase-resistant penicillin, a cephalosporin or clindamycin has been advocated. However, recurrent documented, severe streptococcal tonsillopharyngitis is an indication for tonsillectomy.[38] Usually symptomatic contacts of a GABHS-positive person can be treated without microbial testing. In the case of recurrent infections it is important to take throat cultures

Table 1A.3.4 Suspected causes for recurrent tonsillopharyngitis

GABHS tonsillopharyngitis:
1. Lack of compliance with taking medication
2. Repeated exposure
3. β-lactamase-producing oral microbes inactivate penicillin
4. Eradication of non-pathogenic α-haemolytic streptococci
5. Antibiotic suppression of immunity
6. Carrier state, not disease
7. Tolerance to antibiotic

Chronic infection caused by anaerobes
Chronic infection caused by EBV
Infections of teeth and sinuses

from all family members without paying any attention to whether they are symptomatic or not. Acting like this the therapy can be directed to the right persons. Asymptomatic carriers of GABHS should not be treated unless suspected to be the source of infection in the family. Household pets can rarely be vectors of streptococcal infection.

COMPLICATIONS

The principal non-suppurative complications of group A streptococcal tonsillopharyngitis are acute rheumatic fever (ARF) and glomerulonephritis. Untreated patients may develop ARF and resultant chronic damage to the heart valves. The incidence of ARF has been declining in North America and Western Europe since the early years of the twentieth century.[39] However, in the mid- to late 1980s increases in the numbers of cases of ARF in several geographic areas in the USA have been reported. There are specific M serotypes of GABHS which are most frequently associated with ARF.

Acute glomerulonephritis may follow either a pharyngeal or a skin infection with GABHS. Although most M and T serotypes may result in rheumatic fever, only a limited number are recognized as nephritogenic strains. Adequate treatment of streptococcal tonsillopharyngitis does not necessarily prevent acute glomerulonephritis, if there is infection with a nephritogenic strain.

Infection of the pharynx and tonsils may spread to the surrounding mucous membranes, causing relatively unusual infections (Table 1A.3.5). The aetiological role of GABHS in peritonsillar abscess or in retropharyngeal abscess is prominent, as it is in the aetiology of lymphadenitis, together with *Staphylococcus aureus*.[40] Its role as a causative agent in acute otitis media or in sinusitis is minimal. GABHS bacteraemia is usually not associated with primary pharyngeal infection. Currently suppurative complications are rarely seen in antibiotic-treated patients. Tonsillectomy should be done after the first episode of peritonsillar abscess.

Acute streptococcal tonsillopharyngitis may rarely lead to toxin-associated disease (streptococcal toxic shock-like syndrome) with a high mortality rate. This syndrome occurs most commonly in healthy adults and is usually associated with a soft tissue focus of infection.

Table 1A.3.5   Possible complications of GABHS tonsillopharyngitis

Non-suppurative complications
Acute rheumatic fever
Acute glomerulonephritis
Suppurative complications
Otitis media
Sinusitis or mastoiditis
Peritonsillar abscess or cellulitis
Retropharyngeal abscess

RETROPHARYNGEAL ABSCESS

The retropharyngeal nodes drain both the adenoids and the nasopharynx. The retropharyngeal abscess is usually secondary to severe purulent infections of these areas. GABHS, oral anaerobes and *Staphylococcus aureus* are the most common pathogens. It is most common in children under the age of 3 years.

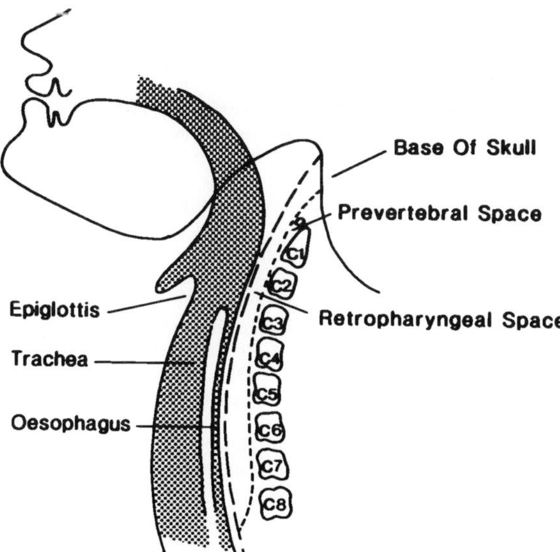

Fig. 1A.3.3 Diagrammatic representation of lateral neck structures.

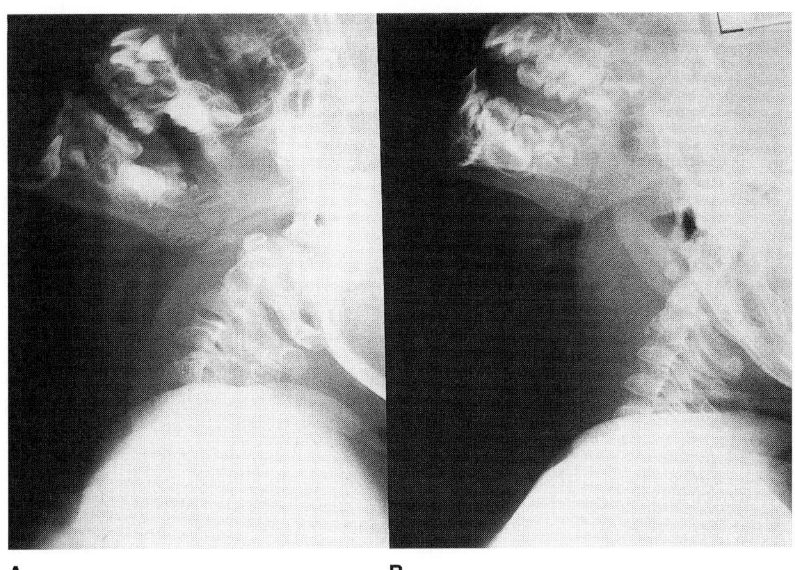

Fig. 1A.3.4 Lateral neck radiographs. **A** Normal. **B** Child with retropharyngeal abscess showing widened retropharyngeal space.

The characteristic features are an abrupt onset of high fever, dysphagia, hyperextension of the neck and noisy respiration. A bulge in the posterior pharyngeal wall is usually apparent, but may not be detectable by simple inspection. A lateral neck X-ray (Fig. 1A.3.4), ultrasound or CT scan of the neck can be used to make the diagnosis.

Intravenous antibiotic therapy should cover GABHS, *Staphylococcus aureus* and anaerobes. An otolaryngologist should be consulted about possible aspiration or drainage of the abscess.

REFERENCES

1 Evans A S, Dick E C. Acute pharyngitis and tonsillitis in University of Wisconsin students. JAMA 1964; 190: 699–708.
2 Glezen W P, Clyde W A Jr, Senior R J, Sheaffer C I, Denny F W. Group A streptococci, mycoplasmas, and viruses associated with acute pharyngitis. JAMA 1967; 202: 455–460.
3 Douglas R M, Miles H, Hansman D, Fadejevs A, Moore B, Bollen M D. Acute tonsillitis in children: microbial pathogens in relation to age. Pathology 1984; 16: 79–82.
4 Putto A. Febrile exudative tonsillitis: viral or streptococcal? Pediatrics 1987; 80: 6–12.
5 Huovinen P, Lahtonen R, Ziegler T et al. Pharyngitis in adults: the presence and coexistence of viruses and bacterial organisms. Ann Intern Med 1989; 110: 612–616.
6 Benjamin J T, Perriello V A Jr. Pharyngitis due to group C hemolytic streptococci in children. J Pediatr 1976; 89: 254–256.
7 Gerber M A, Randolph M F, Martin N J et al. Community-wide outbreak of group G streptococcal pharyngitis. Pediatrics 1991; 87: 598–603.
8 Cimolai N, MacCulloch L, Damm S. The epidemiology of beta-haemolytic non-group A streptococci isolated from throats of children over a one-year period. Epidemiol Infect 1990; 104: 119–126.
9 Hayden G F, Murphy T F, Hendley J O. Non-group A streptococci in the pharynx: pathogens or innocent bystanders? Am J Dis Child 1989; 143: 794–797.
10 McMillan J A, Sandstrom C, Weiner L B et al. Viral and bacterial organisms associated with acute pharyngitis in a school-aged population. J Pediatr 1986; 109: 747–752.
11 Karpathios T, Drakonaki S, Zervoudaki A et al. Arcanobacterium haemolyticum in children with presumed streptococcal pharyngotonsillitis or scarlet fever. J Pediatr 1992; 121: 735–737.
12 Moffet H L, Siegel A C, Doyle H K. Nonstreptococcal pharyngitis. J Pediatr 1968; 73: 51–60.
13 Ruuskanen O, Sarkkinen H, Meurman O et al. Rapid diagnosis of adenoviral tonsillitis: a prospective clinical study. J Pediatr 1984; 104: 725–728.
14 Sumaya C, Ench Y. Epstein–Barr virus infectious mononucleosis in children. 1. Clinical and general laboratory findings. Pediatrics 1985; 75: 1003–1010.
15 McMillan J A, Weiner L B, Higgins A M, Lamparella V J. Pharyngitis associated with herpes simplex virus in college students. Pediatr Infect Dis J 1993; 12: 280–284.
16 Kaplan E L. Group A streptococcal carriers and contacts: (when) is re-treatment with antibiotics necessary? In: Shulman S, ed. Management of pharyngitis in an era of declining rheumatic fever. Ross Conference on Pediatric Research. Columbus, OH, 1984: pp 92–104.
17 Wannamaker L W. Diagnosis of pharyngitis: Clinical and epidemiologic features. In: Shulman S, ed. Management of pharyngitis in an era of declining rheumatic fever. Ross Conference on Pediatric Research. Columbus, OH, 1984: pp 25–42.
18 Ruuskanen O, Meurman O, Sarkkinen H. Adenoviral diseases in children: a study of 105 hospital cases. Pediatrics 1985; 76: 79–83.
19 Alpert J J, Pickering M R, Warren R J. Failure to isolate streptococci from children under the age of 3 years with exudative tonsillitis. Pediatrics 1966; 38: 663–666.
20 Gerber M A. Comparison of throat cultures and rapid strep tests for diagnosis of streptococcal pharyngitis. Pediatr Infect Dis J 1989; 8: 820–824.
21 Mäkelä M, Sintonen H. Rationality and cost-effectiveness of diagnosis and treatment of group A streptococci in primary care patients with pharyngitis. Scand J Infect Dis 1991; 23: 47–53.
22 Holmberg S D, Faich G A. Streptococcal pharyngitis and acute rheumatic fever in Rhode Island. JAMA 1983; 250: 2307–2312.
23 Denny F W Jr. Tonsillopharyngitis 1994. Pediatr Rev 1994; 15: 185–191.
24 El-Daher N T, Hijazi S S, Rawashdeh N M, Al-Khalil I A-H, Abu-Ektaish F M, Abdel-Latif D I. Immediate vs. delayed treatment of group A beta-hemolytic streptococcal pharyngitis with penicillin V. Pediatr Infect Dis J 1991; 10: 126–130.
25 Halonen P, Meurman O, Lövgren T, Hemmilä I, Soini E. Detection of viral antigens by time-resolved fluoroimmunoassay. Curr Topics Microbiol Immunol 1983; 104: 133–146.
26 Sumaya C V, Ench Y. Epstein–Barr virus infectious mononucleosis in children. 2. Heterophil antibody and viral-specific responses. Pediatrics 1985; 75: 1011–1019.
27 Putto A, Meurman O, Ruuskanen O. C-reactive protein in the differentiation of adenoviral, Epstein–Barr viral and streptococcal tonsillitis in children. Eur J Pediatr 1986; 145: 204–206.
28 Markowitz M, Gerber M A, Kaplan E L. Treatment of streptococcal pharyngotonsillitis: reports of penicillin's demise are premature. J Pediatr 1993; 123: 679–685.

29 Gerber M A, Spadaccini L J, Wright L L, Deutsch L, Kaplan E L. Twice-daily penicillin in the treatment of streptococcal pharyngitis. Am J Dis Child 1985; 139: 1145–1148.

30 Pichichero M E. Cephalosporins are superior to penicillin for treatment of streptococcal tonsillopharyngitis: is the difference worth it? Pediatr Infect Dis J 1993; 12: 268–274.

31 Gerber M A, Randolph M F, Chanatry J, Wright L L, Anderson L R, Kaplan E L. Once daily therapy for streptococcal pharyngitis with cefadroxil. J Pediatr 1986; 109: 531–537.

32 Seppälä H, Nissinen A, Järvinen H. Resistance to erythromycin in group A streptococci. N Engl J Med 1992; 326: 292–297.

33 Gerber M A, Randolph M F, Chanatry J, Wright L L, DeMeo K, Kaplan E L. Five vs ten days of penicillin V therapy for streptococcal pharyngitis. Am J Dis Child 1987; 141: 224–227.

34 Macrolides in the treatment of streptococcal pharyngitis. In: Pechere J-C, ed. Acute bacterial pharyngitis. Wellingborough: Sterling Press, 1994: pp 95–100.

35 Snellman L W, Stang H J, Stang J M, Johnson D R, Kaplan E L. Duration of positive throat cultures for group A streptococci after initiation of antibiotic therapy. Pediatrics 1993; 91: 1166–1170.

36 Holm S E. Reasons for failures in penicillin treatment of streptococcal tonsillitis and possible alternatives. Pediatr Infect Dis J 1994; 13: S66–S69.

37 Musser J M, Gray B M, Schlievert P M, Pichichero M E. Streptococcus pyogenes pharyngitis: characterization of strains by multilocus enzyme genotype, M and T protein serotype, and pyrogenic exotoxin gene probing. J Clin Microbiol 1992; 30: 600–603.

38 Bicknell P G. Role of adenotonsillectomy in the management of pediatric ear, nose and throat infections. Pediatr Infect Dis J 1994; 13: S75–S78.

39 Bisno A L. Group A streptococcal infections and acute rheumatic fever. N Engl J Med 1991; 325: 783–793.

40 Shulman S T. Complications of streptococcal pharyngitis. Pediatr Infect Dis J 1994; 13: S70–74.

1A.4 Ears: acute otitis media, recurrent otitis media, glue ear, cholesteatoma, mastoiditis, otitis externa

OTITIS MEDIA: EPIDEMIOLOGY AND PATHOGENESIS

Over 90% of children experience at least one episode of acute otitis media by age 5 years.[1] Nearly one-third will have more than six episodes before entering school. Infants who develop an episode of acute otitis media in the first 6 months of life tend to be otitis prone, and represent a group characterized by multiple episodes of middle ear infection in the ensuing 4–5 years. Risk factors for acute otitis media and recurrent acute otitis media include: (1) male sex; (2) familial predisposition (perhaps due to environmental factors such as exposure to cigarette smoke and/or air pollutants, and also related to Eustachian tube anatomy); (3) bottle-feeding (particularly when infants have their bottle propped); and (4) attendance at day care (where more frequent upper respiratory viral infections are transmitted which predispose to secondary acute otitis media). Acute otitis media reaches a peak incidence between 6 and 24 months of age and then declines. It is less common after 5 years of age. Acute otitis media is most frequently seen in the winter months in temperate climates.

The Eustachian tube protects the middle ear from nasopharyngeal secretions, provides drainage into the nasopharynx of secretions produced within the middle ear, and permits equilibration of air pressure with atmospheric pressure in the middle ear. Obstruction of the Eustachian tube can result from nasopharyngeal infection (usually initially viral), or from an inflammatory response induced by allergy or irritants (e.g. cigarette smoke, air pollutants); middle ear effusion with subsequent acute otitis media may follow. Extrinsic obstruction usually occurs as a consequence of hypertrophied adenoids or, rarely, nasopharyngeal tumours. Obstruction is more common in infants and young children in the first few years of life (the age of greatest incidence of otitis media) because the amount and stiffness of the cartilage support of the Eustachian tube is less than that seen in older children and adults. Eustachian tube obstruction typically results in negative middle ear pressure. If the Eustachian tube is obstructed intermittently, contamination of the middle ear from nasopharyngeal secretions containing bacteria may occur by reflux, and acute (suppurative) otitis media ensues. Alternatively, the Eustachian tube may remain obstructed and a sterile effusion occurs as a consequence of mucus production from middle ear goblet cells.

ACUTE (SUPPURATIVE) OTITIS MEDIA

Clinical manifestations

At the age when children most frequently experience acute otitis media, they are unable verbally to alert their parents as to their discomfort. Thus physicians and parents are left to look for non-specific symptoms of ear tugging, restlessness during sleep, diminished appetite, irritability or fussiness, hearing loss and fever.

When one or more of these symptoms occurs, an examination of the child is appropriate. Classical signs of acute otitis media include a red and bulging ear drum with poor mobility detected during pneumatic otoscopy. Exudate may be visible behind the tympanic membrane, which may be white, yellow or grey in colour. More subtle clinical signs may be present; however, tympanic membrane mobility is the single most useful examination parameter to detect middle ear effusion. Redness of the ear drum is the least reliable sign of acute infection.

Aetiology

The aetiology of acute otitis media based on diagnostic tympanocentesis cultures is summarized from multiple published studies in Figure 1A.4.1. Variations occur in differing geographical regions of the world. *Streptococcus pneumoniae* represents the single most common isolate, followed by *Haemophilus influenzae* and *Moraxella* (*Branhamella*) *catarrhalis*.[2] Together these three bacteria represent the major pathogens to be considered in empirical antimicrobial therapy. *Streptococcus pyogenes* (group A streptococci) and *Staphylococcus aureus* are less common, but require consideration.

In recent years, the emergence of penicillin-resistant pneumococci has complicated empirical antimicrobial management decisions. The prevalence of penicillin-resistant pneumococci in upper respiratory isolates varies from country to country, region to region, community to community, and from one patient population to another. Temporal variations also occur in the same patient population. The prevalence of β-lactamase-producing strains of *Haemophilus influenzae* and *Moraxella catarrhalis* has increased over the last decade. In most communities it should be anticipated that approximately 30–35% of *H. influenzae* and 80–95% of *M. catarrhalis* will produce β-lactamase, thereby rendering these organisms resistant to penicillin and amoxycillin.

The role which respiratory viruses play in otitis media pathogenesis and aetiology is currently not completely established. Respiratory viruses may incite Eustachian tube inflammation and middle ear exudation, thereby establishing a fertile ground for secondary bacterial infection.[3] An exclusive viral aetiology for acute otitis media is uncommon. A failure to respond to antimicrobial therapy might be anticipated in children who have concomitant infection with a virus

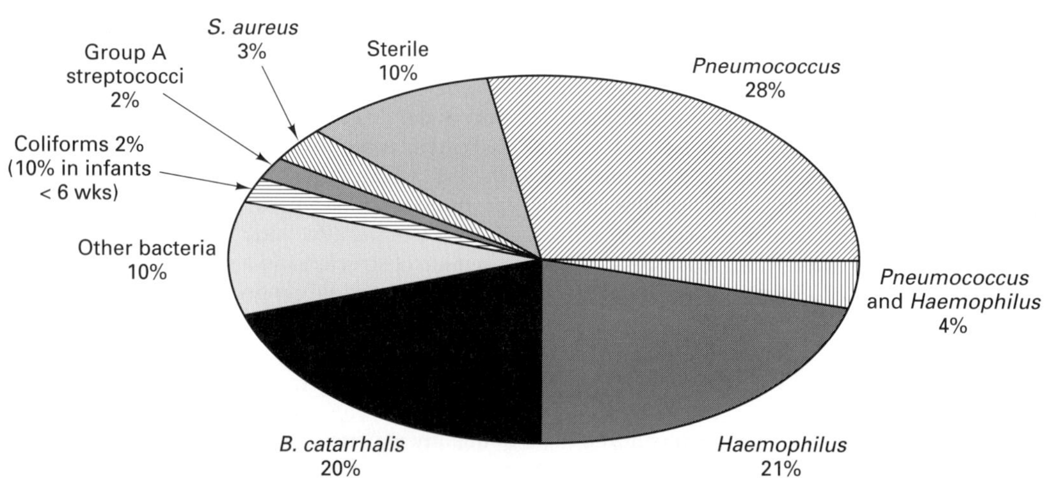

Fig. 1A.4.1   Aetiology of acute otitis media, based on tympanocentesis cultures from published reports in the past decade.

Table 1A.4.1 Spontaneous cure rates in mild-to-moderate acute otitis media[10]

Reference	Patients (n)	Patient's age (years)	Spontaneous cure rate[a] (%)
Halsted et al, 1968	27	0–3	81
Laxdal et al, 1970	48	0–14	46
Howie and Ploussard 1972	116	0–2.5	14
Mygind et al, 1981	77	1–10	69
Van Buchem, 1981	76	2–12	73
Thalen et al, 1989	158	2–15	88
Engelhard et al, 1989	35	0.3–1	23
Burke et al, 1991	118	3–10	86
Appelman et al, 1991	54	0.5–12	81
Kaleida et al, 1991	273	0.5–12	63▲
	86	0.5–12	52▼

[a]Asymptomatic with normal otoscopic results at 10 to 14 days after diagnosis
▲, mild; ▼, moderate.

and a bacteria.[4] When tympanocentesis cultures are obtained and are found to be bacteriologically sterile, this is more often a consequence of host immunity killing the inciting bacteria prior to culture rather than a viral cause or a sterile effusion.

Acute otitis media has a reasonably high spontaneous cure rate, and symptomatic therapy (analgesia) may be satisfactory and appropriate management of some acute otitis media patients.[5,6] A review of controlled trials of acute otitis media which included patients who were not treated with antimicrobials is shown in Table 1A.4.1. Between 14% and 88% of patients (average 60–70%) will experience spontaneous resolution of their middle ear infection within 10–14 days after diagnosis. Higher spontaneous cures are observed when *Haemophilus influenzae* (about 50%) or *Moraxella catarrhalis* (about 80%) are the causative pathogens, in contrast to *Streptococcus pneumoniae* (10–20%).

Treatment

Symptomatic

Acetaminophen (paracetamol), ibuprofen or other analgesics may be useful to relieve pain associated with acute otitis media. Warmed oil containing benzocaine or other anaesthetics applied as ear drops to the affected ear may generate some pain relief. Local heat is also sometimes useful. Decongestants and antihistamines, though widely prescribed, have been repeatedly shown not to produce any benefit in prevention, symptomatic relief or rapidity of resolution of acute otitis media. Nose drops are also of no value, nor are cotton wicks, bed rest or covering the ears.

Antimicrobials

Amoxycillin (40 mg/kg per day in three divided doses) is currently the treatment of choice for most children with acute otitis media. However, the efficacy of amoxycillin in the treatment of relatively resistant and highly penicillin-resistant pneumococci in acute otitis media remains to be evaluated. Levels of antimicrobials in middle ear fluid which can be achieved may be sufficient at least against relatively penicillin-resistant *Streptococcus pneumoniae*. *Haemophilus influenzae* and *Moraxella catarrhalis* strains which produce β-lactamase are not susceptible to amoxycillin, nor are β-lactamase-producing strains of *Staphylococcus aureus*.

Relying on the higher spontaneous cure rate following *Haemophilus influenzae* and *Moraxella catarrhalis* middle ear infections, physicians in some countries utilize penicillin (10–25 mg/kg per day in three divided doses) as treatment mainly targeting *Streptococcus pneumoniae*, which has a much lower spontaneous cure rate. The efficacy of penicillin for treatment of relatively or highly penicillin-resistant pneumococci in acute otitis media has not been studied. Trimethoprim–sulphamethoxazole (8 and 40 mg/kg per day in two divided doses) is often used as an antimicrobial alternative in acute otitis media; however, *Streptococcus pyogenes* is usually resistant, as are 10–30% of *Streptococcus pneumoniae* strains and 1–12% of *H. influenzae*.

Other antimicrobial options available for treatment of acute otitis media are numerous (Table 1A.4.2). When clinical assessment of efficacy is made at the end of treatment or thereafter, the various alternative antimicrobials are generally similar in resolving the signs and symptoms of acute otitis media. Comparative efficacy studies have failed to show significant differences among these agents, largely as a consequence of inadequate sample size in the trials.[7]

Despite the limitations of comparative trials, several general observations have emerged regarding the various antimicrobial alternatives to amoxycillin. The efficacy of cefaclor appears to be lower than that achieved with cefuroxime axetil, cefixime or amoxycillin/clavulanate. A higher incidence of diarrhoea occurs with amoxycillin/clavulanate than with most of the other newer antimicrobial alternatives. This side-effect, however, can be reduced by recommending administration with meals and at 8 h intervals, if possible. The efficacy of cefixime and ceftibuten against *Streptococcus pneumoniae* may not be comparable to that achievable with the second-generation cephalosporins or cefpodoxime proxetil. However, the β-lactamase stability of cefixime and ceftibuten are exceptional, thus affording them consideration as preferred agents when a β-lactamase-producing *Haemophilus influenzae* or *Moraxella catarrhalis* infection is presumed or confirmed by tympanocentesis.

Antimicrobials that produce faster eradication of the bacterial pathogen, or more rapid resolution of middle ear effusion, may offer an advantage in acute otitis media management.[8] The antimicrobial effect on acute otitis media pathogens can most accurately be assessed by comparing pretreatment tympanocentesis cultures with repeat tympanocentesis cultures 2–5 days after starting therapy. This 'in vivo sensitivity test' has been used in several clinical trials and appears to confirm that sensitivity in vitro generally parallels results in vivo in most clinical situations.[9] The spontaneous cure rate from *Streptococcus pneumoniae* infection is low (about 20%) in comparison to that observed with *Haemophilus influenzae* (about 50%). Amoxycillin is effective therapy in eradicating

Table 1A.4.2   Anticipated efficacy of selected antimicrobial agents against acute otitis media pathogens

Agents	*Streptococcus pneumoniae*	*Haemophilus influenzae*	*Streptococcus pyogenes*	*Moraxella catarrhalis*	*Staphylococcus aureus*
Amoxycillin	+	±	+	±	±
Erythromycin and sulphisoxazole	±	±	±	±	±
Trimethoprim and sulphamethoxazole	±	±	–	–	+
Amoxycillin and clavulanate	+	+	+	+	+
Cefaclor	+	±	+	±	±
Cefuroxime axetil	+	+	+	+	+
Cefixime	±	+	+	+	–
Cefprozil	+	+	+	+	+
Loracarbef	+	+	+	+	+
Ceftibuten	±	+	+	+	–
Cefpodoxime proxetil	+	+	+	+	±

+, usually effective; ± may or may not be effective; – not effective.

95% of S. *pneumoniae* if strains are not penicillin resistant, and 95% of *H. influenzae* if the strains do not produce β-lactamase. No data are yet available on the efficacy of amoxycillin for resistant pneumococci, but eradication of β-lactamase-producing *H. influenzae* has been evaluated and shown to be ineffective.

Since the causative organism is rarely known before antimicrobial therapy is prescribed, the circumstances in which an alternative to amoxycillin becomes a preferred therapy for acute otitis media require attention (Table 1A.4.3):

1. Effective antimicrobial therapy in acute otitis media should produce a significant reduction in symptoms within 48 h of initiation. In the absence of such a clinical response, the first selected antibiotic should be discontinued and an alternative prescribed. In the amoxycillin-treated patient, a clinical failure most likely involves β-lactamase-producing strains of *Haemophilus influenzae* or *Moraxella catarrhalis* or possibly penicillin-resistant pneumococci.
2. Patients may appear to respond with clinical improvement on initiation of antimicrobial treatment, but on completion of therapy or shortly thereafter acute otitis media is found to persist. These patients are often infected with resistant microbes and alternative therapy should be used to eradicate infection.
3. Identification of the causative pathogen in acute otitis media is becoming more important with increasing emergence of resistant pathogens. Tympanocentesis should be considered for its diagnostic usefulness for children who unsatisfactorily respond to antimicrobial therapy. If tympanocentesis is performed, bacteria thereby identified can be tested for susceptibility to the antimicrobial alternatives available and therapeutic decisions can be based on these results.
4. Some children develop a pattern of clinical failure with amoxycillin or other first-line therapies. The frequency of failure to be tolerated before abandonment of a first-line agent must be adapted to the specific clinical situation. Two or three failures within a single respiratory season should be sufficient to prompt the use of alternative agents in a particular child.
5. Compliance issues sometimes dictate the selection of an antimicrobial since three times daily dosing can represent a compliance barrier as compared to once- or twice-daily dosing.
6. As the prevalence of penicillin/amoxycillin-resistant pathogens rises, which we expect to occur in the coming years, broader-spectrum, β-lactamase-stable agents may more frequently replace amoxycillin as first-line therapy.[10]

Tympanocentesis. Tympanocentesis is not technically difficult. It is easier to perform than venipuncture or lumbar puncture. Tympanocentesis is a procedure within the purview of primary care physicians who diagnose and treat children with acute otitis media. A simplified method for a myringotomy and tympanocentesis procedure that avoids the use of complicated equipment is presented in the Appendix at the end of this chapter.

Tympanocentesis relieves the pain of the crying child suffering with a bulging

Table 1A.4.3   Indications for alternative antimicrobial agents for acute otitis media

Initial treatment failure
Persistent infection at 10–14 days
Culture-positive susceptible organism
Prior treatment failures
Compliance features
High incidence of resistant organisms in community

tympanic membrane associated with acute middle ear infection. Acute otitis media is essentially an abscess of the middle ear. Polymorphonuclear cells migrate to the middle ear space as part of the natural host defence reaction to bacteria present. In some children, the tympanic membrane bulges to a sufficient degree that on examination its apparent rupture is imminent. In these children, tympanocentesis can preclude spontaneous perforation and its potential complications, while simultaneously providing a culture specimen to direct antimicrobial therapy.

The clinical situation of persistent otitis media and apparent antibiotic failure occurs with some frequency. Subsequent antimicrobial selection is usually empirical. When a child has failed first-line antimicrobial therapy, tympanocentesis can be useful to identify the organisms present and to guide subsequent antimicrobial selection. The value of tympanocentesis is further enhanced when two differing antimicrobial courses have been utilized, one following the other, and still clinical treatment failure is observed. In these circumstances, 50% of children will have a sterile inflammatory effusion.[11,12] An ongoing inflammatory response due to bacterial cell wall fragments mimics clinical failure. In the remaining 50% of children who have failed one or two sequential courses of antimicrobial therapy, an organism can be isolated which guides subsequent antimicrobial selection.[11,12]

The treatment duration with antimicrobials for acute otitis media has not been adequately established by carefully controlled trials. The range of recommendations spans a single injection of ceftriaxone (2–3 days therapy) to 14 days. In most cases 5–7 days therapy is adequate, although the standard in the USA is for a 10-day treatment regimen.

The adverse effects produced by an antimicrobial are an important consideration in prescribing preferences. Overall, the safety of the various oral antimicrobials used for treatment of otitis media is exceptionally good. All have a tendency to produce mild gastrointestinal upset, usually manifest as loosening of the stools. Trimethoprim–sulphamethoxazole is particularly recognized for its greater propensity to produce allergic hypersensitivity reactions and the Stevens–Johnson syndrome. Erythromycin and the newer extended-spectrum macrolides to a lesser degree produce nausea and, in more severe cases, vomiting. Significant alteration of haematological, hepatic or renal chemistries is extremely uncommon with virtually all of these agents. Cefaclor is unique among the various cephalosporins in its propensity to produce a serum sickness-like reaction.

Cost for the various newer antimicrobial agents available for treatment of acute otitis media must be considered (Table 1A.4.4). All of the newer agents are more expensive than penicillin and amoxycillin. Thus, comparisons in an individual community should be sought so the prescribing physician is aware of the antimicrobial expense involved. Consideration of the palatability in suspension formulation is also relevant in selecting among the alternative antimicrobials for treatment.[13]

RECURRENT ACUTE OTITIS MEDIA

Recurrent acute otitis media is a frequent problem for many children. It predominates in males, certain families who are genetically or environmentally predisposed, in bottle-fed infants and in those attending day care. Amoxycillin-resistant bacteria occur more commonly in middle ear effusions in children with recurrences. However, in many cases the bacteria cultured from recurrent acute otitis media effusions by tympanocentesis are susceptible to previously prescribed

Table 1A.4.4 Antimicrobials for treatment of acute otitis media

	Dose per day (mg/kg)	Palatability	Dosing frequency per day	Cost
Amoxycillin	40	Good	×3	Low
Combination agents				
Trimethoprim–sulphamethoxazole	8/40	Brand = good Generic = acceptable	×2	Moderate Low
Erythromycin–sulphisoxazole	50/160	Acceptable	×4	Moderate
Amoxycillin–clavulanate	40/100	Acceptable	×3	High
Cephalosporins				
Cefaclor	30	Excellent	×2	High
Cefuroxime axetil	30	Acceptable	×2	High
Cefprozil	30	Good	×2	High
Loracarbef	30	Good	×2	High
Cefixime	8	Excellent	×1	High
Ceftibuten	9	Good	×1	High
Cefpodoxime proxetil	10	Acceptable	×2	High

antibiotics, suggesting that host factors in addition to antimicrobial susceptibility can be important in predicting recurrent acute otitis media. Significant factors include variations in antimicrobial absorption, bioavailability, penetration into middle ear effusions, activity in the low-pH environment of middle ear pus and host immunity are all contributing factors to in vivo antibiotic efficacy. Tympanocentesis is a useful diagnostic tool in this clinical setting as opposed to a continuation of empirical antimicrobial selection. After two or three treatment courses of different antimicrobials, if clinical resolution has not occurred myringotomy with culture would be recommended.

Antimicrobial prophylaxis is sometimes used to prevent recurrent acute otitis media.[14] Clinical trials have shown that single doses of sulphisoxazole (75 mg/kg per day as a single dose) or amoxycillin (20 mg/kg per day as a single dose) reduce the frequency of recurrent acute otitis media by 50–80%. Antimicrobial prophylaxis therefore may be appropriate in selected children with recurrent acute otitis media. Prophylaxis is usually continued for 6–8 weeks or in some cases for the entire winter respiratory infection season; it should be considered as a therapeutic option in patients who have experienced three recurrent otitis media episodes within a 6-month time frame, or four episodes within 1 year. Prophylaxis should be selectively used, out of concern for promoting emergence of antimicrobial resistance, but it is a preferred approach prior to surgical intervention with the placement of tympanostomy tubes (grommets). Since the occurrence of recurrent acute otitis media is age related and most children will outgrow this problem within 1–2 years, aggressive management should be cautiously undertaken and selectively applied primarily to patients experiencing complications or sequelae.

Tympanostomy tubes (grommets) and adenoidectomy

Surgical prevention of acute otitis media can be achieved in some patients by tympanostomy tube (grommet) insertion. Grommet insertion and antimicrobial prophylaxis are equally effective (about 50–80% success rate) in prevention of recurrent otitis media.[14,15] Grommets have a propensity to produce tympanosclerosis (50% of patients) and tympanic atrophy (20–30% of patients).[16] Adenoidectomy is considered another surgical alternative in children with recurrent acute otitis media and/or chronic otitis media with effusion; however, its value is controversial.

Surgical treatment with myringotomy and grommet insertion has been the most effective treatment for chronic otitis media with effusion. However, 10–15% of children experience progression of disease with accompanying chronic or recurring otorrhoea, and 40–50% require repeat grommet insertion when the initial tubes extrude early.

CHRONIC OTITIS MEDIA WITH EFFUSION ('GLUE EAR')

Otitis media with effusion is recognized clinically in the child who lacks otalgia and fever but on examination shows evidence of effusion, usually with an associated retracted tympanic membrane. The mobility of the ear drum is almost always impaired, the tympanic membrane opaque, and an amber exudate is often observed in the middle ear space through the thickened tympanic membrane. Auditory acuity is usually decreased and as a consequence language acquisition can be delayed and the child's behaviour may reflect disinterest in his or her environment. Most of these effusions resolve spontaneously. However, while they persist, mild to moderate hearing loss may occur. During this time frame, language development may be delayed.

When middle ear effusion persists for 3 months it is termed 'chronic' and more aggressive treatment is usually indicated, particularly if associated with hearing loss in the child. A trial of antimicrobials may be appropriate treatment in these children if one has not recently been used. Bacteria have been found in patients with chronic otitis media with effusion and some studies suggest at least a marginal benefit associated with antimicrobial treatment of 10 days duration. Use of systemic corticosteroids (prednisone, 1 mg/kg per day in two divided doses) has been advocated in some studies and will produce a sufficient reduction in Eustachian tube inflammation to allow drainage in some cases. If these measures are unsuccessful a myringotomy should be performed and consideration should be given to the placement of grommets. Intranasal steroids, vasoconstrictive nose sprays and systemic decongestants/antihistamines are of no benefit. A suggested approach to the child with otitis media with effusion is shown in Figure 1A.4.2.

COMPLICATIONS AND SEQUELAE[17,18]

Hearing loss

Fluctuating or persistent loss of hearing is often associated with acute otitis media and chronic otitis media with effusion. This hearing loss is usually reversible with resolution of the infection and the effusion. However, permanent conductive hearing loss can occur from irreversible changes in the middle ear as a consequence of recurrent acute otitis media or chronic otitis media with effusion (e.g. tympanosclerosis, tympanic atrophy, adhesive otitis, or ossicular discontinuity). Audiometric assessment is usually helpful if the child can cooperate with the examination in order to determine the severity of hearing loss associated with middle ear conditions. As the degree of impairment and duration of the condition lengthens, the necessity for action increases.

Perforation

The tympanic membrane may spontaneously rupture during an episode of acute otitis media. Spontaneous healing usually follows. On occasion, a perforation persists and otorrhoea may occur. Persistent otorrhoea usually represents infection requiring treatment.

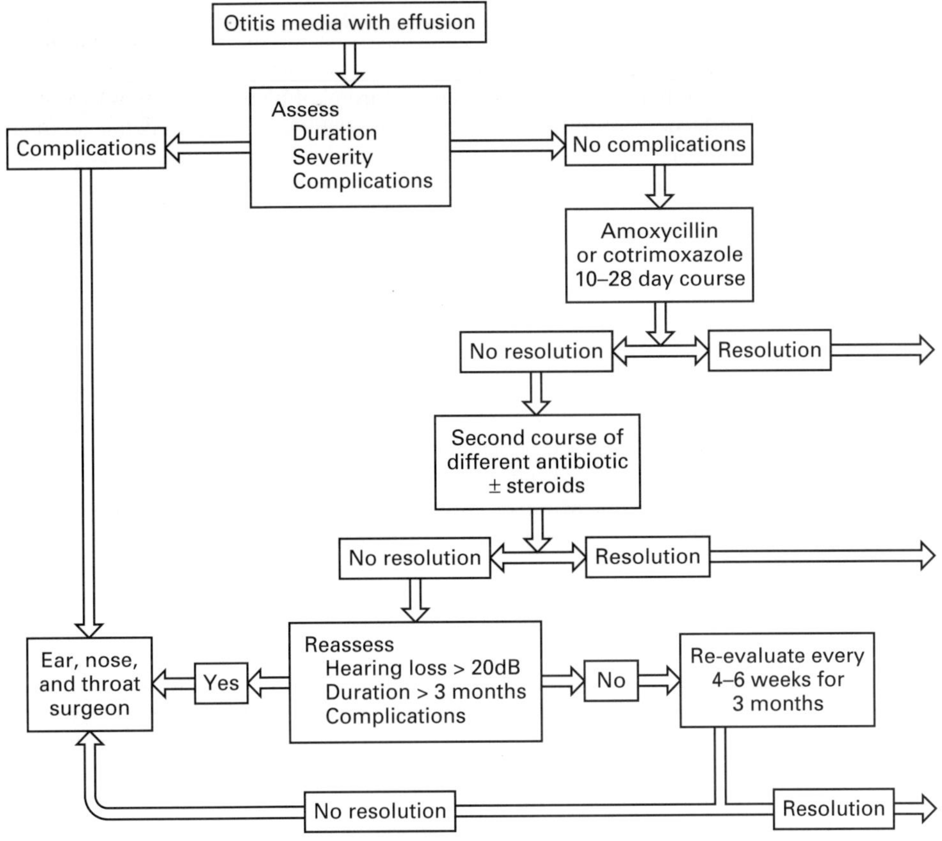

Fig. 1A.4.2 The management of otitis media with effusion. (From Isaacs D. *Goodbye to grommets. Curr Opin Pediatr* 1994; 6: 3–6.

Cholesteatoma

As a consequence of chronic inflammation and particularly in the context of persistent negative middle ear pressure, a cholesteatoma may form. Tympano-mastoid surgery is indicated when this condition is recognized, because if surgery is delayed the condition can progress and destroy other structures in adjacent bone and tissue.

Mastoiditis

Infrequently, acute otitis media is accompanied by mastoiditis. This can be recognized by associated pain, tenderness, erythema and swelling of the post-auricular area. Myringotomy should be performed and antimicrobials prescribed. The same organisms involved in acute otitis media are typically involved in acute mastoiditis. If there is an inadequate clinical response to antimicrobial therapy, then surgical drainage may become necessary. Untreated the infection may advance into adjacent soft tissues, bone or the central nervous system.

Intracranial complications

Meningitis is the most common of the intracranial complications associated with acute otitis media. Dissemination may occur through venous channels, bone erosion or bacteraemia. Brain abscess may result from direct perivascular extension of infection or may develop from an adjacent focus of infection, or from retrograde thrombophlebitis. The lateral sinus lies in the temporal bone in close proximity to the mastoid. Thrombophlebitis may occur, leading to partial or total occlusion of the sinus. Subdural abscess may occur as a result of a direct extension through the dura or from venous thrombophlebitis.

When headache, irritability, lethargy, meningismus or papilloedema occur in the context of acute otitis media, an intracranial process should be suspected. Blood cultures and lumbar puncture should be performed. A CT or MRI scan may be of value diagnostically. Treatment should consist of a diagnostic tympano-centesis and parenteral antimicrobials. Mastoidectomy should be considered if mastoiditis coexists.

CHRONIC SUPPURATIVE OTITIS MEDIA

In association with acute otitis media, particularly recurrent acute otitis media, a chronic tympanic membrane perforation may occur. Drainage of mucus and/or pus from the middle ear through the perforation creates a fertile ground for bacterial superinfection. Mucosal oedema frequently occurs involving the external auditory canal, and eventually a state of chronic inflammation involving the external and middle ear ensues. Most frequently, *Pseudomonas aeruginosa* or other Gram-negative bacilli are involved in pathogenesis. Appropriate culture and sensitivity testing should be undertaken if possible. Empirical therapy with most oral antimicrobials, topical application of antimicrobial ear drops etc. will not be of benefit. Parenterally administered broad-spectrum antimicrobials with activity against *Pseudomonas* spp. and other Gram-negative bacilli may be efficacious. Oral fluoroquinolones have been evaluated and shown to be effective in some patients. Removal of cerumen, exudate and other debris from the external auditory canal through careful suction and gentle irrigation is an important adjunctive therapy. If no response is observed after 6–8 weeks of aggressive medical management with good compliance, referral for tympanic membrane surgery is appropriate.

EXTERNAL OTITIS MEDIA[19]

Aetiology

External otitis is most commonly caused by *Pseudomonas aeruginosa*. Other organisms which less frequently produce external otitis include *Staphylococcus aureus*, streptococci, and various Gram-negative enteric bacilli. External otitis most frequently results from irritation and maceration from excessive moisture in the external auditory canal sometimes referred to as 'swimmer's ear'; the condition is often observed in individuals who have had prolonged exposure to water.

Clinical manifestations

External otitis is easily distinguished from acute otitis media by the presence of increased pain on manipulation of the pinna, and especially by pressure on the tragus. Oedema and inflammation of the external auditory canal may be noted on examination. A creamy or greenish otorrhoea may be apparent. Examination of the tympanic membrane may be difficult due to the pain on insertion of the otoscope. Acute suppurative otitis media rarely accompanies external otitis.

Treatment

Topical installation of otic (or ophthalmic) antimicrobial drops are effective in the treatment of external otitis. Acetic acid solutions (vinegar mixed with water), hydrogen peroxide solutions, or mixtures of the two are probably as effective as antimicrobial ear drop preparations. Cleaning the external auditory canal to remove debris by irrigation with dilute (2%) acetic acid solution will enhance recovery. Oral antimicrobials are usually not necessary. Oral administration of ciprofloxacin or other fluoroquinolone antibiotics may be justified in severe cases since this antimicrobial agent is particularly effective against *Pseudomonas aeruginosa*. It should be kept in mind that fluoroquinolones have been associated with cystic degeneration of developing cartilage in an infant puppy model. The most effective prophylaxis for external otitis is installation of dilute isopropyl alcohol immediately following swimming, bathing or other prolonged exposure to water.

REFERENCES

1 Teele D W, Klein J O, Rosner B and the Greater Boston Otitis Media Study Group. Epidemiology of otitis media during the first seven years of life in children in greater Boston: a prospective, cohort study. J Infect Dis 1989; 160: 83–94.
2 Harrison C J, Marks M I, Welch D F. Microbiology of recently treated acute otitis media compared with previously untreated acute otitis media. Pediatr Infect Dis 1985; 4: 641–646.
3 Arola M, Ruuskanen O, Ziegler T et al. Clinical role of respiratory virus infection in acute otitis media. Pediatrics 1990; 86: 848–855.
4 Chonmaitree T, Owen M J, Howie V M. Respiratory viruses interfere with bacteriologic response to antibiotic in children with acute otitis media. J Infect Dis 1990; 162: 546–549.
5 Van Buchem F L, Peeters M F, Van'T Hof M A. Acute otitis media: a new treatment strategy. Br Med J 1985; 290: 1033–1037.
6 Burke P, Bain J, Robinson D, Dunleavey J. Acute red ear in children: controlled trial of non-antibiotic treatment in general practice.
7 Marchant C D, Carlin S A, Johnson C E, Shurin P A. Measuring the comparative efficacy of antibacterial agents for acute otitis media: the 'Pollyanna phenomenon'. J Pediatr 1992; 120: 72–77.
8 Kempthorne J, Giebink G S. Pediatric approach to the diagnosis and management of otitis media. Otolaryngol Clin North Am 1991; 24: 905–928.
9 Klein J O. Microbiologic efficacy of antibacterial drugs for acute otitis media. Pediatr Infect Dis J 1993; 12: 973–975.
10 Pichichero M E. Assessing the treatment alternatives for acute otitis media. Pediatr Infect Dis J 1994; 13: S27–34.
11 Pichichero M E, Pichichero C L. Persistent acute otitis media. I. Causative pathogens. Pediatr Infect Dis J 1995; 14: 178–183.
12 Pichichero M E, Pichichero C L. Persistent acute otitis media. II. Antimicrobial treatment. Pediatr Infect Dis J 1995; 14: 183–188.
13 Demers D M, Schotik Chan D, Bass J W. Antimicrobial drug suspensions: a blinded comparison of taste of twelve common pediatric drugs including cefixime, cefpodoxime, cefprozil, and loracarbef. Pediatr Infect Dis J 1994; 13: 87–89.
14 Williams R L, Chalmers T C, Stange K C, Chalmers F T, Bowlin S J. Use of antibiotics in preventing recurrent acute otitis media and in treating otitis media with effusion. A meta-analytic attempt to resolve the brouhaha. JAMA 1993; 270: 1344–1351.
15 Le C T, Freeman D W, Fireman B H. Evaluation of ventilating tubes and myringotomy in the treatment of recurrent or persistent otitis media. Pediatr Infect Dis J 1991; 10: 2–11.
16 Casselbrant M L, Kaleida P H, Rockette H E et al. Efficacy of antimicrobial prophylaxis and of tympanostomy tube insertion for prevention of recurrent acute otitis media: results of a randomized clinical trial. Pediatr Infect Dis J 1992; 11: 278–286.
17 Pichichero M E, Berghash L R, Hengerer A S. Anatomic and audiologic sequelae after tympanostomy tube insertion or prolonged antibiotic therapy for otitis media. Pediatr Infect Dis J 1989; 8: 780–787.
18 Teele D W, Klein J O, Chase C, Manyuk P, Rosner B A and the Greater Boston Otitis Media Study Group. Otitis media in infancy and intellectual ability, school achievement, speech, and language at age 7 years. J Infect Dis 1990; 162: 685–694.

19 Fliss D M, Leiberman A, Dagan R. Medical sequelae and complications of acute otitis media. Pediatr Infect Dis J 1994; 13: S34–40.
20 Marcy S M. Infections of the external ear. Pediatr Infect Dis 1985; 4: 192–201.

APPENDIX: TYMPANOCENTESIS

Tympanocentesis is a needle aspiration of middle ear fluid for therapeutic and/or diagnostic purposes. This procedure is performed to relieve pain and/or to identify the pathogens present in acute or persistent otitis media.

Indications

1. Severe ear pain in any child.
2. When tympanic membrane spontaneous rupture appears likely, based on examination.
3. Persistent acute otitis media following empirical antimicrobial therapy.
4. Acute otitis media associated with a suppurative complication such as mastoiditis, meningitis, facial paralysis or brain abscess.
5. Otitis media in the newborn (less than 30 days old).
6. Otitis media in the immunocompromised child (where an unusual organism may produce infection).

Contraindications and precautions

It is difficult to perform tympanocentesis in children below 3 months of age. Visualization of the tympanic membrane is often inadequate as a consequence of the size of the external auditory canal.

The child must be adequately restrained throughout the procedure. This can best be accomplished with the child lying on an examination table in a papoose board with an assisting nurse controlling the head.

Equipment and supplies

1. Otoscope with an operating head.
2. 20 gauge spinal needle bent at a 30° angle approximately one-third from the hub. Bending the needle improves visualization during the procedure because it removes the operator's hand from the visual field at the time of tympanic membrane puncture (see Figs 1A.4.A1–4.A4).
3. 3 ml syringe, tuberculin syringe or senturion collection trap.

Description of the procedure

Proper restraint of the child should be assured by the physician. Local anaesthesia of the tympanic membrane is usually unsuccessful and is not recommended. Sedation or general anaesthesia is not required. The external auditory canal must be completely cleared of cerumen; this can be accomplished by suction or with a blunt curette. Some authorities recommend irrigation of the external auditory canal with betadine or isopropyl alcohol (70%). This is not an essential step because in virtually all cases contamination by *Staphylococcus epidermidis* or other skin commensals is absent or very low in quantity and easily distinguished from growth of middle ear pathogens.

Using the largest speculum that will fit the external canal, visualize the tympanic membrane through the operating head of the otoscope and puncture the inferior portion of the tympanic membrane with a bent 20 gauge spinal needle. As long as the puncture is made in the inferior portion of the tympanic membrane, no harm will come to the patient. The middle ear ossicles and cochlea lie in the superior portion of the middle ear space. It is preferable to puncture the tympanic

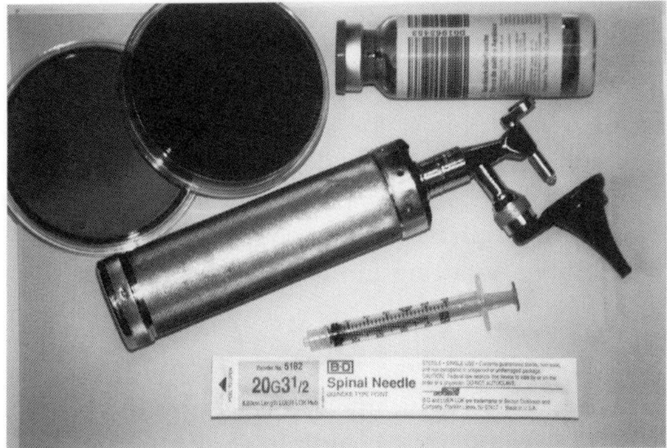

Fig. 1A.4.A1 Equipment and supplies for tympanocentesis: blood and chocolate agar plates; operating head otoscope; 20 G spinal needle and 3 ml syringe.

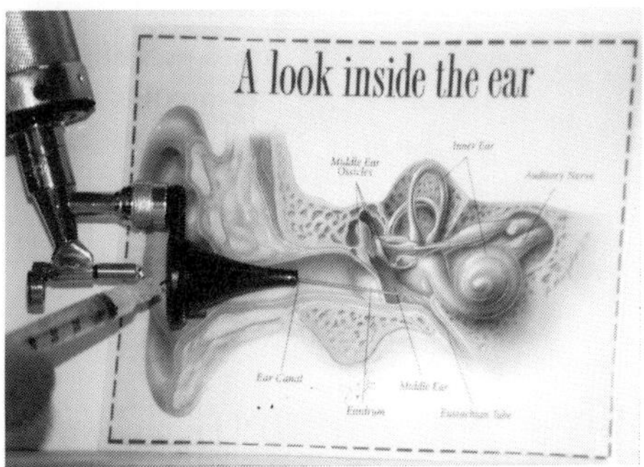

Fig. 1A.4.A2 Two-dimensional simulation of tympanocentesis, showing otoscope and needle/syringe position.

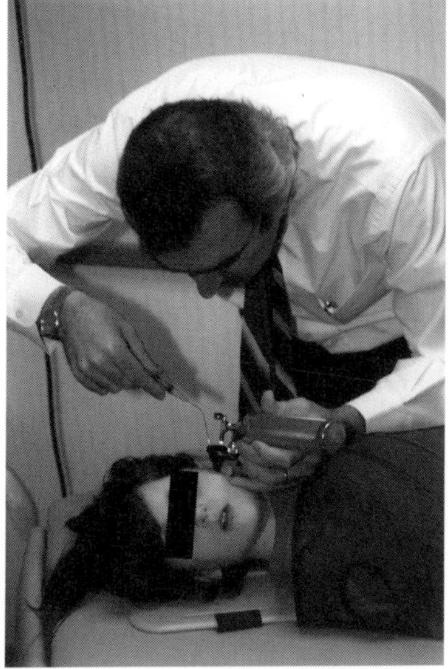

Fig. 1A.4.A3 Child in papoose board undergoing tympanocentesis.

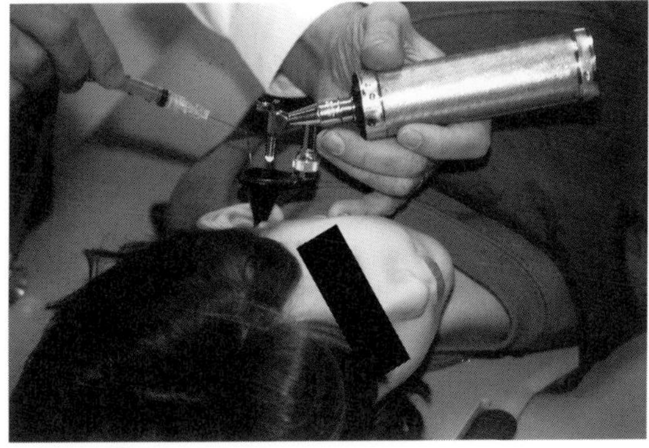

Fig. 1A.4.A4 Close-up of procedure.

membrane in the anterior inferior quadrant because there is more opportunity to push the needle deeper into the middle ear space so that the entire needle bevel is through the tympanic membrane. A common mistake is to only nick the tympanic membrane with the leading edge of the needle. Ensuring that the needle bevel fully penetrates through the tympanic membrane permits more effective suction during aspiration.

Fully aspirate as much of the middle ear fluid as possible. Withdraw the needle. The quantity of the aspirated fluid is usually small (< 0.1 ml). Therefore, it is best to rinse the tympanocentesis needle into blood culture media (trypticase soy broth or similar). One or two millilitres of the culture broth is drawn through the needle and into the attached syringe. The aspirate fluid is flushed back through the needle into the culture bottle to maximize the sensitivity of the collection.

The aspirated middle ear fluid should be cultured in broth and immediately inoculated on blood and chocolate agar plates. Microscopic examination after Gram staining is advisable.

Drainage from the middle ear will persist for approximately 24 h following tympanocentesis. If more prolonged drainage is desired, the tympanocentesis procedure is followed by a myringotomy. After aspiration of the middle ear fluid, the needle is partially withdrawn but with the cutting edge of the tip of the needle still within the tympanic membrane. A cutting motion of 2–3 mm is made across the tympanic membrane.

Side-effects and complications

Tympanocentesis with or without myringotomy typically produces ear fluid drainage sometimes with mild to moderate bleeding. If the petrous bone is struck by the needle after penetration of the tympanic membrane there will be increased bleeding from that periosteum. Persistent otorrhoea usually represents underlying middle ear disease rather than a problem from the procedure itself. Damage to the ossicular chain can be completely avoided with adequate restraint and assuring the needle puncture is made in the bottom half of the tympanic membrane. A persistent perforation of the tympanic membrane or formation of a sclerotic or atrophic scar is rare with tympanocentesis and / or myringotomy.

1A.5   Sinusitis

Upper respiratory infections are the most common organic condition presenting to the primary practitioner who cares for children. It has recently been estimated that approximately 5–10% of upper respiratory infections in early childhood are complicated by acute sinusitis.[1] As children average six to eight colds per year, sinusitis is a very common problem in clinical practice.

PATHOGENESIS

The respiratory mucosa that lines the nose is continuous with the mucosa that lines the paranasal sinuses. The secretions produced within the sinus cavities are delivered via the sinus ostia to the nose by normal mucociliary function. The maxillary, anterior ethmoid and frontal sinuses drain to the middle meatus; the sphenoid and posterior ethmoids drain to the superior meatus.

Three key elements are important to the normal physiology of the paranasal sinuses: the patency of the ostia, the function of the ciliary apparatus and, integral to the latter, the quality of secretions.[2] Retention of secretions in the paranasal sinuses is usually due to one or more of the following: obstruction of the ostia, reduction in the number or impairment in the function of the cilia or over-production or change in the viscosity of secretions.

Most acute sinusitis is thought to be a bacterial complication of a viral upper respiratory infection (URI). The viral infection affects the mucosa of the nose (causing a rhinitis) and often the mucosa of the sinuses as well. In most instances the inflammatory response subsides spontaneously. In some cases, however, the mucositis results in obstruction of the sinus ostia, impairment of the mucociliary apparatus and an alteration in the volume and quality of secretions.

The narrow calibre of the individual ostia that drain the maxillary and ethmoid sinuses sets the stage for obstruction to occur easily and often during the course of a viral URI. When obstruction does occur there is a transient increase in intra-sinal pressure. This is followed quickly by the development of a negative pressure within the sinus cavities as the oxygen component of the intrasinal air is rapidly absorbed by a metabolically active mucosa. When the pressure in the sinuses is negative relative to normal atmospheric pressure in the nose, conditions favour aspiration of mucus heavily laden with bacteria from the nose or nasopharynx into the presumably sterile paranasal sinuses. Alternatively, sneezing, sniffing and nose blowing with altered intrasinal pressure also facilitate bacterial contamination of the paranasal sinuses. Under ordinary circumstances these contaminating bacteria would be swept out again by normal ciliary function. However, when ciliary function is impaired and sinus ostia obstructed, bacteria have a chance to multiply to high density and initiate an intense inflammatory response.

The factors predisposing to ostial obstruction can be divided into those that

Table 1A.5.1 Factors predisposing to sinus ostial obstruction

MUCOSAL SWELLING
  Systemic disorder
    Viral URI
    Allergic inflammation
    Cystic fibrosis
    Immune disorders
    Immotile cilia

  Local insult
    Facial trauma
    Swimming, diving
    Rhinitis medicamentosa

MECHANICAL OBSTRUCTION
  Choanal atresia
  Deviated septum
  Nasal polyps
  Foreign body
  Tumour
  Ethmoid bullae

cause mucosal swelling, consequent either to systemic illness or to local insults, and those due to mechanical obstruction (Table 1A.5.1). Although many conditions may lead to ostial closure, viral URI and allergic inflammation are by far the most frequent and most important.

CLINICAL PRESENTATION (Table 1A.5.2)

During the course of an apparent viral upper respiratory infection, there are two common clinical presentations which suggest that the patient has acute sinusitis. These can be designated as 'persistent' and 'severe'.[3] The most common presentation is with persistent respiratory symptoms. In the context of acute sinusitis, persistent symptoms are those that last more than 10 but less than 30 days and have not begun to improve. The 10-day mark separates simple viral upper respiratory infection from sinusitis and the 30-day mark separates acute from subacute or chronic sinusitis. Most uncomplicated viral upper respiratory infections will last 5–7 days. Although patients may not be asymptomatic by the tenth day they are virtually always improved. The persistence of respiratory symptoms beyond the 10-day mark, without appreciable improvement, suggests a complication of the upper respiratory infection. The nasal discharge may be of any quality (thin or thick; clear, mucoid or purulent) and the cough (which may be dry or wet) must be present in the daytime, although it is often noted to be worse at night. Malodorous breath is often reported by parents of preschoolers. Complaints of facial pain and headache are rare, although occasional, painless, morning eye swelling occurs. The child may not appear very ill, and usually if fever is present it will be low grade. In this case, it is not the severity of the clinical symptoms but their persistence which calls for attention.

Table 1A.5.2 Sinusitis: clinical presentation

Persistent symptoms
  Nasal discharge or cough or both for ≥10 days and not improving

Severe symptoms
  High fever (temperature ≥39°C) and purulent nasal discharge together for ≥3 days

The second less common presentation is a 'cold' that seems more severe than usual. The severity is defined by a combination of high fever (at least 39.0°C) and purulent nasal discharge. The quality of nasal discharge undergoes frequent changes during the course of an uncomplicated viral URI. It begins as a watery discharge which becomes thicker, coloured and opaque after a few days. Most often the nasal discharge will remain purulent for several days and then clear again to a mucoid or watery consistency before resolving. If fever is present at all during the course of a viral URI it is at the outset, in association with other constitutional symptoms such as headache and myalgias. Usually the fever disappears and the respiratory symptoms begin. Accordingly, the combination of high fever and purulent nasal discharge for at least 3–4 days signals a secondary bacterial infection of the paranasal sinuses. This group of patients may suffer from headaches behind or above the eye and occasionally experience periorbital swelling.

Patients with subacute or chronic sinusitis present with a history of very protracted (more than 30 days and not improving) respiratory symptoms. Nasal congestion (obstruction) and cough (day and night) are most common. There is the frequent complaint of sore throat that results from mouth breathing secondary to nasal obstruction. Nasal discharge (of any quality) and headache are less common; fever is rare.

On physical examination the patient with sinusitis may have mucopurulent discharge present in the nose or posterior pharynx. The nasal mucosa is usually erythematous but may on occasion be pale and boggy; the throat may show moderate injection. Examination of the tympanic membranes may show evidence of acute otitis media or otitis media with effusion. This occurs more often in chronic than acute sinusitis. The cervical lymph nodes are usually not significantly enlarged or tender. Occasionally, there will be either tenderness, as the examiner palpates over or percusses the paranasal sinuses, or appreciable periorbital oedema—soft, non-tender swelling of the upper and lower eyelid with discolouration of the overlying skin, or both. Unfortunately, facial tenderness is neither sensitive nor specific. Malodorous breath (in the absence of pharyngitis, poor dental hygiene, or a nasal foreign body) may suggest bacterial sinusitis. None of these characteristics differentiates rhinitis from sinusitis.

DIAGNOSTIC METHODS (Table 1A.5.3)

When the clinical history suggests a diagnosis of sinusitis the following procedures may help confirm the diagnosis.

Table 1A.5.3   Acute sinusitis: diagnostic confirmation

Plain radiographs
(anteroposterior, lateral, occipitomental)
   Complete opacification
   Mucosal thickening (≥4 mm)
   Air–fluid level

CT images: indications
   Recurrent problems
   Persistent infection
   Complicated infection (orbital or CNS)

Sinus aspiration: indications
   Clinical failure
   Complicated infection
   Immunosuppressed patient

Imaging

Radiography has traditionally been used to evaluate the presence of sinus disease. Standard radiographic projections include an anteroposterior, a lateral and for the maxillary sinuses an occipitomental view. Radiographic findings in patients with acute sinusitis are diffuse opacification, mucosal thickening of at least 4 mm or an air–fluid level (Fig. 1A.5.1). While these radiographic findings are not specific for acute sinusitis, they are helpful in confirming the presence of acute sinusitis in patients with suggestive signs and symptoms.

Chronic sinusitis causes an osteoblastic response in the affected sinus walls. Accordingly, in addition to mucosal thickening and complete opacification there may be an actual decrease in sinus size due to increased wall thickness. Foci of irregular bone thinning may also be seen.[5]

Much has been written about the frequency of abnormal sinus radiographs in asymptomatic populations of children; however, most studies have been flawed by either inattention to the presence of symptoms and signs of respiratory inflammation or failure to classify abnormal radiographic findings as major or minor. When children over age 1 year have neither respiratory signs nor symptoms, their sinus radiographs are almost always normal.[6] On the other hand, when children with persistent or severe respiratory symptoms have radiographs demonstrating the presence of an air–fluid level, complete opacification of the sinus cavities or mucosal thickening of at least 4–5 mm, bacteria in high density will be present in a maxillary sinus aspirate 75% of the time.[7]

Sinus radiographs are significantly abnormal in 88% of children less than 6 years of age with persistent respiratory symptoms.[8] Accordingly, sinus radiographs need not be performed in this age group in children with uncomplicated infection. Plain radiographs should be obtained to confirm the presence of sinus infection in children less than 6 years of age who present with severe symptoms and in all children of at least 6 years with suspected sinusitis. The clinician can feel confident that plain radiographs provide sufficient information in patients with signs and symptoms of acute uncomplicated sinus infection.[9]

Several studies have examined the frequency of incidental paranasal sinus abnormalities on computed tomographic (CT) scans of paediatric patients.[10,11] A

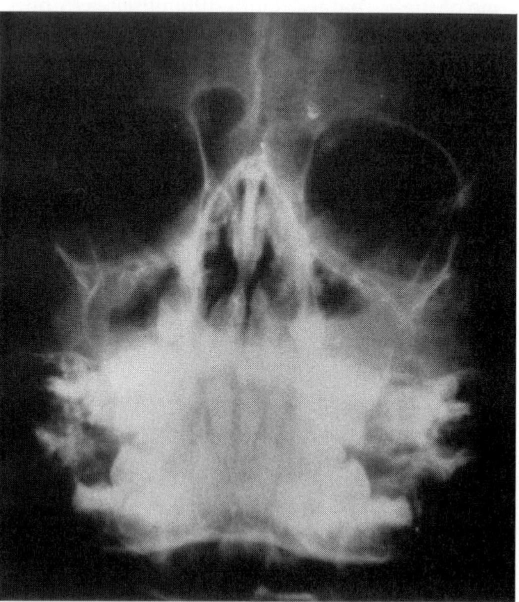

Fig. 1A.5.1 An occipitomental radiograph delineating the maxillary sinuses. Substantial mucosal thickening (distance in millimetres between the bony border and the air–mucosal interface) is seen in the right maxillary sinus. An air–fluid level is seen in the left maxillary sinus.

recent investigation showed frequent abnormalities on CT scan in adult patients with a 'fresh common cold'.[12] These abnormalities indicate inflammation but not necessarily bacterial infection.[13]

The osteomeatal complex is the area of pathology in patients with recurrent acute sinusitis or chronic sinusitis. This area is best examined with the CT scan. However, CT scans are not necessary for the management of children with uncomplicated acute sinusitis; they should be reserved for the evaluation of (1) complicated sinus disease (either orbital or central nervous system complications), (2) patients who experience numerous recurrences, or (3) protracted or non-responsive symptoms (i.e., circumstances in which sinus surgery is contemplated).[13]

Sinus aspiration

Maxillary sinus aspiration can be safely performed by a skilled otolaryngologist in the ambulatory setting using a transnasal approach. Sedation or general anaesthesia may be required for adequate immobilization of the young child. Current indications for maxillary sinus aspiration include (1) failure to respond to multiple courses of antibiotics, (2) severe facial pain, (3) orbital or intracranial complications and (4) evaluation of an immunocompromised host. There must be careful decontamination and anaesthesia of the area beneath the inferior turbinate through which the trocar is passed. Material aspirated from the maxillary sinus should be sent for Gram's stain and quantitative aerobic and anaerobic cultures. The recovery of bacteria in a density of at least 10^4 colony-forming units/ml is considered to represent true infection.[4,7] The finding of at least one organism per high-power field on Gram's stain of sinus secretions correlates with the recovery of bacteria in a density of 10^5 colony-forming units/ml.

MICROBIOLOGY OF SINUSITIS

Data on the microbiology of sinusitis in paediatric patients are best organized according to the duration of clinical symptoms (Table 1A.5.4). However, literature review is complicated by varying definitions of acute, subacute and chronic sinusitis. Several studies done on ambulatory patients with acute (10–30 days) and subacute (30–120 days)[8,14] illnesses have highlighted the important bacterial pathogens as *Streptococcus pneumoniae*, *Haemophilus influenzae* and *Moraxella catarrhalis*. *S. pneumoniae* is most common in all age groups and accounts for 30–40% of isolates. *H. influenzae* and *M. catarrhalis* are similar in prevalence and account for approximately 20% of cases. Both *H. influenzae* and *M. catarrhalis* may be β-lactamase producing and thereby amoxycillin resistant. Other much less frequently recovered bacterial species include group A streptococci, group C streptococci, viridans streptococci, peptostreptococci, *Moraxella* species and *Eikenella corrodens*.[7] Neither staphylococci nor respiratory anaerobes are

Table 1A.5.4   Bacteriology of acute, subacute and chronic sinusitis

Bacterial species	Acute	Subacute	Chronic
Streptococcus pneumoniae	+	+	+
Haemophilus influenzae	+	+	+
Moraxella catarrhalis	+	+	+
Staphylococci			+
Respiratory anaerobes[a]			+

[a] Anaerobic cocci, *Bacteroides* species, *Veillonella*.

commonly recovered from these patients. Respiratory viral isolates include adenovirus, parainfluenza, influenza and rhinovirus in approximately 10% of patients. This number might be higher if diagnostic aspirates were performed earlier in the course of respiratory symptoms.

In patients with very protracted (years) or severe sinus symptoms (requiring surgical intervention) *Staphylococcus aureus* and anaerobic organisms are recovered more frequently. The commonly recovered anaerobes are anaerobic Gram-positive cocci (such as peptococcus and peptostreptococcus) and *Bacteroides* species.[15] In addition viridans streptococci and *Haemophilus influenzae* are occasional aerobic isolates.

MEDICAL TREATMENT

The prescription of antimicrobials is the backbone of the medical management of sinusitis. Table 1A.5.5 shows a list of antimicrobials potentially useful in patients with acute sinusitis. Amoxycillin is acceptable and desirable for the treatment of most cases of uncomplicated sinusitis in children. It is effective most of the time, inexpensive and safe. The latter characteristic is particularly important when treating a condition that has a high spontaneous cure rate.[8]

While amoxycillin is preferred in most cases, there are several clinical situations in which a broader-spectrum regimen is appropriate. These include: (1) failure to improve while being treated with amoxycillin; (2) residence in a geographical area with a high prevalence of β-lactamase-producing *Haemophilus influenzae*; (3) the occurrence of frontal or sphenoidal sinusitis; (4) the occurrence of complicated ethmoidal sinusitis; and (5) presentation with very protracted (more than 30 days) symptoms. Antimicrobials with the most comprehensive coverage for patients with sinusitis are amoxycillin/potassium clavulanate, erythromycin–sulphisoxazole and cefuroxime axetil. For patients with chronic sinusitis, amoxycillin/potassium clavulanate is especially attractive because the mode of amoxycillin resistance of chronic sinus pathogens is β-lactamase production. Six new antimicrobial agents are available for management of respiratory infections but have not been evaluated in published studies of sinusitis in children: cefixime, cefprozil, cefpodoxime, loracarbef, clarithromycin and azithromycin. Studies in patients with acute otitis media have shown these agents to be comparable in efficacy to the older more commonly used antimicrobials. Loracarbef and cefixime have performed well in adult patients with acute sinusitis.[16]

The emerging problem in the antimicrobial management of acute or recurrent sinusitis is infection caused by penicillin-resistant pneumococci.[17] Organisms

Table 1A.5.5   Antimicrobials and dosage schedules for the treatment of sinusitis in children

Antimicrobial	Dosage
Amoxycillin	40 mg/kg per day in 3 divided doses
Amoxycillin/potassium clavulanate	40/10 mg/kg per day in 3 divided doses
Erythromycin/sulphisoxazole	50/150 mg/kg per day in 4 divided doses
Sulphamethoxazole/trimethoprim	40/8 mg/kg per day in 2 divided doses
Cefaclor	40 mg/kg per day in 3 divided doses
Cefuroxime axetil	30 mg/kg per day in 2 divided doses
Cefprozil	30 mg/kg per day in 2 divided doses
Cefixime	8 mg/kg per day in 1 or 2 divided doses
Cefpodoxime proxetil	10 mg/kg per day in 2 divided doses
Loracarbef	30 mg/kg per day in 2 divided doses

are classified as susceptible if the minimal inhibitory concentration (MIC) is less than 0.1 µg/ml, moderately resistant when the MIC is between 0.1 and 1.0 µg/ml and resistant when the MIC $\geq$ 2 µg/ml. The frequency of penicillin-resistant pneumococci varies geographically and many isolates of pneumococci are resistant to other commonly used antimicrobials such as sulphamethoxazole–trimethoprim and erythromycin–sulphisoxazole. Therapeutic options include advanced generation cephalosporins (for some pneumococci with moderate resistance), clindamycin, chloramphenicol and rifampicin. The optimal therapy for these infections is not known; selection should be guided by susceptibility results when available.

Patients with acute sinusitis may require hospitalization because of systemic toxicity or inability to take oral antimicrobials. These patients may be treated with cefuroxime at 50 mg/kg intravenously every 8 h or ampicillin/sulbactam 50 mg/kg per day intravenously every 6 h.

Clinical improvement is prompt in nearly all children treated with an appropriate antimicrobial agent. Patients febrile at the initial encounter will become afebrile, and there is a remarkable reduction of nasal discharge and cough within 48 h. If the patient does not improve, or worsens, in 48 h, clinical re-evaluation is appropriate. If the diagnosis is unchanged, sinus aspiration may be considered for precise bacteriological information. Alternatively, an antimicrobial agent effective against β-lactamase-producing bacterial species and penicillin-resistant pneumococci should be prescribed.

The appropriate duration of antimicrobial therapy for patients with sinusitis has not been systematically investigated. Many patients have a brisk response to antimicrobial intervention and experience dramatic improvement in respiratory symptoms in 3–4 days. For these patients 10 days of treatment is adequate. For patients who respond more slowly, a reasonable recommendation is to treat until the patient is symptom free and then for an additional 7 days.

Adjuvant therapies such as antihistamines, decongestants and anti-inflammatory agents have received little evaluation. Their overall impact on the clinical course of episodes of acute sinusitis has not been reported.

Some children experience recurrent or chronic episodes of sinusitis. The most common cause of recurrent sinusitis is recurrent viral URI, often a consequence of day care attendance or the presence of an older school-age sibling in the household. Other predisposing conditions include allergic and non-allergic rhinitis, cystic fibrosis, an immunodeficiency disorder (insufficient or dysfunctional immunoglobulins), ciliary dyskinesia or an anatomical problem (Table 1A.5.1). Evaluation of children with recurrent or chronic sinusitis should include consideration of consultation with an allergist, a sweat test, quantitative serum immunoglobulins and a mucosal biopsy to assess ciliary function and structure. If specific allergens are identified or an allergic diathesis documented, therapy might include desensitization, antihistamines or topical intranasal steroids. If a treatable immunodeficiency is identified, specific immunoglobulin therapy should be initiated. Antimicrobial prophylaxis has not been studied in patients with recurrent acute sinusitis although it has proved to be a useful strategy in reducing symptomatic episodes of acute otitis media in patients with recurrent ear disease. If patients do not respond to maximal medical therapy, surgical intervention may be appropriate.

The major complications of acute sinusitis are shown in Table 1A.5.6. Subperiosteal abscess of the orbit and intracranial abscesses are the most common. They will be signalled by eye swelling, proptosis and impaired extraocular eye movements in cases of orbital infection and signs of increased intracranial pressure, meningeal irritation and focal neurological deficits in the case of

Table 1A.5.6 Major complications of sinusitis

Orbital
 Inflammatory oedema[a]
  (pre-septal or peri-orbital cellulitis)
 Subperiosteal abscess
 Orbital abscess
 Orbital cellulitis
 Optic neuritis

Osteomyelitis
 Frontal (Pott's puffy tumour)
 Maxillary

Intracranial
 Epidural empyema
 Subdural empyema
 Cavernous or sagittal sinus thrombosis
 Meningitis
 Brain abscess

[a] Inflammatory oedema is not a true orbital complication of sinusitis. Infection is confined to the paranasal sinuses; peri-orbital swelling is due to impedance of venous blood flow.

intracranial pus (Fig. 1A.5.3). CT scan is essential for diagnosis. Antibiotic therapy and surgical drainage are usually required for successful treatment.

SURGICAL THERAPY

Patients with acute sinusitis hardly ever require surgical intervention unless they present with orbital or central nervous system complications. Rarely, sinus aspiration may be required to ventilate a sinus that has not responded to aggressive antimicrobial management.

When patients with recurrent acute or chronic sinusitis fail to improve with maximal medical therapy (including a trial of antimicrobial prophylaxis) sinus surgery should be considered. Early surgical efforts focused on creation of a nasoantral window (an additional dependent ostium) within the maxillary sinus which might facilitate gravitational drainage. A recent retrospective review of the efficacy of nasal antral windows in children showed improvement of only 27% of patients at the 6-month follow-up.[18]

The role of adenotonsillectomy in the management of sinusitis is unclear. Consultation with an otolaryngologist will permit a nasopharyngeal examination to evaluate tonsil and adenoid size. If these structures are enlarged sufficiently to cause obstruction and stasis of secretions, then removal should be considered.[19]

At present, the focus of surgical therapy is on the osteomeatal complex highlighted in Figure 1A.5.2. This is the area between the middle and inferior turbinates which represents the confluence of the drainage areas of the frontal, ethmoid and maxillary sinuses. In the osteomeatal complex there are several areas where two mucosal layers come into contact and thereby are predisposed to local impairment of mucociliary clearance. Using an endoscope, most current surgical efforts attempt enlargement of the natural meatus of the maxillary outflow tract by excising the uncinate process and the ethmoid bullae and performing an anterior ethmoidectomy.[20] A pilot study assessing the safety and efficacy of endoscopic sinus surgery in children with chronic sinusitis reported 71% of patients to be considered normal by their parents 1 year postoperatively.[20] The indications for and success of functional endoscopic surgery in children require further study.

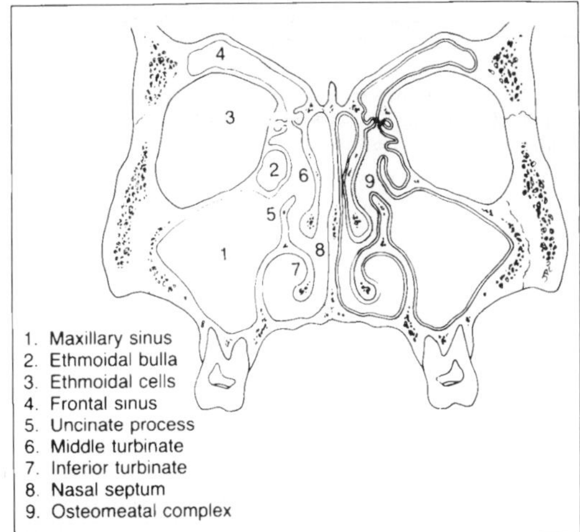

Fig. 1A.5.2 Coronal section of the nose and paranasal sinuses. The stippled area represents the osteomeatal complex. (Reprinted by permission of *the New England Journal of Medicine*, Wald ER, 326, 319–323, 1992. Copyright 1992. Massachusetts Medical Society. All rights reserved.)

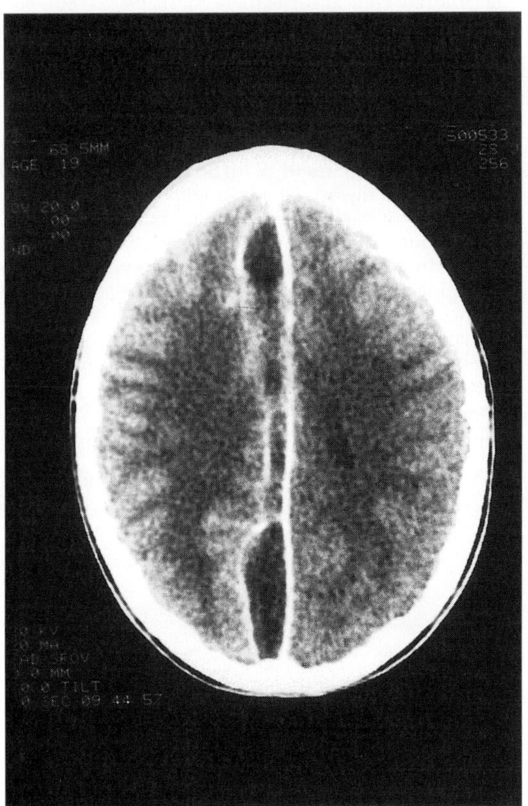

Fig. 1A.5.3 CT scan of the brain showing subdural empyema, extending along the falx, secondary to ethmoid sinusitis in a 12-year-old boy.

REFERENCES

1 Wald E R, Guerra N, Byers C. Upper respiratory tract infections in young children: duration of and frequency of complications. Pediatrics 1991; 87: 129–133.
2 Reimer A, vonMecKlenburg C, Tormalm N G. The mucociliary activity of the upper respiratory tract: III. A functional and morphological study of human and animal

material with special reference to maxillary sinus disease. Acta Otolaryngol 1978; 355 (suppl): 3–20.

3 Wald E R, Reilly J S, Casselbrant M et al. Treatment of acute maxillary sinusitis in childhood: a comparative study of amoxicillin and cefaclor. J Pediatr 1984; 104: 297–302.

4 Evans F O Jr, Sydnor B J, Moore W E et al. Sinusitis of the maxillary antrum. N Engl J Med 1975; 293: 735–739.

5 McAlister W H, Herman T E, Wippold F J. Imaging of sinusitis in infants and children. In: Lusk R P, ed. Pediatric sinusitis. New York: Raven Press, 1992: pp 15–42.

6 Kovatch A L, Wald E R, Ledesma-Medina J, Chiponis D M, Bedingfield B. Maxillary sinus radiographs in children with nonrespiratory complaints. Pediatrics 1984; 73: 306–308.

7 Wald E R, Milmoe G J, Bowen A D, Ledesma-Medina J, Salamon N, Bluestone C B. Acute maxillary sinusitis in children. N Engl J Med 1981; 304: 749–754.

8 Wald E R, Chiponis D, Ledesma-Medina J. Comparative effectiveness of amoxicillin and amoxicillin–clavulanate potassium in acute paranasal sinus infections in children: a double-blind, placebo-controlled trial. Pediatrics 1986; 77: 795–800.

9 Lusk R P, Lazar R H, Muntz H R. The diagnosis and treatment of recurrent and chronic sinusitis in children. Pediatr Clin North Am 1989; 36: 1411–1421.

10 Diament M J, Senac M O, Gilsanz V, Baker S, Gillespie T, Larson S. Prevalence of incidental paranasal sinuses opacification in pediatric patients: a CT study. J Comp Assist Tomogr 1987; 11: 426–431.

11 Glasier C M, Ascher D P, Williams K D. Incidental paranasal sinus abnormalities on CT of children: clinical correlation. AJNR 1986; 7: 861–864.

12 Gwaltney J M, Philips C D, Miller R D, Riker D K. Computed tomographic study of the common cold. N Engl J Med 1994; 330: 25–30.

13 Wald E R. Sinusitis: diagnostic imaging. Report Pediatr Infect Dis 1993; 3: 38–39.

14 Wald E R, Byers C, Guerra N, Casselbrant M, Beste D. Subacute sinusitis in children. J Pediatr 1989; 115: 28–32.

15 Brook I. Bacteriologic features of chronic sinusitis in children. JAMA 1981; 246: 967–969.

16 Gwaltney J M Jr, Scheld W M, Sande M A, Sydnor A. The microbial etiology and antimicrobial therapy of adults with acute community acquired sinusitis: a fifteen year experience at the University of Virginia and review of other selected studies. J Allergy Clin Immunol 1992; 90S: 457–461.

17 Leggiadro R J. Penicillin and cephalosporin-resistant Streptococcus pneumoniae: an emerging microbial threat. Pediatrics 1994; 93: 500–503.

18 Muntz H R, Lusk R P. Nasal antral windows in children: a retrospective study. Laryngoscope 1990; 100: 643–646.

19 Lusk R P. Surgical management of chronic sinusitis. In: Lusk R P, ed. Pediatric sinusitis. New York: Raven Press, 1992: pp 77–125.

20 Lusk R P, Muntz H R. Endoscopic sinus surgery in children with chronic sinusitis: a pilot study. Laryngoscope 1990; 100: 654–658.

P. McIntyre   R. Widmer   A. Cameron

1A.6   Oral and facial infections

Many anatomical structures may be involved in infections of the oral cavity and face. These include the tonsils and adenoids (Ch. 1A.3), the sinuses (Ch. 1A.5), the parotid and other salivary glands (Ch. 1A.7), lymph nodes (Ch. 1A.10), teeth and their supporting structures including bone, skin and soft tissues. Children who have infections of any of these structures may be seen by a wide variety of medical or dental practitioners. These extend from the family doctor or dentist to paediatricians or paediatric dentists, paediatric surgeons, ophthalmologists, ear, nose and throat surgeons or faciomaxillary surgeons. The literature reflects these diverse perspectives, with rather different emphases depending on the specialty. In this chapter, the perspective will be that of the primary clinical presentation, highlighting important aspects of diagnosis, differential diagnosis and treatment for oral and facial infections.

THE TEETH AND ODONTOGENIC INFECTIONS

Dental caries

Dental caries is the most common lesion affecting the teeth and is directly attributable to bacterial infection. Caries is most common on the occlusal surfaces of the posterior teeth, because of deep fissures and grooves in this area.[1] Caries of enamel spreads slowly, symptoms arise when dentine is exposed, and become severe when infection enters the innervated pulp (Fig. 1A.6.1). If the child does not present at the stage of pulpitis, pain disappears once the pulp is destroyed.[1]

Complications of dental caries

If pulpitis is undetected or untreated, infection then progresses to the alveolar bone, causing pain when chewing or on percussion of the affected tooth. Infection usually remains localized; occasionally a proliferative periostitis, manifested as a hard bony swelling in the body of the mandible (Garre's osteomyelitis),[2] or erosion through the periosteum into the mouth or into the soft tissues of the face, may occur (Fig. 1A.6.2).

In children, maxillary root apices are usually above the buccinator muscle, making spread into the canine space, lateral to the nose, or the periorbital fascia more likely (Fig. 1A.6.2).[2] Uncommonly, infections of the mandibular teeth may enter the fascial spaces (masseter, submandibular / sublingual).[1]

Infection of these latter spaces in its most severe form results in Ludwig's angina, leading to oedema of the tongue and respiratory embarrassment (Fig. 1A.6.3). Ludwig's angina due to odontogenic infection is rare in children[2] but a similar clinical syndrome is reported with invasive *Haemophilus influenzae* type b (Hib) infection or due to opportunistic organisms in immunocompromised children.[3] Other complications of odontogenic infections are rare, especially in

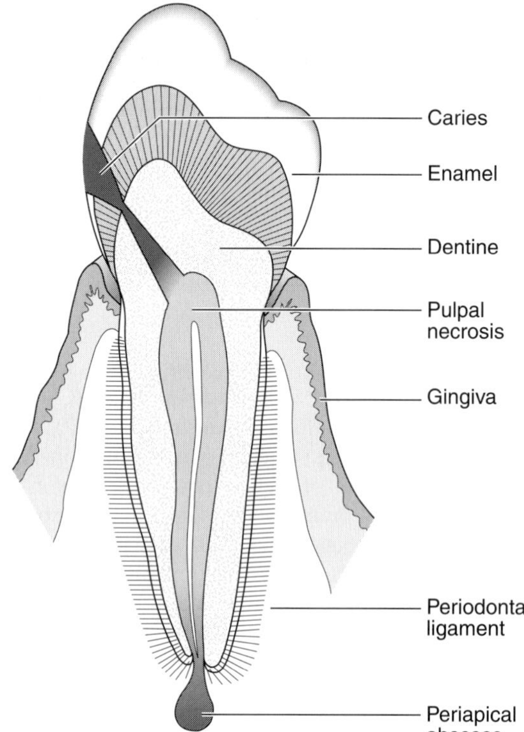

Fig. 1A.6.1   Cross-section of human tooth.

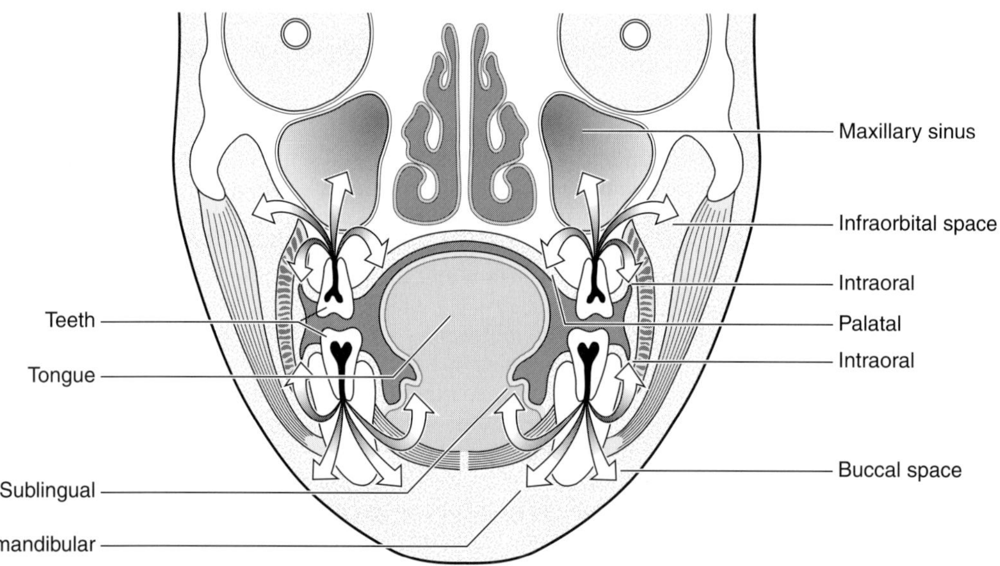

Fig. 1A.6.2   Spread of odontogenic infection along fascial planes.

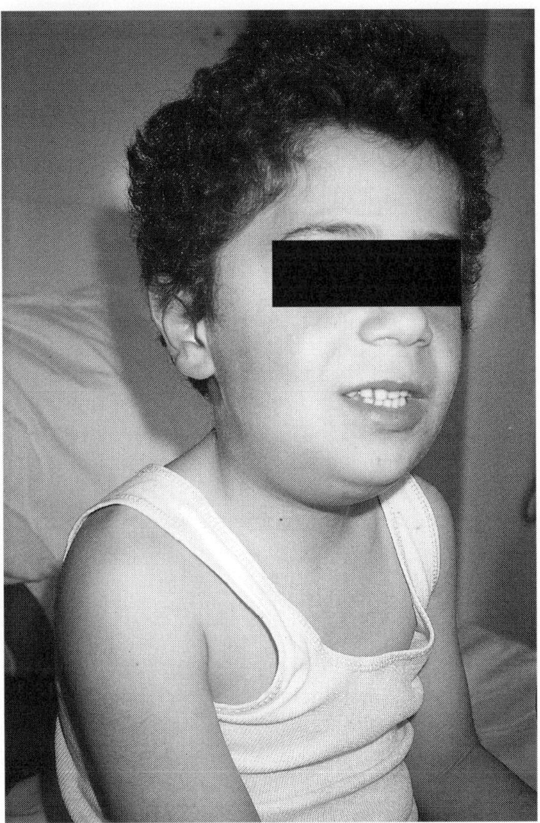

Fig. 1A.6.3   Ludwig's angina.

children. These include rupture into the maxillary sinus or orbital cavity or extension down fascial planes into the retropharyngeal spaces and mediastinum.[1,2,4]

Microbiology

The oral cavity is sterile at birth, but rapidly becomes colonized, initially with streptococci. Anaerobic organisms, which are the most common oral flora in adults, remain in relatively low numbers until the primary teeth appear at 12–24 months of age.[1,2] Odontogenic infections are invariably polymicrobial, with the predominant organisms being anaerobes, particularly *Fusobacterium* and *Bacteroides*, and facultative anaerobic streptococci.[2,4] *Staphylococcus aureus* and enteric Gram-negative bacilli are unusual without underlying factors such as trauma, either accidental or postoperative, or immunocompromise where the normal flora changes during hospitalization.[4]

Therapy

Appropriate dental therapy, with drainage and extraction of diseased teeth, is essential for the successful treatment of odontogenic infections and should not be delayed for a period of antibiotic treatment.[1,2,4] Traditional antibiotic therapy has been with penicillin alone, which is probably still adequate for less severe infection with appropriate surgical treatment. Additional anaerobic cover should be given for more severe infections, as *Bacteroides* species are increasingly β-lactamase producers.[4] This could be with metronidazole or clindamycin. It is essential that penicillin be given with metronidazole as the latter has inadequate activity against streptococci. In less severe infections or as follow-on therapy, the combination of amoxycillin and a β-lactamase inhibitor is also satisfactory. In postsurgical or immunocompromised patients, addition of an aminoglycoside would be prudent for initial treatment.[4]

OTHER INFECTIONS AFFECTING THE DENTITION

Historically, congenital syphilis is the best-known infection affecting the teeth other than dental caries disease. The primary teeth are usually not affected and the dental effects of congenital syphilis are usually not evident until the permanent teeth appear.[1,5] The classical 'mulberry molar' refers to the roughened, hypoplastic appearance of the first permanent molar teeth, while Hutchinson's incisors have crescentic notches on the incisal edge and a conical screwdriver shape. Infection of the developing facial bones will often result in facial deformity in untreated congenital syphilis. Indeed, any severe febrile infection occurring during development of the teeth (10 weeks gestation to 10 years of age) can lead to hypoplasia of either primary or secondary teeth.

GINGIVITIS AND PERIODONTAL DISEASE

Background

The periodontium consists of the gingivae, cementum and the periodontal ligament which attaches the tooth to alveolar bone (Fig. 1A.6.1). Gingivitis resulting from the accumulation of plaque is common in children, with up to 50% of 5–17-year-olds affected in recent surveys.[1] It is, however, usually asymptomatic in younger children and does not reach peak severity until early adolesence. It is reversible once dental hygiene has been improved.[1,2] Periodontitis results from progression of gingival infection to the neck of the tooth, eroding the soft tissue attachments and eventually leading to loosening of the teeth.

Periodontitis is rare before puberty. In a pre-pubertal child, early loss of primary teeth or gingivitis which is more extensive than expected from the level of oral hygiene is a very significant symptom. It may be the first presentation of a primary immunodeficiency state, especially a phagocytic defect,[6] such as chronic granulomatous disease or a neutrophil adhesion defect, or of a genetic disorder, such as hypophosphatasia or Papillon–Lefèvre syndrome.[7] Children with Down syndrome are especially susceptible to severe periodontal disease of early onset.[7] Other possible causes of premature periodontitis are reviewed elsewhere.[7]

ACUTE GINGIVITIS AND ORAL ULCERATION

Diagnosis

Bacterial infection

Acute, necrotizing ulcerative gingivitis or Vincent's infection is rare in children. In severely malnourished children, it may progress to erosion of the soft tissues of the face and jaw (noma), especially after measles or another acute infection.[1,2] Vincent's infection may also occur in adolescence, with extremely poor oral hygiene[1] and in Down syndrome.[9]

A number of other bacterial infections may have oral lesions as part of their presenting symptoms or signs, but these are either rare or oral symptoms are dominated by other aspects of the presentation, so that diagnostic difficulty is unlikely. An extensive discussion of these is available.[5]

Viral infections

Herpes simplex virus (HSV). This is the most common viral cause of acute gingivostomatitis. It is rare before 6 months of age or eruption of primary teeth. The peak incidence is from 10 months to 3 years,[1,2] although cases in older individuals from higher socioeconomic groups have been increasingly recognized, especially university students.[1] Ulcers develop rapidly from vesicles on the lips, gingiva, anterior tongue and hard palate, appearing as shallow grey lesions on an erythematous base (Fig. 1A.6.4). There is often a prodromal phase of 1–2 days with fever and lymphadenopathy. Fever has usually resolved by day 4 and ulcer healing begun by day 5–6, with resolution by 1–2 weeks.[1,2] Acyclovir therapy should probably be reserved for cases in children with eczema, immunocompromised children and for children who are particularly severely affected.

Enteroviral infections. Enteroviruses, most commonly coxsackieviruses and echoviruses, cause two distinctive syndromes of oral ulceration: herpangina, and hand, foot and mouth disease.

Typical herpangina can be relatively easily distinguished from herpetic disease, as ulceration is posterior and there is often an associated papulovesicular cutaneous eruption.[10,11] In contrast to HSV, ulcers are usually limited to two to ten lesions, most commonly on the anterior tonsillar pillars but also the soft palate, uvula and pharyngeal wall. Although tongue and posterior buccal involvement may occur, if the anterior mouth is the main site of ulceration, or if the ulcers are more than 5 mm in diameter, then herpangina is excluded by definition.[11] Although HSV has been reported as a cause of pharyngitis, particularly in adolescents, this is typically a membranous rather than ulcerative pharyngitis and thus infectious mononucleosis is the main differential diagnostic consideration.

Hand, foot and mouth disease (Fig. 1A.6.5) is sometimes difficult to differentiate from herpetic gingivostomatitis. The presenting complaint is often a sore mouth and refusal to eat, the predominant age group is similar and 10–15% of children have only oral lesions, which can have a similar distribution to HSV. Factors which distinguish it from HSV are occurrence in epidemics, rash and absence of cervical adenopathy.[12] The rash may be vesicular or maculopapular and may occur on the buttocks or trunk as well as the hands and feet. Oral

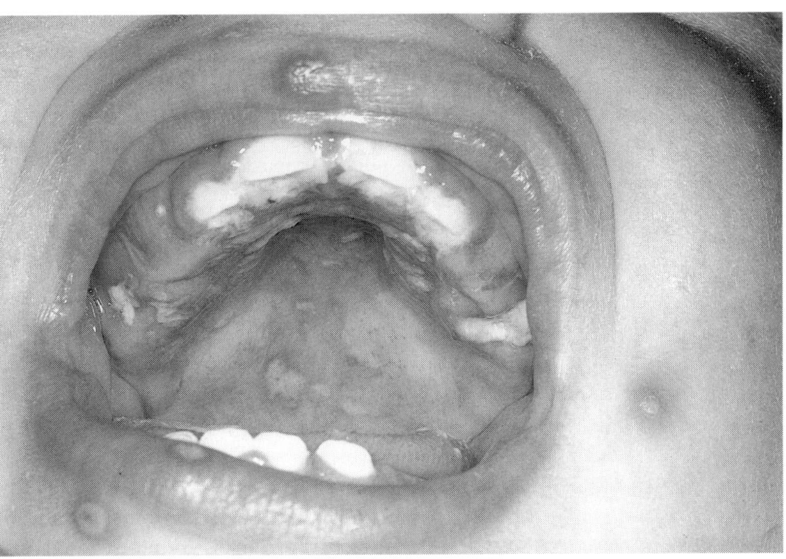

Fig. 1A.6.4 Herpetic gingivostomatitis. See also colour plate.

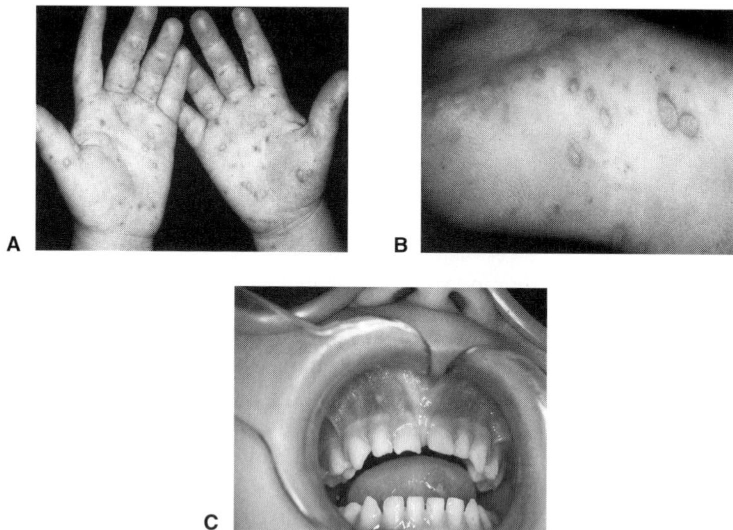

Fig. 1A.6.5   Hand, foot and mouth disease due to Coxsackievirus infection.

involvement most commonly involves the tongue, hard palate and buccal mucosa but ulcers have also been documented on the gingivae and pharynx in culture-confirmed cases.[12]

Other viral infections. It is not surprising that other herpesviruses also cause oral ulceration. Chickenpox may start with oral lesions, most commonly on the hard palate, fauces and uvula, before skin lesions appear.[5,9] As children usually do not complain of discomfort from oral varicella lesions, these are seldom a presenting feature. Purely oral manifestations of Epstein–Barr virus (EBV) infection are uncommon, but both pericoronitis and stomatitis have been reported and may lead to the patient presenting initially to a dental practitioner.[5,7] Cytomegalovirus (CMV) can cause ulceration anywhere in the gastrointestinal tract in immunocompromised patients, but rarely if ever causes oral ulceration in previously well individuals.[13]

Influenza may cause a striking pharyngitis in the first 24 h, and has been reported as causing gingival inflammation and bleeding and very occasionally small herpes-like ulcers.[5] Although oral manifestations occur with a number of other viruses, these are usually part of a systemic illness where the diagnosis is not in doubt, such as measles or mumps.

Fungal and other infections

Candidiasis. Oral candidiasis occurs in two major forms in children: a pseudo-membranous form and an erythematous form. Pseudo-membranous candidiasis appears as loosely adherent cream to grey plaques which when removed leave an erythematous base, which may bleed. Plaques may occur anywhere in the mouth; the most frequent sites are the tongue, soft and hard palates and buccal mucosa.[10,14] At least one episode of oral candidiasis occurs in 2–5% of normal infants and is acquired from the birth canal, usually appearing clinically from 6 to 10 days after birth.[14]

The chronic atrophic form of candidiasis is less common; it may occur de novo or following loss of the overlying plaque. It occurs most commonly in older children with predisposing factors such as antibiotic exposure, chronic illness, surgery, immunosuppression or dental prostheses.[8,14] Severe or recurrent candidiasis is uncommon in infants or children and should prompt a search for other predisposing factors. In the European Collaborative Study of 407 infants at risk for HIV infection, oral candidiasis was present on two examinations at least 2 months apart in 20% of HIV-infected infants but only 0.5% of non-infected infants and was one of the strongest clinical predictors of HIV infection.[15]

Other fungi and other infections. A variety of fungi other than *Candida* can cause oral lesions, but are rare and seen only in immunocompromised hosts or in endemic areas. They are especially uncommon in children and would seldom present with acute symptoms such as pain or difficulty eating.[5]

Non-infectious causes

A number of non-infectious conditions enter the differential diagnosis in a previously well child with acute oral ulceration and difficulty eating. These include severe aphthous ulceration, trauma including non-accidental injury and Stevens–Johnson syndrome (SJS).[10] Enteroviral infections may be confused with SJS, as both can be associated with an extensive rash and ocular involvement. The oral involvement in SJS is typically more diffuse with raw, red areas rather than localized ulcers (Fig. 1A.6.6), but in the absence of typical erythema multiforme differentiation on clinical grounds alone may be difficult.[10]

Laboratory diagnosis

In clinically typical viral syndromes, it is not necessary to obtain specimens for culture. In doubtful cases or in the presence of underlying disease, HSV is readily isolated from oral lesions, with culture usually taking only 3–5 days. Rapid diagnosis of HSV by immunofluorescence is also available in many centres. Enteroviruses can be isolated from the throat or vesicular fluid, but the addition of a stool specimen greatly enhances the yield from viral culture. Enteroviral cultures commonly take 1–2 weeks before results are available — too late for most clinical situations. Serology is available for enteroviruses, but is not group specific and has relatively poor sensitivity compared with culture. Detection of enteroviral RNA by polymerase chain reaction (PCR) methods is available in some research laboratories.

Therapy

Odontogenic infections

Fusobacteria and other oral anaerobes are the predominant organisms and treatment consists of scaling and cleaning of the teeth, together with parenteral penicillin.[1,2,4] An association between severe ulcerative gingivitis or noma and concurrent herpes simplex infection has been described in malnourished children, but the value of concurrent antiviral therapy has not been investigated.[16]

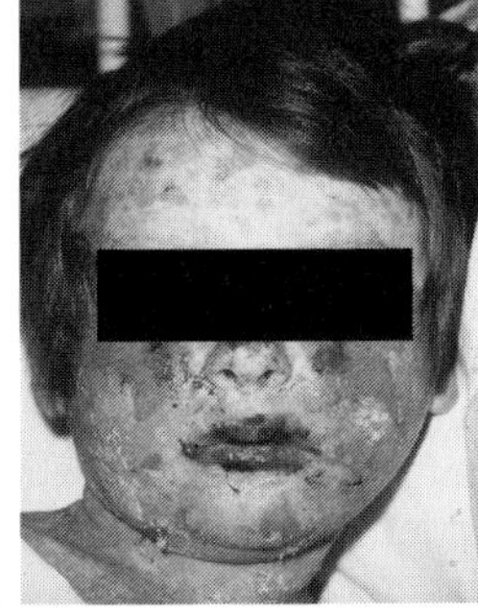
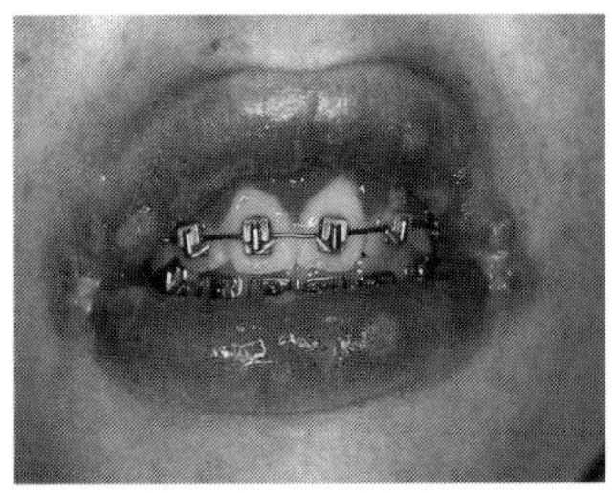

Fig. 1A.6.6 Stevens–Johnson syndrome. **A** Erythema multiforme rash with denuded skin and bullae. **B** Oral ulceration.

Viral infections

Acyclovir, given orally or intravenously, has been shown to be effective for treatment and prophylaxis of genital HSV infection and prophylaxis of oral HSV infection following bone marrow transplant.[17] Acyclovir would be expected to be of benefit for herpetic gingivostomatitis, but efficacy is likely to be limited to early therapy. Japanese investigators studied a nursery school population where 90% of susceptible children under 3 years had developed severe gingivostomatitis in previous outbreaks.[18] Acyclovir given orally as crushed tablets in a dose of 30–60 mg/kg per day in three doses was effective as prophylaxis, reducing the attack rate from 82% in 22 children treated only after symptoms developed to zero in 37 children treated immediately after exposure.[19] These and other data suggest minimal benefit from acyclovir when more than 72 h have elapsed since symptoms developed.

Our current policy is to give acyclovir 5 mg/kg per dose three times daily intravenously, to children who are immunocompromised or require hospital admission for intravenous fluid replacement within the first 48 h of oral symptoms or if new lesions are developing. We do not believe that there are sufficient data to assess the value of early oral acyclovir as an outpatient treatment, but anecdotally have observed some benefit when an adequate dose can be administered by mouth.

Candidiasis

Topical therapy alone is generally adequate for candidiasis; most cases in immunocompetent children will resolve without treatment. We use clotrimazole gel rather than nystatin liquid topically as we have found the latter inconvenient and requiring relatively prolonged therapy. Immunocompromised children usually require systemic therapy with fluconazole or on occasion amphotericin, especially if there is disease extending outside the mouth.[17] For chronic candidiasis associated with a dental prosthesis, at least 8 weeks therapy with topical amphotericin and replacement of the prosthesis are necessary.[8]

Recurrent gingival disease and ulceration

The major clinical problem with recurrent oral ulceration (Table 1A.6.1) is differentiation of HSV-related disease from aphthous ulceration.[10] Recurrent HSV disease is unusual inside the mouth as opposed to the lips; when it occurs it is usually on keratinized epithelium adjacent to bone, such as the gingivae or hard palate. In contrast, aphthous ulcers are uncommon on the gingiva, palate or floor of the tongue, tending to occur on the non-keratinized epithelium of the cheek, tongue, lips or soft palate. Recurrent erythema multiforme may be limited to the mouth[20] and has been strongly linked to HSV infection.[21] Acyclovir is effective as prophylaxis against frequently recurring HSV-related erythema multiforme.[22]

A wide range of conditions are associated with recurrent oral ulceration. These include enteropathies, Behçet's syndrome, Reiter's disease, periodic syndrome associated with pharyngitis, and cyclic neutropenia. The details of diagnosis and management of these diverse conditions are beyond the scope of this chapter and interested readers are referred to more comprehensive texts.[8–10]

Chronic oral ulceration

Tuberculosis may present with a single, painless, indolent ulcer; this is uncommon even in endemic areas and more often seen in children than adults.[5] It is usually on the gingivae and associated with cervical adenopathy. Mucocutaneous leishmaniasis occurs in Central and South America, caused by *Leishmania braziliensis*. A destructive ulcer may present in any part of the mouth or lower in the respiratory tract.[5] In endemic areas, fungal infections such as histoplasmosis and paracoccidiomycosis may cause indolent ulcers which closely resemble those of either tuberculosis or leishmaniasis.[5] Some immunodeficiency disorders, particularly those involving phagocytic cells, are particularly prone to present

Table 1A.6.1   Common or important causes of oral ulceration

Acute	Infective	
		Herpes simplex virus
		Herpangina
		Hand, foot and mouth disease
	Non-infective	
		Aphthous
		Trauma
		Neoplasia
		Langerhans cell histiocytosis
		Leukaemia
		Stevens–Johnson syndrome
Chronic/recurrent	Infective	
		Erythema multiforme (HSV associated)
		HIV
	Non-infective	
		Aphthous ulceration
		Inflammatory bowel disease
		Blood dyscrasias
		Connective tissue disease

with chronic gingivitis and ulceration. These are reviewed elsewhere and include Chediak–Higashi syndrome, leucocyte adhesion defects, thymoma and hyper-IgE syndrome.[6]

FACIAL CELLULITIS

Cellulitis is relatively common in paediatric practice: 50 cases were seen in a 6-month period in a children's hospital accident and emergency department, of which 8 (16%) were facial.[23] Facial cellulitis may usefully be divided into

Table 1A.6.2   Facial cellulitis in infants and children

Site	Age	Origin	Organism	Treatment
Periorbital	Less than 2 years	Haematogenous	Hib, SP	Third-generation cephalosporin
	School age	Sinuses	Hi Streptococci	Third-generation cephalosporin
Infraorbital	Neonate	Haematogenous Maxilla	SA	Flucloxacillin
	School age	Dental	Oral flora	Penicillin ± metronidazole
Buccal	Less than 2 years	Haematogenous	Hib, SP	Third-generation cephalosporin
	School age	Dental	Oral flora	Penicillin ± metronidazole
Submental	Neonate	Haematogenous Lyphadenitis	SA GBS	Ampicillin ± flucloxacillin
	Older children	Dental Infected cyst	Oral floral	Penicillin ± metronidazole
Any site	Trauma		SA	Flucloxacillin
	Animal bite		GAS *Pasteurella Eikenella*	Penicillin/ampicillin

Hib, *Haemophilus influenzae* type b; SP, *Streptococcus pneumoniae*; Hi, *Haemophilus influenzae*; SA, *Staphylococcus aureus*; GBS, group B streptococci; GAS, group A streptococci.

the categories upper (periorbital) and lower (buccal, submandibular) face.[24] As in cellulitis at other sites, an adjacent break in the skin is the most common predisposing factor for facial cellulitis and may occur at any age: *Staphylococcus aureus* or *Streptococcus pyogenes* is almost always the causative organism where a break in the skin is present. Odontogenic origins are frequently overlooked when children present to non-dental practitioners; the causative organisms are outlined above. The likely origin and causative organism of facial cellulitis otherwise differs markedly with age and site (Table 1A.6.2).

Age

Less than 3 months of age

Facial cellulitis is a rare but important problem in this age group. The major causative organisms are *Staphylococcus aureus* and *Streptococcus agalactiae* (group B streptococcus, GBS). GBS cellulitis is most commonly submandibular, but differs from *Staphylococcus aureus*, which also causes infection in this site, in being more diffuse and less likely to require surgical drainage.[25] Hib may cause cellulitis in this age group, although more common from 6 to 24 months of age; it is more commonly buccal and less likely to have an associated lymphadenitis than GBS.[25] Cellulitis in the periorbital area should raise suspicion of underlying osteomyelitis of the maxilla, a rare site of osteomyelitis in any other age group, associated with haematogenous staphylococcal infection. Facial cellulitis in infants is likely to be associated with bacteraemia. Meningitis was present in 2 (12%) cases of GBS cellulitis among 16 infants in a number of case reports.[25]

Preschool age group

Bacteraemic infection remains an important consideration in preschool children, especially under 2 years. Cellulitis due to Hib was first described in the 1950s as especially involving the cheek and having a characteristic violaceous appearance. Subsequent descriptions have emphasized that the violaceous colour is often not present in Hib cellulitis and that pneumococcal cellulitis can appear identical. Both organisms may cause cellulitis in either the buccal (Fig. 1A.6.7) or periorbital (Fig. 1A.6.8) regions and, uncommonly, other sites including the extremities.[23,26]

Meningitis may complicate cellulitis with either of these organisms, and was found in 9/93 (10%) bacteraemic cases in two series.[27,28] Some of these children had minimal clinical evidence of meningitis, leading to a recommendation of routine lumbar puncture.[27] This observation probably resulted from very early presentation due to the obvious external manifestation (cellulitis) and consequent lumbar puncture at a time of minimal cerebrospinal fluid changes.[27,28] Although lumbar puncture should be carefully considered, as in any young child with potential bacteraemia with these organisms, routine lumbar puncture for all cases of facial cellulitis is not justified.

Sinus radiographs are difficult to interpret in this age group; sinusitis cannot be diagnosed by sinus opacity alone. From 3 to 5 years, bacteraemia in association with facial cellulitis is uncommon and occasional cases of sinus or dental origin occur, but remain uncommon.

School-age and older children

Bacteraemia is almost never documented in this age group, even in severe infections such as orbital cellulitis. Breaks in the skin, odontogenic and sinus infection are the most common causes of facial cellulitis.

Site of involvement

The upper face was almost four times as common as the lower face as a site of cellulitis in a hospital series of 113 children under 15 years of age.[24] The teeth were

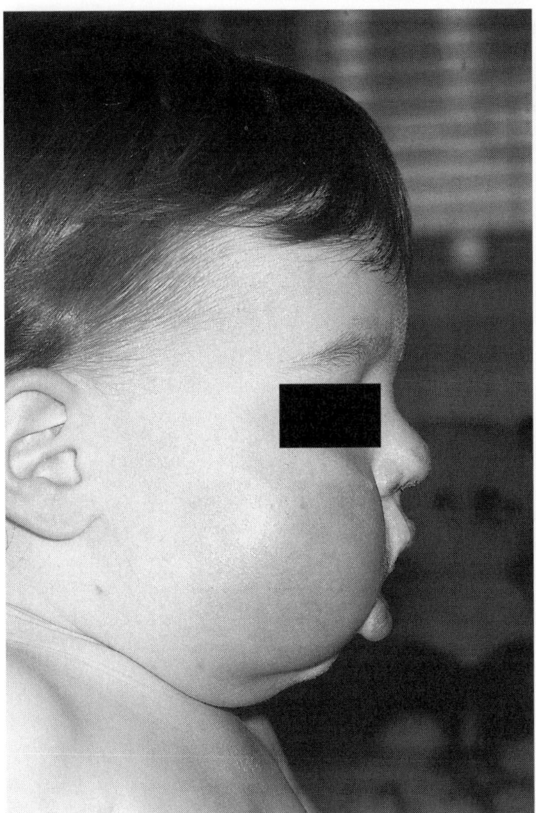

Fig. 1A.6.7 Buccal cellulitis due to *Haemophilus influenzae* type b.

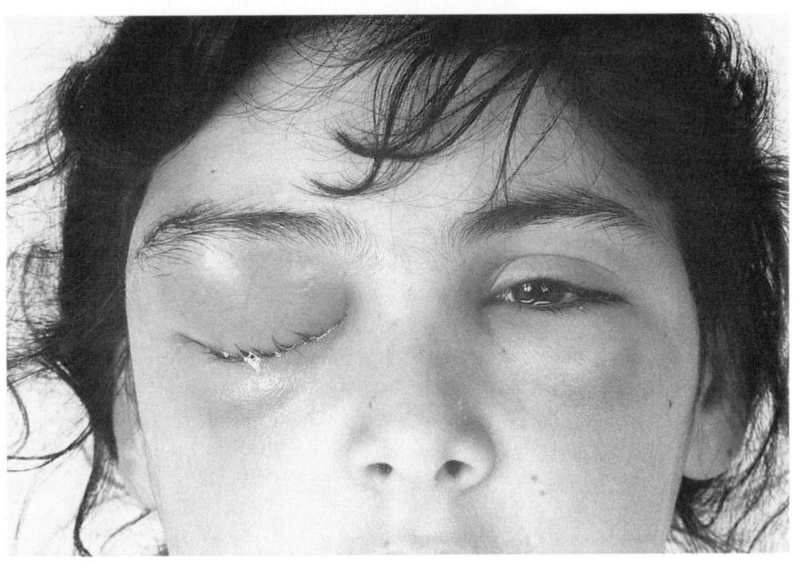

Fig. 1A.6.8 Periorbital cellulitis due to *Haemophilus influenzae* type b. See also colour plate.

the most common source identified in lower facial infections, while infections of the upper face were most commonly related to trauma.[24,29] Series confined to periorbital cellulitis, on the other hand, seldom report a dental origin, but

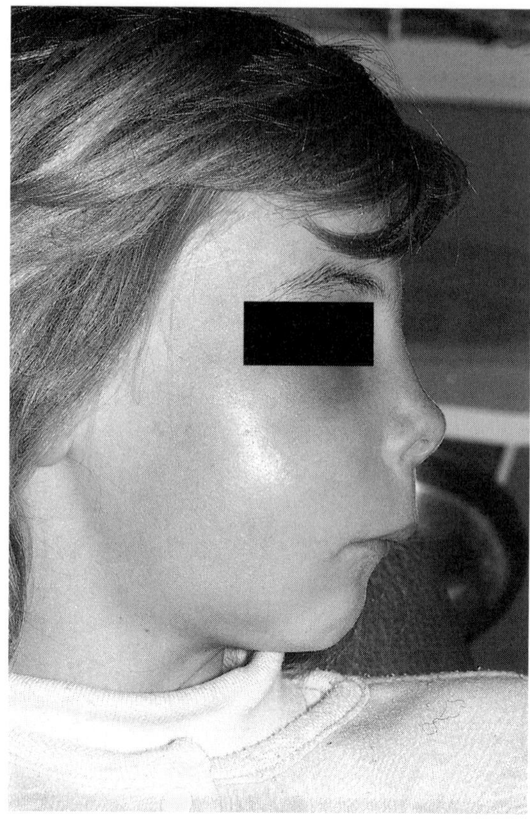

Fig. 1A.6.9 Infraorbital cellulitis due to maxillary dental abscess.

commonly report sinusitis, especially where infection has extended beyond the orbital septum.[30] Differentiating features of dental versus other causes are a slower onset and infraorbital (Figs 1A.6.9, 1A.6.10), rather than periorbital, location. A dental cause is not excluded when there is no history of dental problems, as children who have never been to a dentist may have non-vital teeth from causes such as trauma or congenital defects.[8] If clinical examination shows teeth which are obviously restored or obviously decayed, they are the most likely source of infection.

Unusual organisms causing facial cellulitis

Nocardia species can cause facial cellulitis in previously well and immuno-compromised children. Initial trauma is common, presumably related to inoculation of the organism from soil.[31] Unless the laboratory is alerted to this possibility, specimens for culture may be discarded too early for *Nocardia* to be detected. Although uncommon, the possibility of *Nocardia* should be considered in facial cellulitis which is not responding or which relapses after standard therapy for *Staphylococcus aureus* infection.

Cervicofacial actinomycosis can occur either as an acute, painful pyogenic infection or as a more indolent, painless swelling; both tend to occur in the submandibular area or neck. Cases in children are unusual but reported.[32] Osteomyelitis due to *Actinomyces* can also occur, following either dental infection or trauma such as a compound fracture of the mandible.[2] In general, osteomyelitis is extremely rare in the mandible and maxilla and should not be diagnosed only on the basis of dental rarefactions in the periapical area on radiographs.

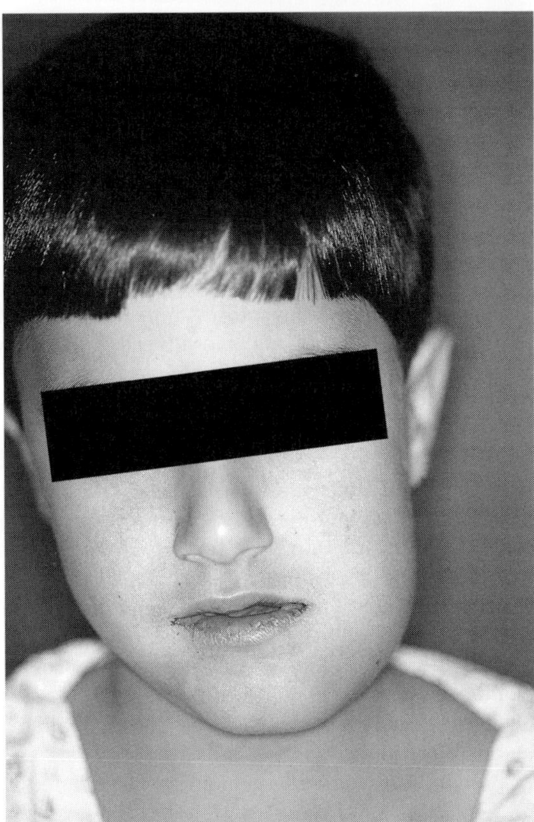

Fig. 1A.6.10 Buccal cellulitis due to mandibular molar abscess.

Infections following bites or trauma

Human or animal bites to the face, head and neck are not uncommon. The potential for serious complications, including cosmetic appearance, justifies empirical antibiotic therapy.[34]

Management

Children below the age of 2 years who have a unilateral facial cellulitis without an obvious entry site are likely to be bacteraemic, more so with decreasing age. Management should include blood culture; lumbar puncture should be performed according to the usual criteria. A third-generation cephalosporin is the most appropriate empirical therapy, even in the post-Hib vaccine era, as penicillin-resistant *Streptococcus pneumoniae* remains an important consideration. In neonates, specific antistaphylococcal therapy should also be given.

Older children with apparently spontaneous facial cellulitis should be evaluated for a dental cause and for sinusitis. The authors have personal experience of children discharged from hospital without consideration of a dental cause for facial cellulitis who re-presented with complications. A CT scan will often be required if periorbital swelling precludes adequate examination of the eyes and to assess the extent of sinus disease. The antibiotic therapy of odontogenic infection has been discussed above; a third-generation cephalosporin is adequate for all the likely pathogens causing complications of sinus disease in children.

If there is an adjacent break in the skin, flucloxacillin in a dose of 100 mg/kg per day intravenously is adequate for both streptococcal and staphylococcal infection. An exception to this is bites, where *Eikenella corrodens* is of particular importance in human bites and *Pasteurella multocida* in animal bites.[33,34] Both these organisms require therapy with ampicillin or penicillin and will not respond to flucloxacillin, other isoxazoyl penicillins or clindamycin. Amoxycillin with a β-lactamase inhibitor is appropriate oral therapy. Surgical therapy is often essential in dental disease. The need for surgical drainage is based on imaging and response to therapy in facial cellulitis from other causes.

IMMUNOCOMPROMISED PATIENTS

Human immunodeficiency virus (HIV) infection

The oral manifestations of HIV infection are manifold and extensive reviews are available.[35] In children, candidiasis is the most common oral infection, but recurrent or persistent HSV infection can also be a management problem. Although varicella zoster virus also causes recurrent and persistent infection in HIV-infected children, oral involvement appears to be an infrequent clinical problem.[36] Oral hairy leucoplakia (OHL) is closely related to EBV infection and was initially described in association with HIV infection, but also occurs with other causes of cell-mediated immunosuppression, such as bone marrow or cardiac transplantation.[35,36] Clinically, OHL appears as a vertically corrugated, white surface alteration, differentiated from candidiasis by its characteristic location (the lateral or ventral surface of the tongue) and by not being removable. OHL had occurred in only 2% of children with HIV by the age of 5 years, but may become more prevalent with increasing length of follow-up.[37] By contrast, salivary gland enlargement is relatively more common in children, occurring in 15–30% of cases, as compared with some 5% of adult males.[37] In a longitudinal study of outcome in HIV, oral candidiasis was significantly associated with earlier death, while parotid enlargement was associated with prolonged survival.[37]

Children with cancer

The oral cavity is important as a reservoir and portal of entry for potential infectious agents.[38] Some 40% of a series of 214 children with cancer in Tennessee followed for 2.5 years developed at least one oral complication.[39] Not surprisingly, the complications were most common among children with the most severe disease and most intensive therapy. The exception was gingivitis, which was more common among children with leukaemia. Initial dental assessment is important, as many children with cancer require dental treatment when first seen.[38,39] Candida and HSV are the most important infectious agents.[38,39] HSV is of particular importance in bone marrow transplant patients, where its frequency and severity justifies prophylactic intravenous acyclovir, often given in high dose to provide protection against reactivation of CMV disease.[38]

REFERENCES

1 Wright J M, Taylor P P, Allen E P, Byrd R L. A review of the oral manifestations of infections in pediatric patients. Pediatr Infect Dis 1984; 3: 80–83.
2 Piecuch J F, Topazian R G. Infections of the oral cavity. In: Feigin R D, Cherry J D, eds. Textbook of pediatric infectious diseases. Philadelphia: W B Saunders, 1987: 168–179.
3 Barkin R M, Bonis S L, Enghammer R M, Todd J K. Ludwig angina in children. J Pediatr 1975; 87: 563–565.
4 Megan D W, Scheifele D W, Chow A W. Odontogenic infections. Pediatr Infect Dis J 1984; 3: 257–265.
5 McFarlane T W, Samaranayaka L P. Systemic infections. In: Jones J H, Mason D K, eds. Oral manifestations of systemic disease, 2nd ed. Baillière Tindall, 1990: 339–386.

6 Porter S R, Scully C. Oral manifestations in the primary immunodeficiency disorders. Oral Surg Oral Med Oral Pathol 1994; 78: 4–13.

7 Lesco B A, Brownstein M P. Recognition of periodontal disease in children. Pediatr Clin North Am 1982; 2: 457–474.

8 Hall R K. Paediatric orofacial medicine and pathology. London: Chapman & Hall, 1994.

9 Kinene D F, Davies R M. Periodontal manifestations of systemic disease In: Jones J H, Mason D K, eds. Oral manifestations of systemic disease, 2nd ed. Baillière Tindall, 1990: 339–386.

10 Dilley D H, Blozis G G. Common oral lesions and oral manifestations of systemic illness and therapies. Pediatr Clin North Am 1982; 29: 585–609.

11 Cherry J D. Herpangina. In: Feigin R D, Cherry J D, eds. Textbook of pediatric infectious diseases. Philadelphia: W B Saunders, 1987: 261–263.

12 Adler J L, Mostow S R, Mellin H, Janney J H, Joseph J M. Epidemiologic investigation of hand, foot and mouth disease. Am J Dis Child 1970; 120: 309–313.

13 Eversole L R. Viral infections of the head and neck among HIV seropositive patients. Oral Surg Oral Med Oral Pathol 1992; 73: 142–144.

14 Fitzpatrick R E, Newcomer V D. Dermatophytosis and candidiasis. In: Feigin R D, Cherry J D, eds. Textbook of pediatric infectious diseases. Philadelphia: W B Saunders, 1987: 843–855.

15 European Collaborative Study. Children born to women with HIV-1 infection: natural history and risk of transmission. Lancet 1991; 337: 253–259.

16 Whittle H C, Smith J S, Kogbe O I, Dossetor J, Duggan M. Severe ulcerative herpes of the mouth following measles. Trans R Soc Trop Med Hyg 1979; 73: 66–69.

17 Lee J W, Pizzo P A. Management of specific problems in children with leukaemias and lymphomas. In: Patrick C C, ed. Infections in immunocompromised infants and children. Edinburgh: Churchill Livingstone, 1992: 207.

18 Kuzushima K, Kimura H, Kino Y et al. Clinical manifestations of primary herpes simplex type 1 infection in a closed community. Pediatrics 1991; 87: 152–158.

19 Kuzushima K, Kudo T, Kimura H, Kido S et al. Prophylactic oral acyclovir in outbreaks of primary herpes simplex virus type 1 infection in a closed community. Pediatrics 1992; 89: 379–383.

20 Bean S F, Quezada R K. Recurrent oral erythema multiforme. JAMA 1983; 249: 2810–2812.

21 Weston W L, Brice S L, Jester J D et al. Herpes simplex virus in childhood erythema multiforme. Pediatrics 1992; 89: 32–34.

22 Green J A, Spruance S L, Wenerstrom G, Piepkorn M W. Post-herpetic erythema multiforme prevented with prophylactic oral acyclovir. Ann Intern Med 1985; 102: 632–633.

23 Fleisher G, Ludwig S, Campos C. Cellulitis: bacterial etiology, clinical features, and laboratory findings. J Pediatr 1980: 591–593.

24 Dodson T B, Perrott D H, Kaban L B. Pediatric maxillofacial infections: a retrospective study of 113 patients. J Oral Maxillofac Surg 1989: 328–330.

25 Baker C J. Group B streptococcal cellulitis–adenitis in infants. Am J Dis Child 1982; 136: 631–633.

26 Powell K R, Kaplan S B, Hall C B, Nasello M A et al. Periorbital cellulitis. Am J Dis Child 1988; 142: 853–857.

27 Baker R C, Bausher J C. Meningitis complicating acute bacteremic facial cellulitis. Pediatr Infect Dis J 1986; 5: 421–423.

28 Ciarallo L R, Rowe P C. Lumbar punctures in children with periorbital and orbital cellulitis. J Pediatr 1993; 122: 355–359.

29 Carter S, Feldman W E. Etiology and treatment of facial cellulitis in pediatric patients. Pediatr Infect Dis J 1983; 2: 222–224.

30 Israele V, Nelson J D. Periorbital and orbital cellulitis. Pediatr Infect Dis J 1987; 6: 404–410.

31 Lampe R M, Baker C J, Septimus E J. Cervicofacial nocardiosis in children. J Pediatr 1981; 99: 593–595.

32 Drake D P, Holt R J. Childhood actinomycosis: report of three recent cases. Arch Dis Child 1976; 51: 979–981.

33 Chow A W. Infections of the oral cavity, neck and head. In: Mandell G L, Douglas R G, Bennett J E. Principles and practice of infectious diseases, 3rd ed. Edinburgh: Churchill Livingstone, 1990.

34 Marcy S M. Infections due to dog and cat bites. Pediatr Infect Dis 1982; 1: 351–356.

35 Greenspan J S, Barr C E, Sciubba J J, Winkler J R. Oral manifestations of HIV infection. Oral Surg Oral Med Oral Pathol 1992; 73: 142–225.

36 Leggott P J. Oral manifestations of HIV in children. Oral Surg Oral Med Oral Pathol 1992; 73: 187–191.
37 Katz M H, Mastrucci M T, Leggott P J, Westenhouse J et al. Prognostic significance of oral lesions in children with perinatally acquired HIV infection. Am J Dis Child 1993; 147: 45–48.
38 Hopkins K P. Predental antibiotic prophylaxis in the immunocompromised child. In: Patrick C C, ed. Infections in immunocompromised infants and children. Edinburgh: Churchill Livingstone, 1992: 761–769.
39 Childers N K, Stinnet E A, Wheeler P, Wright J T et al. Oral complications in children with cancer. Oral Surg Oral Med Oral Pathol 1993; 75: 41–47.

1A.7 Parotitis

Inflammatory swelling of the parotid gland may be acute, recurrent or chronic. Clearly mumps is the most important cause of acute parotitis. However, other causes of facial swelling, such as facial cellulitis and even facial oedema due to allergy or nephrotic syndrome, can mimic parotid swelling.

The syndrome of recurrent parotitis is a relatively common yet ill-understood childhood disease, frequently mistaken for suppurative parotitis. Chronic parotid swelling may be due to a number of different causes, of which HIV infection is a new but important cause.

ANATOMY

It is usually easy to diagnose neck swelling as being parotoid in origin because of the characteristic anatomical position of the parotid gland is shown in Figure 1A.7.1. A tongue of the parotid is present in front of the ear, but a large amount behind the ear, so that parotid swelling often pushes the ear lobe upwards and outwards. The parotid gland extends inferiorly as far as the lower angle of the mandible. Swelling outside the anatomical distribution of the parotid gland may be due to the simultaneous involvement of other glands, as for example the mandibular glands in mumps, or alternatively swelling in the region may be due to a process not involving the parotid, such as facial cellulitis or oedema. The opening of the parotoid duct is adjacent to the third upper molar, and pus or white exudate may be expressed from the duct by pressure on the parotoid gland or purulent and non-purulent parotitis respectively (Fig. 1A.7.2).

ACUTE PAROTITIS

Although mumps is by far the commonest cause of acute parotitis in an un-immunized population, the widespread use of measles/mumps/rubella vaccine in many industrialized countries has increased the importance of other causes of parotitis. A list of possible causes of acute swelling of the parotid or in the parotid region is given in Table 1A.7.1.

MUMPS

Parotitis is a complication of mumps virus infection, rather than a sine qua non: serological studies suggest that up to 30% of children with mumps virus infection have a mild upper respiratory infection as the sole manifestation or are asymptomatic, and that only about two-thirds have parotitis. Most mumps parotitis

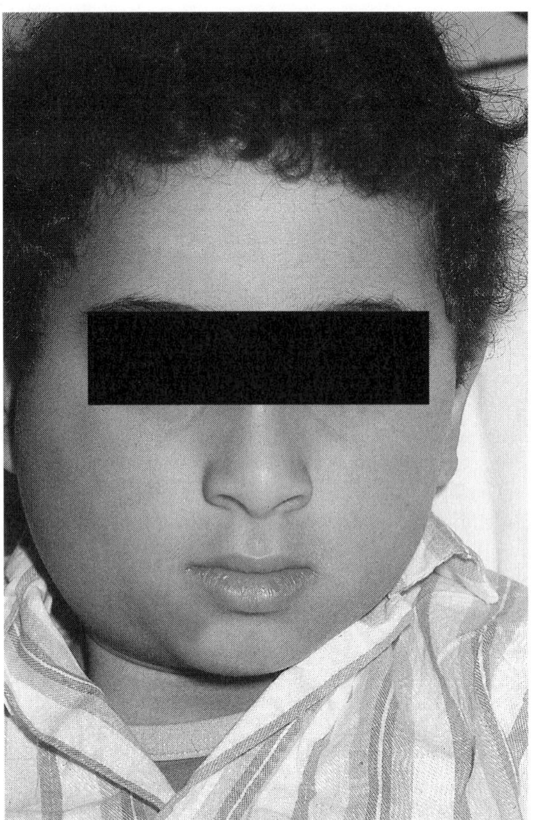

Fig. 1A.7.1 Acute parotitis. Child with unilateral parotid gland swelling. This child subsequently had recurrent episodes of parotitis.

Table 1A7.1 Causes of acute parotitis or parotid swelling

Viral	Mumps virus
	Coxsackie A and echovirus
	Cytomegalovirus (immune compromised)
	Lymphocytic choriomeningitis
	Parainfluenza virus types 1 and 3
Bacterial	*Staphylococcus aureus*
	Streptococcus pyogenes
	Gram-negative bacilli (neonate)
	Mycobacterium tuberculosis
	Atypical mycobacteria
	Cat-scratch disease
Idiopathic	Recurrent parotitis
Collagen vascular	Systemic lupus erythematosus, juvenile chronic arthritis
Mechanical	Salivary calculus
	Cystic fibrosis
Tumours	Lymphoma (Hodgkin and non-Hodgkin), leukaemia, lymphosarcoma

is bilateral, although one side may be involved a day or two before the other. Unilateral parotitis can be due to mumps, but its presence should alert the clinician to other possible diagnoses.

Mumps is an ancient disease: Hippocrates described acute parotitis compli-

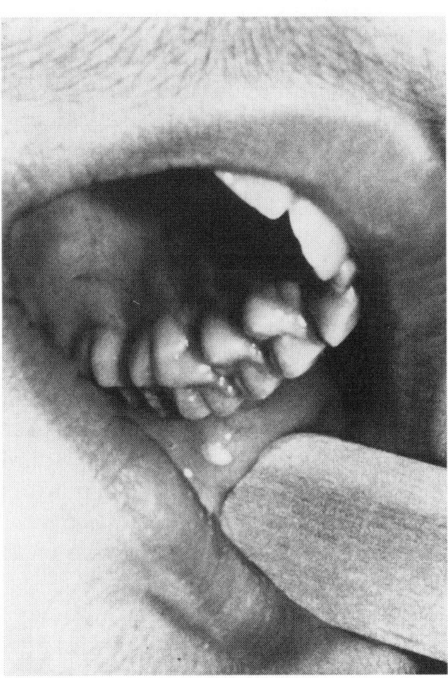

Fig. 1A.7.2 Child with recurrent parotitis. White exudate being expressed from Stensen's duct. See also colour plate.

cated by orchitis in the fifth century BC. The virus was first grown in 1934, and is an enveloped RNA paramyxovirus with only one known serotype.

In unimmunized populations mumps is an endemic disease, primarily of urban children. Virus can be cultured from saliva and urine of infected children (as well as from the cerebrospinal fluid of subjects with mumps meningitis). Spread is probably mostly by airborne droplets, although direct person-to-person spread via hands, fomites and even urine can also occur.

Parotid swelling may represent the inflammatory response to infection, since viral replication has been demonstrated in the monkey parotid gland for several days before the advent of parotid swelling. Histopathologically, mumps virus causes damage mainly to epithelial cells lining parotid ducts rather than to acini.

The incubation period of mumps is 14–24 days. The infectious period is from up to 6 days before to 9 days after the appearance of parotid gland swelling. There is usually no prodromal period, and fever with tender enlargement of one or both parotid glands is the commonest initial presentation. Parotid swelling is said to begin at the upper pole, between the mandible and mastoid, and then extend downwards and forwards. Up to 20% of children may be afebrile. Involvement of the submandibular glands or occasionally the sublingual glands leads to a more diffuse swelling.

The diagnosis of mumps is primarily clinical. The virus can readily be cultured from throat swabs and often from urine during mumps infection. Serum antibodies to the 'S' antigen of the virus appear early in most patients, and persist for up to 12 months. Antibodies to the 'V' antigen are detectable later, reach a peak after a month, and wane to low levels which persist for life. This anti-V is a typical IgG response, but anti-S is not a typical IgM response. The parotitis of mumps usually resolves within 7 days, and parotid swelling that lasts longer than this may have a different aetiology. In mumps, the opening of Stensen's duct may be red and swollen. If pus can be expressed from the duct by pressure on the gland, the diagnosis is bacterial parotitis, although a white fluid can sometimes be expressed in recurrent parotitis (see Fig. 1A.7.2). Mumps virus infection generally confers lifelong protection. Patients who have been diagnosed as having more than one episode of mumps may actually be suffering from repeated episodes of lympadenopathy or from the syndrome of recurrent parotitis.

BACTERIAL PAROTITIS

True acute suppurative parotitis is very rare in childhood. Over a 20-year period, 16 children, 14 of them boys, were seen at the Mayo Clinic with this condition: 7 were under a year old, of whom 3 were neonates, 2 were aged 1–5 years, 2 aged 6–10, and 5 aged 11–15 years. Four patients had suppurative parotitis in association with a terminal illness.[1]

The hallmark of this disease is tender, unilateral enlargement of the parotid gland, usually with fever and overlying redness. Pus can be expressed from Stensen's duct, the parotid duct, which is adjacent to the third upper molar (see Fig. 1A.7.1).

The organisms that have been cultured in pure or mixed growth from the parotid duct during bacterial parotitis are *Staphylococcus aureus*, pyogenic streptococci and, in the neonatal period, Gram-negative bacilli such as *Escherichia coli* and *Pseudomonas aeruginosa*.

In the past, many children with the syndrome of recurrent parotitis have been misdiagnosed as having suppurative parotitis, probably because in the latter condition white or even mucopurulent fluid can be expressed from Stensen's duct by palpating the gland. However, only normal mouth flora can be cultured from the fluid in recurrent parotitis. For example, the Mayo Clinic series, mentioned above, also describes 30 children with what they call 'recurrent suppurative parotitis'. However, viridans streptococci were the only organisms cultured from these children.[1] Similarly, in Feigin and Cherry's textbook, the chapter on 'Suppurative Parotitis'[2] includes recurrent parotitis as a form of recurrent suppurative parotitis, despite quoting normal mouth flora as the organisms responsible for 'suppuration'.

RECURRENT PAROTITIS

The syndrome of recurrent parotitis is a poorly understood entity, sometimes thought to be autoimmune in origin, in which children have recurrent attacks of painful parotid swelling. The attacks are usually unilateral, although either side may be affected at different times. Bilateral swelling is not rare. Most studies have found recurrent parotitis to be more common in boys. The peak age of onset is 3–6 years and usually in the first decade, although rare cases have started in infancy or after 10 years old.[3] Constitutional symptoms, including fever, are usually minimal or absent. Pain and swelling usually resolve within 2–7 days, though may rarely take up to 3 weeks. Most children have one to five attacks per year, although some children have been described with more than 20. The natural tendency is to resolution with time, and over 90% of patients no longer have symptoms by early adult life.[3]

The aetiology of recurrent parotitis is unknown. Evidence for autoimmune involvement is provided by a small number of cases with immunological disorders associated with immune deficiency.[4,5] However, there is no consistent immunological defect in affected children and very little evidence of other autoimmune disorders, while the tendency to remission is atypical of most autoimmune conditions.[6] It is probably wise to measure serum immunoglobulin levels, as there is a recognized though rare association between immunoglobulin deficiency and recurrent or chronic parotitis.[5]

There is no specific test for recurrent parotitis but almost all affected patients have unilateral or bilateral sialectasia demonstrated if a sialogram is performed. Ultrasound of the parotid gland sometimes shows a markedly dilated parotid duct. It is doubtful whether a sialogram is necessary in every case, but it is often performed to exclude a calculus or a stricture.

The treatment is with gentle massage and analgesia. There are anecdotal reports of ligation of the parotid duct and of parotidectomy, but these are extremely invasive procedures for a condition which nearly always resolves spontaneously.

CHRONIC PAROTITIS

A number of disorders can lead to the relatively uncommon condition of chronic parotid swelling. Some of these have already been considered in Table 1A.7.1 under acute parotid swelling, since acute swelling may become chronic. Disorders more likely to cause chronic parotitis are given in Table 1A.7.2.

While most of these are rare, there has been a recent increase in the number of children with chronic parotid swelling due to HIV infection. Parotid swelling in HIV is often associated with generalized lymphadenopathy and is a relatively good prognostic sign, being more common in long-term survivors.[7] It is thought that the involvement of lymphoid and salivary tissue represents a vigorous cellular immune response, which may in itself be protective against HIV infection.

Table 1A.7.2 Causes of chronic parotid swelling

Infections	HIV infection Cat-scratch disease
Collagen vascular	Sjögren syndrome Systemic lupus erythematosus Polyarteritis nodosa
Sarcoidosis	
Drugs	Anticholinergics Phenothiazines Antihistamines Gentamicin (by aerosol)
Mechanical	Cystic fibrosis Calculi
Benign tumours	Haemangioma, lymphangioma, lipoma, adenoma, congenital cyst
Malignant tumours	Leukaemia, Hodgkin and non-Hodgkin lymphoma, primary tumour

REFERENCES

1 David R D, O'Connell E J. Suppurative parotitis in children. Am J Dis Child 1970; 119: 332–335.
2 Inlaterer D. Suppurative parotitis. In: Feigin R D, Cherry J D, eds. Textbook of pediatric infectious diseases, 3rd ed. Philadelphia: W B Saunders, 1992: 236–238.
3 Geterud A, Lindvall A-M, Nylen O. Follow-up study of recurrent parotitis in children. Ann Otol Rhinol Laryngol 1988; 97: 341–346.
4 Friis B, Karup Pedersen F, Schiodt M, Wiik A, Hoj L, Andersen V. Immunological studies in two children with recurrent parotitis. Acta Paediatr Scand 1983; 72: 265–268.
5 Mulcahy D, Isaacs D. Recurrent parotitis. Arch Dis Child 1992; 67: 1036–1037.
6 Konno A, Ito E. A study on the pathogenesis of recurrent parotitis in childhood. Ann Otol Rhinol Laryngol 1979; 88 (suppl 63): 1–20.
7 Italian Register for HIV Infection in Children. Features of children perinatally infected with HIV-1 surviving longer than 5 years. Lancet 1994; 343: 191–195.

1A.8   Epiglottitis

INTRODUCTION

Epiglottitis, like bronchiolitis, is a pathological term which is also used as a clinical diagnosis. As supraglottic tissues other than the epiglottis are usually also involved, the term supraglottitis is preferred by some. Usually due to infection with *Haemophilus influenzae* type b (Hib), it is a relatively uncommon, rapidly progressive septic disease which causes life-threatening respiratory obstruction. It is often hard to diagnose and requires expert emergency care to minimize mortality. Routine infant vaccination against Hib has the potential of making epiglottitis a rare condition.

EPIDEMIOLOGY

Although Hib is the causative organism in over 95% of children, a similar clinical course can result from other infections. Streptococci and viruses[1,2] make up most of the remainder. Acute epiglottitis has been reported as a thermal injury. Chronic epiglottitis has been described in association with immunodeficiency and with sarcoidosis.

Epiglottitis has been described in very young infants, though most commonly affects children between 9 months and 4 years of age, with peak incidence at 2–3 years, somewhat later than the peak incidence for Hib meningitis. It only occasionally affects older children and occurs rarely in early and middle adult life. Typical acute epiglottitis is a severe infection which almost always leads to hospital admission, though milder forms may occur and remain undiagnosed, self-limiting or responding to empirical antibiotic therapy. Untreated or poorly treated, it has a high mortality. In developed countries high levels of training and awareness combined with high standards of acute care have reduced deaths to a low level but deaths still occur.

The incidence of epiglottitis varies considerably and inexplicably between various countries[3] and even within the same country. The incidence is high in Sweden, Finland and Australia and lower in the USA and the UK. The ratio of epiglottitis to meningitis and other systemic Hib infections also varies considerably. Aboriginal children in northern Australia, and native North American Indians and Eskimos experience a far higher incidence of Hib infection overall, most of this occurring in the first 12 months as meningitis, with very little epiglottitis at any age.

Epiglottitis occurs throughout all seasons, though usually with a higher incidence in winter. With the introduction of infant vaccination against Hib, epiglottitis quickly falls in incidence and with high vaccine uptake rates soon becomes a rare disease.

PATHOGENESIS AND PATHOLOGY

Epiglottitis usually occurs in association with bacteraemia or septicaemia. Blood cultures are positive for Hib in 80–90% of children at the time of diagnosis. Clinical manifestations of bacteraemia or septicaemia often precede airway obstruction. With both viral and bacterial infections the throat may represent the primary site of ingress of infection.

The supraglottic tissues, especially the epiglottis and aryepiglottic folds, become grossly inflamed and oedematous. The epiglottis loses its normal shape, becoming globular and many times its usual size. It may appear pale, or red due to inflammatory hyperaemia. Copious thin secretions may be present. The respiratory tract below the larynx is usually normal, though with prolonged severe airway obstruction pulmonary oedema may be present.

IMMUNITY

The presence of passive maternal IgG may explain why Hib infections are less common in early infancy but does not explain why meningitis, the most frequent serious infection due to Hib, tends to occur earlier than epiglottitis.

Infants may not develop immunity to Hib after epiglottitis, and second episodes of epiglottitis are known but are very rare. Most children develop humoral immunity against Hib by the age of 5 years without suffering severe infection, and the falling incidence with age is an indication of increasing rates of immunity.

Unusual causative organisms, e.g. *Candida*, may be seen in children with immunodeficiency disorders.

SPREAD

Haemophilus infections are usually acquired via droplet spread, presumably often from relatively healthy carriers. Non-immune children under 4 years old in close proximity, either in a family or child care setting, are at increased risk when one child has any form of invasive Hib infection. A contact of a child with epiglottitis may suffer meningitis or any other systemic Hib infection and vice versa. Such spread of infection can be prevented by the use of rifampicin in all children and adults in the immediate group.

CLINICAL FEATURES

Sore throat and fever usually appear first, sometimes rapidly followed by drooling, due to reluctance to swallow. The voice may sound muffled and the child may be reluctant to talk. The child appears lethargic and toxic, and fever between 38°C and 40°C is common. Symptoms and signs of upper airway obstruction often begin insidiously but may then progress rapidly. Stridor is often absent and if present tends to be soft and wheezy. Cough is usually not present. The child takes up a posture to optimize the airway; this may be sitting or supine, with a fixed, unusual head retraction. Children with epiglottitis almost always appear apprehensive and may resist any attempt to change their posture or to carry out throat examination. Chest retractions are increasingly present as obstruction progresses, but respiratory rate is usually slow, and signs of toxicity may distract the observer from signs of respiratory difficulty. Profound airway obstruction may develop within several hours of the first symptom or may develop progressively over 12–24 h. Where severe airway obstruction has been prolonged, pulmonary oedema may complicate the clinical picture.[4] Without treatment to overcome airway obstruction, many children with epiglottitis will die from hypoxaemia due to upper airway obstruction.

DIAGNOSIS

Because epiglottitis is relatively rare, and because it initially causes symptoms which are both common and non-specific, initial misdiagnosis is common. Unlike croup, which 'bespeaks its name', the early features of epiglottitis are subtle and, with progression, the overall impression of an extremely unwell child may direct attention away from the upper airway. The correct diagnosis is usually suspected on the clinical features (described above) by one who is aware of the condition, either from adequate instruction or from experience.

When epiglottitis is suspected clinically it is not appropriate to examine the throat during initial assessment. Occasionally, however, the diagnosis is made inadvertently on physical examination of the throat, from visualizing the epiglottis during an induced 'gag' manoeuvre. The epiglottis will usually appear bulbous and intensely inflamed. Direct visual examination can more safely be done during the procedure to relieve the obstruction, as described below. Lateral airways X-rays often demonstrate a 'classical' appearance diagnostic of epiglottitis.[5] This is sometimes seen when the diagnosis has not been suspected clinically. However, lateral airways X-rays in children with epiglottitis are potentially dangerous because of postural changes which may be forced upon the child, for instance neck extension. This may dramatically worsen the degree of obstruction. Such X-rays, then, are generally not advised though it is valuable to be able to recognize the X-ray changes of the various causes of airway obstruction. Where upper airway obstruction is the dominant clinical appearance, other causes of acute

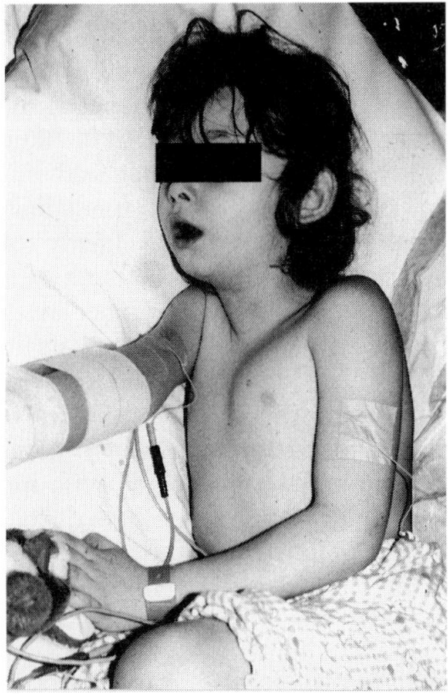

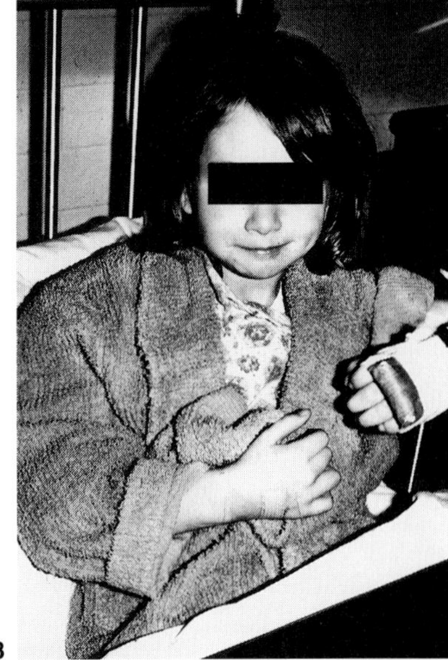

Fig. 1A.8.1 Five-year-old girl with acute epiglottitis (**A**) and 48 h later (**B**), after treatment.

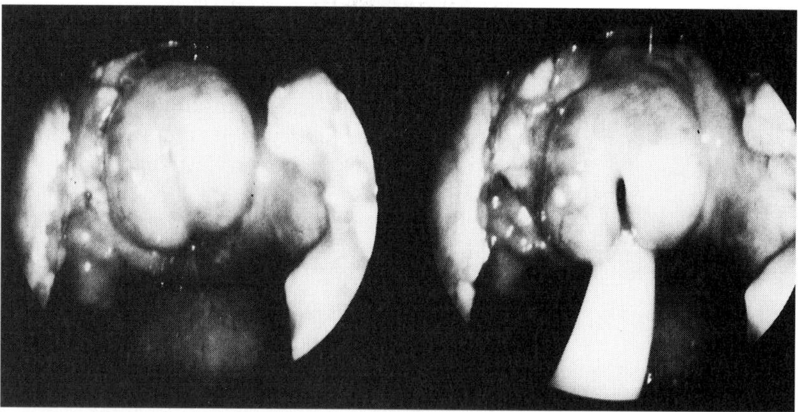

Fig. 1A. 8.2 Acute epiglottitis due to *Haemophilus influenzae* showing the gross swelling and inflammation of the epiglottis and other supraglottic structures. In the right-hand photograph, a fairly small-diameter endotracheal tube has been passed. It is noteworthy that the airway is not only through the lumen of the endotracheal tube, but the tube itself splints open and separates the swollen structures.

upper airway obstruction must be distinguished from epiglottitis (see p. 83). Blood culture taken during initial assessment and/or urinary antigen studies will usually confirm Hib as the causative organism.

ASSESSMENT OF SEVERITY

Though 'mild' cases of epiglottitis may occur and remain undiagnosed, in general it is assumed that epiglottitis will progress to severe airway obstruction and that almost all children are likely to need an artificial airway for this. Because of this all children suspected of having epiglottitis must be urgently admitted to hospital and urgently assessed for the need for airway intubation. On the infrequent occasion when it is felt that intubation is not warranted, extremely close observation of the subsequent need for this must be maintained, in a paediatric intensive care unit.

TREATMENT

Relief of airway obstruction

Optimal management consists of short-term nasotracheal intubation, and requires skills in paediatric anaesthesia, experience with difficult tracheal intubation and subsequent intensive care facilities. Intubation is most safely and humanely achieved by adding an inhalational anaesthetic (e.g. halothane) to oxygen and carrying out intubation once the child is adequately anaesthetized. Where airway obstruction is profound and the child already collapsed, oxygenation and intubation must be achieved at once by the most experienced person present. Muscle relaxants must *never* be used. When no anaesthetist is available, an attempt at intubation would still be preferable to an unskilled attempt at tracheotomy. Tracheal intubation is required for 24–36 h. Early extubation, e.g. within 8–12 h, is associated with an unacceptable rate of requiring re-intubation. Epiglottitis can be successfully managed with tracheotomy, though the morbidity and length of hospital stay are much greater than with intubation. During intubation it is essential that the child does not attempt to dislodge the tube. This can be achieved with a combination of adequate strapping of the tube to the face, arm splints and good nursing care.

Antibiotics

Depending upon known local sensitivities of Hib, either chloramphenicol or a third-generation cephalosporin (cefotaxime or ceftriaxone) are effective, if given intravenously in the upper limits of conventional dosage. Treatment is given for 5 days intravenously, or 2–4 days intravenously, until systemic toxicity is absent, followed by up to several days of oral therapy. The choice between chloramphenicol and a third-generation cephalosporin has been the subject of some controversy.[6,7] The toxicity of chloramphenicol is to be weighed against the greater cost of the cephalosporins. We prefer to use cefotaxime, initially, followed by oral amoxycillin or amoxycillin–clavulanic acid, depending on sensitivity.

Supportive

Oxygen should be administered by mask if airway obstruction is present. Assisted ventilation with positive end-expiratory pressure may be required in extremely sick children, for instance those with pulmonary oedema. It is not our practice to use more than mild sedation in intubated children, except those requiring ventilatory assistance.

PREVENTION

Widespread infant vaccination against Hib will greatly reduce the occurrence of epiglottitis in children. Where this has not yet been achieved, the use of rifampicin prophylaxis in close contacts of children with epiglottitis or other systemic Hib infection will produce a significant further reduction in the number of cases occurring.

REFERENCES

1 Grattan-Smith T M, Gillis J, Kilham H A. Viral supraglottitis. J Pediatr 1987; 110: 434–435.
2 Narasimhan N, van-Stralen D W, Perkin R M. Acute supraglottitis caused by varicella. Pediatr Infect Dis J 1993; 12: 619–620.
3 Clements D A, Booy R, Dagan R et al. Comparison of the epidemiology and cost of Haemophilus influenzae type b disease in five western countries. Pediatr Infect Dis J 1993; 12: 362–376.
4 Lang S A, Duncan P G, Shephard D A, Ha H C. Pulmonary oedema associated with airway obstruction. Can J Anaesth 1990; 37: 210–218.
5 Rothrock S G, Pignatiello G A, Howard R M. Radiologic diagnosis of epiglottitis: objective criteria for all ages. Ann Emerg Med 1990; 19: 978–982.
6 Shann F. Which antibiotic for epiglottitis? J Paediatr Child Health 1992; 28: 217–218.
7 Knight G J, Harris M A, Parbari M et al. Single daily dose ceftriaxone therapy in epiglottitis. J Paediatr Child Health 1992; 28: 220–222.

1A.9   Croup

INTRODUCTION

Applied strictly, the term *croup* refers to a symptom complex of harsh barking cough, stridor and respiratory distress. In common usage, and in this section, croup is used as a 'shorthand' term to imply a diagnosis of either acute viral laryngotracheitis, or 'spasmodic croup', or the much less common entity, bacterial tracheitis ('pseudo-membranous croup'). A disadvantage of this 'shorthand' term is that it implies a firm diagnosis, with the result that serious alternative causes of the croup symptom complex such as diphtheria or subglottic foreign body are less likely to be considered.

Croup is an extremely common illness of young children, usually mild and self-limiting, though occasionally it may cause severe, even fatal respiratory obstruction.

It is controversial as to whether acute laryngotracheitis and spasmodic croup are separate conditions. It has been argued that they represent different ends of the 'spectrum' of one condition, and that as management is the same the distinction is irrelevant. We believe there are clinical and epidemiological differences which are outlined below.

EPIDEMIOLOGY

Laryngotracheitis can result from infection with a variety of respiratory tract viruses, including parainfluenza, influenza, measles and respiratory syncytial virus.[1] Croup mostly affects children aged between 6 and 36 months though it can occur at any age. Boys slightly outnumber girls. Croup occurs in all seasons though in most countries far more cases occur in autumn and winter. At times of high incidence, one particular virus will often be identifiable as causing most cases.

Spasmodic croup affects a similar population, though is believed to be allergic. It is more likely to be associated with a family history of croup or asthma and is more likely to recur. Children who suffer spasmodic croup are more likely to suffer asthma over subsequent years and some episodes of spasmodic croup evolve into asthma.

Bacterial tracheitis is a rare condition which may be a primary bacterial infection or which may represent bacterial infection complicating viral laryngotracheitis.[2] It is most often due to *Staphylococcus aureus* (or *Haemophilus influenzae* type b).[3]

Children with congenital or acquired subglottic stenosis are more likely to suffer severe croup and are more likely to require hospital admission. However, overall only a very small proportion of children with croup will require hospital treatment.

PATHOGENESIS AND PATHOLOGY

In *acute laryngotracheitis* the respiratory tract from the nasal mucosa to the bronchi is involved in direct viral infection, with hyperaemia, increased secretions and mucosal oedema. In more severe cases tracheobronchial secretions may be copious, varying from almost clear to purulent. The infection probably commences in the nose or throat and extends contiguously. It may be largely a 'surface' infection though at times there is significant systemic toxicity. As the subglottic trachea is the narrowest part of the airway in children, inflammatory oedema at this level, once sufficiently severe, will cause croupy cough, stridor and respiratory difficulty.

In *spasmodic croup* mucosal oedema is more localized to the subglottic trachea. As with viral laryngotracheitis, the normally ovoid cross-section of the airway immediately below the larynx is altered by oedema pressing inwards from both sides, giving an appearance at endoscopy of a fore-and-aft 'slit'. In spasmodic croup, tracheobronchial secretions are much less increased than with viral croup.

In *bacterial tracheitis* there is direct bacterial invasion of the tracheobronchial mucosa, with copious purulent secretions. A thick layer of secretions may mimic the appearance of the trachea in diphtheria, leading to the earlier nomenclature 'pseudo-membranous croup'. However, in diphtheria, the 'membrane' is tougher and more adherent. As bacterial tracheitis is caused by pyogenic bacteria, it is not surprising that systemic toxicity is usually present.

IMMUNITY

Passive maternal IgG may explain why croup is relatively uncommon in the first few months of life. Otherwise, so many viruses may cause croup that recurrent viral croup with different organisms is not uncommon.

SPREAD

Viral croup is not considered particularly contagious. Spread of viral respiratory infection is usually via droplet, with the exception of respiratory syncytial virus infection which is often spread by direct contact with nasal secretions.

CLINICAL FEATURES

In *viral laryngotracheitis*, coryzal symptoms may be present for a few days, followed by development of a harsh barking cough, hoarse voice, inspiratory difficulty and variable respiratory difficulty. Most children have a spiking fever. The symptoms are usually worse at night, though in some severe cases the symptoms are inexorably progressive over 12–36 h, leading to the need for intubation. Symptoms associated with severe croup are described below, under 'Assessment of severity'. In the overwhelming majority of children with croup the illness lasts for a few days and requires no treatment. With improvement the cough becomes less croupy and may sound productive.

Spasmodic croup is similar to viral croup, but with the absence of fever and coryzal symptoms. In spasmodic croup there is more likely to be a family history of asthma or atopy and episodes of spasmodic croup sometimes evolve into asthma. Spasmodic croup is often recurrent and in some older children, especially boys, an alarming degree of respiratory difficulty may develop within a very short time, precipitating the need for urgent treatment. In most children, respiratory distress is only mild and transient and only a small proportion of children require hospital management.

Bacterial tracheitis is a rare condition, initially similar to acute viral laryngo-tracheitis. In some cases it may represent bacterial infection complicating viral croup. It is associated with high spiking fever, systemic toxicity and progressive respiratory distress. At intubation copious thick secretions are aspirated from the trachea, often Gram stain positive for pyogenic organisms. It should be noted that in severe viral croup tracheobronchial secretions are also copious and may be thick, and a diagnosis of bacterial tracheitis is made partly on clinical features and partly on positive culture of a bacterial pathogen known to be associated with the condition.

DIAGNOSIS

Croup is a clinical diagnosis, made on signs and symptoms. When the croup symptom complex is present it is most important to exclude other conditions which may require different management. Other causes of acute upper airway obstruction are listed in Table 1A.9.1, with an indication of those conditions which may produce the croup symptom complex. The most important differential diagnosis is acute epiglottitis, a dangerous cause of upper airway obstruction, though its features are usually quite distinct (Ch. 1A.8).

In the differential diagnosis, *diphtheria* should be considered in any unimmunized child with the croup symptom complex. Progression of airway obstruction may be rapid. Marked halitosis is usually present. A grey adherent membrane is often present in the pharynx or on the tonsils. A *foreign body* in the larynx, subglottis or lower trachea or oesophagus may produce the croup symptom complex. A choking episode is not always witnessed. Foreign body should be suspected whenever clinical features are atypical or when history has indicated the availability of likely objects, especially nuts. Lateral airways X-rays are occasionally useful in demonstrating foreign bodies, though if the index of suspicion is

Table 1A.9.1   Differential diagnosis of acute upper airway obstruction

Supraglottic
   *Acute epiglottitis
    Acute tonsillar enlargement
    Retropharyngeal abscess
   *Foreign body
   *Acute angioneurotic oedema

Laryngeal/subglottic
   *Acute laryngotracheitis
   *Spasmodic croup
   *Bacterial tracheitis
   *Foreign body
   *Diphtheria
   *Thermal/chemical injury
   *Intubation trauma
   *Laryngospasm (neural, hypocalcaemia, reflux-induced)

Tracheal
   *Trauma (haematoma)
   *Tumour (anterior mediastinal lymphoma)
   *Foreign body (oesophageal, tracheal).

* May cause some or all of the symptoms of croup.

sufficiently high endoscopy must be done. Foreign body should be considered even when fever is present, fever being common in children generally. Reflex laryngospasm associated with gastro-oesophageal reflux may cause acute stridor and croupy cough.[4]

Rarely, recurrent croup symptoms may be an indication of a congenital abnormality (e.g. vascular ring) or an acquired condition (e.g. subglottic haemangioma) or hypocalcaemia. Acute angioneurotic oedema may occasionally mimic croup in older children; in this condition, face and neck swelling will usually suggest the diagnosis, though these features are not invariably present.

ASSESSMENT OF SEVERITY

Although infrequent, severe airway obstruction is the major clinical concern in croup. Assessment of the degree of airway obstruction is, therefore, the most important aspect of assessment. It relies almost entirely on clinical signs, and is one of the most difficult assessments in paediatric medicine. Because airway obstruction in croup can worsen rapidly, repeated careful clinical assessment is essential. In severe croup, the critical clinical questions are need for, and timing of, tracheal intubation. Both unnecessary intubation and delayed, urgent intubation will increase morbidity and mortality. The most reliable assessment is that of the skilled observer, 'from the end of the bed', as opposed to auscultatory findings, pulse and respiratory rates, etc.

Mild airway obstruction

This can be assumed where the infant or child appears happy and is prepared to drink, eat, play and take an interest in the surroundings. There may be some chest wall retractions and mild tachycardia.

Moderate airway obstruction

This is indicated by more marked chest wall retractions, use of accessory muscles of respiration and increasing heart rate. The infant or child may begin to appear worried, preoccupied or tired. He or she may still sleep for short periods. Such a child requires close, continuing observation, and progression in signs indicates the need for tracheal intubation.

Severe airway obstruction

As airway obstruction increases the appearance will be that of increasing tiredness and exhaustion. Marked tachycardia is usually present. Restlessness, agitation, irrational behaviour, decreased conscious level, hypotonia, cyanosis and marked pallor are 'late' signs indicating that dangerous airway obstruction is now present and that tracheal intubation is urgently required.

Clinical scoring systems

A variety of points-scoring systems have been devised to attempt to grade severity with greater objectivity. These give a cumulative score, grading for the degree of stridor, retractions, air entry, cyanosis, dyspnoea, conscious level, etc. Such systems are of value in research studies involving croup, but are usually of little or no value in ordinary clinical practice.

Oximetry

Pulse oximeters are increasingly used in hospital management of croup. Oximetry can never substitute for good clinical assessment. It has been shown that oxygen saturation may be near normal in severe croup and yet significantly lowered in some children with mild to moderate croup.[5] Oximetry has poor predictive value, in assessing the need for intubation. However, unexpectedly low oxygen saturations may occasionally alert observers to airway obstruction more severe than assessed clinically.

TREATMENT

Home management

Most children with croup have only mild airway obstruction and can be managed at home. Reassurance of the parents, observation and comforting of the child by the parents are the important features of home care. The need for hospital treatment will be indicated by increasing respiratory distress, agitation and retractions. Steam inhalation is associated with a risk of scalds.[6]

Hospital management

Avoiding harm from airway obstruction is the main aim of hospital management. As detailed above, assessment of severity and timing of intervention depend almost entirely on clinical judgement.

Mist tent therapy

This should not be used. There is no evidence that it is beneficial. It can be harmful, by impeding adequate observation and by impeding optimal comforting of the child by a parent.

Parental comforting

The value of this cannot be overestimated.

Oxygen

Children with mild or mild-to-moderate croup rarely need additional oxygen. Oxygen should not be withheld from any child with severe croup. It has been argued that the use of oxygen in severe croup is dangerous because it may prevent cyanosis and hypoxic agitation. However, additional oxygen will improve the general condition of any child with severe croup whilst definitive management is arranged. Any child considered sick enough to require additional oxygen also requires very close observation for the need for intubation.

Nebulized adrenaline

Nebulized adrenaline will often dramatically reduce the degree of upper airway obstruction in croup, though the effect is often transient, with return of severe obstruction within 20–40 min.[7] Adrenaline can be repeated, often with benefit, but it should be used only when severe airway obstruction is present, under very close supervision, and the need for repeated doses is usually an indication of the need for intubation. Excessive adrenaline can cause pallor and tachycardia, and mimic respiratory failure.

Corticosteroids

Either oral steroids (e.g. prednisone or dexamethasone) or inhaled steroids (budesonide) may reduce the severity of croup and shorten the illness.[8,9] Such treatment should be restricted to children with severe acute or troublesome recurrent croup.

Intubation

Tracheal intubation is required when airway obstruction is particularly severe, as described above under 'Assessment of severity'. This should be carried out by an experienced anaesthetist. Except when collapse has occurred and resuscitation is needed, giving a light inhalational anaesthetic prior to intubation is both more humane and safer. The intubated child is cared for in an intensive care ward. Avoiding accidental extubation is a high priority.

Treating pulmonary oedema   Any child with profound airway obstruction may suffer acute pulmonary oedema. This is usually apparent at the time of intubation, and will require additional oxygen, constant positive airways pressure or assisted ventilation with positive end-expiratory pressure.

Antibiotics   Antibiotics are given only to children with bacterial tracheitis or to those intubated children with severe croup in whom secondary bacterial infection is suspected.

REFERENCES

1 Phelan P D, Landau L I, Olinsky A. Respiratory illness in children, 3rd ed. Blackwell, Oxford: 1990: pp 54–55.
2 Henry R L, Mellis C M, Benjamin B. Pseudomembranous croup. Arch Dis Child 1983; 58: 180–183.
3 Donnelly B W, McMillan J A, Weiner L B. Bacterial tracheitis: report of eight new cases and review. Rev Infect Dis 1990; 12: 729–735.
4 Burton D M, Pransky S M, Katz R M, Kearns D B, Seid A B. Pediatric airway manifestations of gastroesophageal reflux. Ann Otol Rhinol Laryngol 1992; 101: 742–749.
5 Stoney P J, Chakrabarti M K. Experience of pulse oximetry in children with croup. J Laryngol Otol 1991; 105: 295–298.
6 Greally P, Cheng K, Tanner M S, Field D J. Children with croup presenting with scalds. Br Med J 1990; 301: 113.
7 Waisman Y, Klein B L, Boenning D A et al. Prospective randomised double-blind study comparing L-epinephrine and racemic epinephrine aerosols in the treatment of laryngotracheitis (croup). Pediatrics 1992; 89: 302–306.
8 Kairys S W, Olmstead E M, O'Connor G T. Steroid treatment of laryngotracheobronchitis: a meta-analysis of the evidence from randomised trials. Pediatrics 1989; 83: 683–693.
9 Klassen T P, Feldman M E, Watters L K, Sutcliffe T, Rowe P C. Nebulised budesonide for children with mild–moderate croup. N Engl J Med 1994; 331: 285–289.

1A.10 Cervical lymphadenopathy

Enlargement of the cervical nodes may be due to the involvement of the nodes in a generalized infectious, inflammatory or malignant process, or may be due to a localized infection of the head or neck with enlargement of the draining nodes.

ANATOMY

Lymphocytes are made in the primary lymphoid organs, B cells in the bone marrow and T cells in the bone marrow, but 'educated' in the thymus. The B and T lymphocytes then circulate in the bloodstream until they reach one of the secondary lymphoid organs, these being the lymph nodes, spleen, tonsils, adenoids and Peyer's patches. In the lymph node they leave the bloodstream through high endothelial venules and enter the cortex of the node (see Fig. 1A.10.1).

Antigenic material and antigen-presenting cells such as macrophages enter the lymph node via afferent lymphatic channels. Antigenic material is phagocytosed by macrophages or by specialized follicular dendritic cells, both of which can act as antigen-presenting cells. These cells can degrade antigen into peptides in

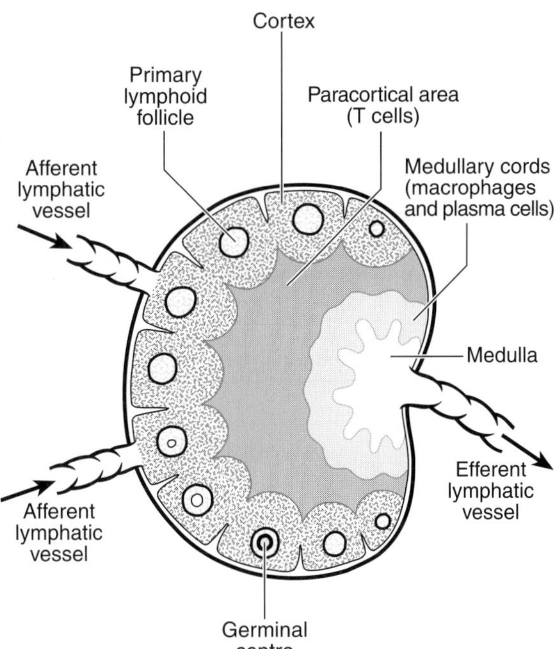

Fig. 1A.10.1 Schematic drawing of a lymph node.

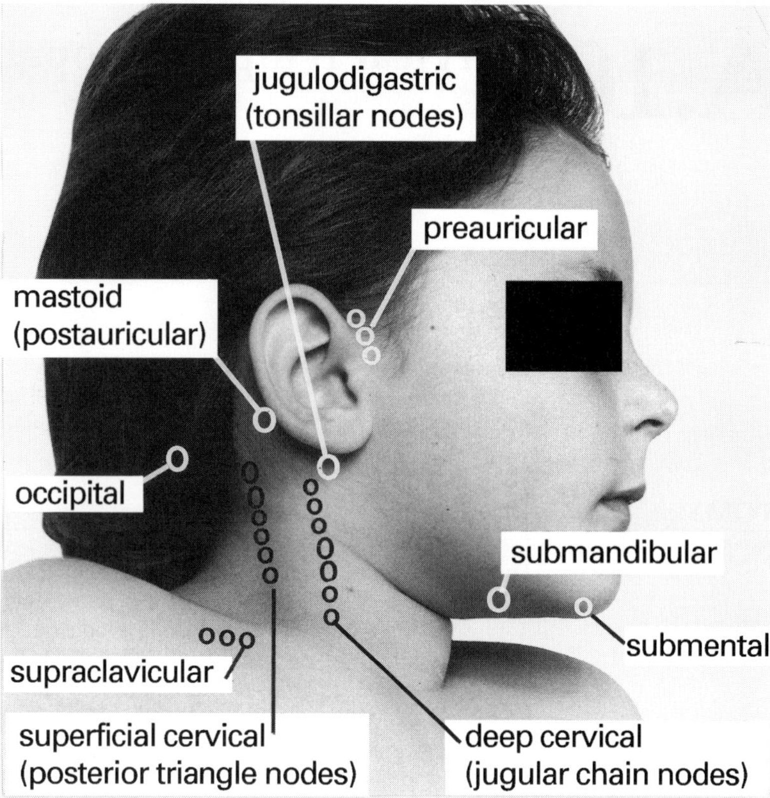

Fig. 1A.10.2 Distribution of cervical lymph nodes.

their cytoplasm. The degraded peptides are transported to the cell surface, in conjunction with major histocompatibility complex (MHC) molecules and presented to T cells. T cell activation by antigen generally takes place in the paracortex.

B cells respond to soluble antigen by becoming antibody-producing plasma cells, which occurs in the germinal centres of the lymphoid follicles.

Activated B and T cells leave the lymph node via the efferent lymphatics and enter the bloodstream. There are about 300 lymph nodes in the head and neck area. The distribution of the lymph nodes is shown in Figure 1A.10.2, and the areas drained by each group of nodes is given in Table 1A.10.1.

Most lymphatic drainage goes to the deep cervical and submandibular/

Table 1A.10.1 Areas drained by lymph nodes of the neck

Groups of glands	Areas drained
Deep cervical	
Jugulodigastric	Tonsil
Lower deep cervical	Larynx, trachea, thyroid, oesophagus
Superficial cervical	Skin, mastoid, parotid
Mastoid (postauricular)	Parietal scalp, inner surface of pinna
Occipital	Occipital scalp, neck
Submental	Tongue, chin, lower lip
Submandibular	Lower lip, nose, cheek, forehead, eyelids
Submaxillary	Mouth, gums, tongue

submaxillary groups, which are most commonly involved in cervical lymphadenopathy in childhood.

Cervical lymphadenitis is extremely common in children. It may be of infectious or non-infectious origin. Infections associated with cervical lymphadenitis include local respiratory viral infections, generalized viral infections (e.g. Epstein–Barr virus (EBV), cytomegalovirus (CMV), human immunodeficiency virus (HIV)), granulomatous bacterial (e.g. cat-scratch), pyogenic bacterial (group A streptococcal, staphylococcal), mycobacterial (atypical and tuberculous) and protozoal infections (e.g. toxoplasmosis).

Non-infectious causes include collagen vascular diseases (e.g. systemic Still's) and malignancy (e.g. leukaemia, Hodgkin, non-Hodgkin lymphoma). The lymphadenopathy of Kawasaki disease may be an inflammatory one in response to a bacterial toxin. Rarely a congenital neck lesion may mimic cervical lymphadenitis: branchial cleft cysts and thyroglossal cysts may become infected, while cystic hygromas may appear in the first 2 years of life.

Clearly, the finding of cervical lymphadenitis in childhood is non-specific, and evaluation of the child will depend on the clinical and epidemiological setting.

EPIDEMIOLOGY

The biggest epidemiological divide, albeit an over-simplistic one, is between childhood cervical lymphadenitis occurring in industrialized and non-industrialized countries. The causes found will also depend on referral patterns: hospital-based studies in industrialized countries show that group A streptococcal infection is the commonest cause, followed by staphylococcal infection, and that these two organisms cause 60–80% of hospital cases.[1] Tuberculous lymphadenitis is far less common in industrialized countries than adenitis caused by atypical mycobacteria. In contrast, tuberculosis is probably the commonest cause of cervical lymphadenitis presenting to medical attention in non-industrialized countries.

Age is an important factor: atypical mycobacterial infection, group A streptococcal suppurative lymphadenitis and Kawasaki disease are all more common in preschool children than in children 5 years or older, while malignancy rarely presents with cervical lymphadenopathy in children under 5 years old.

PATHOPHYSIOLOGY

Lymph nodes may become enlarged due to lymphocyte accumulation in viral and non-infectious inflammatory conditions and due to malignant cells in leukaemia and lymphoma. Accumulation of neutrophils and suppuration may be the cause of lymphadenitis in some children with group A streptococcal infection, but frank suppuration is the exception, and in most children with adenitis and a 'strep' sore throat the adenitis resolves with oral antibiotic therapy.

CLINICAL PRESENTATION

The clinical presentation of cervical lymphadenitis is a strong pointer to aetiology. Important considerations are age, duration, presence of fever and other systemic symptoms, history of tonsillitis, tenderness, firmness and overlying redness (Table 1A.10.2). The nodes are usually unilateral in cat-scratch fever and Kawasaki disease, and bilateral in generalized infections such as EBV, CMV, HIV or toxoplasmosis, in association with lymphadenopathy elsewhere in the body, and often

Table 1A.10.2   Significance of different factors in children with cervical lymphadenopathy

Age	Suppurative lymphadenitis, atypical mycobacterial infection disease and Kawasaki disease more common < 5 years old; malignancy more common > 5 years
Fever	Present in streptococcal and staphylococcal infections, cat-scratch disease, Kawasaki disease. Absent in TB (usually) and atypical mycobacterial infection
Tenderness	Nodes are usually tender in suppurative adenitis and cat-scratch disease; characteristically non-tender in mycobacterial infections
Redness	Overlying redness suggests suppuration
Firmness	Malignant nodes particularly firm
Duration	Acute: bacterial, viral, Kawasaki disease Subacute or chronic: mycobacterial, cat-scratch disease, malignancy

with splenomegaly and hepatomegaly. The nodes may be unilateral or bilateral in pyogenic infection and malignancy.

Important questions in the history include contact with tuberculosis (TB), ingestion of unpasteurized milk and possibly contaminated water, contact with cats, drug use (e.g. phenytoin) and foreign travel.

Matted, non-fluctuant, unilateral lymphadenitis with fever tends to be diagnosed as bacterial infection. However, if the fever persists despite antibiotics, a diagnosis of Kawasaki disease should be considered. The teeth should always be examined carefully, as dental abscesses may be relatively silent in young children.

CAT-SCRATCH DISEASE

Cat-scratch disease almost always occurs in children with a cat, usually a kitten, in the family.[2] There may be a history of a scratch, and even an indurated sore, but the organisms can also be inoculated into the conjunctiva by a lick. Unilateral axillary or epitrochlear node involvement, secondary to a scratch on the hand, is more common, but about 25% of children with cat-scratch disease have isolated cervical involvement. The incubation period is about 2 weeks from the scratch. Despite the oldname '*cat-scratch fever*', the majority of patients are in fact afebrile. The nodes suppurate in about 10% of patients. Rare, but well-recognized complications of cat-scratch fever are Parinaud's oculoglandular syndrome, which is due to conjunctival inoculation of the organism, an encephalopathy with normal cerebrospinal fluid, pneumonitis, hepatitis and polyneuritis.

Most cases of cat-scratch fever are caused by *Bartonella* (previously *Rochalimaea*) *henselae*,[3] a Gram-negative rod, although *Afipia felis*, another Gram-negative rod, has been implicated in a minority of cases. The histopathology of the lymph nodes is of epithelioid cell granulomas and microabscesses, not pathognomonic, but suggestive. Silver stains, notably the Warthin–Starry stain, will reveal characteristic dark-staining rods. Serological tests for *Bartonella* and polymerase chain reaction (PCR) tests on tissue are now available in some laboratories.

Often antibiotic therapy is unnecessary, but if indicated then oral cotrimoxazole and rifampicin is an effective oral combination, while intravenous gentamicin can be used in severe cases.

KAWASAKI DISEASE

Cervical lymphadenitis is the least constant clinical feature of Kawasaki disease, and is often absent (see Ch. 11). However, some patients present with unilateral neck swelling due to matted nodes. These children are often misdiagnosed as having suppurative lymphadenitis, because of the tender nodes, fever and blood film suggestive of bacterial infection, with neutrophil leucocytosis and toxic granulation.

Other features suggestive of Kawasaki disease are lips which are dry and cracked, or bright red as if the child is wearing lipstick (the 'lipstick sign'); strawberry tongue and/or marked pharyngitis; non-exudative conjunctivitis with characteristic halo appearance of limbal sparing (Fig. 11.2.1); non-specific truncal rash; peeling in the napkin area; redness or non-pitting oedema of the hands and feet; and, less commonly, arthralgia, arthritis, aseptic meningitis and/or enlarged, palpable, tender gall-bladder due to hydrops. Children with Kawasaki disease are often excessively irritable and miserable.

ATYPICAL MYCOBACTERIAL INFECTION

Cervical lympadenopathy due to atypical mycobacteria is fairly common in industrialized countries.[4,5] Most children are 1–4 years old, of Caucasian origin, well, afebrile, and have unilateral, painless lymphadenopathy. Chest radiography is normal. Occasionally, the nodes will discharge spontaneously, or erode into bone. Diagnosis is by positive (>10 mm) intradermal skin test to *Mycobacterium avium-intracellulare* (MAI). There may be some cross-reaction with purified protein derivative (PPD). Usually surgical excision of the nodes is necessary and sufficient for treatment, although some authorities advocate no treatment at all, given that spontaneous resolution occurs with time. Treatment with conventional antituberculous drugs is generally unsatisfactory, but there are encouraging although anecdotal reports of the use of clarithromycin to treat atypical mycobacterial infections.

TUBERCULOSIS

In contrast to atypical myobacterial infections, children with tuberculous cervical adenitis may be of any age, may have systemic symptoms such as weight loss, may have bilateral or generalized adenitis, and may have an abnormal chest X-ray. The incidence of fever is no different from in atypical mycobacterial infections. On the other hand, affected children may be well, with no symptoms.

The main distinguishing feature in industrialized countries is that almost all children with TB were born in a country with a high incidence of TB, or are part of a family from such a country, or have a history of contact with an adult with TB. Occasionally children, however, will have TB with no apparent risk factors.

DIAGNOSIS

There is an aphorism that there is no substitute for a tissue diagnosis. On the other hand, there are a number of conditions causing cervical lymphadenitis for which lymph node biopsy is unnecessary. A differential Mantoux test, i.e. skin testing with PPD in one arm and MAI in the other arm, can be useful in distinguishing between TB and atypical mycobacterial infection or in excluding these diagnoses. There is often cross-reaction between the PPD and MAI responses:

a child with atypical mycobacterial infection may, for example, have a 20 mm MAI response and a 15 mm PPD response. If there is any doubt, excision of affected nodes is advised, as white children with no systemic symptoms and no history of contact with TB may nevertheless have TB.

Needle aspiration may be diagnostic in pyogenic neck abscesses, and may obviate the need for operation.

Computed tomographic scan or magnetic resonance imaging can be useful in delineating the anatomy in complicated cases.

SUMMARY

Cervical lymphadenitis is a common condition in childhood. The causes range from trivial viral infections, requiring no treatment, through treatable bacterial infections and inflammatory conditions such as Kawasaki disease, to malignancy. The optimal management of cervical lymphadenitis is clearly dependent on a high degree of skill and clinical acumen.

REFERENCES

1 Baker C J. Cervical lymphadenitis. In: Feigin R D, Cherry J D, eds. Textbook of pediatric infectious diseases, 3rd ed. Philadelphia: Saunders, 1992: pp 220–230.
2 Zangwill K M, Hamilton D H, Perkins B A et al. Cat-scratch disease in Connecticut. N Engl J Med 1993; 329: 8–13.
3 Adal K A, Cockerell C J, Petro W A. Cat-scratch disease, bacillary angiomatosis, and other infections due to Rochalimaea. N Engl J Med 1994; 330: 1509–1515.
4 Margileth A M, Chandra R, Altman R P. Chronic lymphadenopathy due to mycobacterial infection. Am J Dis Child 1984; 138: 917–922.
5 Spark R P, Fried M L, Bean C K, Digueroa J M, Crowe C P, Campbell D P. Non-tuberculous mycobacterial adenitis of childhood: the ten-year experience at a community hospital. Am J Dis Child 1988; 142: 106–108.

1B.1 Bronchiolitis

INTRODUCTION

Bronchiolitis is a pathological description that has come to be used as a clinical diagnosis. This has engendered much confusion. In Europe and Australia the term bronchiolitis is used to describe children under 1 year of age with a febrile pneumonitis characterized by cough, crepitations and hyperinflation. In the USA, the term has been used for children up to 2 or more years old, often with wheezing, resulting in considerable overlap with asthma.

EPIDEMIOLOGY

Bronchiolitis is caused primarily by respiratory syncytial virus (RSV). At least 70% of cases in epidemic months are RSV positive.[1] Passively acquired maternal antibodies are poorly protective against RSV, so babies may be affected in the first weeks after birth. RSV causes winter epidemics in temperate climates and although these outbreaks may vary in severity they occur every year. There are occasional isolates in the summer months, but it is a mystery where the virus spends the summer. In tropical climates RSV epidemics tend to occur in the rainy season, although there is a less clearcut seasonality (see Fig. 1B.1.1).[2]

Over 90% of children have been infected with RSV by the end of their second winter, and of these about 40% will have lower respiratory tract involvement. Only about 1% of these will need hospitalization.[1] Reinfections, of decreasing severity, are common throughout life. Older children may develop wheeze, pneumonia or otitis media. Adults tend to get a febrile cold with sore throat.

Bronchiolitis occurring outside the RSV season is usually due to parainfluenza virus infection, although a similar clinical picture can also be caused by other viruses such as adenoviruses, rhinoviruses and enteroviruses.

The overall mortality from primary RSV infection in previously healthy infants has been estimated at from 1 in 5000 to 1 in 20 000.[3] The mortality in all hospitalized children is about 1%. Mortality is increased, to about 3.5%, for children with cyanotic congenital heart disease or chronic lung disease (bronchopulmonary dysplasia, cystic fibrosis).[4] Children with immune deficiency[5] and babies born preterm[1] have more severe RSV infection and a greatly increased mortality.

There are two main subtypes of RSV: A and B. These can circulate concurrently during epidemics, or one or other subtype may predominate. There are contradictory data on whether or not subtype A causes more severe disease than subtype B.

PATHOGENESIS AND PATHOLOGY

RSV infects epithelial cells, entering the cells via unknown cell receptors, and

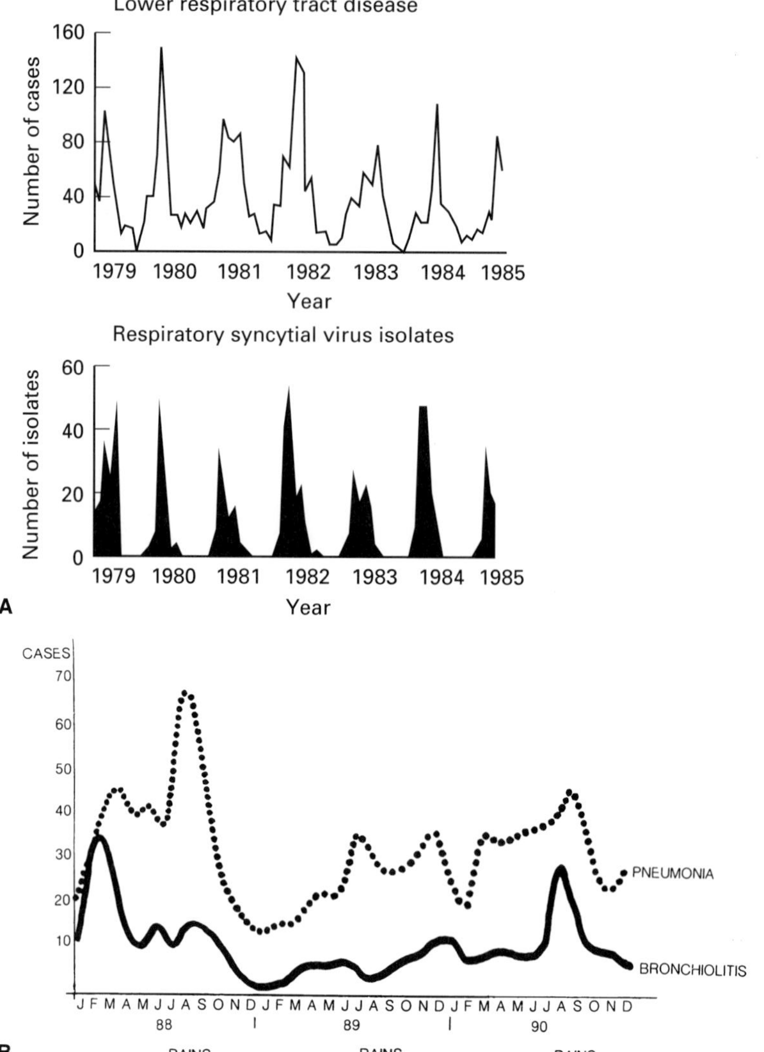

Fig. 1B.1.1 Seasonality of RSV bronchiolitis. **A** In temperate climate: USA. **B** In tropical climate: The Gambia (data courtesy of Dr David Brewster, Queen Victoria Hospital, Banjul, The Gambia).

spreading cell to cell. The cells may fuse to form syncytia (giant cells). RSV is not classically a viraemic illness, although about 15% of circulating mononuclear cells can be shown to be RSV positive by immunofluorescence.

In severe bronchiolitis there is necrosis of the respiratory epithelium, affecting mainly the bronchioles and other small airways, and lymphocytic peribronchial infiltration. Oedema and cellular debris obstruct small airways causing hyperinflation. If the alveolar debris is extensive it can cause pneumonia.

IMMUNITY

The presence of IgG antibody, whether passive maternal IgG or serum IgG from past infection, does not protect absolutely against RSV infection.[1] For this reason babies can be infected from birth onwards, and reinfections are common. However, babies under 2 months old appear to be relatively protected against RSV infection, in that the incidence is lower than from 2 to 6 months. This protection may be due to high levels of maternal antibody or to reduced exposure to infection. Breast-feeding affords relative protection against RSV infection.

T lymphocytes are critical in recovery from RSV infection. Children with impaired T cell function, whether congenital as in severe combined deficiency, or acquired, as in HIV infection or children on cytotoxic therapy, develop persistent symptomatic RSV infection with wheezing. Such children have an increased mortality from RSV.

Infection with one RSV subtype, A or B, appears to confer little or no immunity against infection with the other type, and indeed only transient immunity against reinfection with the same type.

SPREAD

RSV is spread mainly by direct contact with nasal secretions, usually via hands but also by fomite spread on inanimate objects, since the virus can survive some hours. Droplet spread seems to be rare.[6] Spread within wards, child care facilities and homes can thus be minimized by handwashing, and in hospitals by nursing affected babies in separate wards or a separate area on each ward (cohorting).[7] Babies usually catch RSV from an older school-age sibling, but on hospital wards infected adult staff are an important source.

CLINICAL FEATURES

The baby characteristically starts with a cold with rhinitis or nasal congestion, followed within 1–2 days by a febrile illness characterized by an intermittent, spluttering, bubbly cough and sometimes audible wheeze. Clinically the most notable features are hyperinflation with a barrel chest associated classically with diffuse, fine, scattered crepitations and often also with wheeze (Fig. 1B.1.2). Babies are usually tachypnoeic, and often have intercostal recession or sternal retraction. Cyanosis is rare, and indicates severe infection. Fever is usual, although fever >40°C is rare in uncomplicated RSV infection.

The typical age is 2–6 months, although bronchiolitis does occur up to 12 months of age. Babies older than this who wheeze with a viral infection may well have asthma.

Babies who were born preterm and develop RSV are likely to present with apnoea, often with no other respiratory signs or symptoms. Early on, it can be impossible to distinguish such babies from those with pertussis infection, although later the preterm babies with RSV will often develop the classical signs of bronchiolitis. In contrast, the babies with pertussis develop paroxysmal apnoea and cyanosis, but generally have no respiratory signs between paroxysms. However, it may be very difficult to distinguish the two infections.[8]

The X-ray appearance in bronchiolitis is not pathognomonic, but can vary from being normal, to showing patchy, subsegmental consolidation with hyperinflation, and sometimes more extensive consolidation. Lobar collapse/consolidation can occur, and unilateral or bilateral upper lobe collapse is common following endotracheal intubation.

DIAGNOSIS

The diagnosis of bronchiolitis can be made clinically with a fair degree of

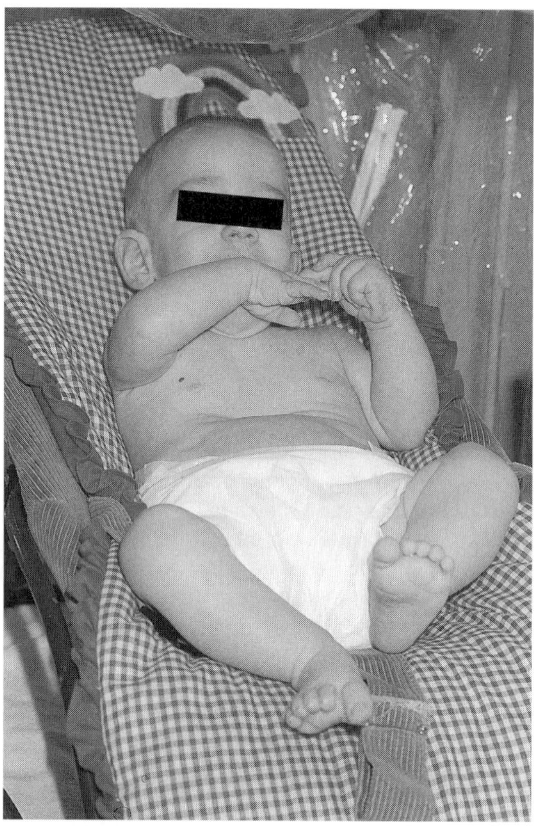

Fig. 1B.1.2 Bronchiolitis. Note sternal retraction in child with mild disease.

confidence, particularly during the RSV season. When a baby with bronchiolitis requires hospital admission it is important to know whether the baby is RSV positive. RSV was the first virus for which rapid viral diagnosis was used routinely. RSV-positive babies should be admitted to a separate room, an isolation ward or an RSV area within a ward,[7] whereas to nurse an RSV-negative baby with other RSV-positive babies runs the risk of infecting the former with RSV. Nasopharyngeal secretions, aspirated using a mucus extractor or catheter, are tested for the presence of RSV-infected cells using antisera labelled with fluorescein (immunofluorescent assay) or an enzyme (enzyme-linked immunosorbent assay, ELISA). The result is usually available the same day, although at weekends specimens may wait until Monday, and a decision on where to send the baby has to be made on clinical grounds.

ASSESSMENT OF SEVERITY

When a clinical diagnosis of bronchiolitis has been made, the first question is whether or not hospital admission is required. Any baby with difficulty feeding due to respiratory distress should be admitted, as should any baby with apnoea. Babies with risk factors for severe RSV infection, namely those born with congenital heart disease, chronic lung disease, immune deficiency or Down syndrome, and those born preterm, should all be admitted as they may deteriorate rapidly. Cyanosis is an indicator of severe disease, and tachypnoea of over 50 breaths/min is also a danger sign, and a reasonable indicator for admission to hospital.[9] Pulse oximetry should be performed in casualty to assess the baby's oxygen saturation,[10] and a pulse oximeter reading below 92% (provided the trace is satisfactory) is an indication for admission and oxygen therapy.

A single measurement of respiratory rate may be misleading, since the natural history of bronchiolitis is for the respiratory rate to rise to a peak, plateau, and then subside with resolution. Thus a single reading may be when the respiratory rate is rising or falling. Not surprisingly, therefore, the admission respiratory rate does not correlate well with outcome.[10] Oxygen saturation on admission, measured by pulse oximetry, does correlate with severity, and need for supplemental oxygen.[10] Clinical predictors of severity are tachypnoea (>70 breaths/min), age less than 3 months, preterm delivery (particularly before 34 weeks), and an 'ill' or 'toxic' appearance.[11]

Babies with mild bronchiolitis, who can be managed at home, will generally have been born at term, will be over 3 months old, feeding well and have a respiratory rate below 50 breaths/min.[9] Even these babies should be reviewed to ensure they do not deteriorate.

When children with bronchiolitis are admitted to hospital, it is important that sequential observations be made, to follow the progress of the infection. Ideally, inpatients should have oxygen saturation measured by pulse oximetry at least once a day, even if there are insufficient pulse oximeters available for continuous monitoring. Where pulse oximetry is unavailable, a rising respiratory rate may indicate the need for respiratory support. Although death from bronchiolitis is rare, babies with bronchiolitis occasionally collapse suddenly, probably due to unrecognized, progressive hypoxia. Monitoring of oxygen saturation is the single most important investigation in bronchiolitis. If such monitoring is not available, babies can usually be safely nursed in 40% oxygen.

TREATMENT

Ribavirin

The antiviral agent ribavirin has modest activity against RSV. Its use is not, I believe, indicated in normal children with RSV infection, in whom the mortality is less than 0.1%.[3] Nebulized ribavirin should be considered for high-risk babies with RSV infection, preferably given early in the course of the infection into a head-box, since there are problems with precipitation of ribavirin in ventilator tubing which make ribavirin difficult to administer to ventilated babies. The main indication for ribavirin is for immune-deficienct children awaiting bone marrow transplant,[12] since this is often the only way they can clear the virus from the respiratory tract. We virtually never use ribavirin other than for this last indication.

Antibiotics

Secondary bacterial infection is rare in RSV infection, occurring in less than 1% of hospitalized children.[13] Bacteraemia, when it does occur, is usually due to *Streptococcus pneumoniae* or untypable *Haemophilus influenzae*, so that cefotaxime or ceftriaxone is the antibiotic of choice. Antibiotics have not been shown to speed recovery in RSV infection in general, and in some studies they have actually been shown to be deleterious.

Bronchodilators

In some studies bronchodilators such as salbutamol have been shown to be helpful,[14] but in others they have been ineffective or even caused deterioration.[15,16]

It is possible that the former studies contained a number of babies with asthma. We do not routinely use bronchodilators in bronchiolitis, but there may be a role for their use when wheezing predominates and/or there is a strong atopic family history.

Supportive

Children hospitalized with bronchiolitis may require no treatment if they are feeding well and oxygen saturation is normal. If they have difficulty feeding they are at risk of aspiration, and should be fed by nasogastric tube or given intravenous fluids. Oxygen by head-box or nasal prongs should be given to hypoxic babies. Apnoea may respond to continuous positive airway pressure (CPAP), but babies with apnoeic episodes often need artificial ventilation.

PREVENTION

There is no effective vaccine against RSV. Prevention of hospital-acquired infection depends on recognizing that most RSV is spread by direct contact with nasal secretions or by fomite spread.[6] Spread can be limited by 'cohorting' infected babies (and infected carers) into RSV areas, by reducing contact with infected older siblings and by encouraging handwashing (see Fig. 1B.1.3).[7]

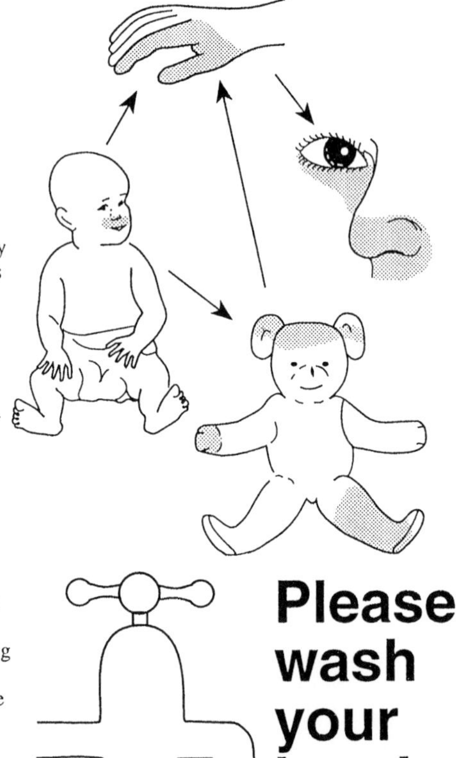

* Your baby is in hospital with a condition called bronchiolitis.

* This is caused by a virus called respiratory syncytial virus (RSV).

* The disease is very infectious and is passed on by infected nasal secretions carried on hands or toys but not usually by coughing. The secretions are rubbed into the nose or eyes to cause infections.

* The best way of preventing spread of RSV infection is, therefore, by washing your hands after handling your baby. If you have a cold yourself try to wash your hands before handling other children.

* Many children on the ward have conditions such as heart disease which can be made much worse by RSV infection. To prevent these children being infected please wash your hands. If you have an older child with a cold do not let them play in the play areas on the ward until they are better. Thank you

Fig. 1B.1.3   Information leaflet handed out to parents of children with bronchiolitis.

REFERENCES

1 Hall C B. Respiratory syncytial virus. In: Feigin R D, Cherry J D, eds. Textbook of pediatric infectious disease, 3rd ed. Philadelphia: Saunders, 1992.
2 Brewster D R, Greenwood B M. Seasonal variation of paediatric diseases in The Gambia, West Africa. Ann Trop Paediatr 1993; 13: 133–146.
3 Hall C B, Geimann J M, Biggar R, Kotok D I, Hogan P M, Douglas R G Jr. Respiratory syncytial virus infection within families. N Engl J Med 1976; 294: 414–419.
4 Navas L, Wang E, de Carvalho V, Robinson J and the Pediatric Investigators Collaborative Network on Infections in Canada. Improved outcome of respiratory syncytial virus infection in a high-risk hospitalised population of Canadian children. J Pediatr 1992; 121: 348–354.
5 Hall C B, Powell K R, MacDonald N E et al. Respiratory syncytial viral infection in children with compromised immune function. N Engl J Med 1986; 315: 77–81.
6 Hall C B, Douglas R G Jr. Modes of transmission of respiratory syncytial virus. J Pediatr 1981; 99: 100–103.
7 Isaacs D, Dickson H, O'Callaghan C, Sheaves R, Winter A, Moxon E R. Handwashing and cohorting in prevention of hospital acquired infections with respiratory syncytial virus. Arch Dis Child 1991; 66: 227–231.
8 Nelson A L, Hopkins R S, Roe M H, Glode H P. Simultaneous infection with Bordetella pertussis and respiratory syncytial virus in hospitalized children. Pediatr Infect Dis 1986; 5: 540–544.
9 Isaacs D. Bronchiolitis. Br Med J 1995; 310: 4–5.
10 Mulholland E K, Olinsky A, Shann F A. Clinical findings and severity of bronchiolitis. Lancet 1990; 335: 1259–1261.
11 Shaw K N, Bell L M, Sherman N H. Outpatient assessment of infants with bronchiolitis. Am J Dis Child 1991; 145: 151–155.
12 Gelfand E W, McCurdy D, Rao C P et al. Treatment of viral pneumonitis with ribavirin in severe combined immunodeficiency. Lancet 1983; ii: 732–733.
13 Hall C B, Powell K R, Schaubel K C et al. Risk of secondary bacterial infection in infants hospitalized with respiratory syncytial virus infection. J Pediatr 1988; 113: 266–271.
14 Schuh S, Canny G, Reisman J J et al. Nebulised albuterol in acute bronchiolitis. J Pediatr 1990; 117: 633–637.
15 Ho L, Coilis G, Landau L I, Le Souef P N. Effect of salbutamol on oxygen saturation in bronchiolitis. Arch Dis Child 1991; 66: 1061–1064.
16 Wang E E L, Milner R, Allen U, Maj H. Bronchodilators for treatment of mild bronchiolitis: a factorial randomised trial. Arch Dis Child 1992; 67: 289–293.

1B.2 Cough

INTRODUCTION

Cough is one of the most common presenting symptoms in children. Although there are a vast number of possible causes, most children with troublesome coughing will have either acute viral bronchitis or asthma (Table 1B.2.1). The age of the child has a major influence on the likely cause of cough, as shown in Table 1B.2.2. Whether an individual develops troublesome, recurrent coughing illnesses

Table 1B.2.1 Causes of cough

1. *Very common*
   Acute viral bronchitis
   Asthma

2. *Common*
   Tobacco smoke
      Passive smoking (infants)
      Active smoking (adolescents)

   Primary bacterial bronchitis
      Bordetella pertussis
      Mycoplasma pneumoniae
      Other
         Chlamydia (*C. trachomatis* and *C. pneumoniae*)
         Mycobacterium tuberculosis

   Secondary bacterial bronchitis[a]
      Streptococcus pneumoniae
      Haemophilus influenzae

3. *Uncommon*
   Inhaled foreign body
   Recurrent pulmonary aspiration
      Secondary to abnormal swallowing
      Secondary to gastro-oesophageal reflux

   'Attention-seeking' (hysterical) cough

4. *Rare*
   Suppurative lung disease
      Cystic fibrosis
      Immune deficiency syndromes
      Immotile cilia syndrome

   Focal lesions of (or compressing) the airways
      Mediastinal glands, tumours, cysts, blood vessels
      Bronchial adenomas
      Tracheomalacia (1^0 and 2^0) and bronchomalacia
      Pulmonary aspiration due to anatomical communication
      (e.g., H-type tracheo-oesophageal fistula or laryngeal cleft)

[a] Complicating acute viral bronchitis.

Table 1B.2.2   Age and likely cause of cough

Neonate (0–4 weeks)
Congenital airway malformations
   Congenital lobar emphysema
   Primary tracheomalacia
   Tracheo-oesophageal fistula / laryngeal cleft

Pulmonary aspiration, secondary to:
   Meconium aspiration
   Gastro-oesophageal reflux (GOR)
   Incoordinate swallowing

Chronic lung disease of prematurity
Familial bronchiectasis
   Cystic fibrosis
   Primary ciliary dyskinesia

Infants (1–12 months)
Viral bronchitis / bronchiolitis (esp. RSV)
Infantile asthma
Chronic lung disease of prematurity
Infantile 'atypical' bronchopneumonia
   e.g. *Chlamydia*; *Ureaplasma*; *Mycoplasma*; CMV
Pulmonary aspiration
   e.g. GOR, incoordinate swallowing
Familial bronchiectasis
Passive smoking

Toddlers/preschoolers (1–4 years)
Asthma
Recurrent viral bronchitis (incl. viral 'croup')
Pertussis ('whooping cough')
Inhaled foreign body

Primary school (5–12 years)
Asthma
Recurrent viral bronchitis
Mycoplasma pneumoniae bronchitis

High school/adolescent (13–18 years)
Asthma
Active smoking
'Attention-seeking' (psychogenic) cough

during early childhood depends upon a number of host and environmental factors (Fig. 1B.2.1).

THE COUGH REFLEX

The act of coughing is a complex, protective reflex designed to rid the airway of unwanted secretions or irritants.[1] In the presence of increased secretions, cough results from the mucociliary escalator being 'overloaded'. Thus, cough is best considered abnormal, rather than physiological. The cough reflex is shown schematically in Figure 1B.2.2.

1. *The afferent limb*: nerve endings ('irritant' or cough receptors) on the mucosal surface of the intrathoracic airways, which can be blocked by inhalation of local anaesthetic agents (e.g. xylocaine).[2]
2. *The cough centre*: situated in the brain stem, and responsible for coordinating the integrated series of activities which constitute an effective cough. This portion of the reflex can be suppressed by narcotic drugs (which also depress

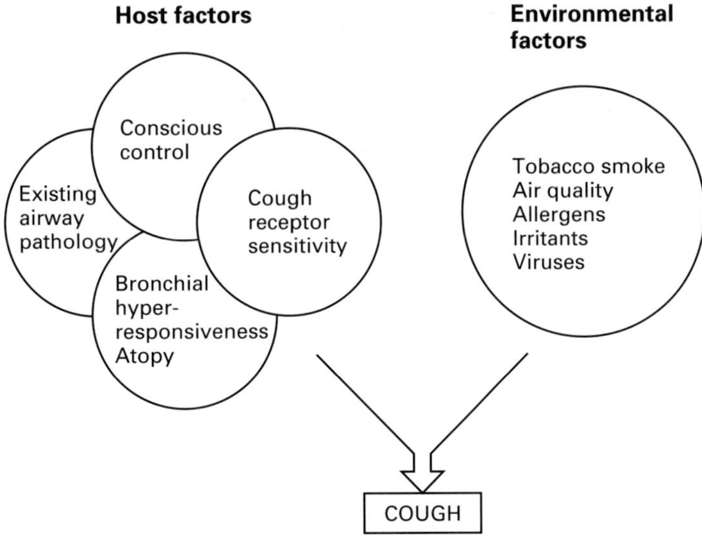

Fig. 1B.2.1 Predisposing factors for cough.

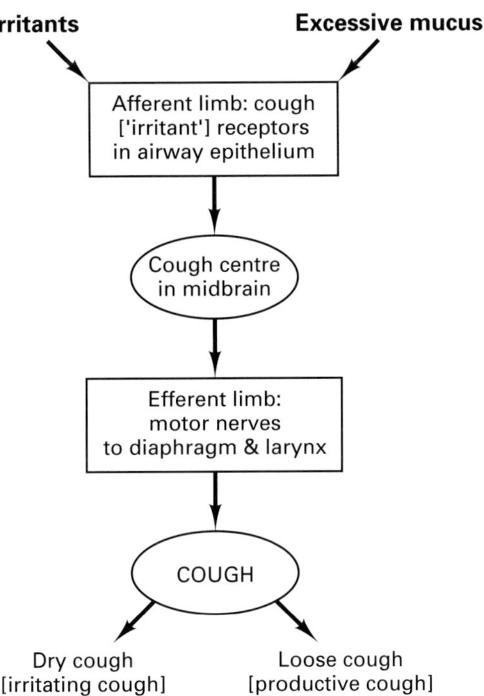

Fig. 1B.2.2 Cough reflex.

respiration). Central control can also be overridden consciously, either by suppressing the reflex cough or by consciously generating an 'attention-seeking' cough.

3. *The efferent limb*: via the vagus, phrenic and spinal motor nerves, to the larynx, diaphragm and abdominal wall. This part of the cough reflex can be blocked by inhalation of anticholinergics (e.g. atropine or ipratropium bromide ('Atrovent')).[2]

COUGH RECEPTOR SENSITIVITY

Children with asthma (recurrent wheeze) have bronchial hyperresponsiveness (BHR), which can be demonstrated by excessive bronchoconstriction to various non-specific stimuli (e.g. exercise; inhalation of histamine or methacholine). Children with recurrent or persistent cough (due to either viral bronchitis or 'cough-variant asthma') may have hyperresponsive cough receptors.[3,4]

This inherent sensitivity of the cough reflex can be measured by various irritant challenges (e.g. inhalation of citric acid, acetic acid or capsaicin). Studies of cough receptor sensitivity in adults show those with a chronic, non-productive cough have an abnormally sensitive cough reflex, compared to either normals or those with a chronic, productive cough.[5,6]

Although few paediatric studies of cough receptor sensitivity have been performed, this measurement could have a role in improving our understanding and management of coughing children.[3,7,8]

THE PROCESS OF COUGHING

The act of coughing is initiated by a short inspiration, followed by closure of the glottis (inspiratory phase). Contraction of the diaphragm, pelvic and abdominal muscles (compressive phase) follows. This results in a marked increase in intrathoracic pressure, causing a sudden opening of the glottis and the immediate release of the trapped intrathoracic gas at very high velocity (expiratory phase). The end result is removal of the unwanted material from the respiratory tract.

EPIDEMIOLOGY

Most children with troublesome cough are suffering from either recurrent viral bronchitis or asthma. Both conditions are common, although their exact frequency is difficult to ascertain. This is because of difficulties defining asthma, particularly when cough is the major symptom. Moreover, it is unclear what is a 'normal' number of bouts, and duration, of acute viral bronchitis.

Given these difficulties, the rate of 'recent' (i.e. during the previous 12 months) cough plus wheeze (asthma) in a state-wide survey of Australian 7-year-old children was 15%, while a further 30% reported a 'recent' bout of non-asthmatic bronchitis.[9] Five per cent of the children reported four or more episodes of non-asthmatic bronchitis per year — a rate of bronchitis which is arbitrarily considered abnormal.[10] Thus, approximately 1 in 20 children have 'frequently recurrent' acute viral bronchitis, while 1 in 5 have asthma, many of whom present predominantly with cough (Table 1B.2.3). By comparison, all other causes of cough are rare.

Table 1B.2.3   Spectrum of vulnerablity to lower respiratory symptoms

Normal	Recurrent viral bronchitis	Asthma
Cough only with major pathogens (e.g. influenza A)	Troublesome COUGH, with most viral respiratory infections	WHEEZE and/or cough Shortness of breath Other atopy
70–80%	5–10%	15–20%

PATHOGENESIS AND PATHOLOGY

Cough is the usual response to the acute mucus hypersecretion and epithelial damage caused by a respiratory virus. Clinically, the result is a typical bout of acute viral bronchitis, or laryngotracheobronchitis ('viral croup'). Of particular importance are respiratory syncytial virus (RSV) in infants; parainfluenza viruses in toddlers and preschoolers; and influenza viruses in school-age children. While a variety of bacterial pathogens can complicate acute viral bronchitis ('secondary' bacterial bronchitis), 'primary' bacterial bronchitis typically occurs with *Mycoplasma pneumoniae* and *Bordetella pertussis* infection.

Cough in asthma results from stimulation and sensitization of afferent (irritant) receptors in the airway epithelium. The typical pathology of asthma is a chronic desquamating eosinophilic bronchitis, which exposes the superficial nerve fibres to the usual airway insults; for example, drying or cooling of the airway epithelium with exercise or hyperventilation, resulting in troublesome cough (and/or wheeze).

ASTHMA VERSUS ACUTE VIRAL BRONCHITIS

Although in some children this differential diagnosis can be very difficult, there are a number of characteristic features which should enable accurate distinction in most (see Ch. 1B.3). However, it is likely that there is an overlap between these two syndromes: asthma (presenting as cough) and recurrent viral bronchitis. Indeed, these two conditions may simply represent different parts of a 'spectrum of vulnerability' to lower respiratory tract symptoms (Table 1B.2.3).

DIAGNOSIS OF CAUSE OF COUGH

The standard method of arriving at a clinical diagnosis involves 'pattern recognition', an appropriate method for diagnosing the underlying cause of cough in children. Although the history alone may enable accurate diagnosis, ideally the cough should be observed directly during the course of history taking and physical examination. Alternatively, if the cough is infrequent or episodic, the parents should make a tape or video recording of the child's typical cough.

RECOGNIZABLE PATTERNS OF COUGH

Dry, irritating cough

Recurring bouts of dry, irritating cough are most commonly due to the early stages of acute, uncomplicated viral bronchitis. This dry cough is usually of short duration (2–5 days), followed by a more productive cough, which gradually subsides over the next 7–10 days. Many infants and toddlers have frequent recurrences with respiratory viruses during the winter months — especially those attending full-time day care.

If a dry, irritating cough persists for prolonged periods (months), it is most likely due to underlying asthma, especially if the cough is predominantly at night.[11] This 'asthma cough' often has a wheezy or 'tight' quality, and many will admit to a history of recurrent wheezing when specifically asked.

A similar wheezy cough is seen in infants with acute viral bronchiolitis, and can persist for up to 6–8 weeks after resolution of the acute wheeze and breathlessness.

Loud, barking cough

This is most commonly seen during acute viral laryngotracheobronchitis ('viral croup' or LTB). The cough is particularly prominent at night, and is usually accompanied by intermittent inspiratory stridor. Duration of this barking cough is relatively short (7–10 days).

A persistent form of this cough is seen in infants and children with primary tracheomalacia (congenitally soft, 'floppy' trachea). Compression of the large, central intrathoracic airways produces a similar cough ('secondary' tracheomalacia). This can result from tumours, cysts, enlarged hilar nodes, abnormal blood vessels (vascular ring), or large, congested pulmonary arteries (especially with large ventricular septal defects).

Children with an 'attention-seeking' cough (hysterical or psychogenic cough) may have the same quality cough. This cough typically has an unusual 'honking' quality, often accompanied by unusual posturing movements (e.g. hand to throat; flexing of the neck). This cough conveniently worsens at opportune times (e.g. mealtimes, school classroom) — but dramatically disappears when the child is asleep!

Uncontrollable paroxysms ('fits') of coughing

This cough is classically seen in children with pertusstis ('whooping cough'). These 'fits' of coughing are accompanied by flushed face or central cyanosis, and followed by an inspiratory 'whoop' or vomiting. Paroxysms can last for several minutes, and recur every 30–60 min, both day and night. Typically, the child is strikingly well between these spasms of coughing. The cough can persist for 8–12 weeks, although the paroxysms progressively improve over this time. Other specific forms of bronchitis can result in a cough with similar features to pertussis (e.g. *Bordetella parapertussis*, *Chlamydia*, *Mycoplasma*). Generally, however, the cough is less severe and less prolonged than that produced by *Bordetella pertussis*.

Immediately after inhalation of a foreign body (e.g. peanut), similar paroxysms of cough with cyanosis may occur. This cough is usually of short duration (several minutes only), even though the foreign body may be retained in a major airway. Infants with cystic fibrosis, complicated by persistent viral or bacterial bronchitis/bronchiolitis, can develop a similar, distressing cough.

Moist, productive but 'effective' cough

This is typically seen in the later stages of acute, uncomplicated viral bronchitis. Sputum is generally swallowed rather than expectorated. If the cough is slow to settle (persists for more than 3 weeks) it may indicate a complication of viral bronchitis, such as segmental collapse, lobar collapse or secondary bacterial bronchitis. Alternatively, persistence may indicate that a specific infective agent, such as *Mycoplasma pneumoniae*, is responsible.

Some infants and toddlers with asthma will have chronic hypersecretion of mucus, resulting in a 'rattle' in the chest and a loose, productive cough, rather than wheeze and laboured respirations.

If a loose, productive cough persists for a prolonged period (months) it suggests serious underlying suppurative lung disease (bronchiectasis) — particularly if there is expectoration of purulent sputum. This scenario must not be dismissed lightly. Suppuration can result from a retained inhaled foreign body, a previous severe infective injury (e.g. adenoviral necrotizing bronchiolitis/bronchitis), or as a consequence of one of the familial forms of this disease (e.g. cystic fibrosis, primary ciliary dyskinesia, or an immune deficiency syndrome).

Children with chronic or recurrent pulmonary aspiration will generally have a loose, productive cough. Aspiration can result from either inhaling feeds during swallowing or as a consequence of gastro-oesophageal reflux (GOR). These infants have either obvious feeding difficulties (indicating poorly coordinated swallowing) or frequent effortless vomiting after feeds (indicating GOR). Rarely, aspiration is due to an anatomical communication between the tracheobronchial tree and gastrointestinal tract (such as an H-type tracheo-oesophageal fistula or a laryngeal cleft).

Moist, 'rattly' cough, but weak and 'ineffective'

This cough is classically seen in infants and children with significant neurological handicap, such as severe cerebral palsy, severe mental retardation, or bulbar palsy. The cough is often accompanied by drooling of saliva, regurgitation of feeds into the nose, and obvious inhalation during feeding.

Children with severe muscle weakness, with involvement of the respiratory muscles (diaphragm), also have this type of cough. Both acute and reversible (e.g. Guillain–Barré syndrome) and chronic and irreversible (e.g. congenital muscular dystrophy) forms can occur in children.

Throat clearing, 'hawking' cough

This is not a true, explosive cough. It is commonly seen in children with perennial allergic rhinitis (hay fever). Many of these atopic children will have persistently abnormal paranasal sinuses (chronic sinusitis), and increased postnasal secretions (postnasal drip). However, this is not a genuine 'cough', and it is inappropriate to attribute a true cough to a postnasal drip. Excessive upper airway secretions will not spill into the lower respiratory tract, provided the child is neurologically normal. In many situations, there is similar pathology in the upper and lower airways (e.g. viral infection of both upper and lower airways; asthma and allergic rhinitis), suggesting a 'causal' relationship. Some children will have a 'habitual' throat-clearing manoeuvre, and some use it as an 'attention-seeking' device for secondary gain.

TREATMENT OF COUGH

Management of the symptom of cough depends upon the underlying cause. Most coughing children will have either asthma or viral bronchitis, and the treatment of these two conditions is considered in detail elsewhere (see Ch. 1B.3 and 1B.4).

Cough due to asthma is managed with a crescendo of inhaled bronchodilators and preventive medications (cromoglycate and inhaled corticosteroids), or a short course of oral corticosteroids, depending upon severity and response to initial therapy. The general principles of drug therapy for uncomplicated viral bronchitis are as follows: for a dry, irritating cough — a simple cough suppressant syrup; for a moist, productive cough — a simple expectorant and/or chest physiotherapy.[12] In most cases, however, no therapy apart from a full explanation of the cause and likely natural history of the cough (to the child and parent) will be necessary. Antibiotics have no role in either asthma or uncomplicated viral bronchitis.

CONCLUSION

Although the number of possible causes of cough are legion, most cases of troublesome cough are due to either acute viral bronchitis or asthma. In most children, taking a full history and physical examination will reveal the underlying cause of cough. Although laboratory investigations have a limited role, a chest X-ray should be performed when there is doubt about the diagnosis. The most difficult age group are young infants, in whom the possibility of a serious congenital malformation, unusual infection, or pulmonary aspiration needs to be considered.

REFERENCES

1 Kamei R. Chronic cough in children. Pediatr Clin North Am 1991; 38: 593–615.
2 Editorial. Cough and wheeze in asthma: are they interdependent? Lancet 1988; i: 447–448.
3 Mitsuhashi M, Mochizuki H, Tokuyama K et al. Hyperresponsiveness of cough receptors in patients with bronchial asthma. Pediatrics 1985; 75: 855–858.
4 Choudry N, Fuller R. Sensitivity of the cough reflex in patients with chronic cough. Eur Respir J 1992; 5: 296–300.
5 O'Connell F, Thomas V, Pride N, Fuller R. Capsaicin cough sensitivity decreases with successful treatment of chronic cough. Am J Respir Crit Care Med 1994; 150: 374–380.
6 Fujimura M, Sakamoto S, Kamio Y, Matsuda T. Cough receptor sensitivity and bronchial responsiveness in normal and asthmatic subjects. Eur Respir J 1992; 5: 291–295.
7 Riordan M, Beardsmore C, Brooke A, Simpson H. Relationship between respiratory symptoms and cough receptor sensitivity. Arch Dis Child 1994; 70: 299–304.
8 Cloutier M, Loughlin G. Chronic cough in children: a manifestation of airway hyperreactivity. Pediatrics 1981; 67: 6–12.
9 Hall G, Gandevia B, Silverstone H et al. The inter-relationships of upper and lower respiratory tract symptoms and signs in seven year old children. Int J Epidemiol 1972; 1: 389–403.
10 Phelan P D, Landau L I, Olinsky A. Cough. In: Respiratory illness in children, 3rd ed. Oxford: Blackwell, 1990: pp 169–179.
11 Thomson A, Pratt C, Simpson H. Nocturnal cough in asthma. Arch Dis Child 1987; 62: 1001–1004.
12 Taylor J. Efficacy of cough suppressants in children. J Pediatr 1993; 122: 799–802.

C. Mellis

1B.3 Bronchitis

INTRODUCTION

Infective bronchitis is very common in children and is generally seen in association with an acute viral upper respiratory infection. The illness is due to inflammation of the trachea and/or major bronchi, and the clinical hallmark is cough. Typically, the cough is dry and irritating, but becomes loose and productive as the illness runs its natural course over 7–10 days. While the usual cause is a respiratory virus, many other organisms can cause bronchitis (Table 1B.3.1).[1]

Virtually all children suffer occasional bouts of mild, uncomplicated acute viral bronchitis. However, a substantial proportion of otherwise normal children complain of either frequent, severe or prolonged episodes. Such children are sometimes described as having 'chronic' bronchitis, a poorly defined entity in paediatrics (Table 1B.3.2).[2,3]

There are a large number of conditions which can mimic infective bronchitis, particularly asthma when it presents as predominantly cough (Table 1B.3.3). An important group to detect are the very small proportion of children presenting as 'bronchitis', who have a serious underlying condition.

Table 1B.3.1 Causes of infective bronchitis

1. Viruses
    RSV (respiratory syncytial virus)
    Parainfluenza (types 1, 2 and 3)
    Influenza (A and B)
    Adenovirus
    Measles

2. Bacteria
    Primary (specific)
        Bordetella pertussis
        Mycobacterium tuberculosis
    Secondary (non-specific)
        Streptococcus pneumoniae
        Group A streptococcus
        Haemophilus influenzae
        Staphylococcus aureus
        Branhamella (Moraxella) catarrhalis

3. Non-viral/non-bacterial
    Mycoplasma pneumoniae
    Chlamydia species:
        C. trachomatis
        C. pneumoniae (TWAR agent)

Table 1B.3.2   Definitions of infective bronchitis

Acute bronchitis
Acute, self-limiting lower respiratory infection, in which the major symptom is cough. Most commonly due to a respiratory virus.

Chronic bronchitis (paediatric)
No universally accepted definition. Term often used to describe the following 'cough syndromes', provided asthma and other specific, or serious underlying conditions are excluded:[2,3]

1. 'Adult' chronic bronchitis
   Cough and sputum, most days for 3 months, for two consecutive years. Very rare in children.

2. 'Frequently recurrent' bronchitis
   Four (or more) episodes of acute bronchitis per year. Occurs in approximately 5% of young children.

3. 'Persistent' acute bronchitis
   Episode of acute bronchitis persisting for more than 3 weeks. Very common in children. Cumulative prevalence between 15% and 25% by late childhood.

Table 1B.3.3   Conditions mimicking 'infective bronchitis'

1. Asthma

2. Retained foreign body

3. Chronic, familial suppurative lung diseases
   Cystic fibrosis
   Primary ciliary dyskinesia ('immotile cilia syndrome')
   Congenital hypogammaglobulinaemia

4. Chronic pulmonary aspiration
   Secondary to gastro-oesophageal reflux
   Secondary to poorly coordinated swallowing
   Secondary to anatomical communications (see item 5 below)

5. Congenital lung/airway malformations
   H-type tracheo-oesophageal fistula
   Laryngeal cleft
   Lung sequestration
   Bronchogenic cyst

6. Acquired lung/airway abnormalities
   Bronchiectasis (secondary to chronic airway damage)
   Chronic atelectasis (secondary to mucus impaction)
   Obliterative bronchiolitis (secondary to acute infection)

7. 'Psychogenic' cough
   Other names: 'attention-seeking', habit or 'hysterical' cough

EPIDEMIOLOGY

Almost all children, especially infants and toddlers, suffer at least one bout of acute viral bronchitis annually. While it is difficult to arbitrarily define the 'normal' frequency, large population studies in Australia indicate that only 5% of 7-year-old children have four or more bouts of acute bronchitis per year.[4] The cumulative (i.e. 'ever') frequency of at least one episode of prolonged bronchitis (persisting for 3 weeks or more) is between 15% and 25% in Australian secondary school children.[5] However, large measurement errors in these epidemiological studies are likely, due to the lack of precise definitions for either acute or 'chronic' bronchitis (severe, persistent or prolonged), difficulty distinguishing asthma from recurrent infective bronchitis using questionnaires, and recall bias (parents forgetting early childhood problems).

RISK FACTORS FOR BRONCHITIS

It is clear that a significant proportion of apparently healthy children are excessively vulnerable to repeated, prolonged or severe bouts of bronchitis. This abnormal susceptibility can be due to a number of identifiable host and environmental factors (Fig. 1B.3.1).[6]

The likelihood of an episode of bronchitis in a normal child is largely dependent upon the specific infecting agent. For example, all unimmunized children infected with measles virus have a significant cough. Age of the child also predicts bronchitis: the younger the child, the more likely the viral infection will spread to the lower respiratory tract. Genetic susceptibility to recurrent viral bronchitis is also a key host factor, and long-term cohort studies of children with this predisposition show they are abnormally prone to chronic bronchitis and chronic airflow limitation as adults.[7] Those environmental factors which reflect heavy exposure to viral infections, such as attendance at full-time day care and over-crowded housing, are also strong predictors of recurrent viral bronchitis.

PATHOLOGY

Viral inflammation of the lower respiratory tract is characterized by mucosal oedema and shedding of the respiratory epithelium, causing a dry cough, due to stimulation of airway cough receptors. The subsequent mucus hypersecretion results in the typical loose, productive cough.[8]

The pathology of 'chronic' bronchitis in children has recently been investigated in studies of non-asthmatic children with either recurrent or persistent bronchitis. Evidence of severe, chronic epithelial damage has been found. Findings include increased airway inflammatory cells (predominantly lymphocytes), abnormalities

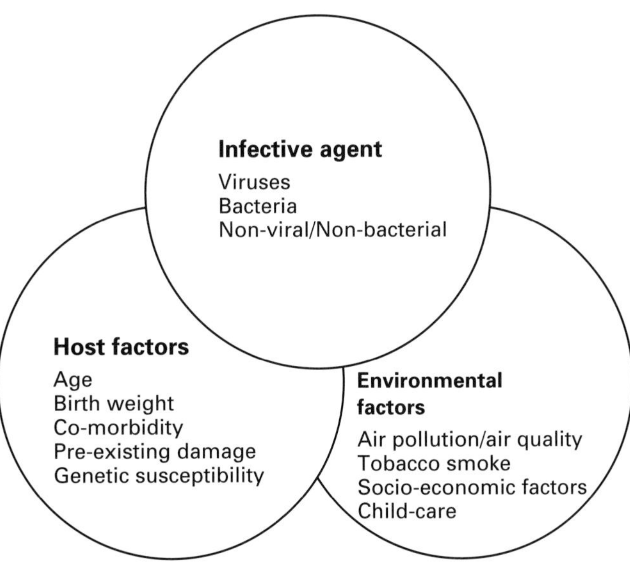

Fig. 1B.3.1 Risk factors for infective bronchitis.

of mucus content (increased protein), reduced ciliary beat frequency, and delayed mucociliary clearance.[9,10] These findings imply long-term respiratory problems for these children.

SPREAD

Respiratory viruses are generally spread by direct contact with nasopharyngeal secretions, transmitted via the hands, to the mucous membranes of the recipient. By contrast, primary bacterial bronchitis is normally by droplet spread, as a consequence of coughing.

DIAGNOSIS

Correct diagnosis of mild, acute viral bronchitis is simple. The real difficulty is determining the cause of bronchitis when it is either severe, prolonged or frequently recurrent. Severe bronchitis usually indicates a specific, potent pathogen, such as influenza A virus, or *Bordetella pertussis*. Specific bacterial forms of bronchitis have features which assist their recognition:

Bordetella pertussis: this organism produces 'whooping cough', a readily identifiable coughing syndrome. These children have an acute illness with repeated spasms of uncontrollable cough, accompanied by facial flushing and sometimes central cyanosis. The coughing spasms are followed either by an inspiratory 'whoop' or a vomit — after which the child is apparently perfectly well, until the next spasm. These spasms continue until the illness finally resolves 6–12 weeks later. Typically, several other members of the household, including adults, will have a similar cough. The diagnosis is made clinically, although this can be confirmed bacteriologically.[11]

Mycoplasma pneumoniae: classically causes a low-grade bronchopneumonia in school-age children, most of whom present with persistent cough. Other features include fever, widespread crackles on chest auscultation, diffuse inflammatory changes on chest X-ray, and failure to respond to antibiotics (other than erythromycin). Although serological methods can provide proof, the diagnosis is usually made clinically, by a combination of the typical clinical picture plus knowledge that *Mycoplasma* is currently in the community.

Chlamydia pneumoniae (previously known as TWAR agent): produces a very similar clinical illness to *Mycoplasma*, and is a relatively common cause of community-acquired acute bronchitis and bronchopneumonia in school-age children. However, it is not clinically important to differentiate between *M. pneumoniae* and *C. pneumoniae*, since optimal therapy for both is oral erythromycin.[12]

Prolonged bronchitis could mean a complication of viral bronchitis, such as segmental/lobar atelectasis, or secondary bacterial bronchitis. The latter follows a typical bout of acute viral bronchitis, and is usually heralded by a relapse of fever, moderate constitutional upset, loose cough and purulent sputum.

A severe or prolonged bout of bronchitis could also indicate a pre-existing airway abnormality, which may be either congenital or acquired (Table 1B.3.3). Distinguishing those children with a serious or specific underlying disorder is obviously an important diagnostic issue. Features which suggest serious lower respiratory pathology include: a history of persistent expectoration of purulent sputum; haemoptysis; finger clubbing; persistent localized crackles (crepitations) on auscultation; differential breath sounds (air entry); abnormal growth parameters (especially underweight); chronic chest deformity (e.g. chest asymmetry or pectus carinatum); and persistent or focal chest X-ray abnormalities.

BRONCHITIS VERSUS ASTHMA

A common diagnostic difficulty is distinguishing asthma from infective bronchitis (Table 1B.3.4). Since respiratory viruses are the usual trigger for both acute exacerbations of asthma and acute bronchitis, and since cough is a striking symptom of both conditions, this distinction can be very difficult. The hallmarks of asthma are recurrent bouts of cough, wheeze and difficulty breathing. However, a substantial proportion of children with asthma have cough as their only symptom ('cough-variant asthma'). This cough is generally worse at night, is dry and irritating, and can persist for months. However, the 'asthma cough' may be more episodic, loose and productive, and accompanied by a 'rattle' in the chest — particularly in infants and toddlers ('allergic bronchitis' or 'hypersecretory asthma').

Table 1B.3.4 Differentiating asthma from recurrent viral bronchitis (RVB)

Asthma		RVB
	History	
Yes	Persistent night cough	No
Yes	Wheeze	No
Yes	Difficulty breathing	No
Yes	Other clinical atopy	No
Yes	Family history of asthma (or atopy)	No
No	Family history RVB	Yes
	Examination	
Yes	Wheeze	No
Yes	Increased work of breathing	No
No	Coarse crackles: clears after cough	Yes
Yes	Clear chest: wheeze after cough	No
	Other clinical atopy	
Yes	Eczema or allergic rhinitis	No
	Investigations	
Yes	Positive allergen skin tests (IgE)	No
Yes	Reversible airflow obstruction	No
Yes	Responds to antiasthma therapy	No
No	Responds to chest physiotherapy	Yes
Yes	Normal chest X-ray[a]	Yes

[a] Asthma may cause hyperinflation, while both asthma and RVB may cause areas of segmental lung collapse.

TREATMENT

No drug therapy is indicated for acute, uncomplicated viral bronchitis. If there is high fever, an antipyretic such as paracetamol may be useful. If the cough is dry, irritating and causing disruption of sleep, then a simple cough suppressant or demulcent syrup may help. However, since cough is a primitive, protective reflex, cough suppressants are of limited efficacy. Bronchodilators or other antiasthma drugs are only indicated if wheeze is present, or asthma is considered likely. Antibiotics are useless, unless primary or secondary bacterial bronchitis is likely.

Specific bacterial causes of primary bronchitis, such as *Mycoplasma pneumoniae*, *Chlamydia* species and *Bordetella pertussis* should be treated with an oral course of erythromycin. However, the clinical response is variable, and in the case of *Bordetella* the purpose of the antibiotic is to eliminate the organisms to prevent spread.[13,14]

Children suspected of secondary bacterial bronchitis should be given a broad-spectrum antibiotic which covers the most likely organisms (Table 1B.3.1). Amoxycillin, amoxycillin–clavulanic acid, co-trimoxazole or cefaclor are appropriate. If there is an area of atelectasis and/or a very productive cough, chest physiotherapy may also be beneficial.

PREVENTION

While effective vaccination is available for measles virus, the value of influenza virus vaccine in children is unclear,[15] and there are no vaccines available for the remainder of the respiratory viruses. Thus, prevention of viral bronchitis is aimed at limiting spread by reducing exposure and improved personal hygiene. The only relevant immunization for primary bacterial bronchitis is pertussis vaccine. Although not 100% effective, pertussis vaccine has been extremely efficient in reducing the community prevalence of whooping cough. This was well documented in several countries when vaccine programmes were temporarily suspended, due to concern about possible brain damage in infants.[16,17]

Early diagnosis and appropriate antibiotics for *Bordetella pertussis*, *Mycoplasma pneumoniae* and *Chlamydia* species are highly effective in stopping person-to-person transmission of these forms of bronchitis.[12]

CONCLUSION

Bronchitis in children is usually due to a potent respiratory virus, and no specific treatment is required. The major diagnostic problem is distinguishing asthma from infective bronchitis. A significant proportion of otherwise normal children are abnormally prone to recurrent, or severe, or persistent bronchitis. These children are at increased risk of developing chronic bronchitis in adulthood — especially if they become cigarette smokers. There are a small number of children, presenting as 'bronchitis', who have a serious underlying problem as the cause.

REFERENCES

1 Phelan P, Landau L, Olinsky A. Clinical patterns of acute respiratory infection. In: Respiratory illness in children, 3rd ed. Oxford: Blackwell, 1992: pp 47–88.
2 Taussig L, Smith S, Blumfeld R. Chronic bronchitis in childhood: what is it? Pediatrics 1981; 67: 1–5.
3 Morgan W, Taussig L. The chronic bronchitis complex in children. Pediatr Clin North Am 1984; 31: 851–863.
4 Hall G, Gandevia B, Silverstone H et al. The interrelationships of upper and lower respiratory tract symptoms and signs in seven-year-old children. Int J Epidemiol 1972; 1: 389–403.
5 Peat J, Woolcock A, Leeder S et al. Asthma and bronchitis in Sydney schoolchildren. I. Prevalence during a six year study. Am J Epidemiol 1980; 111: 721–726.
6 Graham N. Respiratory infections. In: Pless I B, ed. The epidemiology of childhood disorders. Oxford: Oxford University Press, 1994: Ch. 7, pp 173–206.
7 Colley J, Douglas J, Reid D. Respiratory disease in young adults: influence of early

childhood lower respiratory tract illness, social class, air pollution and smoking. Br Med J 1973; 3: 195–198.

8 Lundgren J, Shellamer J. Pathogenesis of airway mucus hypersecretion. J Allergy Clin Immunol 1990; 85: 399–417.

9 Gaillard D, Jouet J-B, Egreteau L et al. Airway epithelial damage and inflammation in children with recurrent bronchitis. Am J Respir Crit Care Med 1994; 150: 810–817.

10 Heino M, Juntenen-Backman K, Leijala M, Rapola J, Laitinen L. Bronchial epithelial inflammation in children with chronic cough and early lower respiratory tract illness. Am Rev Respir Dis 1990; 141: 428–432.

11 Editorial. Pertussis: adults, infants and herds. Lancet 1992; 339: 526–527.

12 Stark J. Lung infections in children. Curr Opin Pediatr 1993; 5: 273–280.

13 Bass J. Erythromycin for treatment and prevention of pertussis. Pediatr Infect Dis J 1986; 5: 154–157.

14 Bergquist S, Bernander S, Dahnsjo H et al. Erythromycin in the treatment of pertussis: a study of bacteriologic and clinical effects. Pediatr Infect Dis J 1987; 6: 458–461.

15 Isaacs D. Influenza immunization: time to stop the charade. Current Opinion Pediatr 1995; 7: 3–5.

16 Romanus V, Jonsell R, Bergquist S. Pertussis in Sweden after the cessation of general immunisation in 1979. Pediatr Infect Dis J 1987; 6: 364–371.

17 Sato Y, Kimura M, Fukumi H. Development of a pertussis component vaccine in Japan. Lancet 1984; 122–126.

1B.4   Viral-induced asthma

INTRODUCTION

Asthma and viral respiratory tract infections (URI) represent the top of the paediatric 'league table', being the most common chronic and acute medical conditions, respectively, in childhood. Moreover, there is a close interaction between the two. The single most common identifiable trigger for acute episodes of asthma in childhood are viral respiratory tract infections.[1] Not only are viruses the commonest triggers for acute exacerbations of asthma, but the clinical onset of asthma often follows a viral respiratory tract infection, suggesting the disease can be induced by a virus.[2] There is also evidence that some cases of persistent, severe asthma in childhood are a direct consequence of a single acute, but persisting, viral infection.[3]

Although all respiratory viruses are capable of triggering an attack of asthma, age has an influence on the specific viral agent responsible. In infants, respiratory syncytial virus (RSV) is the most important; in older children, human rhinovirus (HRV) or the 'common cold' virus is the major culprit.[4] Whether or not a specific viral URI will trigger a wheezy episode is dependent on the type of virus, the age of the child, plus other viral and host factors (Fig. 1B.4.1).

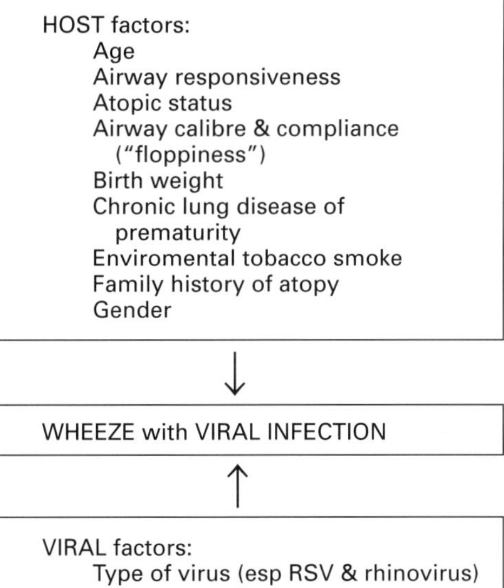

Fig. 1B.4.1 Factors associated with viral induced wheezing.

DEFINITIONS

Asthma

There is no universally accepted definition of asthma. However, the classical clinical features of asthma are wheeze (often associated with difficulty breathing) and/or chronic cough (typically a dry, nocturnal cough). These two symptoms are now used as an operational definition of asthma, especially in infants and pre-school children — provided other, rarer causes of cough and/or wheeze have been ruled out.[5] In school-age children, lung function tests can provide objective evidence of asthma.[6]

In questionnaire surveys, asthma is usually defined as wheezing in the past 12 months (i.e. 'current' or 'recent' wheeze).[7] Terms such as 'ever wheezed' or 'ever diagnosed as asthma' suffer from major errors in misclassification.

The characteristic airway pathology in asthma is well documented, at least in adults; namely, a chronic, desquamating eosinophilic bronchitis.[8] There is an excess of airway inflammatory cells (particularly eosinophils, mast cells and lymphocytes), disruption of the respiratory epithelial lining, and a characteristic thickening of the respiratory epithelial basement membrane.

'Wheezy bronchitis'

This is a term used to describe young children who wheeze only in association with intercurrent viral respiratory tract infections. The episodes are generally mild, and many outgrow the tendency to wheeze by early to mid-childhood. This is presumably due to lung and airway growth plus acquisition of immunity to the common respiratory viruses. Other terms used to describe this entity include 'wheezing-associated respiratory infection' (WARI) and 'virus-associated wheeze' (VAW).[9] The natural history of wheezy bronchitis is largely dependent on whether or not atopy (IgE antibodies) develops since this is the strongest risk factor for ongoing asthma (Fig. 1B.4.2). However, rather than being a separate

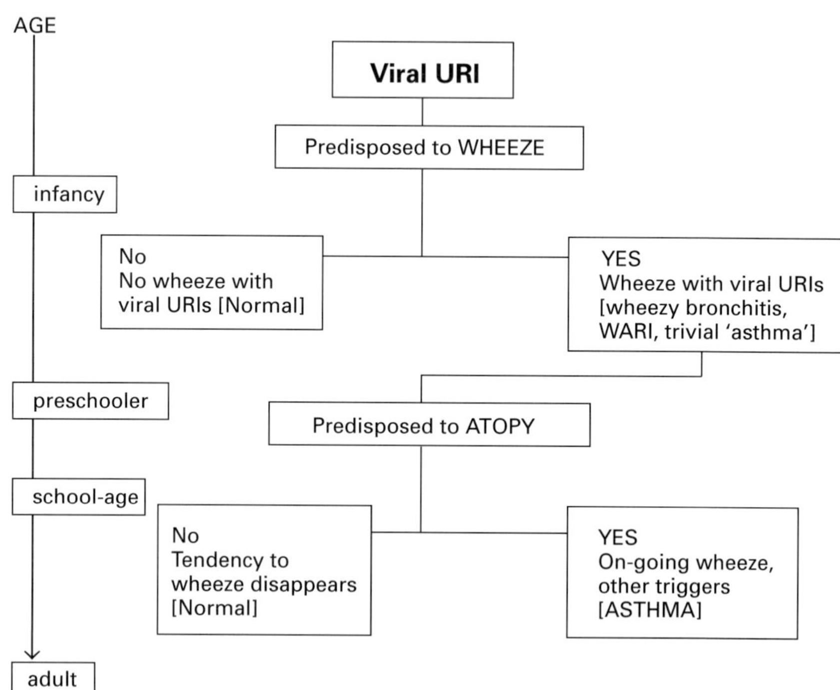

Fig. 1B.4.2 Natural history of wheeze in infants.

entity, many view 'wheezy bronchitis' as simply the mildest end of the asthma spectrum.[10] Such children are usually classified as having 'trivial' asthma.[11]

Irrespective of what terminology is used, it is clear that bronchodilators, and not antibiotics, are the preferred treatment. Medications should only be given if the wheeze is causing significant morbidity (e.g. wheeze interfering with normal activities, or wheeze accompanied by significant breathlessness). If not, then 'no drug treatment' is the preferred option.

Bacterial infection in the respiratory tract does not generally trigger acute exacerbations of wheezing, either in asthmatic or normal children. Thus, antibiotics are inappropriate treatment for uncomplicated wheeze. The two exceptions are chronic bacterial sinusitis[12] (which may cause worsening of asthma) and *Mycoplasma pneumoniae* infection, which can trigger acute wheezing.[13] However, antibiotics should be given only if *Mycoplasma* infection is proven.

EPIDEMIOLOGY

The first reports of asthma triggered by viral infection were in the late 1950s, when frequent asthma attacks were observed in children during influenza A epidemics. Since then, there have been numerous cross-sectional and cohort studies examining the relationship between acute bouts of wheeze and the isolation of respiratory viruses from the upper airway.[1]

In cross-sectional studies of children presenting with acute wheeze, the rate of positive viral isolations is approximately 25%. However, this is clearly an underestimate of the true rate of viral infection as the time course is against positive isolation. Typically, the coryzal symptoms of the viral infection precede the acute exacerbation of wheezing by approximately 48 h.

Using the more accurate cohort (longitudinal) study of children with asthma, the rate of positive virus isolation with acute episodes of wheeze in some studies is as high as 50%, with the average from all published studies of over 30%. In similar cohort studies in adults with asthma, the rate of positive viral isolation during acute episodes of wheezing is 15%.[1]

However, when an asthmatic child has a *proven* respiratory virus, acute wheezing will occur in 60%–80%.[1] Results in adults are almost identical. These studies suggest a strong causal relationship between viral respiratory tract infections and acute bouts of wheezing, both in children and adults.

PATHOGENESIS

The mechanisms whereby a respiratory virus triggers an acute exacerbation of asthma are unclear. However, direct epithelial damage resulting from the respiratory virus is the most likely cause. Additional mechanisms include release of inflammatory mediators (such as histamine) and pro-inflammatory cytokines. Nasal obstruction and resultant mouth breathing could also exacerbate the situation, since the normal filtering and air-conditioning function of the nose is bypassed.[4]

Rhinovirus is the commonest virus associated with wheeze (except in infants) and the pathogenesis of acute wheeze with this infection deserves special mention.[14] It is now clear that the receptor site for rhinovirus is a cell surface receptor, ICAM-1. This receptor is an adhesion molecule which plays a key role in promoting airways inflammation, especially in allergic reactions. ICAM-1 causes adhesion, and subsequent migration of polymorphs (especially eosinophils) from the circulation into inflamed tissues. ICAM-1 also facilitates the interaction between T lymphocytes and antigen-presenting cells. Thus, rhinovirus infection, by upregulating ICAM-1 expression, further exacerbates airways inflammation.

IMPORTANT RESPIRATORY VIRUSES

All of the respiratory viruses are capable of triggering acute bouts of wheeze. However, in the first 2 years of life respiratory syncytial virus (RSV) is the virus most likely to be responsible. In older children, rhinovirus (the 'common cold' virus) is most likely. This is not simply because there are so many strains (over 100) of rhinovirus, but also because of specific features of this virus which make it more 'asthmogenic' (see above).[14] Coronavirus also has a high likelihood of triggering wheeze, although this virus has not been studied as well as the others. Adenovirus, parainfluenza and influenza virus (A and B) are also important, although the exact rate of acute wheeze with each of these specific infections varies from study to study.

Mycoplasma pneumoniae can trigger wheeze, particularly in older children and adolescents, and is the only specific bacterial pathogen which is clinically relevant to acute wheeze.[13]

'PROTECTIVE' EFFECT OF VIRUSES

There has been a recent suggestion that recurrent infections in early infancy could protect against the development of atopy and asthma.[15,16] This is based on ecological data comparing populations with high and low rates of infections in early infancy. Most Third World countries have very high rates of 'infective' airways disease (bronchiectasis), but very low rates of 'reactive' airways disease (asthma), while the reverse is true in developed countries. The reunification of Germany has enabled comparisons between 'affluent' West German children and 'less affluent' East German children, the majority of whom attend full-time day care from a very early age. These studies support this hypothesis.[17] There is also evidence that smaller family size (and presumably fewer early infections) increases the risk of atopy and asthma.[18] Birth order also has an influence on clinical atopy. First-borns are less likely to have frequent infections in early infancy, but are more likely to develop clinical atopy, than subsequent born children.

The proposed mechanism for this protective effect of recurrent infection is the 'switching', in early life, of T helper lymphocytes into either TH_1 or TH_2 clones.[15,16] TH_1 subtypes promote 'tolerance' of airborne allergens, while TH_2 subtypes promote 'sensitization'. Thus, a predominance of TH_2 clones results in abnormal IgE production (atopy) and a high risk of subsequent clinical atopy — especially asthma. Recurrent infection in early infancy (either viral or bacterial) promotes the switch to favourable TH_1 clones. Clearly, further proof and the exact timing of this 'switch' will need to be determined. If these findings are confirmed, we have a paradoxical situation where early and frequent viral infections 'protect' against asthma; but if the child has asthma, viral infections are the major trigger responsible for acute attacks of wheeze (Fig. 1B.4.2).

ASSESSING SEVERITY OF CHILDHOOD ASTHMA

There is international consensus that severity of childhood asthma can be divided

Table 1B.4.1 Categories of asthma severity (including diagnostic criteria)

Asthma category	Frequency of episodes (per year)	Severity of episodes	Triggers of episodes	Interval symptoms
Trivial (wheezy bronchitis)	1–3	Trivial	Viral URI	Nil
Mild (infrequent episodic)	3–6	Mild	Viral URI	Nil
Moderate (frequent episodic)	6–12	Moderate	Several (including URI)	1–3 per week (especially with exercise)
Severe (persistent)	>12	Severe	Numerous (including URI)	Daily

Table 1B.4.2 Proportions in each category of asthma and treatment

Asthma	Treatment	Percentage of total asthma
Trivial (wheezy bronchitis)	Nil	45
Mild (infrequent episodic)	p.r.n. bronchodilator	30
Moderate (frequent episodic)	Regular cromoglycate and p.r.n. bronchodilator	20
Severe (persistent)	Regular inhaled corticosteroids and p.r.n. bronchodilator	5

into discrete clinical categories.[19,20] This arbitrary classification is based on frequency and severity of episodes, plus whether or not there are symptoms between attacks (interval symptoms). The details of each category, the recommended treatment for each category, and the relative proportions of asthmatic children in each category are outlined in Tables 1B.4.1 & 1B.4.2.

It is clear that most childhood asthma belongs to the mild end of the asthma spectrum.[11] This includes both 'infrequent episodic' (or mild) asthma and 'trivial' asthma ('wheezy bronchitis' or 'WARI'). The two striking features of this end of the asthma spectrum are the absence of symptoms between acute attacks, and that viral upper respiratory infections are the only trigger for attacks. 'Trivial' asthma is particularly common in preschool children, reflecting the frequency of viral infections in this age group. It is also likely that the small size of the very young child's airways predisposes them to wheeze, and this will improve with lung and airway growth.

TREATMENT

If there is no significant breathlessness associated with the wheeze, then no treatment is indicated. If any drug therapy is prescribed then a bronchodilator on an 'as required' basis is optimal. This should be a beta agonist by inhalation, which can be either via a metered dose inhaler and spacer device (either mouthpiece or face mask depending upon the age of the child) or a nebulizer. Oral bronchodilators are less appropriate due to frequent side-effects, particularly hyperactivity.

If the episodes are more troublesome, accompanied by definite shortness of breath, and requiring bronchodilators, or if the episodes are more frequent (four to six bouts per year) or more prolonged then the term 'infrequent episodic asthma' (mild asthma) is preferable. These episodes should be treated with bronchodilators by inhalation, on an as required (p.r.n.) basis. Those with 'frequent episodic' (moderate asthma) or 'persistent' (severe asthma) require long-term maintenance treatment with cromoglycate ('Intal') or inhaled corticosteroids respectively.[20]

If an acute bout of wheeze is associated with severe shortness of breath, which does not respond promptly to 4-hourly inhaled bronchodilators, then a short course of oral prednisolone (in a dose of 1–2 mg/kg per day for 2–3 days) may be indicated. This is a very effective measure for preventing progression of the attack, and for reducing the need for hospitalization.[21]

CONCLUSION

Viral respiratory infections (URIs) are by far the most important identifiable triggers for acute attacks of asthma in children. Thus, treatment of acute wheeze with antibiotics is inappropriate. The emphasis of treatment should be relief of any breathing difficulties with appropriate inhaled bronchodilators, and if severe, possibly a short course of oral prednisolone. Whether viral infections can actually induce, or permanently worsen asthma, is less clear. There is recent evidence suggesting that viral URIs occurring at a specific, critical time in early infancy may protect against the development of asthma. Unfortunately, at present we are unable to reduce the frequency of viral URIs in children who already have asthma. Moreover, should it be proven that early viral URIs can prevent asthma, it is difficult to see how this information could be implemented practically.[16]

REFERENCES

1 Pattemore P, Johnston S, Bardin P. Viruses as precipitants of asthma symptoms. I. Epidemiology. Clin Exp Allergy 1993; 22: 325–336.
2 Busse W. Respiratory infections: their role in airway responsiveness and the pathogenesis of asthma. J Allergy Clin Immunol 1990; 85: 671–683.
3 Macek V, Sorli J, Kopriva S, Marin J. Persistent adenoviral infection and chronic airway obstruction in children. Am J Respir Crit Care Med 1994; 150: 7–10.
4 Bardin P, Johnston S, Pattemore P. Viruses as precipitants of asthma symptoms. II. Physiology and mechanisms. Clin Exp Allergy 1992; 22: 809–822.
5 Warner J O, Gotz M, Landau L I et al. Management of asthma: a consensus statement. Arch Dis Child 1989; 64: 1065–1079.
6 Le Soeuf P. Validity of methods used to test airway responsiveness in children. Lancet 1992; 339: 1282–1284.
7 Toelle B, Peat J, Salome C, Mellis C, Woolcock A. Towards a definition of asthma for epidemiology. Am Rev Respir Dis 1992; 146.
8 Kay A B. Asthma and inflammation. J Allergy Clin Immunol 1991; 87: 893–910.
9 Wilson N. Wheezy bronchitis revisited. Arch Dis Child 1989; 64: 1194–1199.
10 Williams H, McNicol K. Prevalence, natural history, and relationship of wheezy bronchitis and asthma in children: an epidemiological study. Br Med J 1969; 4: 321–325.
11 Rosier M J, Bishop J, Nolan T, Robertson C F et al. Measurement of functional severity of asthma in children. Am J Respir Crit Care Med 1994; 149: 1434–1441.
12 Friedman R, Ackerman M, Wald E et al. Asthma and bacterial sinusitis in children. J Allergy Clin Immunol 1984; 74: 185–189.
13 Mertsola J, Zeigler T, Ruuskanen O et al. Recurrent wheezy bronchitis and viral respiratory infections. Arch Dis Child 1991; 66: 124–129.
14 Johnston S, Bardin P, Pattemore P. Viruses as precipitants of asthma symptoms. III. Rhinoviruses: molecular biology and prospects for future intervention. Clin Exp Allergy 1993; 23: 237–246.
15 Holt P, McMenamin C, Nelson D. Primary sensitisation to inhalant allergens during infancy. Pediatr Allergy Immunol 1990; 1: 3–13.

16 Holt P. A potential vaccine strategy for asthma and allied atopic diseases during early infancy. Lancet 1994; 344: 456–458.
17 Von Mutius E. Prevalence of asthma and allergic disorders among children in United Germany: a descriptive comparison. Br Med J 1992; 305: 1395–1399.
18 Strachan D. Hay fever, hygiene, and household size. Br Med J 1989; 299: 1259–1260.
19 National Heart, Lung and Blood institutes. International Consensus Report on Diagnosis and Treatment of Asthma. Eur Respir J 1992; 5: 601–641.
20 Isles A, Robertson C. Position statement: treatment of asthma in children and adolescents; the need for a different approach. Med J Aust 1993; 158: 761–763.
21 Brunette M G, Lands L, Thibodeau L P. Childhood asthma: Prevention of attacks with short-term corticosteroid treatment of upper respiratory tract infection. Paediatrics 1988; 81: 624–629.

1B.5 Whooping cough

INTRODUCTION

Whooping cough or pertussis syndrome is a term for a clinical condition characterized by paroxysmal cough with an inspiratory whoop and/or lymphocytosis. The name pertussis is preferred by some authors because not all patients have a whoop. The main aetiological agent for whooping cough is *Bordetella pertussis* bacterium. *B. parapertussis* can cause similar but often milder symptoms. The global annual incidence of whooping cough is estimated to be 60 million cases, with 600 000 deaths yearly.[1]

EPIDEMIOLOGY

Humans are the only known reservoir of *Bordetella pertussis*. Whooping cough occurs all over the world in all seasons. The highest incidence rates are seen in regions where immunization coverage is low. This has been clearly demonstrated also in developed countries like the UK, Germany, Sweden and Japan, where immunization levels have fallen or immunization has been withdrawn.[1] The important factors that influence the transmission of this disease are infectivity of the organisms, the number of contacts exposed and the level of immunity in the contact persons. The secondary attack rate in susceptible household contacts is from 70% to 100%. Vaccinated children at day care centres are usually well protected. The immunity provided by the vaccination declines, however, with time, and school-aged children (even if vaccinated in infancy) and adolescents are again at risk of whooping cough.

Whooping cough is both an endemic and epidemic disease. Traditionally epidemics occurred with a cycle of 3–4 years. Whole-cell pertussis vaccines have been effective in controlling the disease but have not eliminated the spread of *Bordetella pertussis* bacteria. Infants and unimmunized children are at risk of severe disease, whereas older children and adults might have milder and atypical disease. These vaccinated persons with waning immunity serve as important disseminators and reservoirs of the *B. pertussis* organisms.[2] Whooping cough may not be suspected in these patients until they have transmitted the disease to a young infant, who develops a classic whooping cough.

There is no chronic carriage of *Bordetella pertussis*, but short colonization during outbreaks is common in partially immune contact persons, as shown in studies using modern serological and polymerase chain reaction (PCR) techniques.[2,3]

PATHOGENESIS

Bordetella pertussis causes a superficial infection, and no systemic septic manifestations directly caused by these organisms have been reported. The pathogenesis includes three key phases: attachment, local damage, and development of systemic disease, which are made possible by evasion and failure of host defence mechanisms. Several virulence factors, such as filamentous haemagglutinin (FHA), pertussis toxin (PT), 69 kDa outer membrane protein and some agglutinogens (especially 2 and 3/6) appear to be important for the attachment of *B. pertussis* to ciliated respiratory epithelial cells. Tracheal cytotoxin disturbs mucociliary clearance, allowing better anchoring of the bacteria. PT and adenylase cytotoxin inhibit phagocyte function of the host, facilitating propagation of the infection.

PT is an exotoxin protein which is responsible for the major systemic manifestations of pertussis. In animals it causes lymphocytosis, sensitization to histamine and enhancement of insulin secretion. The exact pathogenesis of the paroxysmal cough, typical of whooping cough, has, however, not been resolved. Neurogenic effects of PT have been suspected, but local damage and irritation of the airways might also be the primary stimulus to cough attacks.

IMMUNITY

The immunological mechanisms responsible for protection against whooping cough are not fully known. Passive transfer of antibodies against PT, FHA and some other components of *Bordetella pertussis* can protect experimental animals in challenge tests. However, most clinical studies have failed to find a significant correlation between serum antibody levels and protection. It is proposed that antibodies play a role in preventing colonization and combating toxin-mediated disease, but complete clearance of *B. pertussis* organisms requires cellular immune responses mediated by Th_1 cells.[4]

SPREAD

Transmission of *Bordetella pertussis* occurs by close contact via respiratory secretions. The spread is highest during the first 2 weeks of illness. Patients with pertussis should be excluded from day care, school or other setting during the first 3 weeks of illness, or until they have stopped coughing or until they have received erythromycin for 5 days, whichever comes first.[5] If treated in the hospital the patient should be placed in respiratory isolation during the first 3 weeks of whooping cough, if not treated with erythromycin for at least 5 days.[6] Occasionally, immunized children and adults who are in close contact with a pertussis patient will be transiently colonized with *B. pertussis* but do not develop symptoms. There are no data indicating that these asymptomatic persons could transmit the disease.

CLINICAL FEATURES

The incubation period of whooping cough is 6–20 days, but usually less than 14 days. During the catarrhal stage, non-specific upper respiratory symptoms such as rhinorrhoea, low-grade fever and mild cough predominate. After 1–2 weeks cough gradually increases in severity and other symptoms subside. The patient is usually afebrile and appears to be rather healthy between the paroxysms. This paroxysmal stage lasts up to 4 weeks. During the paroxysm the patient is almost exhausted, before the first opportunity to inspire is offered. The paroxysm terminates by crowing, inspiratory whoop followed by vomiting. In young infants apnoea is common, whereas whoop can be absent. Also in older, partially immune children and adults whooping cough is often atypical. Most of them do not whoop but have only prolonged paroxysmal cough. Symptoms wane gradually during the convalescent stage. In China this disease is called 100-day cough, stressing the long duration of symptoms. Even 1 year after the active disease the paroxysmal cough may recur during viral respiratory infections.

Whooping cough is most severe in young infants. The case fatality rate was 1.3% in children less than 2 months of age in the USA in 1980–1989.[7] In children less than 12 months of age the rate was 0.6%. Pneumonia occurred in 22%, seizures in 3% and encephalopathy in 0.9% of these children. This rate of mortality and morbidity is more than 1000 times greater than any risk attributed to the whole-cell pertussis vaccine.

DIAGNOSIS

In unimmunized infants the clinical diagnosis of whooping cough is relatively easy. Because atypical or mild clinical cases are often encountered, laboratory diagnosis is highly important. Culture of *Bordetella pertussis* is the diagnostic 'gold standard'. The specimens should be taken from the posterior nasopharynx, either by intranasal aspiration or by a swab. Calcium alginate swabs are better than dacron, rayon or cotton wool swabs.[8] Because the organism is fastidious and slow growing, selective media with antibiotics are needed. Regan–Lowe or Bordet–Gengou medium and incubation at 35°C for 7 days are recommended. Usually *B. pertussis* grows in 4 days whereas *B. parapertussis* grows faster. If direct plating is not possible, special transport media could be used. Semi-solid media are usually recommended but we have found a solid Regan–Lowe medium as a slant in a tube very useful for direct plating before transportation (Fig. 1B.5.1). The advantage of these tubes is that they retain humidity and can be stored for months before use. If transport time exceeds 1 day, incubation of transport

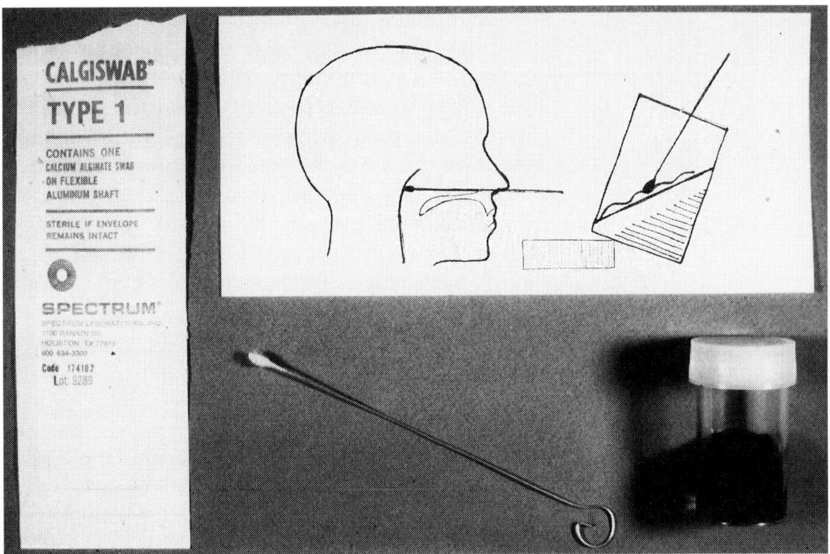

Fig. 1B.5.1 Calcium alginate swab for pernasal swab.

medium at 35°C for 1–2 days prior to shipping may improve culture yield. The culture positivity is highest during the first 2 weeks of illness, and cultures are seldom positive if cough has lasted more than 4 weeks. Usually the sensitivity of culture is less than 50% and false negative cultures are common, especially in vaccinated children.

The direct fluorescent assay (DFA) from nasopharyngeal secretions is a rapid test but has variable sensitivity and specificity. The antibodies used in DFA tend to cross-react with other bacteria and an experienced microscopist is needed if this test is used.

Enzyme immunoassay (EIA or ELISA) for detection of IgM, IgA and IgG antibodies to *Bordetella pertussis* was developed for serological diagnosis of whooping cough in the early 1980s. EIA is particularly useful in diagnosis during the late stage of the disease (cough longer than 4 weeks) when other tests are negative. In those cases the diagnosis often has to be made from a test of a single serum specimen. Currently EIA is mainly used in research laboratories. If it is used in routine diagnosis of whooping cough, the assay has to be well standardized for the local conditions. This often results in such strict criteria of seropositivity that the sensitivity is decreased to a level of 50–70%. Even with various purified antigen preparations no single test is shown to be highly sensitive. Although EIA has its limitations, it is shown to be a practical aid in diagnosis of small local outbreaks in countries with high vaccine acceptance rate but where atypical whooping cough occurs in older children with waning immunity.[2,9]

PCR is a new method for diagnosis of early whooping cough from nasopharyngeal swabs or aspirates.[3] Several different assay systems have been reported.[10] PCR results are ready within 24 h and the number of diagnosed patients is increased by about four-fold when compared to culture. The high sensitivity of the assay, however, makes it vulnerable to contamination problems.

TREATMENT

All children who have severe paroxysms with apnoea and cyanotic episodes should be treated in hospital. This is particularly the case with infants less than 6 months of age. Treatment with erythromycin should be given unless the symptoms have persisted more than 3 weeks. The recommended dose is 40–50 mg/kg per day, maximum 2 g per day, and duration of therapy is 14 days.[6] Erythromycin eliminates *Bordetella pertussis* from the nasopharynx and decreases the symptoms of the patients if started during the first 2 weeks of illness. Later, during the paroxysmal stage the antimicrobials usually have no discernible effect on the course of whooping cough. Trimethoprim–sulphamethoxazole is an alternative for those who do not tolerate erythromycin. There is no convincing evidence of the efficacy of cough suppressants, salbutamol or corticosteroids in the treatment of whooping cough. Limited recent data, however, indicate that early treatment with high-dose specific immunoglobulin with high antitoxin titre is beneficial in young infants.[11]

CHEMOPROPHYLAXIS

Erythromycin prophylaxis (same dose and duration as in treatment) is recommended in the USA and Canada to all household and other close contacts of whooping cough patients irrespective of their vaccination status.[5,6] If the mother has whooping cough at the time of labour, she and the infant should be treated with erythromycin, but the mother can safely be allowed to nurse her infant.[12] Early prophylaxis to families with a case of whooping cough and children younger than 6 months of age is important, because young infants are at risk of serious illness. Widespread chemoprophylaxis in day care centres and schools, however, is not without problems and needs further studies with cost–benefit analysis.

PREVENTION

Vaccinations are the most important measure in the prevention of whooping cough. Usually immunizations are started at 2 or 3 months of age. On special occasions, during an epidemic in the community, vaccinations can be started as early as 4 weeks of age.[6] Immunization from birth is not recommended as it may lead to tolerance, and a reduced response. The protection induced by whole-cell pertussis vaccines is often estimated to be from 80% to 90%.[1] This degree of protection lasts only about 3 years and then declines rapidly. Children older than 6 years are often not reimmunized, because adverse reactions are considered to be more common in older age groups. Therefore *Bordetella pertussis* circulates among older children and adults, even in countries with very high vaccination acceptance rates.[3] New, less reactogenic acellular vaccines are good candidates for boosters in older age groups.

REFERENCES

1 Cherry J D, Brunell P A, Golden G S, Karzon D T. Report of the task force on pertussis and pertussis immunization — 1988. Pediatrics 1988; 81 (Suppl): 939–984.
2 Mertsola J, Ruuskanen O, Eerola E, Viljanen M K. Intrafamilial spread of pertussis. J Pediatr 1983; 103: 359–363.
3 He Q, Viljanen M K, Nikkari S, Lyytikäinen R, Mertsola J. Outcomes of Bordetella pertussis infection in different age-groups of an immunized population. J Infect Dis 1994; 170: 873–877.
4 Mills K H G, Redhead K. Cellular immunity in pertussis. J Med Microbiol 1993; 39: 163–164.
5 National Advisory Committee on Immunization, Advisory Committee on Epidemiology and Canadian Pediatric Society. Management of people exposed to pertussis and control of pertussis outbreaks. Can Med Assoc J 1990; 143: 751–753.
6 Committee on Infectious Diseases, American Academy of Pediatrics. Pertussis. In: Report of the Committee on Infectious Diseases, 23rd ed. Elk Grove Village, IL: American Academy of Pediatrics, 1994: pp 355–367.
7 Farizo K M, Cochi S I, Zell E R et al. Epidemiological features of pertussis in the United States, 1980–1989. Clin Infect Dis 1992; 14: 708–719.
8 Hoppe J E, Weiss A. Recovery of Bordetella pertussis from four kinds of swabs. Eur J Clin Microbiol 1987; 6: 203–205.
9 Lawrence A J, Parton J C. Efficacy of enzyme-linked immunosorbent assay for rapid diagnosis of Bordetella pertussis infection. J Clin Microbiol 1987; 25: 2101–2104.
10 Meade B D, Bollen A. Recommendations for use of the polymerase chain reaction in the diagnosis of Bordetella pertussis infections. J Med Microbiol 1994; 41: 51–55.
11 Granström M, Olinder-Nielsen A M, Holmblad P, Mark A, Hanngrenn K. Specific immunoglobulin treatment of whooping cough. Lancet 1991; 338: 1230–1233.
12 Granström G, Sterner G, Nord C E, Granström M. Use of erythromycin to prevent pertussis in newborns of mothers with pertussis. J Infect Dis 1987; 155: 1210–1214.

1B.6   Pneumonia

EPIDEMIOLOGY

Pneumonia is a disease of great importance worldwide. UNICEF report pneumonia was the cause of 3.1 million deaths in children under the age of 5 in 1992. This is a small decrease over 10 years (3.3 million).[1] In the developed world the incidence of pneumonia is approximately 40 per 1000 children in the preschool age, falling to 9 per 1000 in the age group 9–15 years.[2] Pneumonia may be caused by bacteria, viruses, mycoplasmas, other atypical organisms and tuberculosis. The predominant organism changes with age and season of the year (Figs 1B.6.1 and 1B.6.2). As with all respiratory infections, males have a higher incidence than females.

There is an increased incidence of pneumonia in situations which confer vulnerability. Children from poor socioeconomic backgrounds, with a large number of other siblings, whose parents smoke and those who were born preterm are therefore at increased risk. In addition, children with any condition which alters local defences by, for example,

- decreasing or suppressing the cough reflex
- impairing mucociliary activity
- impairing immunological responses

are more prone to lung infection.

PATHOGENESIS

The lung can be infected by aspiration, inhalation, colonization of a diseased

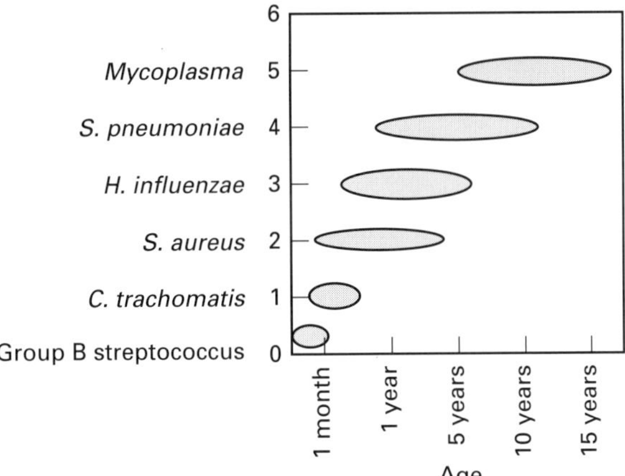

Fig. 1B.6.1 Diagrammatic representation of bacterial causes of pneumonia at different ages.

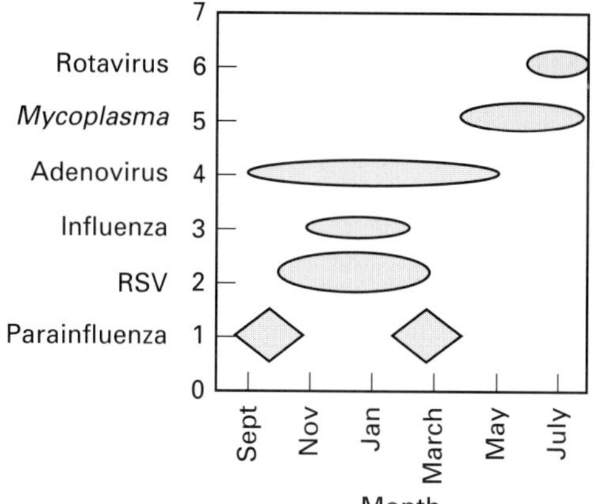

Fig. 1B.6.2   Diagrammatic representation of peak viral seasons in the UK and other countries with a temperate climate.

lower respiratory tract, or by blood spread. In normal healthy children inhalation is the normal method of infection. Many of the bacterial organisms involved in pneumonia exist as commensals in the oropharynx and their entry to the lower respiratory tract is often facilitated by a previous viral infection. Viruses increase susceptibility by causing an increase in secretions, a decrease in ciliary activity and a decrease in local immune responses in the lung. More than 50% of children with bacterial pneumonia have concurrent viral infection.

DIAGNOSIS

There is a great overlap in signs and symptoms between bacterial and viral pneumonias which often makes a specific diagnosis difficult. It is important, however, to try to identify the aetiological agent. Overall, blood cultures are said to be positive in between 10% and 50% of bacterial pneumonias. Identification of the agent from the pleural fluid is at least as high. Children rarely produce sputum for culture and in severe infections it is worth considering lung puncture as a relatively easy technique for obtaining samples for analysis (Appendix 1).

Viruses are generally identified from nasopharyngeal aspirates and rapid techniques such as immunofluorescence can often give an early diagnosis. However, as viral and bacterial infections frequently coexist, it may still be important to look for further aetiological agents.

Bacterial antigen detection methods including counterimmune electrophoresis are attractive as they can be performed in urine or serum or pleural fluid. Antigen can be detected several days after bacteraemia. However, both false positive and negative results have been reported so results need to be interpreted cautiously.[3,4]

Chest X-ray changes are important in making a diagnosis of pneumonia. If the pneumonia is lobar or segmental, *Streptococcus pneumoniae* or *Haemophilus influenzae* is the likely organism. If pneumatoceles or abscesses are present, *Staphylococcus aureus* is the most likely organism. If a large pleural effusion is present, a viral pneumonia is unlikely. If the chest X-ray changes are patchy, diffuse or perihilar, viral or *Mycoplasma* infection is probable. Non-infectious causes of pulmonary infiltrates should always be considered if the clinical features and chest X-ray appearances do not fit together.

GENERAL TREATMENT

In any child with respiratory distress, supportive care to maintain oxygenation is paramount. Blood gas estimation should be done in any child who is severely ill and oxygenation thereafter monitored to maintain oxygen saturation above 92%. Full ventilatory support may be needed. Hydration should be maintained but intravenous fluids should be given at only approximately 80% of basal levels, as inappropriate antidiuretic hormone secretion is a recognized complication in severe pneumonia.[5]

SPECIFIC TREATMENTS

In most cases the physician will wish to start treatment before a specific organism has been identified. A 'best guess' treatment regime will be based on the information from

- patient age
- sign and symptoms
- chest X-ray appearances

A suitable approach is presented in Table 1B.6.1.

Lack of response to conventional treatment should make one consider whether there is an effusion and empyema present, whether there is a lung abscess,

Table 1B.6.1   Clinical approach to pneumonia syndromes

Age	Signs and symptoms	Chest X-ray appearance	Likely organism	Therapy
1. Neonate	Respiratory distress Lethargy Fever	Reticular pattern or lobar	Group B streptococcus *Listeria*	Ampicillin + gentamicin
2. Infant	Cough Tachypnoea Minimal fever	Hyperinflated, bilateral infiltrates	Viral or chlamydia	Supportive ± erythromycin ± flucloxacillin
3. Infant	High fever Cough Tachypnoea	Lobar/segmental ± effusion	Pneumococcus, *Haemophilus influenzae,* *Staphylococcus aureus*	Third-generation cephalosporin
4. Child	Abrupt onset High fever Cough Tachypnoea	Lobar	Pneumococcus	Ampicillin/penicillin G
5. Child	Postviral Fever Tachypnoea Bilateral signs	Patchy consolidation	Pneumococcus, *Haemophilus influenzae,* *Staphylococcus aureus,* viral	Third-generation cephalosporin
6. Child	Postviral Fever Tachypnoea Unilateral or bilateral signs Hypoxic	Lobar/segmental effusion	Pneumococcus, *Haemophilus influenzae,* *Staphylococcus aureus*	Third-generation cephalosporin + flucloxacillin (or equivalent anti- staphylococcal)
7. Child	Malaise, cough, wheeze, mild fever, myalgia	Segmental or patchy consolidation, reticular shadowing	Mycoplasma, viral	Erythromycin

whether there is a foreign body in the airway or whether there is superinfection by another organism.

NEONATAL PNEUMONIA

Pneumonia presenting in the first few days after birth is likely to have been acquired in utero or from organisms present in the birth canal. By far the commonest cause is group B streptococcal infection but other infections such as Gram-negative enteric bacilli, *Listeria, Chlamydia* or viral pneumonias must be considered.

Group B streptococcus

Group B streptococcus is a common commensal of the birth canal, and where there has been prolonged rupture of the membranes or evidence of a maternal fever or amnionitis the baby can be infected before birth by aspiration of infected amniotic fluid. Intrauterine infection may trigger preterm delivery.

Clinical features

Clinical symptoms in the first 6–12 h are fever, evidence of respiratory distress with tachypnoea, nasal flaring, intercostal recession and grunting or apnoea. This may progress to cardiovascular collapse. Persistent pulmonary hypertension may develop. In some infants, however, there is a more insidious course with non-specific features such as lethargy, irritability and decreased tone.

Diagnosis

The diagnosis is both clinical and on X-ray appearances. Chest X-ray changes in approximately 40% of group B infections will be lobar but in the other 60% there is a diffuse reticular pattern, with air bronchograms making differentiation from hyaline membrane disease difficult.

A Gram stain of gastric aspirate can be helpful if it is loaded with Gram-positive cocci. Cultures of blood, cerebrospinal fluid, skin and gastric aspirate should be taken where there is a suspicion of infection.

Treatment

A combination of ampicillin and an aminoglycocide can be used in neonatal infections to cover all likely invading organisms including *Listeria* (see below), e.g. ampicillin 150–300 mg/kg per 24 h, gentamicin 7.5 mg/kg per 24 h. Intensive supportive care, including ventilation and inotropic circulatory support, may be needed.

Listeria monocytogenes

Listeria monocytogenes is a Gram-positive coccobacillus. In pregnant women it causes a non-specific influenzal or gastrointestinal illness but may gain transplacental access to the fetus, resulting in preterm delivery with an ill infant. The infection is often disseminated and the infant may have severe lung disease with grunting, retractions and cyanosis.

Listeria is a fastidious organism which may be slow growing and identification is dependent on meticulous culture of routine samples.

INFANCY

Chlamydia infection

Infection occurs during vaginal delivery through an infected cervix. The incidence of maternal infection varies in different populations but is highest in poor, non-white, adolescent populations. Rate of transmission is high, with evidence of an antibody response in 60–70% of the infants of infected mothers. An inclusion conjunctivitis develops in 33–50% of infants and pneumonia occurs in 10–20%.[6,7] Approximately 90% of infants with chlamydia pneumonia present between the ages of 4 and 11 weeks.

Pathogenesis and pathology

Chlamydia trachomatis is a small coccus-shaped bacterium containing both DNA and RNA. It is an obligatory intracellular parasite and primarily infects columnar epithelium. It causes a diffuse intra-alveolar infiltrate of histiocytes, lymphocytes, plasma cells, eosinophils and neutrophils, with a necrotizing bronchiolitis, alveolitis and airway plugging with atelectasis.

Clinical features

The illness starts with a rhinitis and nasal pharyngitis, often with some nasal obstruction. The infants are afebrile. The main respiratory symptoms are a cough, often staccato in nature, and tachypnoea. There are scattered crackles on auscultation and 10–20% have an expiratory wheeze. There is a decrease in oral intake, with some severely infected infants presenting as failure to thrive. Conjunctivitis is present in 40–50% of the infants with pneumonia.[7]

Diagnosis

Chest X-ray shows bilateral hyperinflation with bilateral and symmetrical interstitial pulmonary infiltrates. The white blood count is usually normal but the absolute eosinophil count is raised ($>300/mm^3$) in approximately 70%, and immunoglobulins M, A and G are raised in 80–100% of cases. There may be moderate hypoxaemia with normal carbon dioxide tension.

In infants with conjunctivitis the diagnosis can be confirmed by the identification of inclusion bodies in a conjunctival scrape. In others, nasopharyngeal secretions can be cultured using tissue culture techniques, or more commonly antigens can be detected by direct fluorescent antibody assay. The diagnosis can also be made by serology.

Management

Erythromycin has been shown to shorten the course of the disease[8] and is usually given for 14 days in a dose of 50 mg/kg per day. Parents should also be

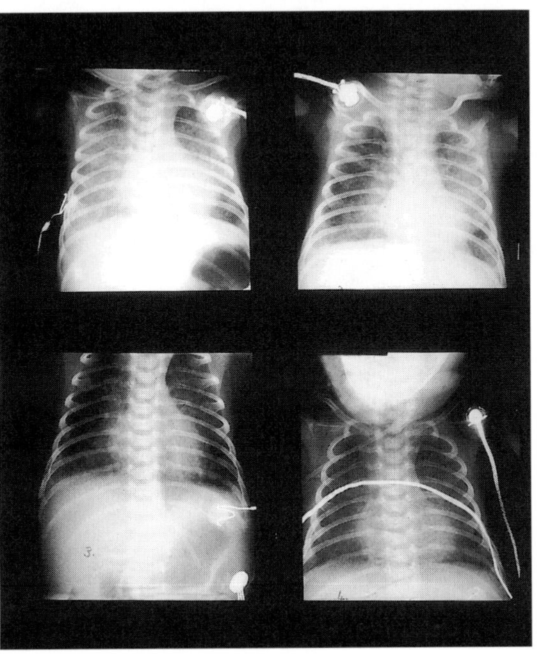

Fig. 1B.6.3 Chlamydia pneumonia. Bilateral infiltrates, gradually resolving.

treated. Supportive care with oxygen therapy and supplemental feeding may be necessary. Chest X-ray changes may persist for months. Long-term studies have demonstrated increased symptoms of cough and wheeze and reversible airflow obstruction 7–8 years after the recovery from the acute illness.[9]

Viral pneumonia

Viral pneumonias are most frequent in infancy (less than 1 year) and thereafter the frequency falls throughout childhood. They spread in an epidemic manner with a seasonal distribution. The commonest viruses involved are respiratory syncytial virus (RSV), parainfluenza viruses, influenza A and B viruses and adenovirus.

Pathology

The virus enters the upper respiratory tract and spreads to the lower respiratory tract. In small airways it involves the respiratory epithelium, causing loss of ciliary function and increased secretion, leading to partial or complete obstruction of the airways with air trapping or atelectasis. There is a general mononuclear or polymorph infiltrate.

Clinical features

The illness starts with a mild upper respiratory tract infection and fever for several days, then specific respiratory signs of cough, tachypnoea, tachycardia, nasal flaring and intercostal recession develop. Apnoea may occur, particularly with RSV. On examination the infant is hyperinflated with signs of respiratory distress, and on auscultation may have widespread crackles with a prolonged expiratory phase and/or expiratory wheeze. The infant may be hypoxic.

Diagnosis

On chest X-ray the lungs are usually hyperinflated and there may be bilateral, scattered, interstitial infiltrates or a perihilar infiltrate. There are frequently small subsegmental areas of atelectasis.

The white cell count may be normal or raised. On blood gas estimation, hypoxia is frequent but carbon dioxide retention only occurs in severe cases.

Nasopharyngeal aspirates permit rapid identification of viruses using fluorescent antibody or ELISA techniques. If these are negative the aspirate should be put up for culture. The virus may be identified retrospectively by serology.

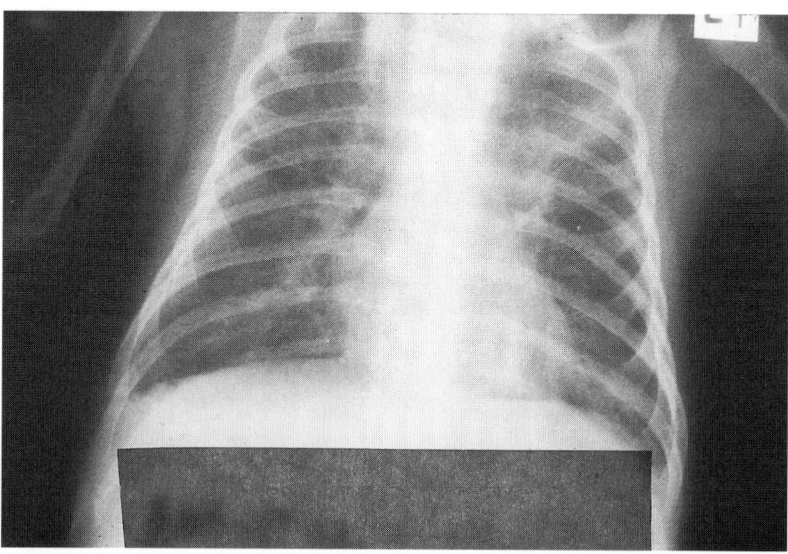

Fig. 1B.6.4 RSV pneumonia. Hyperinflation and patchy shadowing.

Management

Supportive care to maintain good oxygenation is essential. Some infants will require ventilation. Supplemental feeding by orogastric tube may be necessary to maintain hydration. Very rarely, in severely compromised infants with pre-existing conditions, specific antiviral agents such as amantadine in influenza A infection or ribavirin for RSV infections may be considered.

Complications

Most infants make a full recovery with no sequelae from their viral pneumonia. There is, however, an increased incidence of wheeze with subsequent viral infections. Adenovirus has a higher incidence of long-term problems. Adenovirus types 3, 7, 11 and 21 are well recognized as being responsible for a life-threatening obliterative bronchiolitis with chronic lung changes but this can also occur with other serotypes. Measles pneumonia has a high incidence of complications including bronchiectasis in poorly nourished and in immunosuppressed patients.

Prevention

RSV spreads by direct inoculation of secretions and by fomites, and cohorting of infants with handwashing by attendants are major preventive techniques for use in hospitals. All children should be vaccinated against measles and pertussis, and influenza vaccine should be given annually in the autumn to any child more than 6 months old with chronic respiratory disease, haemodynamically significant heart disease, sickle cell disease or any child who is HIV positive.

INFANCY AND CHILDHOOD: BACTERIAL INFECTIONS

Pneumococcus

Seventy per cent of the population are asymptomatic carriers of pneumococcus in their nasopharynx. It is the commonest invasive organism when respiratory defences have been compromised by previous viral infections. There are 80 types of *Streptococcus pneumoniae* identified by the antigenicity of their polysaccharide capsules, but approximately a dozen infective types are responsible for 75% of pneumonia. Type 3 is particularly virulent. Children with functional asplenia are particularly susceptible.

Pathology

In pneumococcal pneumonia the first stage is an inflammatory congestion where the alveoli fill with a fluid and haemorrhagic exudation. The exudate coagulates and the lung becomes solid (red hepatisation). There is invasion by neutrophils and then macrophages which remove cellular and bacterial debris. The process is spread by the infected bronchial fluid. The effect of consolidation is to decrease compliance of the lung and decrease the vital capacity. Physiologically there is a right-to-left shunt with ventilation–perfusion mismatch, leading to hypoxia.

Clinical features

There is often a mild coryza, then abrupt onset of high fever, sometimes accompanied by rigors. The child has a dry cough, is tachypnoeic and tachycardic and may look flushed and ill. Pleuritic pain is common and in lower lobe pneumonia the pain may be referred to the abdomen and the child mistaken for a surgical emergency. Similarly, upper lobe pneumonia can present with neck pain and stiffness and be mistaken for meningitis. On examination there may be mild intercostal recession, and classically there is a decreased percussion note, with bronchial breathing, and a few inspiratory crackles over the area of consolidation.

Diagnosis

Chest X-ray classically reveals a lobar pneumonia. Lower lobes are most frequently affected. Chest X-ray changes follow the clinical signs by approximately 12 h, so the chest X-ray may be normal at presentation.

The white cell count is raised, with a polymorphonuclear leucocytosis. Blood culture will be positive in somewhere between 10% and 50% of cases. Bacterial antigen may be detected by counterimmune electrophoresis in urine, serum or pleural fluid.[3]

Treatment

When the organism is known to be penicillin sensitive, benzyl penicillin is appropriate. Otherwise, it may be necessary to cover other bacterial infections such as *Staphylococcus* and *Haemophilus influenzae*.

Course

Clinical response to antibiotics is fast, with a prompt and dramatic fall in fever. Pleural effusions occur in up to 25%, but empyema only in 1% of cases. Disseminated infection with meningitis, peritonitis or septic arthritis is rare if treatment is commenced promptly. Chest X-ray clearing is usually complete in 3–5 weeks.

Prevention

A vaccine containing polysaccharide antigens of pneumococcal types responsible for over 80% of pneumococcal infection is available and should be used for vulnerable children, for example those with sickle cell disease, or post splenectomy. These children should also take oral penicillin lifelong as prophylaxis.

Staphylococcus aureus

Up to 30% of individuals carry *Staphylococcus aureus* in their nasopharynx. Staphylococcal pneumonia may follow viral infection or may occur secondary to bacteraemia at a distant site, for example infected intravenous cannulae or endocarditis.

Pathology

Staphylococcus aureus produces toxins and extracellular proteins resulting in extensive tissue necrosis and abscess inflammation in the lungs. Necrosis may be aided by small vessel thrombosis.

Clinical features and X-ray appearances

Fever and respiratory distress develop rapidly. Signs may be bilateral. Effusions occur in up to 55% of staphylococcal pneumonia. Pneumothorax may occur. Empyema occurs in approximately 10%. Pneumatoceles which are thin-walled, air-containing pseudocysts may appear on the chest X-ray, often after the first few days of the illness as clinical resolution takes place (Fig. 1B.6.5). Blood cultures are positive in 25% of cases; pleural fluid should always be examined both for culture and bacterial antigens.

Treatment

The treatment is intravenous flucloxacillin (or equivalent antistaphylococcal antibiotic) in a dose of 25–50 mg/kg 6-hourly. Rifampicin may be used as adjunctive treatment. Vancomycin is the antibiotic of choice for methicillin-resistant *Staphylococcus aureus* (MRSA). Response to antibiotics may be slow, with intermittent spikes of fever continuing. This is partly due to decreased penetration into necrotic areas of the lung and also to the incidence of empyema or lung abscess if treatment is delayed.

Haemophilus influenzae

Type b capsulated *Haemophilus influenzae* can cause bacteraemia, epiglottitis and pneumonia. Non-capsulated *H. influenzae* is a commensal in the upper respiratory tract, and frequently causes disease where host defences are decreased, for example in cystic fibrosis and in children in developing countries. Previously 83% of *H. influenzae* type b (Hib) pneumonia occurred in the under 2-year age group,[10] but with the introduction of Hib vaccine the incidence of Hib pneumonia is decreasing.

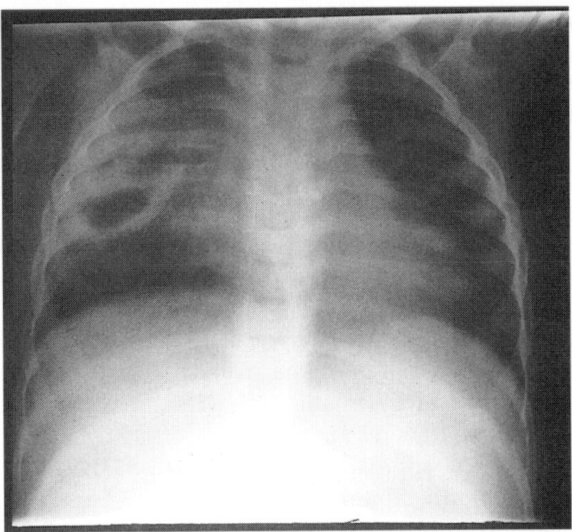

Fig. 1B.6.5 Staphylococcal pneumonia. Large right-sided pneumatocele.

Clinical features

There are no features specific to *Haemophilus influenzae* pneumonia. The chest X-ray shows a consolidated lobe or lobes. Non-capsulated *H. influenzae* more commonly causes patchy bronchopneumonia on chest X-ray. Evidence of pleural fluid is common (up to 75%).

Diagnosis is by culture of blood or pleural fluid and by detection of Hib antigen in the urine, although false positives can occur.[3]

Treatment

There is now widespread ampicillin resistance, so treatment should be with a third-generation cephalosporin, or with amoxycillin–clavulanic acid.

SCHOOL AGE

Mycoplasma pneumoniae

Mycoplasmas are the smallest living organisms known to survive outside host cells. They are pleomorphic and lack a cell wall. Adherence to and penetration of respiratory epithelium are necessary for infection.

Epidemiology

Mycoplasma infection is sporadic and endemic throughout the year but peak epidemics occur every 3–4 years. It is relatively more common in summer. It is spread by droplets and requires relatively close contact. Incubation period is 10–14 days.[11] Pneumonia occurs in only 10% of those infected. Infection is highest in 5–9-year-olds and second highest in 10–14-year-olds. Primary infection may be asymptomatic and reinfection is common.

Pathology

The primary process is of bronchitis and bronchiolitis with intraluminal exudation of neutrophils and macrophages and a submucosal and peribronchial infiltrate of inflammatory cells. Cilial motility is markedly impaired.

Clinical features

There is a wide range of clinical features. The illness often starts with a mild upper respiratory tract infection, then progressive symptoms of malaise, fever, cough, headache, pyrexia and mild myalgia. The cough is often paroxysmal and initially non-productive. There may be substernal discomfort or other chest pain. Other systemic features and extrapulmonary disease may occur (Table 1B.6.2).[12] *Mycoplasma pneumoniae* may precipitate severe exacerbations of asthma in children with previously mild or well controlled disease. Wheeze and cough can last for many weeks. On examination the child may look relatively well, with few clinical signs. Bilateral crackles or wheeze may be heard, and occasionally there are local signs of consolidation.

Diagnosis

Chest X-ray findings are very variable. There may be reticular, interstitial, patchy shadowing which is unilateral in 65%. Segmental or patchy consolidation may be present. Pleural effusions which are small, transient and unilateral occur in 10–20%. Nodular shadowing or enlargement of hilar lymph nodes may occur. The chest X-ray appearance classically looks worse than the child appears on clinical examination.

The white cell count is usually normal, but there may be a lymphopenia. Erythrocyte sedimentation rate (ESR) may be raised. Cold agglutinins which are IgM autoantibodies are positive in 50% of children with mycoplasma pneumonia and appear approximately 7 days from the onset of the illness, with a peak 4 weeks into the illness. Specific serum IgM antibodies can be detected early in the infection and rapid kit tests are now available. Definitive diagnosis is by serology.

Treatment

The treatment is a 14-day course of erythromycin. Supportive care may be necessary in severe infections, with oxygen therapy and bronchodilators if wheeze is a significant factor. The mycoplasma carriage rate is not affected by treatment and there is therefore a high infection rate in families.

Complications

Accompanying arthralgia and rashes are common. Mycoplasma infections may predispose long term to reactive airway disease, and persistent abnormalities of the small airways have been demonstrated.[13]

Table 1B.6.2   Manifestations of *Mycoplasma pneumoniae* infection

Common	Rare
Arthralgia	Stevens–Johnson syndrome
Myalgia	Bullous myringitis
Anorexia	Haemolytic anaemia
Vomiting	(Coombs positive)
Diarrhoea	Hepatitis
Skin rashes	Splenomegaly
Erythematous	Pancreatitis
Maculopapular	Neurological disease/convulsions
Vesicular	Guillain-Barré syndrome
	Cerebellar ataxia
	Transverse myelitis
	Meningoencephalitis

OTHER ATYPICAL PNEUMONIAS

Legionella pneumophilia

Legionella as a cause of pneumonia is rare in childhood and most, but not all, cases have occurred in the immunocompromised.[14]

Clinical features

The child may have a non-specific viral-like prodrome but then become acutely unwell with a high fever, rigors, nausea, vomiting and a dry cough. There may be neurological involvement, with unsteadiness, confusion and slurring of speech. As the disease progresses, breathlessness and a productive cough become prominent features.

Diagnosis

The chest X-ray shows a patchy bronchopneumonia with rounded opacities or perihilar densities which progress to a lobar or multilobar consolidation. The organism can be cultured from respiratory secretions, or direct fluorescent stains of lung secretions can identify the organism in about 60% of cases.

Treatment

Erythromycin (50 mg/kg per day) is the drug of choice. Most patients respond within 48 h. Treatment should continue for 2 weeks.

Chlamydia pneumoniae **(TWAR)**

This recently recognized organism was accepted as a new strain of chlamydia in 1989. Pneumonia is the disease most often associated with the organism but it seems that many infective episodes are mild and antibody conversion can occur in asymptomatic children. During childhood, pneumonia caused by *Mycoplasma pneumoniae* is at least five times more common than that caused by *Chlamydia pneumoniae*.[15]

Clinical findings

A gradual onset of sore throat, headaches and mild fever is common. Cough with signs of lower respiratory illness develop slowly. Approximately 60% of children cough for more than 3 weeks when infected with this organism. Crackles and wheeze may be heard on auscultation.

Diagnosis

A chest X-ray may show an unilateral segmental area of pneumonitis. The ESR is often high. Techniques for isolation and specific serology are specialized and may not be readily available.

Treatment

Erythromycin is the drug of choice.

RECURRENT PNEUMONIA

Recurrent pneumonias are likely to occur in children who have lowered host defences. Aspiration pneumonia may occur in children who are comatose, neurologically impaired, have nasogastric tubes in place, suffer from seizures, or have major gastrointestinal reflux. Pneumonias in these conditions are commonly caused by anaerobic or Gram-negative bacteria.

Cystic fibrosis, immune deficiencies and HIV infection are conditions which need to be actively ruled out where a child suffers from recurrent pneumonia.

Recurrent pneumonia in the same lung or lung segment suggests a local problem such as a sequestered lobe or foreign body in the airway and requires full investigation.

REFERENCES

1 UNICEF. The state of the world's children 1994. Oxford: Oxford University Press, 1994.
2 Glezen W P, Denny F W. Epidemiology of acute lower respiratory disease in children. N Engl J Med 1973; 288: 498–505.
3 Isaacs D. Problems in determining the etiology of community acquired childhood pneumonia. Pediatr Infect Dis J 1989; 8: 143–148.
4 Ramsay B W, Marcuse E K, Foy H M et al. Use of bacterial antigen detection in the diagnosis of paediatric lower respiratory tract infections. Paediatrics 1986; 78: 1–9.
5 Shann F, Germer S. Hyponatraemia associated with pneumonia or bacterial meningitis. Arch Dis Child 1985; 60: 963–966.
6 Hammerschlag M R. Chlamydial infections. J Pediatr 1989; 114: 727–734.

7 Tipple M A, Beem M O, Saxon E M. Clinical characteristics of the afebrile pneumonia associated with Chlamydia trachomatis infection in infants less than 6 months. Pediatrics 1979; 63: 192–197.
8 Beem M O, Saxon E, Tipple M A. Treatment of chlamydial pneumonia of infancy. Pediatrics 1979; 63: 198–203.
9 Weiss S G, Newcombe R W, Beem M O. Pulmonary assessment of children after chlamydial pneumonia in infancy. J Pediatr 1986; 108: 659–664.
10 Ginsburg C W, Howard J B, Nelson J D. Report of 65 cases of Haemophilus influenzae b pneumonia. Pediatrics 1979; 64: 283–286.
11 Foy H M, Kenny G E, Cooney M K, Allan I D. Longterm epidemiology of infections with Mycoplasma pneumoniae. J Infect Dis 1979; 139: 681–687.
12 Broughton R A. Infections due to Mycoplasma pneumoniae in childhood. Pediatr Infect Dis J 1986; 5: 71–85.
13 Mok J Y Q, Waugh P R, Simpson H. Mycoplasma pneumoniae infection: a follow up study of 50 children with respiratory illness. Arch Dis Child 1979; 54: 506–511.
14 Carlson N C, Kuskie M R, Dobyns E L, Wheeler R N, Roe M H, Abzug M J. Legionellosis in children: an expanding spectrum. Pediatr Infect Dis J 1990; 9: 133–137.
15 Grayston J T. Chlamydia pneumoniae (TWAR) infections in children. Pediatr Infect Dis J 1994; 13: 675–685.

APPENDIX 1: LUNG PUNCTURE TECHNIQUE

A 20 gauge needle is attached to a 10 ml syringe containing 1 ml of sterile isotonic saline. The lung is punctured into an area of consolidation. The intercostal space is anaesthetized with 2% lignocaine and then the technique is a quick stab through the space across the pleura and into the lung to a depth of 2–3 cm. The saline is injected and immediate suction applied to the syringe as the needle is withdrawn. The needle is in the lung only for a few seconds and the contents of the needle in the syringe may be used for culture, antigen detection and viral detection. Although there are theoretical risks of a small pulmonary haemorrhage or a pneumothorax, complications are exceedingly rare.

A. Thomson

1B.7   Pleural effusion/empyema

INTRODUCTION

The two layers of the pleura must slide easily over one another to permit the thorax to move the lungs with minimal energy loss. Lubrication is provided by a layer of surfactant absorbed onto the pleural surfaces. A single layer of meso-thelial cells covers the pleural surfaces. These cells have numerous microvilli which greatly increase the surface area for the absorption of pleural fluid.

The pleural membranes are permeable and the mechanisms concerned with the transfer of fluids across the pleural membranes are

1. transcapillary exchange
2. lymphatic drainage

The net effects of hydrostatic capillary pressures, osmotic pressures and elastic recoil pressures are approximately 6 mmHg (0.8 kPa), encouraging transudation of fluid from the parietal pleura, and a larger pressure, approximately 13 mmHg (1.7 kPa), encouraging resorption of fluids by the visceral pleura.

The accumulation of any fluid in the pleural space is termed a pleural effusion. It is often forgotten that once an effusion is formed it is in a dynamic state with a turnover of 30–75% per hour.[1]

PATHOGENESIS

Pleural effusions are characterized by whether the fluid is a transudate or an exudate. Differentiation is usually easy. Transudates are caused by systemic conditions which alter the hydrostatic pressures or osmotic forces across the pleural membranes. They are therefore usually bilateral. If the cause is corrected the fluid is very quickly reabsorbed and complete resolution is the norm. Typical causes are cardiac failure, nephrotic syndrome and hepatic cirrhosis.

Exudates are due to local disease causing increased capillary permeability or lymphatic obstruction. The protein content of the pleural fluid is increased. The mechanism of increased capillary permeability is not fully understood but may be an effect of bacterial toxins or related to deposition of immune complexes and the release of inflammatory mediators. Exudates resolve more slowly than transudates because the removal depends on protein reabsorption by lymphatics, which is slow compared with the transfer of fluid across the normal pleura. Exudates are commonly unilateral and there may be residual pleural thickening and adhesions on resolution.

Examination of the pleural fluid permits differentiation of transudates from exudates (Table 1B.7.1).

Table 1B.7.1

Transudates	Exudates
Clear	Turbid
Straw coloured	Purulent/bloody
Non-viscous	Viscous
Do not smell	Sometimes offensive
Do not clot	Can clot
Protein < 30 g/l in 90%	Protein > 30 g/l in 90%
WBC < 1000/ml³	WBC > 10 000/ml³
Lactic dehydrogenase (LDH) < 200 IU	LDH > 200 IU/ml

The pleural response to infection consists of:

1. pleurisy (dry) with pain or pleural rub
2. serous exudate (parapneumonic effusion)
3. empyema
   - (a) exudate phase (thin fluid), progressing to
   - (b) fibropurulent (thicker with many white cells and fibrin strands), progressing to
   - (c) organizing phase (with lung entrapment)

Transition from parapneumonic effusion to empyema involves the appearance of organisms in the fluid, an increase of polymorphs, and a fall in pH and glucose, probably reflecting a breakdown in local defence mechanisms. Practically speaking, the term empyema is often reserved for fluid with a naked eye appearance of pus. Infection of the pleura most commonly occurs secondary to pneumonia but can occur as a complication of a subphrenic abscess or surgery.

CAUSATIVE ORGANISMS AND EPIDEMIOLOGY

An effusion occurs in up to 40% of bacterial pneumonias. In a large study of parapneumonic effusions and empyema, Freij found that 70% occurred in the first 2 years of life. *Staphylococcus aureus* was the major pathogen in the first 6 months of life and *Haemophilus influenzae* and *Streptococcus pneumoniae* were responsible for over 50% of the cases aged 7–24 months. Pleural fluid culture was positive in two-thirds of the cases. There was a preponderance of males.[2] Virus infections rarely cause effusions. Effusions occur in up to 20% of mycoplasma pneumonias but are usually small. In developing countries effusions secondary to tuberculosis are common, particularly in school-age children, with a peak in adolescence.

The chances of an empyema developing vary with the cause of the pneumonia. Pneumococcus is the most common cause of pneumonia and effusions are common, but the development of empyema is less common than with pneumonia due to *Staphylococcus aureus* or *Haemophilus influenzae*.[3] A high proportion of anaerobic, coliform or *Pseudomonas* pneumonias spread to the pleura.

CLINICAL FEATURES

Effusion

The effects of accumulation of fluid in the pleural space depend on the cause and the amount of the fluid. Small effusions are often symptomless and even large effusions, if they accumulate slowly, may cause little or no discomfort.

If the effusion is secondary to infection, pleuritic pain may be an early feature, followed by shortness of breath, cough and aching pain on the side of the effusion.

Most effusions are in the dependent part of the pleural space, so on clinical examination there is decreased movement, stony dull percussion note and diminished or absent breath sounds at the base of the lungs. Bronchial breath sounds may be heard immediately above an effusion. Large effusions may cause mediastinal shift.

Empyema

In a child with pneumonia the development of an empyema should be suspected if the clinical state is slow to improve and/or there is persistent or recurrent fever. The child often has no energy, has a poor appetite (often with associated weight loss) and may complain of dull chest pains. On examination there are the signs of pleural effusion and, if left untreated, clubbing and anaemia may develop within weeks.

RADIOLOGICAL FEATURES

Small amounts of fluid in the pleural space result in blunting of the costophrenic angle on chest radiographs. Larger effusions are most dense at the base, obscuring the diaphragm, but as the fluid rides up around the edges of the lung the attenuation of the X-rays decreases so the effusion appears higher in the axilla than anteriorly or posteriorly on the chest X-ray. Occasionally effusions may be encysted, e.g. interlobar effusion appearing like a mass or tumour, and can cause diagnostic difficulties.

Ultrasound examination is very valuable where there is doubt about the size or position of an effusion. It is also extremely useful to characterize the fluid viscosity and determine if the effusion is loculated.

DIAGNOSIS

The diagnosis of effusion or empyema is suspected clinically and on radiological appearances Figs 1B.7.1 and 1B.7.2. All children with significant effusions (clinically detectable) should have a diagnostic pleural aspiration. The characteristics of the fluid help in diagnosis (Table 1B.7.1). The fluid should be sent for

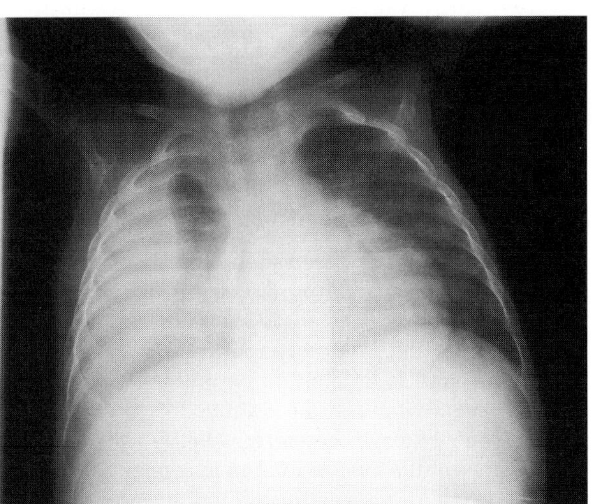

Fig. 1B.7.1   Chest X-ray demonstrating right lower lobe pneumonia with a large D-shaped effusion.

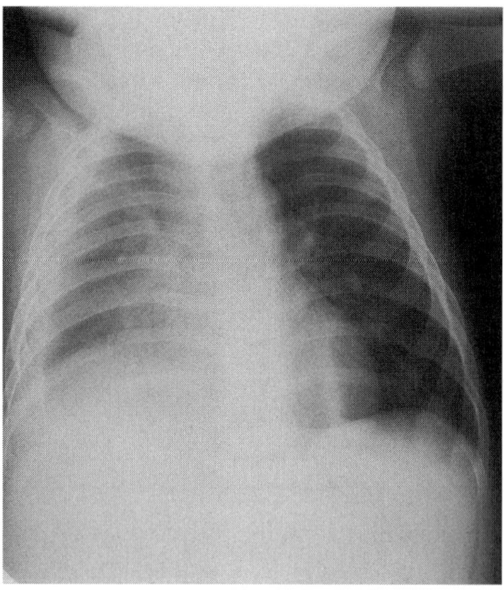

Fig. 1B.7.2   Supine X-ray of a 10-month-old boy with a right-sided empyema (line parallel to ribs).

microscopy and culture (aerobic and anaerobic) as well as for bacterial antigen detection if infection is a likely cause.

PLEURAL ASPIRATION

Large pleural effusions can be aspirated blind. Small effusions should be aspirated under ultrasonic guidance. Depending on the age and state of the child, sedation may be necessary for the procedure. Local anaesthetic should always be used. For large effusions the child is best positioned sitting up with arms forward over pillows. Aspiration should be performed in the sixth intercostal space or one space below the upper level of dullness to percussion in the scapular line using an 18 gauge needle or cannula attached to a three-way tap and syringe. If thick pus is suspected a larger gauge needle should be chosen. It is reasonable to remove as much fluid as possible.

MANAGEMENT

Transudate

A transudate will resolve with treatment of the primary problem.

Exudate

Parapneumonic effusion

The effusion associated with bacterial pneumonia is initially sterile but may frequently be invaded by the causative bacteria, leading to empyema. Antibiotics are much less effective in the management of pleural infection compared with lung infection. Polymorph function in the pleural space is normal and persistence of infection is unlikely to be due to inadequate antibiotic activity. Recent work suggests that depletion of antibodies and complement in the empyema fluid may be contributory. Therefore aspiration of as much fluid as possible at the time of presentation is optimal management. The underlying pneumonia should be treated vigorously with antibiotics.

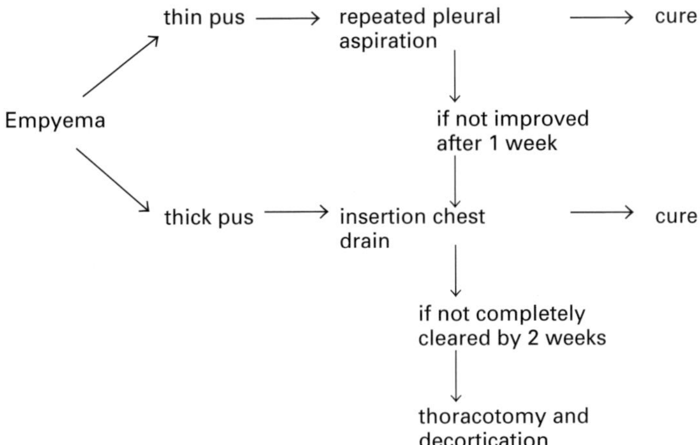

Fig. 1B.7.3 Management of empyema.

Empyema

Where the pleural fluid is clearly infected, adequate drainage is essential. A plan of management is outlined in Figure 1B.7.3. Antibiotic therapy should be continued in high dosage. Early loculation of an empyema may prevent aspiration or a chest tube from providing full drainage. If chest aspiration is dry or chest tube drainage decreases, ultrasound examination may be helpful in guiding needle or tube drainage. The instillation of urokinase, as a fibrinolytic agent, has been reported in loculated empyema in children but needs further evaluation before it can be recommended.[4] However, if the empyema is not draining satisfactorily there should be no delay in proceeding to decortication. Early decortication may hasten recovery.[5] By the end of the third week organization within an empyema is well established and the lung becomes trapped. The inflammatory adhesions become extremely vascular and thereafter decortication is a more difficult procedure. The objects of decortication are (1) to remove all infected material, including the visceral and parietal pleura, and (2) to allow the underlying lung to unfold and expand fully and prevent a long-term restrictive deficit.

FURTHER INVESTIGATION

In any child with a severe or complicated pneumonia, further investigation to exclude local or systemic disease such as structural abnormalities, immune deficiency or cystic fibrosis should be considered.

LONG-TERM OUTLOOK

Long-term follow-up studies have shown complete recovery and normal long-term lung function in the vast majority of children.[6]

REFERENCES

1 Black L F. Pleural effusion. In: Staub N C, Taylor A E, eds. Edema. New York: Raven Press, 1984: p 695.
2 Freij B J, Kusmiesz H, Nelson J D, McCracken G H. Parapneumonic effusions and empyema in hospitalised children: a retrospective review of 127 cases. Pediatr Infect Dis J 1984; 3: 578.
3 Ginsburg C M, Howard J B, Nelson J D. Report of 65 cases of Haemophilus influenzae b pneumonia. Pediatrics 1979; 64: 283.
4 Handman H P, Reuman P D. The use of urokinase for loculated thoracic empyema in children: a case report and review of the literature. Pediatr Infect Dis J 1993; 12: 958–959.
5 Hoff S J, Neblett W W, Edwards K M et al. Parapneumonic empyema in children: decortication hastens recovery in patients with severe pleural infections. Pediatr Infect Dis J 1991; 10: 194–199.
6 Reading G J, Walun D L, Wellun D, Jones J W, Stamey D C, Gibson R L. Lung function in children following empyema. Am J Dis Child 1990; 144: 1337–1342.

1B.8 Lung abscess

INTRODUCTION

A lung abscess is a cavitated, infected, necrotic lesion of the lung parenchyma. Lung abscesses can be divided into primary lung abscess occurring in otherwise healthy children, and secondary lung abscess occurring in children with some underlying predisposition, for example immunosuppressed or neurologically abnormal children. Secondary lung abscesses are more common than primary lung abscess.

EPIDEMIOLOGY

Lung abscess has become a rare condition in the developed world since antibiotic treatment became available. An incidence has been reported from Canada of 0.7 per 100 000 paediatric admissions per year[1] and even in Zimbabwe only 24 cases were seen over a 10-year period in a large hospital.[2] Lung abscess is rare in the neonatal period. It is more common in boys than girls.

PATHOGENESIS

The lung may become infected from a number of sources (Table 1B.8.1). In children with neurological disorders, aspiration of small amounts of saliva is common. Poor dental hygiene will favour the growth of anaerobic bacteria in the saliva and increase the risk of infection. Lung abscess secondary to aspiration occurs in the dependent segments of the lung, i.e. the posterior segment of the right upper lobe or the apical segments of either lower lobe.

Conditions which prevent normal clearance of pulmonary secretions will favour development of infection:

Table 1B.8.1 Predisposing causes for lung abscess

1. Aspiration of oropharyngeal contents
2. Pneumonias
3. Bloodborne infection/septic emboli
     Gram-negative sepsis
     Endocarditis
     Infected skin
     Infected intravenous cannula
4. Immunodeficiency
5. Abdominal sepsis (transdiaphragmatic)
6. Bronchial obstruction
7. Trauma

- Mechanical clearance
  - Cilial dysmotility
  - Foreign body
  - Bronchiectasis, cystic fibrosis
- Immunocompetence
  - Primary immune deficiencies
  - Immunosuppressed

Infection with lung abscess formation is more common following a viral infection such as influenza and, in the Third World, measles.

PATHOLOGY

A lung abscess begins as an area of pneumonia in which small zones of necrosis or micro-abscesses develop. Some of these areas coalesce and when they reach an arbitrary size of 1–2 cm are referred to as abscesses.

If this process is interrupted by appropriate antibiotic treatment, healing may be complete without residual damage seen on a chest X-ray. However, if treatment is delayed or inadequate the inflammatory process proceeds and enters a more chronic phase. Fibrosis occurs in or around the abscess cavity so that it becomes loculated and enclosed by dense scar tissue.

In some abscesses the bronchi adjacent to the area of inflammation become eroded so that some of the purulent contents of the abscess can spill into the bronchial tree. This is usually expectorated as sputum but can cause disseminated lung infection. When there is a communication with the bronchial tree, air enters the cavity and an air-fluid level is visible on chest radiography.

If treated with appropriate antibiotics the abscess cavity becomes sterilized and heals with granulation of fibrous tissue. Occasionally a cavity may become epithelialized by epithelial cells from the adjacent bronchus and remains as a lung cavity with bronchial communication.

MICROBIOLOGY

Almost any organism can be involved in a lung abscess, including *Mycobacterium tuberculosis* and fungi. In secondary lung abscess it is common for more than one organism to be involved. *Staphylococcus aureus* is by far the leading cause of lung abscess in children.[1,3] Other reported organisms in primary lung abscess are *Haemophilus influenzae*, *Streptococcus viridans*, group A streptococcus and rarely *Streptococcus pneumoniae*. Gram-negative organisms such as *Klebsiella*, *Escherichia coli* and *Pseudomonas* have been reported. Anaerobic organisms are particularly common in lung abscesses associated with aspiration, when it is common for more than one organism to be involved.[4]

CLINICAL FEATURES

Lung abscess secondary to pneumonia usually presents as an acute illness with high fever, cough, tachypnoea and sometimes chest pain. Older children may produce sputum which occasionally is blood stained.

Lung abscess resulting from aspiration may present with a more insidious onset and the child may have malaise, fever and weight loss over days or weeks. Signs and symptoms in the very young or immunosuppressed may be non-specific.

If the lung abscess is secondary to pneumonia, signs of consolidation may be present. A pleural rub is occasionally heard. In some children there may be minimal signs of chest disease.

DIAGNOSIS

Radiographic features

The diagnosis is suggested by characteristic radiographic features of one or more spherical areas of homogeneous density seen on chest radiographs (Fig. 1B.8.1). Air–fluid levels may be seen within the cavity. Abscess cavities may be multilocular. It can be difficult to distinguish a pleural collection of pus (empyema) from a lung abscess. A lateral chest X-ray may help to localize the lesion (Fig. 1B.8.2) but if doubt remains a computed tomographic (CT) scan of the lung will be helpful in defining the shape and extent of the lung abscess (Fig. 1B.8.3).

Blood tests

The white blood cell count is usually increased, with a polymorphonuclear leucocytosis. There may be a mild normochromic, normocytic anaemia. The erythrocyte sedimentation rate (ESR) is usually raised. Blood cultures are usually sterile but an organism may be identified if the lung abscess is secondary to haematogenous spread.

Microbiology

It is often difficult to identify the responsible organism in children. Adults with

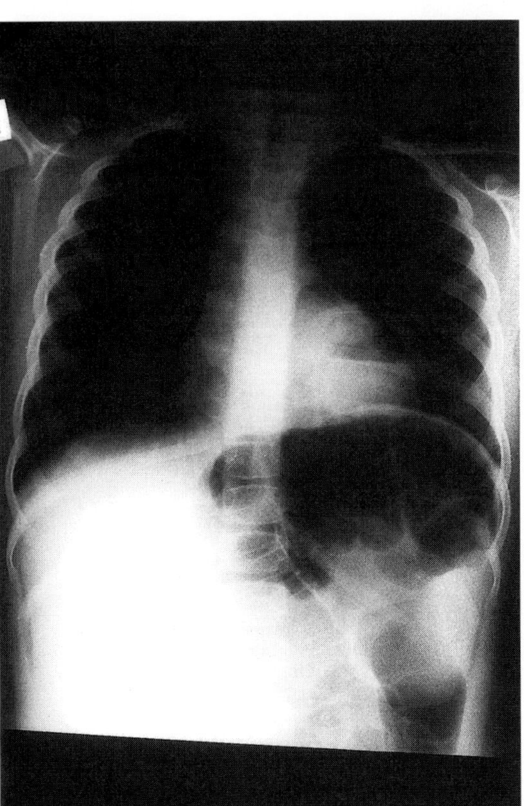

Fig. 1B.8.1 Lung abscess. Seen behind heart on chest radiograph. This occurred secondary to inhalation from a dental abscess.

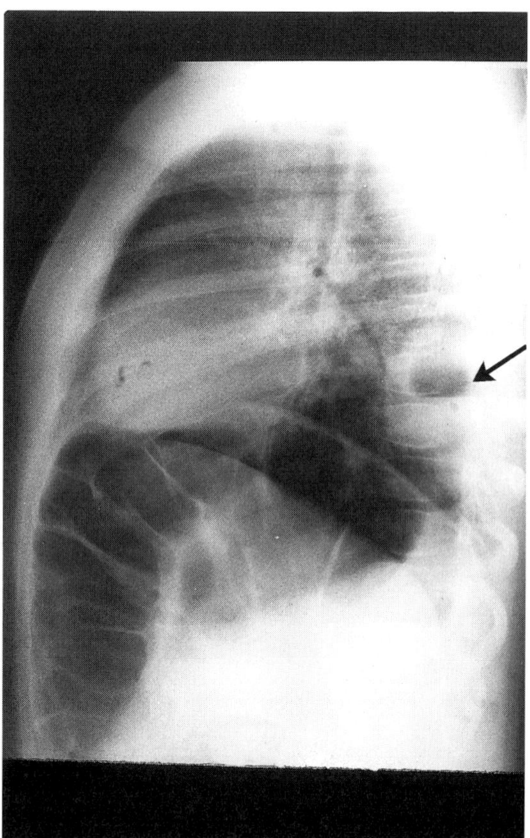

Fig. 1B.8.2   Lung abscess. Fluid level seen on lateral radiograph (abscess arrowed).

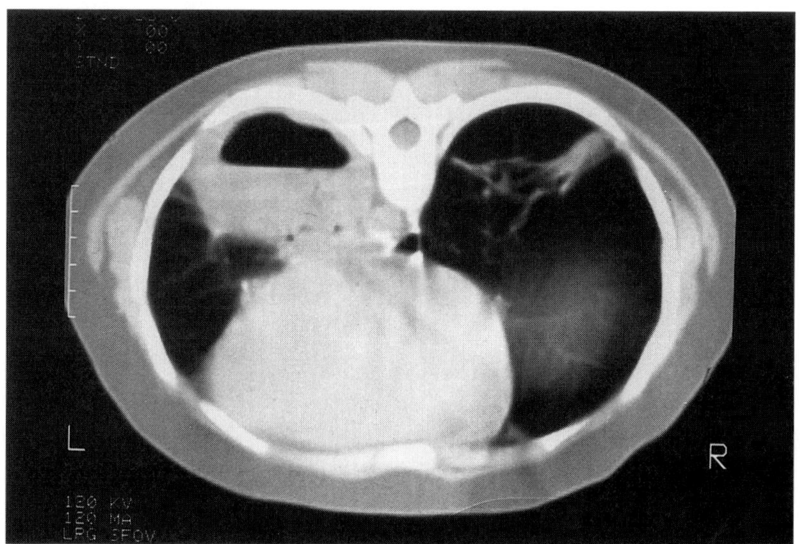

Fig. 1B.8.3   Lung abscess. CT scan appearance.

lung abscess frequently produce purulent sputum and when anaerobic organisms are present the spit has a characteristic foul smell. Where sputum is not available, treatment is usually started with an empirical choice of antibiotics to treat the most likely organisms. Invasive methods for obtaining specimens for culture from lung abscess are rarely attempted in children unless first-choice antibiotics fail. The most reliable method for identifying the aetiological agent is by direct percutaneous aspiration of the material in the abscess. This can be performed under ultrasound or CT control but is technically difficult unless the abscess is peripherally placed in the lung. Peribronchial sampling with a fibre-optic bronchoscope has been reported in adults but puncturing a lung abscess from the bronchi may release thick pus into the bronchial tree. When specimens are obtained they should be carefully cultured for both anaerobic and aerobic organisms.

DIFFERENTIAL DIAGNOSIS

Congenital pulmonary lesions

Bronchogenic and other congenital foregut cysts, cystadenomatous lesions or sequestered segments may all have to be considered. If any of these congenital abnormalities become infected it may be impossible to differentiate from a lung abscess unless previous films are available for comparison.

Infected hydatid cyst

Hydatid cysts may resemble lung abscesses and should be considered in endemic areas.

Solid lesions

If the lesion on chest X-ray is homogeneous without an air–fluid level, other solid lesions such as pneumonia, loculated empyema, pulmonary haematoma or tumour should be considered.

Hollow organs

A gas–fluid level seen in oesophagus, stomach or bowel may occasionally be misleading.

MANAGEMENT

Antibiotics are the mainstay of treatment. If the organism is unknown, broad-spectrum antibiotics which have good activity against *Staphylococcus aureus* should be chosen, e.g. flucloxacillin. If there is any suggestion that anaerobic organisms may be involved, metronidazole should be added. Treatment should be intravenous initially, but oral therapy, using probenecid to achieve good blood levels, can be used when the child is afebrile. Treatment should be continued for at least 6 weeks, otherwise there is a high rate of recurrence. In the majority of abscesses an air–fluid level is seen, suggesting that there is some communication with the bronchial tree. Drainage is probably provided by this route. Physiotherapy and postural drainage are conventional treatments but it is not known whether they are beneficial.

Most children respond well to antibiotic therapy. However, if fever persists for longer than 10 days despite what seems appropriate antibiotic therapy it is reasonable to consider means for obtaining cultures from the abscess cavity and providing drainage.[5] This can be attempted either peribronchially or percutaneously.[6] Very occasionally lobectomy may be the treatment of choice for a chronic abscess with persisting symptoms or one causing significant haemoptysis.

PROGRESS

When treatment is successful the first indication is resolution of the child's fever, which settles within a week in most children. The cavity then slowly closes, but full radiological clearance may take many months. In one adult study, 13% of cavities had disappeared in 2 weeks, 44% were gone within 4 weeks and 70% had disappeared by 3 months.[7]

Subsequent pulmonary function in children with primary lung abscess is entirely normal.[1]

COMPLICATIONS

Complications are extremely rare but the following have been reported:

- Empyema
- Haemoptysis (erosion of blood vessels)
- Rapid necrosis spreading through the lung (immunosuppressed)
- Persistent cavity which can become reinfected or colonized with aspergillus
- Embolic cerebral abscess
- Amyloidosis secondary to chronic suppuration.

REFERENCES

1 Asher M I, Spier S, Beland M, Coates A L, Beaudry P H. Primary lung abscess in childhood. Am J Dis Child 1982; 136: 491.
2 Tumwine J K. Lung abscess in children in Harare, Zimbabwe. East Afr Med J 1992; 69: 547–549.
3 Mark P H, Turner J A P. Lung abscess in childhood. Thorax 1968; 23: 216.
4 Brook I, Finegold S M. Bacteriology and therapy of lung abscess in children. J Pediatr 1979; 94: 10.
5 Powell K R. Primary pulmonary abscess. Am J Dis Child 1982; 136: 489.
6 Kosloske A M, Ball W S, Butler C, Musemeche C A. Drainage of paediatric lung abscess by cough, catheter, or complete resection. J Pediatr Surg 1986; 21: 596.
7 Weiss W. Cavity behaviour in acute, primary non specific lung abscess. Am Rev Respir Dis 1973; 108: 1273.

1B.9   Pulmonary tuberculosis

INTRODUCTION

Tuberculosis (TB) is a controversial subject, clouded by many fallacies (Table 1B.9.1). One popular misconception is that TB is no longer a significant medical problem. Unfortunately, however, TB is 'out of control' in the developing world and the rate of new cases in many western countries is increasing.[1,2] TB now infects more than one-third of the world's population and is the leading cause of death from a single infectious agent.[1]

Since TB in children can present in many different and subtle ways, the possibility of this infection must be borne in mind when evaluating any ill child, particularly the very young (0–4 years).[3] The confusing terminology regarding TB is summarized in Table 1B.9.2.[4]

DIFFERENCES BETWEEN 'ADULT' AND 'CHILDHOOD' TUBERCULOSIS

The key differences are listed in Table 1B.9.3. These can be summarized as follows. Children are suffering from their first exposure to *Mycobacterium tuberculosis*

Table 1B.9.1   Facts and fallacies about pulmonary TB in children

A. Fallacies
1. Children with primary TB are infectious to other children and/or hospital staff.
2. BCG vaccination results in subsequent inability to use Mantoux testing in that individual.
3. The minimum duration of treatment and/or chemoprophylaxis is 12 months.
4. Pyridoxine should be used in conjunction with isoniazid therapy in children.
5. Regular monitoring of liver function is necessary to detect/prevent the development of liver damage from anti-TB drug therapy in children.

B. Facts
1. Primary pulmonary TB in children is non-communicable. Children in paediatric hospitals are much more likely to be infected with *Mycobacterium tuberculosis* from adult hospital staff than the reverse.
2. Previous BCG vaccine does not affect the utility of subsequent Mantoux testing in that individual. The Mantoux reaction after BCG is generally small and wanes rapidly with time. The only exception to this is that with repeated use of BCG vaccines it is possible to have Mantoux greater than 10 mm, particularly if the repeat BCG was given recently.
3. The current recommended duration of drug therapy for both chemoprophylaxis and treatment of pulmonary tuberculosis is 6–9 months, provided the infective strain of *Mycobacterium tuberculosis* is sensitive to the first-line drugs (particularly isoniazid and rifampicin). The only exception to this is disseminated TB, where the minimum treatment period should be 12 months.
4. Pyridoxine is only recommended for adults receiving isoniazid. This is due to the fact that many adults, particularly those who have abused alcohol, have borderline liver function and pyridoxine deficiency and can develop symptoms of polyneuropathy unless pyridoxine is given.
5. Hepatotoxicity is uncommon from anti-TB drugs in childhood. The current recommendation is not to do serial liver function tests, but to do these only in the presence of symptoms (particularly jaundice).

Table 1B.9.2   Definitions/terminology

TB infection

Positive Mantoux test ONLY. No symptoms, no signs, and normal chest X-ray.

Infection, without disease. Also known as TB 'contact', Mantoux 'conversion' or 'subclinical' TB.

TB disease ('Tuberculosis')

Positive Mantoux test PLUS either abnormal chest X-ray or clinical symptoms, or clinical signs of pulmonary or extrapulmonary tuberculosis.

Also known as TUBERCULOSIS

In children, usually means 'complicated' primary TB or 'progressive' primary TB. Rarely, a disseminated form of TB (e.g., miliary TB, TB meningitis).

In adults usually means 'reactivation' TB ('active TB' or 'sputum-positive pulmonary TB').

Table 1B.9.3   Differences in adult versus paediatric pulmonary TB

	Adult	Child
Infection	Reactivation	Primary
No. of organisms	Large	Small
Bacteriology proof	Easy	Difficult
Infectivity	High	Very low
Risk of blood spread	Low	High (age 0–4 years)
Cause of lung lesion	Rampant infection	Immune response

and develop a 'primary' lung infection. The lung manifestations of this primary infection are predominantly those of delayed hypersensitivity to *M. tuberculosis* (cell-mediated immunity). The bacterial load is small, but the immunological reaction can be very marked. By contrast, adults are generally suffering from 'reactivation' of a previous primary infection. Adult TB is characterized by large numbers of *M. tuberculosis* and little immunological response.

EPIDEMIOLOGY

In 1993 the World Health Organization declared TB a 'global emergency'. In the developed world, TB is now making a resurgence, reversing the declining rates of previous decades.[5] Health care workers are particularly at risk. In the USA, the rate of new TB infection amongst medical students now exceeds 1% per year, and in some medical schools it is as high as 5% per year.[6] The explanations for the increase include the appearance of HIV infection, widespread migration and travel from underdeveloped (high-prevalence) countries to developed (low-prevalence) countries, the appearance of multi-resistant strains of *Mycobacterium tuberculosis*, and the dismantling of many of the previous public health surveillance measures for TB.

PATHOGENESIS

Children are infected with *Mycobacterium tuberculosis* when they come into contact with an adult who has sputum-positive, reactivation pulmonary TB. There are large numbers of microorganisms in the sputum of these adults, which are then inhaled by the child. The timetable and sequence of events in the child following contact are outlined in Figure 1B.9.1.[7] Once infected, the child will mount an immune response to the organisms. This results in a primary lung focus of which there are two components: a small parenchymal (subpleural) component and a regional lymph node (hilar node) component. Both components are small, asymptomatic and invisible on chest X-ray. Less commonly, there is progression of the primary complex, with increasing enlargement of either, or both, the parenchymal or hilar component. The pathogenesis of these complications of the primary is outlined in Figure 1B.9.2.[7] A complicated primary will produce symptoms, especially cough and fever. If bronchial obstruction occurs, wheeze and shortness of breath may result. Within 4–8 weeks of the initial infection, the child develops delayed hypersensitivity to *M. tuberculosis* and will have a positive Mantoux test (see below). Since complications of the primary complex occur after this time, there will be a marked local immunological response should there be sudden spillage of tubercular protein into airways or pleural cavity (see Fig. 1B.9.2).

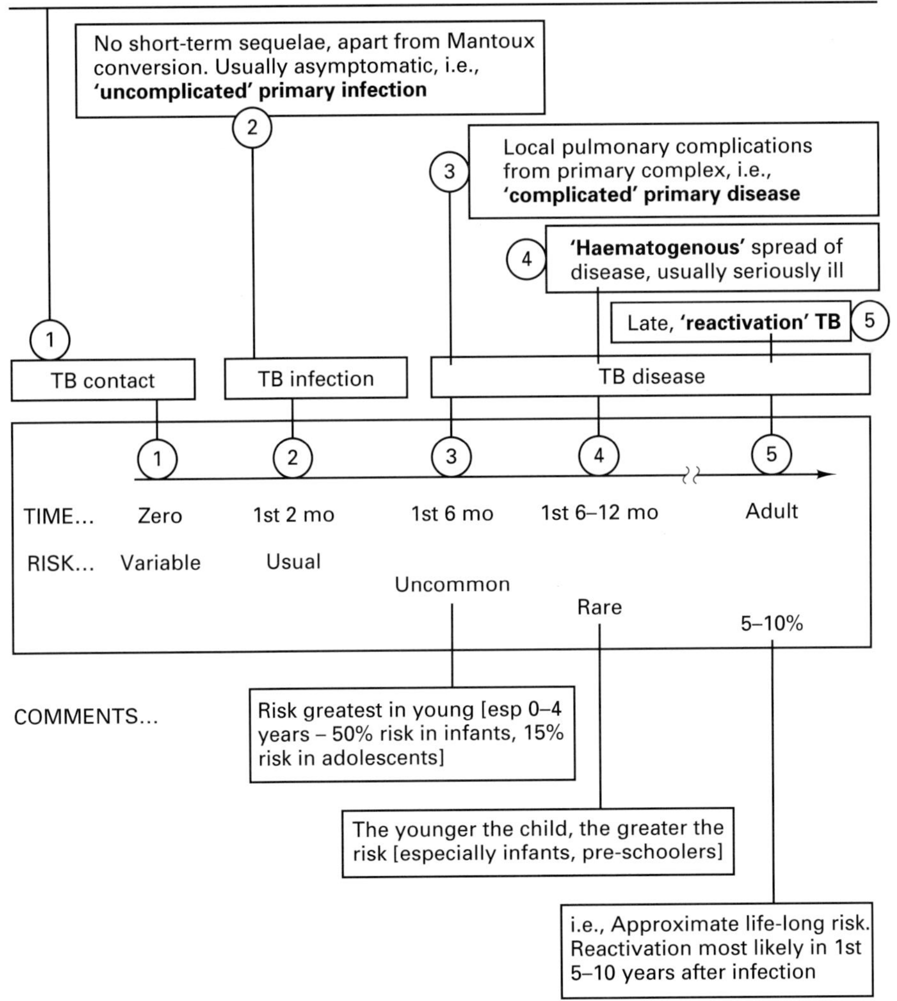

Fig. 1B.9.1   Sequence of events in a child, and usual timing, following contact with infectious (adult) TB.

1 HILAR LYMPH NODE COMPONENT

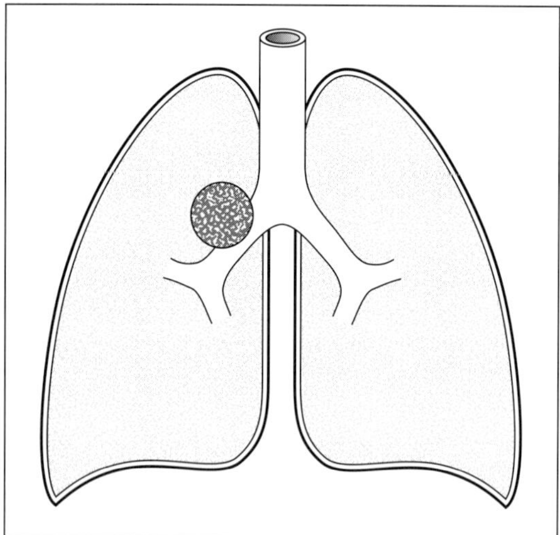

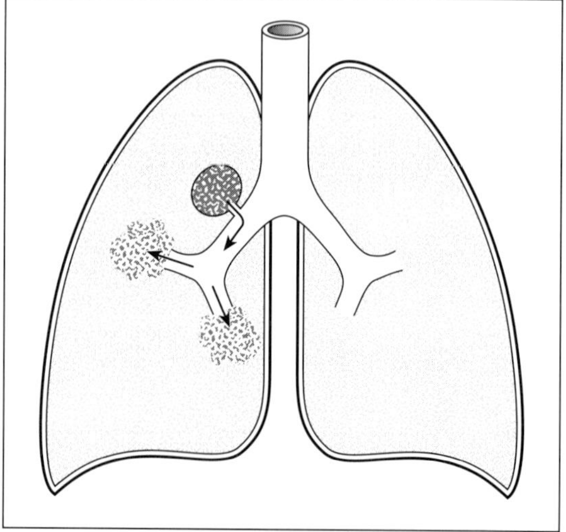

A **Obstruction of major bronchus.**
Causes cough, localised wheeze, and possible shortness of breath.

B **Rupture into major bronchus.**
Causes acute bronchitis, and possible broncho-pneumonia

2 LUNG PARENCHYMAL COMPONENT

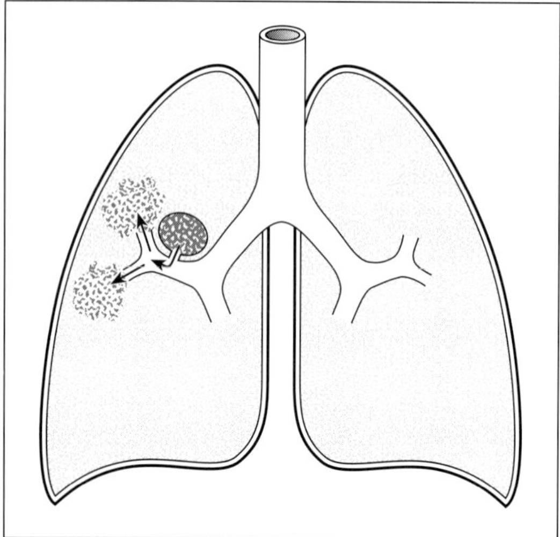

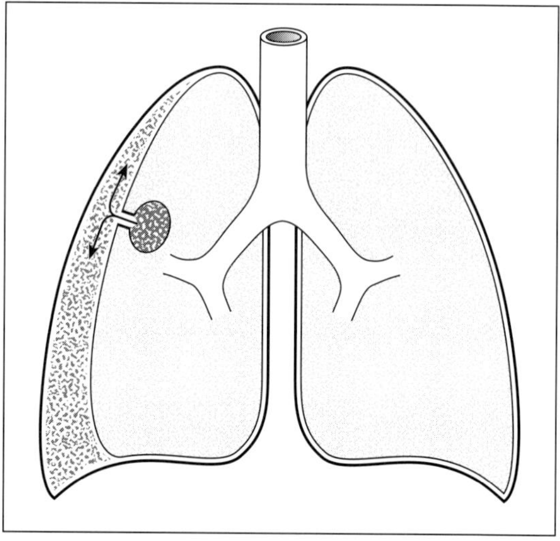

A **Rupture into peripheral bronchus.**
Causes peripheral bronchopneumonia.

B **Rupture into pleural cavity.**
Causes acute pleurisy with effusion.

Note : These complications of the primary complex occur **after** the development of delayed hypersensitivity to *Mycobacterium tuberculosis*. Thus, the response to the release of tubercular protein into the lung, or pleura, is due to a marked **hypersensitivity reaction**. Very few viable organisms are present.

Fig. 1B.9.2   Local complications of primary TB. **1** Hilar lymph node component. **A** Obstruction of major bronchus. Causes cough, localized wheeze and possible shortness of breath. **B** Rupture into major bronchus. Causes acute bronchitis and possible bronchopneumonia. **2** Lung parenchymal component. **A** Rupture into peripheral bronchus. Causes peripheral bronchopneumonia. **B** Rupture into pleural cavity. Causes acute pleurisy with effusion.

Rarely, the organisms will enter the bloodstream, resulting in disseminated ('haematogenous') tuberculosis. This is particularly likely to occur in infants and young children (0–4 years), with devastating results. Possible sequelae include miliary tuberculosis, tuberculous meningitis, or TB infection of bones, joints or kidneys.

However, the usual consequence of infection is an uncomplicated primary lung complex. This results in a small area of fibrosis (scarring), which may calcify over the subsequent 1–2 years, and become visible on chest X-ray. This is more commonly seen in the hilar component of the primary complex.

In the long term, there is an approximate 5–10% risk of reactivation of the healed primary complex.[8] This results in 'open', sputum-positive, cavitating, pulmonary TB, which is highly infectious. Reactivation is particularly likely to occur at the time of significant intercurrent illnesses, particularly those associated with weight loss, debility or the use of immunosuppressive drugs.

CLINICAL FEATURES

Uncomplicated primary TB infection in a child is most likely to be asymptomatic. Should there be progression (or a complication) of the lung primary, symptoms such as cough, wheeze, shortness of breath and fever are likely (Fig. 1B.9.2).

With haematogenous spread, the child may become acutely ill, particularly if miliary tuberculosis ensues. The usual source of the organisms into the bloodstream is a hilar lymph node. The characteristic symptoms are fever, weight loss and general debility (apathy, loss of appetite). Multiple small focal lung lesions produce a 'miliary' picture on chest X-ray. The miliary lung lesions do not usually cause any specific respiratory symptoms, and cough is an uncommon feature. On examination there may be hepatosplenomegaly and choroidal tubercles may be seen in retinal blood vessels. Without treatment, miliary TB will progress, with a high case fatality rate. Untreated cases are usually complicated by tuberculous meningitis.

Unlike bacterial meningitis, TB meningitis develops slowly and insidiously. The initial symptoms are vague, such as weight loss, night sweats and lethargy. Later, there is progression to the more typical symptoms and signs of meningeal irritation, namely headache, neck stiffness, convulsions, altered conscious level and raised intracranial pressure (bulging fontanelle in infants; blurred optic discs in older children). Lumbar puncture reveals a predominantly lymphocytic response with an elevated protein and low glucose level. Visible *Mycobacterium tuberculosis* (acid-fast bacilli) are seen in approximately a third of cases, while between 50% and 90% will grow *M. tuberculosis* on culture.[9] Approximately half of the children with TB meningitis have abnormalities visible on chest X-ray.

Diagnosis of tuberculous meningitis is difficult, and a high index of suspicion is essential for early recognition. Treatment must be commenced promptly if the disease is suspected. Tuberculous meningitis has a high morbidity and mortality, which is directly related to the delay in diagnosis and treatment.

DIAGNOSIS

Paediatric TB infection (and TB disease) rates are highest amongst those children who are in contact with adults from high-risk populations for tuberculosis (Table 1B.9.4). The greatest risk is in socially deprived, racial and ethnic minorities, particularly in children born in countries with a high prevalence of TB. Health

Table 1B.9.4 Risk of TB infection and TB disease

Increased risk of exposure to an infectious adult
Born overseas in high-prevalence region (Africa, South East Asia, India, South America)
Family contact
Lower socioeconomic groups, ethnic and racial minority groups

Increased likelihood of TB disease after infection
Infants and preschool children (age 0–4 years)
Malnutrition
Acquired immunodeficiency, e.g. HIV, post-measles
Immunosuppressive therapy (including oral corticosteroids)

---

care professionals are also at high risk for TB, with many acquiring the infection in medical school or during their hospital residency. Young age is a strong predictor for the development of TB disease following infection. Thus, the possibility of TB should be borne in mind when seeing children with a wide assortment of symptoms, particularly if they belong to a high-risk category.[5]

THE TUBERCULIN SKIN TEST (MANTOUX TEST)

The hallmark of primary infection with *Mycobacterium tuberculosis* is a positive tuberculin test.[10] Multiple puncture techniques (e.g. Heaf test) are no longer recommended because of poor repeatability and difficulty determining the exact dose injected.[1,4] Thus, the only currently recommended method is the Mantoux test. This is an intradermal test of delayed hypersensitivity to tuberculin. Either 5 or 10 units of purified protein derivative (PPD) tuberculin is generally used. Following injection, into the forearm, the diameter of skin induration (measured in millimetres) is read 48–72 h later.

Interpretation of the result is highly dependent on the population of children being tested (Table 1B.9.5).[5] If the child is at high risk of infection then anything greater than 5 mm should be considered a positive reaction. For those assessed to be at medium risk, 10 mm (or greater) is considered positive. If a child is unlikely to be infected with *Mycobacterium tuberculosis*, then a Mantoux test should not generally be performed. However, if the test is performed on children without a defined risk factor for tuberculous infection, a reaction of 15 mm is generally considered positive.

Table 1B.9.5 Mantoux 'cut-off' and 'risk' of tuberculosis infection[a]

High risk: positive > 5 mm
Close contacts of infectious adult (especially age 0–4 years)
HIV infection

Medium risk: positive > 10 mm
Overseas born from high TB prevalence regions
Socially deprived, ethnic or racial minorities
Other locally identified high-risk populations
Infants and young children (< 4 years)

Low risk: positive > 15 mm
No risk factors (should not generally be Mantoux tested)

---

[a] *Note*: Previous BCG vaccination should generally be ignored when applying these rules.

EFFECT OF PRIOR BCG VACCINATION

The above recommendations for assessing Mantoux skin test reactions do not take into account prior BCG vaccination. As yet, there is no totally reliable method of distinguishing a tuberculin reaction caused by BCG vaccine from that due to *Mycobacterium tuberculosis*. However, most children who receive BCG vaccine (particularly when vaccinated in the newborn period) are unlikely to have induration exceeding 5–10 mm as a result of BCG vaccine alone.[11,12] Further, there is progressive waning of the induration within several years of the vaccine being given. Thus, if the risk of TB infection is considered high, then the Mantoux result should be read according to Table 1B.9.5 and any prior BCG vaccination should be ignored. The only exception is if BCG was given recently, and it was a repeat BCG vaccination.[13]

An additional consideration in interpreting the Mantoux size is the possibility of non-tuberculous mycobacterial infection ('atypical' or 'anonymous' TB). These organisms are prevalent in many regions of the world. Infection in childhood generally causes localized, unilateral cervical adenitis. These organisms very rarely infect the lungs of immunologically competent children. Children with 'atypical' mycobacterial infection of a cervical node will usually have a weakly positive Mantoux reaction (to tuberculin), but a substantially larger reaction to atypical strains (e.g. 'Batty' Mantoux, avian, or 'MAIS complex' Mantoux). Therefore, when there is a diagnostic dilemma, dual 'Mantoux' testing with *Mycobacterium tuberculosis* and an 'atypical' organism is appropriate.

BACTERIOLOGICAL PROOF OF DIAGNOSIS

Since there are very few organisms present in children with pulmonary TB, it is usually necessary to rely on the results of cultures and sensitivities of specimens taken from the adult source of infection. If, after contact tracing, a source of infection cannot be found, then microbiological proof may be possible using early-morning gastric washings, bronchoscopic specimens (bronchoalveolar lavage), or induced sputum. This is especially indicated if a drug-resistant strain is considered likely.

TREATMENT

There are two forms of treatment of TB in children: chemoprophylaxis and chemotherapy. For the child who has had TB infection only, chemoprophylaxis (or preventive therapy) is warranted. This is given to prevent subsequent reactivation of TB many years later, is a highly effective measure, and an important public health initiative to reduce TB in the future. All children considered to have a positive tuberculin test (Table 1B.9.5) should be given chemoprophylaxis. The usual recommendation is isoniazid only for either 6 or 9 months.[5,8] Isoniazid is given in a dose of 10–20 mg/kg per day (maximum daily dose 300 mg). Significant side-effects from isoniazid in children are uncommon (Table 1B.9.6).

Children with pulmonary TB disease (Fig. 1B.9.1) should be treated along similar lines to adults with pulmonary TB, namely, a 6-month regimen consisting of three or four drugs depending upon the child's age (Table 1B.9.7). All three (or four) antituberculous drugs are given for 2 months, then two drugs (isoniazid and rifampicin) are given for 4 months. Alternatively, a 9-month course of two drugs (isoniazid and rifampicin) is effective.[5,8] The appropriate choice and dosage

Table 1B.9.6   Anti-TB drugs for paediatric use

Drug	Dose	Comments
Isoniazid	10–20 mg/kg per day Max. daily = 300 mg	Single daily dose No need for pyridoxine [a]S/E: skin rashes and hepatotoxicity (rare in children)
Rifampicin	10–20 mg/kg per day Max. daily = 600 mg	Single daily dose Colours body fluids orange [a]S/E: gastrointestinal upset; skin rashes and hepatotoxicity (rarely)
Pyrazinamide	15–30 mg/kg per day	[a]S/E: gastrointestinal intolerance; skin rashes; hepatotoxicity
Ethambutol	15–25 mg/kg per day	NOT to be given to children unless visual acuity can be measured (age approx. 7–8 years) [a]S/E: ocular effects (blurred vision, scotomata, colour-blindness).

[a]S/E: commonest side-effects.

Table 1B.9.7   Treatment options

Disease category and drugs[a]	Duration (months)
TB infection (i.e. chemoprophylaxis) Isoniazid	6 months (9 months, USA)
TB disease (i.e. chemotherapy)	

● Pulmonary TB
   Option 1: isoniazid and rifampicin
   Option 2:
       (a) I + R + E + Z
 	
       (b) I + R + Z
	6–9 months
	
	(a) 2 months all four drugs, then 4 months I + R only
	(b) 2 months all three drugs, then 4 months I + R only

● Disseminated TB Choose either option 2(a) or 2(b) above, depending upon child's age. Total duration of treatment should be 12 months	Three (or four) drugs for 2 months, then I + R for 10 months

[a]I, isoniazid; R, rifampicin; E, ethambutol; Z, pyrazinamide.
[b]Choose 2(a) only if age > 7 years.

of these medications and the common side-effects are listed in Tables 1B.9.6 and 1B.9.7. For disseminated (miliary) disease and TB meningitis, at least 12 months therapy is recommended. Many children require supervised medication to ensure compliance. Since these children are commonly from ethnic minorities, with poor English, and low socioeconomic status, the likelihood of non-adherence to prolonged drug therapy is high. Supervision is easier if a twice-weekly schedule of medications is used, rather than daily. Appropriate regimens are available for this purpose using the same drugs (but in slightly higher doses than listed in Table 1B.9.6).

The usual, first-line anti-TB drugs are relatively free of side-effects in children. However, ethambutol should not be used unless visual acuity can be reliably monitored. Thus, it is recommended that ethambutol be avoided in children less than 7 years of age. Rifampicin, isoniazid and pyrazinamide are all capable of producing hepatotoxicity. However, since it is uncommon, it is not recommended that routine liver function tests be performed. Rather, the child should be reviewed clinically, and if there is any evidence of hepatic complication (especially jaundice) investigations should be performed and the drug therapy revised accordingly.

Systemic corticosteroids are currently advocated for children with TB meningitis[9] and for progressive primary pulmonary TB where there is significant bronchial obstruction[14] (Fig. 1B.9.2 (1A)). The usual dose is 1–2 mg/kg per day as prednisolone (or equivalent).

PREVENTION

The role of BCG vaccination in preventing TB has been surrounded by controversy. The effectiveness of BCG vaccine in various trials throughout the world has ranged from no protection to 80% protection. A recent meta-analysis[15] demonstrated that BCG vaccine has reasonable efficacy (Table 1B.9.8). While BCG vaccine reduces the risk of TB by approximately 50%, protection from the more serious forms of disseminated TB is substantially greater. However, unless the annual TB conversion rate (new infections) exceeds 1%, BCG vaccine is not considered cost effective.[16]

To reduce the burden of TB in the future, it may be necessary to reintroduce TB surveillance in high-risk communities. This should be linked to widespread chemoprophylaxis of TB infection, to reduce the prevalence of TB disease in the future. Thus, control of TB will need to be a multi-faceted approach combining Mantoux surveillance of appropriate groups, BCG vaccine, chemoprophylaxis (preferably under supervision) and effective treatment of those with TB disease. Unfortunately, eradication of TB does not appear to be feasible at present, given the worldwide prevalence of the disease.

Table 1B.9.8 Efficacy of BCG vaccine

Protection against DISSEMINATED TB = 80%
Protection against DEATH from TB = 70%
Protection against TB MENINGITIS = 65%
Protection against TB INFECTION = 50%

CONCLUSIONS/SUMMARY

Tuberculosis has not disappeared. It must be considered in the differential diagnosis of a variety of clinical presentations in young children, particularly infants and preschoolers with fever and cough. A high index of suspicion is essential, particularly when dealing with children who belong to well-known high-risk categories for TB. In a very young child, if tuberculosis is suspected treatment should be commenced forthwith, particularly if one of the disseminated forms of TB is considered possible. If subsequent investigations disprove the diagnosis, TB therapy can be ceased without any adverse consequences.

REFERENCES

1 Godlee F. Tuberculosis: 'a global emergency'. Br Med J 1993; 306: 1147.
2 American Policy Statement of Pediatrics. Screening for tuberculosis in infants and children. Pediatrics 1994; 93: 131–134.
3 Vallejo J G, Ong L T, Starke J R. Clinical features, diagnosis, and treatment of tuberculosis in infants. Pediatrics 1994; 94: 1–7.
4 American Thoracic Society: Official Statement. Diagnostic standards and classification of TB. Am Rev Respir Dis 1990; 142: 725–735.
5 Starke J R. Resurgence of TB in children. J Pediatr 1992; 120: 839–852.
6 Nolan C. Tuberculosis in health care professionals: assessing and accepting the risk. Ann Intern Med 1994; 120: 964–965.
7 Phelan P, Landau L, Olinsky A. Tuberculosis in children. In: Respiratory illness in children, 3rd ed. London: Blackwell, 1990: Ch 2.
8 American Thoracic Society: Official Statement. Treatment of tuberculosis and tuberculosis infection in adults and children. Am J Respir Crit Care Med 1994; 149: 1359–1374.
9 Newton R W. Tuberculosis meningitis. Arch Dis Child 1994; 70: 364–366.
10 Cetron K. Tuberculin positive children. Thorax 1992; 47: 768–769.
11 Ormerod L, Palmer C. Tuberculin reactivity after neonatal percutaneous BCG immunisation. Arch Dis Child 1993; 69: 155.
12 Tan K K. Significance of the tuberculin test in Singapore. Singapore Med J 1989; 30: 159–163.
13 Menzies R. Effect of BCG vaccination on tuberculin reactivity. Am Rev Respir Dis 1992; 145: 621–625.
14 Toppet M. Corticosteroids in primary TB with bronchial obstruction. Arch Dis Child 1990; 65: 1222–1226.
15 Colditz G, Brewer T, Berkey C, Wilson M et al. Efficacy of BCG vaccine in the prevention of tuberculosis: meta-analysis of the published literature. JAMA 1994; 271: 698–702.
16 Conway S. BCG vaccination in children. Routine vaccination of schoolchildren is not cost effective and could be stopped. Br Med J 1990; 301: 1059–1060.

A. Thomson

1B.10 Bronchiectasis

INTRODUCTION

Bronchiectasis is the description given to a condition where there is chronic dilatation of one or more bronchi. It is the end result of a number of disorders where there is chronic bronchial sepsis.

EPIDEMIOLOGY

In the developed world, with ready access to antibiotics for respiratory infection, vaccination against pertussis and measles, and improved socioeconomic conditions, the prevalence of bronchiectasis has fallen. True prevalence figures for the 1990s are unknown but it has become a rare disorder in general paediatric practice, and in a recent report only 1% of tertiary referrals with respiratory disease had bronchiectasis (excluding cystic fibrosis).[1]

PATHOGENESIS

It seems clear from experimental work that both obstruction to a bronchus and infection distal to the obstruction are essential requirements for the production of bronchiectasis.[2,3] It is suggested that the airway wall may be damaged by both the direct effects of microorganisms and the secondary effects of the host's inflammatory response.[4]

PATHOLOGY

Macroscopic

Dilatation of subsegmental airways is found. The airways may appear flabby or tortuous and may be partially or totally obstructed by secretions.

Microscopic

There is chronic inflammation of the bronchial wall and replacement of ciliated epithelium with squamous or columnar epithelium. The elastin layer of the bronchial wall is deficient, the muscle and cartilage often show signs of destruction and there is a variable amount of fibrosis. There are peribronchial pneumonic changes and areas of atelectasis.

Immunopathology

T lymphocyte number is increased in epithelial, lamina propria and submucosal layers. These cells are mainly suppressor/cytotoxic CD8-positive activated cells. Activated macrophages are also present.

AETIOLOGY

Bronchiectasis is the end result of a number of disorders in the lung, any of which can lead to obstruction of the bronchi with bronchial infection distal to the obstruction (Table 1B.10.1).

The most common cause of bronchiectasis is postinfective bronchial damage. In a large series, reported in 1966, 33% of cases were seen after a pneumonic illness and a further 14% after measles or pertussis.[5] A much smaller series, reported in 1978, attributed 38% of cases to pneumonia and 17% to measles,[6] and recently 12 of 41 cases were reported after pneumonia, two after measles and one after pertussis.[1] Adenovirus (particularly type 1, 3, 4, 7 and 21) can cause a severe pneumonia with a high incidence of residual lung damage including bronchiectasis.[7]

Table 1B.10.1   Causes of bronchiectasis

1. Postinfective bronchial damage
     Pneumonia (particularly adenovirus)
     Measles
     Pertussis
     Tuberculosis
2. Secondary to mechanical obstruction
     Inhaled foreign body
     Aspiration
     Postinfective bronchial stenosis (TB)
3. Mucociliary clearance defects
     Primary or secondary ciliary dyskinesia
4. Cystic fibrosis
5. Immunodeficiency
     Panhypogammaglobulinaemia
     Selective IgG deficiencies
6. Congenital abnormalities
     Deficiency of bronchial cartilage
     Pulmonary sequestration

DIAGNOSIS

The diagnosis is suggested by the history of a chronic cough with purulent sputum. A small proportion (~10%) of children will report haemoptysis, and a similar proportion wheeze. Rarely there is a history of episodic fever, malaise and dull chest pain with minimal sputum production. In many children and adults (~30%) there is associated chronic upper respiratory tract symptoms.

Examination of the chest may be entirely normal, especially if performed shortly after expectoration. However, a localized area of respiratory crackles is an important sign if found. Clubbing may not be present with early disease but is an indicator of chronic intrathoracic sepsis.

INVESTIGATION

Investigation has two components: (1) To confirm the diagnosis and to define the extent of the disease; and (2) to seek a cause.

Confirm the diagnosis

Sputum culture   There may be a variety of low-virulence organisms but one often predominates.

Uncapsulated non-typable *Haemophilus influenzae* is the commonest, *Streptococcus pneumoniae* is frequent and *Pseudomonas aeruginosa* (usually mucoid) is not uncommon. Sputum should be cultured for acid-fast bacilli.

Sputum volume/weight

It may be helpful to establish the daily volume of sputum produced.

Lung function tests

Most children have entirely normal lung function. Some have evidence of airflow obstruction with air trapping and this may be reversible with bronchodilator treatment.

Chest X-ray

Severe bronchiectasis may be seen on a plain film (Fig. 1B.10.1A). Thickened bronchial walls are seen with volume loss and crowding of vessels in affected areas and sometimes the cystic lesions of saccular bronchiectasis are clear. Early bronchiectasis cannot be excluded on a plain film.

High-resolution computed tomographic scanning

This has become the investigation of choice for confirming the site of bronchiectasis and defining the extent of the disease.[8] It has largely replaced bronchography.

Seek a cause

The history may give a clue to the aetiology. If the history is from birth or early infancy, then congenital abnormalities and inherited disorders such as cystic fibrosis should be considered. An associated history of chronic serous otitis media ± nasal discharge from early life suggests primary ciliary dyskinesia as a possible cause. The chest X-ray may reveal the diagnosis. Investigations may then include:

1. Sweat test.
2. Serum immunoglobulins including IgG subsets and other immunology.[1]
3. Mucociliary clearance assessment:
   a. If the patient is of school age, use the saccharin test as a screen (Appendix 1).
   b. Nasal ciliary brushing for ciliary beat frequency and ultrastructure.
4. Fibre-optic bronchoscopy:
   a. To exclude bronchial obstruction.
   b. Bronchogram of selected area by direct injection of contrast media is possible.

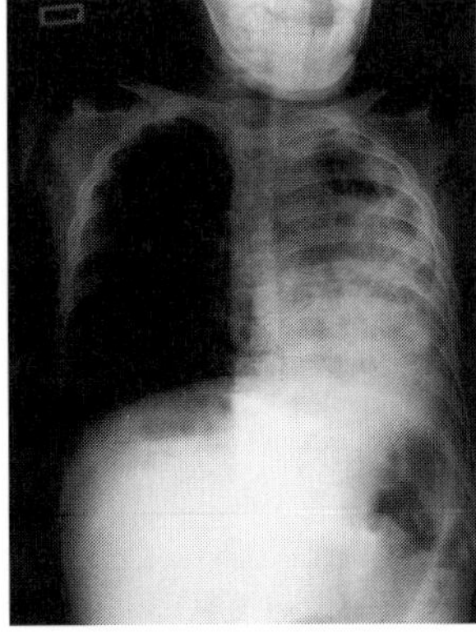
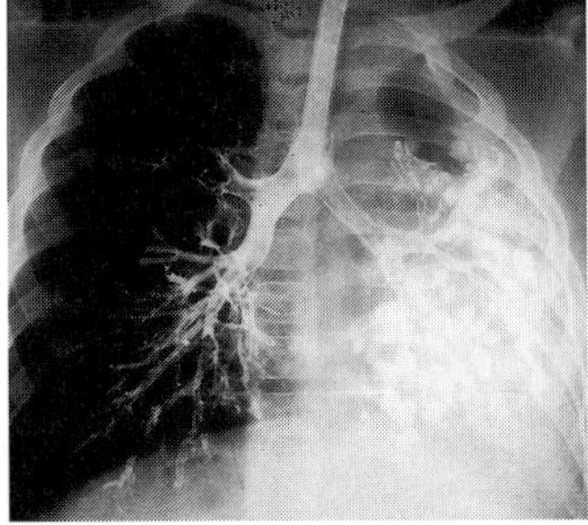

Fig. 1B.10.1 **A** Bronchiectasis. Plain chest radiograph showing left lung collapse. **B** Bronchiogram showing extensive left-sided bronchiectasis.

MANAGEMENT

1. Treat a treatable cause, e.g. immunodeficiency.
2. Consider surgery as a cure for localized disease. Surgery is the only curative treatment for bronchiectasis and should be considered if it is clear that there is localized, resectable disease with no detectable underlying disease likely to cause recurrence.
3. Medical management consists of treatment to prevent further infection and to improve bronchial clearance:

Antibiotics

Antibiotics should be used promptly and in high dosage for any respiratory exacerbations. Some patients find it beneficial to be on long-term continuous oral antibiotic therapy. Other strategies are continuous nebulized antibiotics or intermittent intravenous antibiotic courses. The clinical disease varies much from patient to patient, so that it is probably best to adopt an individual treatment regime. The aim is to keep infection and hence further lung destruction to a minimum.

Physiotherapy

The importance of regular physiotherapy cannot be over-emphasized. Physiotherapy assists bronchial clearance and should be performed at least twice daily. In small children physiotherapy consists of classical postural drainage and percussion but as children become older they can be taught regimes such as the active cycle of breathing and/or use of positive expiratory pressure (PEP) masks which allow them to be completely independent.

Bronchodilators

Where there is evidence of reversible airflow obstruction, optimal lung function should be obtained using bronchodilators and corticosteroids.

4. Long-term follow-up to detect any increase in symptoms, spread of the disease or deterioration in lung function.

OUTCOME

Severe or rapid progression of bronchiectasis is rare (other than in cystic fibrosis). A 20-year follow-up study from 1961 reported that there was a tendency for symptoms in medically treated patients to improve in the teenage years and then remain stable.[9] A more recent study showed that 91% of medically treated patients were unchanged over a 10-year period, but patients suitable for surgery did better, with 40% completely well and 60% improved.[10] It is likely that early diagnosis and prompt treatment will improve these figures further.

REFERENCES

1 Nikolaizik W H, Warner J O. Aetiology of chronic suppurative lung disease. Arch Dis Child 1994; 70: 141–142.
2 Tannenberg J, Pinner M. Atelectasis and bronchiectasis: an experimental study concerning their relationship. J Thorac Surg 1942; 11: 571.
3 Lapa e Silva J R, Guerreiro D, Noble B, Poulter L W, Cole P J. Immunopathology of experimental bronchiectasis. Am J Respir Cell Mol Biol 1989; 1: 297.
4 Cole P J. Host–microbial interactions in chronic respiratory disease. In: Reeves D,

Geddes A, eds. Recent advances in infection, Vol 3. Edinburgh: Churchill Livingstone, 1989: p 141.

5 Glauser E M, Cook C D, Harris G B C. Bronchiectasis: a review of 187 cases of children with follow up pulmonary function studies in 58. Acta Paediatr Scand (Suppl) 1966; 165: 1.

6 Fernald G W. Bronchiectasis in childhood: a 10 year survey of cases treated at North Carolina Memorial Hospital. NC Med J 1978; 39: 368–372.

7 Simila S, Linna O, Lanning P. Heikkinen E, Ala-Houhala M. Chronic lung disease caused by adenovirus type 7: a ten year follow up study. Chest 1981; 80: 127–131.

8 Kornreich L, Horev G, Ziv N, Grunebaum M. Bronchiectasis in children: assessment by CT. Pediatr Radiol 1993; 23: 120–123.

9 Field C. Bronchiectasis: a long-term follow-up of medical and surgical cases from childhood. Arch Dis Child 1961; 36: 587–603.

10 Wilson J F, Decker A M. The surgical management of childhood bronchiectasis. Ann Surg 1982; 195: 354–363.

11 Stanley P, McWilliam L, Greenstone M, Mackay I S, Cole P J. Efficacy of a saccharin test for screening to detect abnormal mucociliary clearance. Br J Dis Chest 1984; 78: 62.

APPENDIX 1: ASSESSMENT OF MUCOCILIARY CLEARANCE BY SACCHARIN TEST[11]

1. Blow the nose.
2. Check the patient can taste saccharin by placing a little on the tongue.
3. Place a 1 mm cube of saccharin under direct vision on the inferior turbinate on an unobstructed nostril 1 cm behind its anterior margin.
4. Sit with head in normal position. Do not sniff, sneeze, eat or drink.
5. The time from placing the particle to the patient tasting the saccharin is measured (normally < 30 min).
6. If the time is > 60 min there is a gross defect in mucus transport and further investigation is necessary.

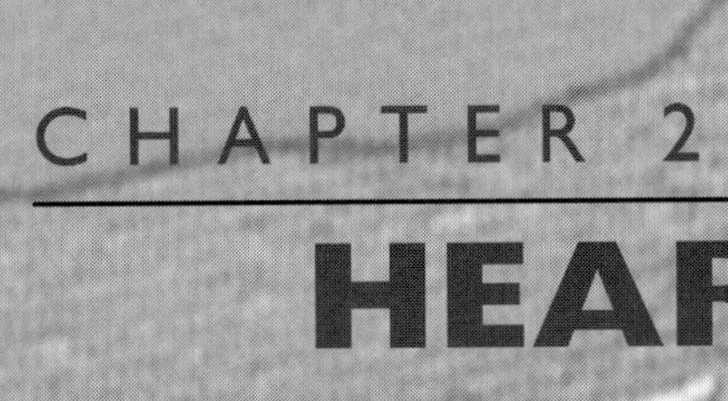

CHAPTER 2

HEART

2.1. Infections involving the heart

S. T. Shulman   W. Hanekom

2.1   Infections involving the heart

INTRODUCTION

Several infections directly or indirectly lead to important cardiac disorders. These include acute rheumatic fever (ARF) following group A streptococcal pharyngo-tonsillitis, which may result in chronic rheumatic heart disease (RHD). Infective endocarditis, usually occurring in the setting of pre-existing cardiac disease and/or cardiac surgery, is an important illness. Acute myocarditis and pericarditis are most often viral in aetiology, and each can be associated with substantial morbidity and mortality. Kawasaki disease, which leads primarily to coronary artery abnormalities, sometimes with serious complications, is discussed in Chapter 11.

ACUTE RHEUMATIC FEVER AND RHEUMATIC HEART DISEASE

Epidemiology

In the early decades of the twentieth century, ARF was an extraordinarily common childhood illness, and resultant RHD accounted for much morbidity and mortality. From 1925 to 1950, ARF was the leading cause of death in Americans 5–19 years of age and the leading cause of heart disease below the age of 40 years. There was a very striking predilection for ARF to afflict individuals from lower socioeconomic classes, directly paralleling tuberculosis. Coincident with less crowded living conditions, improved sanitation and general societal improvements, ARF in the developed world declined steadily throughout the twentieth century, especially following the Second World War. This decline clearly began before both Lancefield's classification of streptococci in 1933 and antimicrobial therapy. In addition, a slower but highly significant decline in death rates from chronic RHD has occurred. By 1980, very low rates of ARF were documented in many areas of Western Europe and the USA. The severity of ARF also decreased substantially during this period, antedating the widespread use of penicillin or corticosteriods.

ARF was thought to have virtually disappeared from the USA by the early 1980s, but an unexpected resurgence of cases with classic manifestations was noted in several areas of the USA beginning in 1985–1986. That these were focal outbreaks was suggested by a nationwide survey indicating slowly declining numbers of hospitalized ARF patients from 1984 to 1990. This pattern suggests that highly rheumatogenic strains of group A streptococci in a region may account for focal outbreaks against a background of declining endemic cases. Group A streptococci from ARF outbreak areas tended to be highly mucoid (heavily encapsulated) strains of serotypes previously linked epidemiologically to ARF, including M1, M3, M5, M6 and M18. By 1994, ARF rates had returned to baseline low levels in almost all areas of the USA.

Several epidemiological features are highly characteristic of ARF. The acute illness primarily affects school-age children 5–15 years old, being much less common in younger children and in adults. There is a clear peak occurrence in spring. ARF does not follow group A streptococcal skin infection, but exclusively occurs after untreated group A streptococcal infection of the upper respiratory tract. Both sexes are affected equally, with some tendency for multiple cases in an extended family. The recent US outbreaks uniquely lacked the classic association with lower socioeconomic status. Racial differences also affect the prevalence of ARF, as shown by the much higher attack rates in the New Zealand Maori and Pacific Islander population compared to the remainder of the New Zealand population, in proportions far exceeding that accounted for by socioeconomic factors.

Pathogenesis

ARF results from an interaction between group A streptococci and a genetically susceptible host, but details concerning both host and bacterial factors remain obscure. Strains of group A streptococci clearly differ in their rheumatogenic potential, with more rheumatogenic strains being rich in M-protein, heavily encapsulated, serum opacity factor negative and often of specific M-types noted above. The concept of a genetic predisposition to ARF is supported by a limited number of family studies, and associations with HLA-DR antigens and two possible non-HLA B cell allotypic markers.

The lack of an adequate animal model for ARF has contributed to the difficulty of proving specific immunopathogenetic mechanisms. The clinical similarity of ARF to other immunopathogenetic illnesses, the latent period between streptococcal infection and ARF, and the antigenicity of many streptococcal products and constituents support an immunopathogenesis. Immunological cross-reactivities between group A streptococcal components and mammalian tissues further suggest that 'molecular mimicry' is a central feature of the immunopathogenesis.

Clinical features

Because no clinical or laboratory finding is pathognomonic for ARF, T. Duckett Jones established guidelines to aid in its diagnosis in 1944. The Jones Criteria as revised in 1992 by the American Heart Association are shown in Table 2.1.1 and are now used only to diagnose the initial attack of ARF. ARF can be diagnosed

Table 2.1.1   Jones Criteria for diagnosis of first attack of rheumatic fever

I   Major criteria
  A. Carditis
  B. Polyarthritis
  C. Chorea
  D. Erythema marginatum
  E. Subcutaneous nodules

II   Minor criteria
  A. Clinical findings
    1. Arthralgia
    2. Fever
  B. Laboratory findings
    1. Elevated acute-phase reactants (ESR, C-reactive protein)
    2. Prolonged P–R interval

III Supporting evidence of antecedent group A streptococcal infection
  A. Positive throat culture or rapid antigen test *or*
  B. Elevated or rising streptococcal antibody titre

using the Jones Criteria when a patient fulfils two major criteria, or one major and two minor criteria, with the absolute requirement for evidence (microbiological or serological) of a recent group A streptococcal infection. Patients with pure Sydenham's chorea may not fulfil the Jones Criteria, often lacking fever and elevated acute-phase reactants.

ARF typically develops 2–4 weeks after acute streptococcal pharyngitis, and pharyngitis is no longer present. In one-third, history of a specific pharyngitis illness cannot be elicited at the time of presentation with ARF. As Osler noted in 1892, one of the most characteristic features of ARF is its propensity to recur. Those who have had an attack of ARF are susceptible to recurrent attacks following reinfection of the upper respiratory tract by group A streptococci, and therefore they require long-term continuous antistreptococcal prophylaxis to prevent recurrences (see below).

Major manifestations

Migratory polyarthritis

This occurs in about 75% of ARF patients, classically involving larger joints, particularly the knees, ankles, wrists and elbows. Involvement of the spine, the small joints of the hands and feet, or hips is rather infrequent. Arthritis (defined as objective evidence of joint inflammation) is often the earliest manifestation of ARF. Affected joints and periarticular tissues are very tender, generally hot, red and swollen, and pain may precede the other findings, appearing disproportionate to the objective findings. Most characteristic is migratory arthritic involvement, so that an involved joint becomes normal within 1–3 days without treatment, as one or more other large joints become inflamed. Monoarthritis is unusual unless anti-inflammatory therapy has been started prematurely, aborting the progression of polyarthritis. Very characteristic of the arthritis of ARF is its dramatic response to even small doses of salicylates. The lack of a prompt and dramatic response to salicylates raises substantial doubt about the diagnosis of ARF. The arthritis of ARF is not deforming. Synovial fluid in ARF yields 10 000–100 000 WBC/mm^3, with a predominance of neutrophils, protein about 4 g/l, normal glucose and good mucin clot. Frequently an inverse relationship exists between the severity of arthritis and cardiac involvement in ARF. Often, the most important diagnostic manoeuvre in a child with fever and arthritis suspected possibly to have ARF is to withhold salicylates in order to allow the migratory polyarthritis to manifest.

Carditis

Carditis occurs in 50–60% of ARF, and resultant chronic RHD accounts for essentially all of the long-term morbidity and mortality associated with ARF. Rheumatic carditis is characterized by pancarditis, with inflammation of myocardium, pericardium and endocardium, and varies in severity from a fulminant, potentially fatal, exudative pancarditis to very mild transient cardiac involvement. Endocarditis, manifested by one or more cardiac murmurs of valvar insufficiency, is always present with rheumatic carditis, while pericarditis and myocarditis are much more variable. Patients with myocarditis and/or pericarditis, without evidence of endocarditis, rarely if every suffer from ARF. Isolated mitral valve disease or aortic and mitral disease comprise the vast majority of RHD. The threat of chronic rheumatic valvular disease as a sequel to an attack of ARF, and worsening RHD with recurrent attacks, makes ARF a serious illness. During the acute and convalescent phases of ARF, valvulitis and valvular insufficiency occur, with valvular stenosis developing only years or decades later. In developing areas of the world, mitral stenosis and aortic stenosis develop sooner after ARF and may occur in young children. RHD predisposes patients to infective endocarditis (see below).

Acute rheumatic carditis is manifested by tachycardia and murmurs of valvar insufficiency, with or without transient rhythm disturbances reflecting myocardial involvement, or a friction rub, muffled heart tones and/or tamponade reflecting pericarditis. Moderate to severe rheumatic carditis results in cardiomegaly and congestive heart failure with hepatomegaly, peripheral oedema and pulmonary oedema. Echocardiographic findings include pericardial effusion, decreased ventricular contractility, and aortic and/or mitral regurgitation.

Chorea

Sydenham's chorea, also known as St Vitus dance, occurs in 10–15% of patients with ARF. This manifests as emotional lability, incoordination, poor school performance, uncontrollable choreoathetoid movements and facial grimacing, all frequently exacerbated by stress. Chorea occasionally is unilateral, and movements disappear with sleep. The onset of chorea is often insidious. Chorea usually begins many months after the inciting acute streptococcal infection and may develop some months following the onset of arthritis or carditis. Although very distressing, Sydenham's chorea rarely if ever leads to permanent neurological sequelae. However, as many as 25% of chorea patients ultimately develop chronic RHD because of recurrent attacks of ARF, emphasizing the need for continuous antistreptococcal prophylaxis. Clinical manoeuvres to elicit chorea include the milkmaid's grip with irregular contractions of the hand muscles, spooning and pronation of the hands when the patient's arms are extended, and wormian tongue movements upon protrusion. An association between Sydenham's chorea and obsessive-compulsive personality characteristics and behaviour has been described recently.

Erythema marginatum

This is a characteristic but rare rash of ARF, consisting of erythematous, serpiginous, macular lesions that are non-pruritic and have pale centres. Erythema marginatum is seen in fewer than 3% of patients with ARF, occurs primarily on the trunk and extremities but never on the face, and is accentuated by warming the skin.

Subcutaneous nodules

These are firm, approximately 1 cm nodules seen in 1% of ARF patients that are palpated along the extensor surfaces of tendons near bony prominences. Patients with these nodules usually have significant RHD.

Minor manifestations

These are less specific clinical or laboratory criteria commonly present in ARF. The two clinical minor manifestations are (1) arthralgia, i.e. subjective joint pain without objective arthritis, utilized only in the absence of polyarthritis as a major manifestation, and (2) fever, typically 39°C or greater.

Laboratory minor manifestations include (1) elevated acute-phase reactants such as the erythrocyte sedimentation rate and C-reactive protein, and (2) prolonged P–R interval on electrocardiogram (first-degree heart block). Prospective studies have demonstrated that prolonged P–R intervals per se do not correlate with other manifestations of carditis nor predict long-term cardiac sequelae of ARF.

Recent streptococcal infection

Because of the interval between pharyngitis and ARF, a positive throat culture or rapid streptococcal antigen test provides evidence of recent streptococcal infection in only 10–20% of cases. Residual pharyngitis is not present; therefore, the diagnosis of ARF generally requires demonstration of elevated antibody titres to group A streptococci , usually to extracellular products such as anti-streptolysin-O (ASO), anti-deoxyribonuclease B (anti-DNaseB), anti-hyaluronidase, and anti-streptokinase. Antibody responses peak approximately 3 weeks after the inciting infection, so that ARF generally coincides with peak responses. Patients with pure Sydenham's chorea may present when antibody titres have returned to normal.

Two important points should be noted regarding the interpretation of streptococcal antibody tests. First, an elevated streptococcal antibody titre may be unrelated to the particular illness in question. This is most often true in children, many of whom have streptococcal impetigo in the summer or unrelated streptococcal pharyngitis during the winter/spring months. Therefore, the Jones Criteria should be used to establish the diagnosis of ARF. Secondly, only 80–85% of ARF patients manifest elevated titres of a specific antibody, but 95–100% will demonstrate elevation of at least one titre if three different antibodies are measured. Therefore, one should perform several streptococcal antibody tests when ARF is suspected clinically.

Differential diagnosis

The differential diagnosis of ARF includes those illnesses that commonly present with fever and arthritis or fever and carditis. These include collagen vascular diseases, serum sickness, pyogenic arthritis, Lyme disease, reactive arthritis and gonococcal tenosynovitis. Infective endocarditis may resemble ARF. In younger patients, Kawasaki disease also may enter the differential diagnosis.

Treatment

The therapy of ARF is divided into (1) prevention of the primary attack, (2) treatment of the ARF episode, (3) prevention of recurrent ARF, and (4) management of chronic RHD, including prevention of infective endocarditis.

Primary prevention of ARF refers to preventing the first attack by appropriate diagnosis and treatment of group A streptococcal pharyngitis. An appropriate antibiotic, instituted by the ninth day of pharyngitis and continued for 10 days, is highly effective in preventing ARF.

Treatment of an ARF episode includes antistreptococcal therapy, anti-inflammatory therapy and cardiac medications as indicated. Ten days of oral penicillin or erythromycin or a single injection of 1.2 million units of benzathine penicillin intramuscularly is given whether or not group A streptococci are found in the throat. Anti-inflammatory therapy with salicylates or corticosteroids is important. The arthritis of ARF is self-limited and almost always responds very dramatically to salicylates at 50–100 mg/kg per day in four divided doses. This is also adequate for carditis that is not associated with congestive heart failure or with moderate or severe cardiomegaly. Salicylates are generally continued for 2–4 weeks and then gradually tapered and discontinued over the subsequent 4–6 weeks. Prednisone at 2 mg/kg per day is given only to those ARF patients with more serious carditis, i.e. with moderate to severe cardiomegaly and/or congestive heart failure. In these circumstances, prednisone can improve cardiac function dramatically. Typically prednisone is given at full dose for 2–4 weeks, then tapered over the subsequent month, with salicylates added as the steroids are being withdrawn. Although steroids are highly effective in controlling the activity of ARF, they do not alter the long-term prevalence of residual valvular disease. Other supportive therapies for moderate to severe carditis include digoxin, fluid and salt restriction, diuretics and oxygen. Digitalization should be instituted carefully because myocarditis increases cardiac irritability. Bed rest may be useful in the very acute stage of illness, but prolonged bed rest is no longer recommended. Patients with Sydenham's chorea, which is self-limited, occasionally benefit from confinement to a quiet room and administration of phenobarbitone or haloperidol in moderate doses, with variable response.

Secondary prophylaxis for ARF refers to long-term administration of antibiotics to prevent streptococcal pharyngitis in rheumatic patients and thus prevent subsequent attacks of ARF. The greatest risk for recurrence is within 5 years of an attack of ARF. Rheumatic patients with or without cardiac disease should receive one of three standard prophylactic regimens: 1.2 million units of benzathine penicillin G intramuscularly every 4 weeks, 1 g sulphadiazine orally daily, or penicillin V 250 mg orally twice daily. For patients who cannot tolerate penicillin or sulfa, erythromycin is the recommended alternative and the cephalosporins also are probably effective. The duration of ARF prophylaxis is somewhat controversial, with the American Heart Association recommending lifetime prophylaxis for patients with RHD. Prophylaxis probably can be discontinued safely at age 21 years in patients without cardiac involvement, or at least 5 years after the last attack of ARF.

Patients with chronic RHD, i.e. mitral and/or aortic valve insufficiency and/or stenosis, need long-term cardiac follow-up. With successful prevention of recurrent attacks of ARF, many patients resolve auscultatory and even echocardiographic evidence of valvar disease, particularly mitral insufficiency. Others, however, progress eventually to develop stenotic valvular lesions; some of these patients ultimately require valvuloplasty or prosthetic valve placement because of valvar dysfunction. In addition, patients with RHD should be instructed regarding infective endocarditis prophylaxis; i.e. antibiotic administration prior to dental procedures or genitourinary/gastrointestinal surgery or instrumentation, as recommended by the American Heart Association and the British Working Party (see below).

INFECTIVE ENDOCARDITIS

Epidemiology

Infective endocarditis (IE) in children has increased in incidence because of the improved survival of children with cardiac disease, in great measure related to improved surgical techniques for managing complex forms of congenital heart disease. Additional factors that affect the overall frequency of childhood IE are the declining numbers of patients with rheumatic heart disease and the great increase in use of prosthetic indwelling intravascular devices. Neonatal IE is particularly often associated with use of central vascular catheters. The mean age of postneonatal IE in childhood has risen over several decades, reflecting primarily the large number of survivors of curative or palliative cardiac surgical procedures.

Pathogenesis

IE generally results from the concurrence of two factors: predisposing heart disease with resulting endothelial injury; and bacteraemia (or fungaemia). From experimental animal studies it has been learned that the sequence of events in the development of IE is initial vascular endothelial injury, then formation of non-bacterial thrombotic endocarditis comprised of fibrin and platelets but not leucocytes at the site of that injury, and subsequent entrapment of circulating microorganisms, with resultant IE. Transient bacteraemia is virtually a daily occurrence, occurring with chewing hard foods, toothbrushing, and dental and surgical procedures that involve colonized mucosal surfaces.

The cardiac conditions that most commonly predispose children to IE include those associated with a pressure gradient and resulting turbulent blood flow.

Jet lesions such as small ventricular septal defects may damage endothelium directly. Other commonly associated cardiac lesions are bicuspid aortic valve, rheumatic mitral and/or aortic dysfunction, patent ductus arteriosus, complex congenital heart disease with surgically constructed shunts and conduits (especially those with systemic–pulmonary connections), mitral valve prolapse with regurgitation, prosthetic heart valves and others. About 10% of paediatric patients with IE have no apparent underlying heart defect.

The microorganisms implicated most frequently in IE are Gram-positive cocci, although other bacteria and fungi also are isolated from relatively small numbers of patients. Virtually every bacterial species isolated from man has been associated with IE at some time. However, about 90% of paediatric IE is caused by Gram-positive cocci, with 75% of the total related to oral viridans (α-haemolytic) streptococci or to *Staphylococcus aureus*. Much less common are enterococci, pneumococci, and β-haemolytic streptococci. Coagulase-negative staphylococci are of increasing importance, particularly in the patient who has undergone cardiac surgery. The most common Gram-negative organisms are the members of the HACEK group (non-influenza *Haemophilus*, *Actinobacillus*, *Cardiobacterium*, *Eikenella* and *Kingella*). Enteric Gram-negatives and *Neisseria* are quite unusual causes of childhood IE. Fungal IE, which is often an autopsy diagnosis, is usually due to *Candida* species or to *Aspergillus*.

Clinical features

Endocarditis should be considered in any child with an underlying cardiac condition who presents with fever that is not readily explained or with an obscure deterioration in cardiac function.

Although IE may present in a variety of ways, two major syndromes predominate. Acute endocarditis (usually due to *Staphylococcus aureus*) is characterized by a toxic, febrile course of short duration, and subacute endocarditis (usually due to streptococci or coagulase-negative staphylococci), by an insidious onset of low-grade fever, malaise, headache, myalgias and arthralgias. The clinical features may differ by anatomical site of infection, and this explains why paediatric IE, which most often involves the right heart, is somewhat different from adult IE, which is most often left-sided. Left-sided IE may be associated with systemic

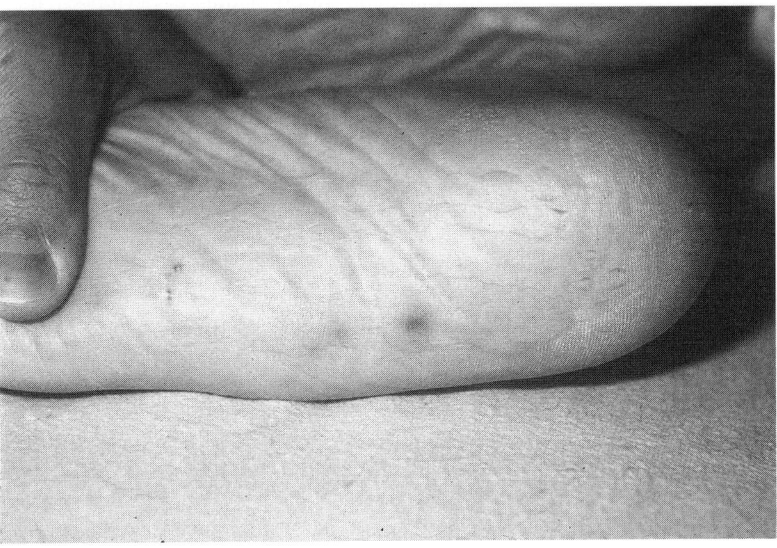

Fig. 2.1.1 Infective endocarditis. Janeway lesion: necrotic macule on sole of foot.

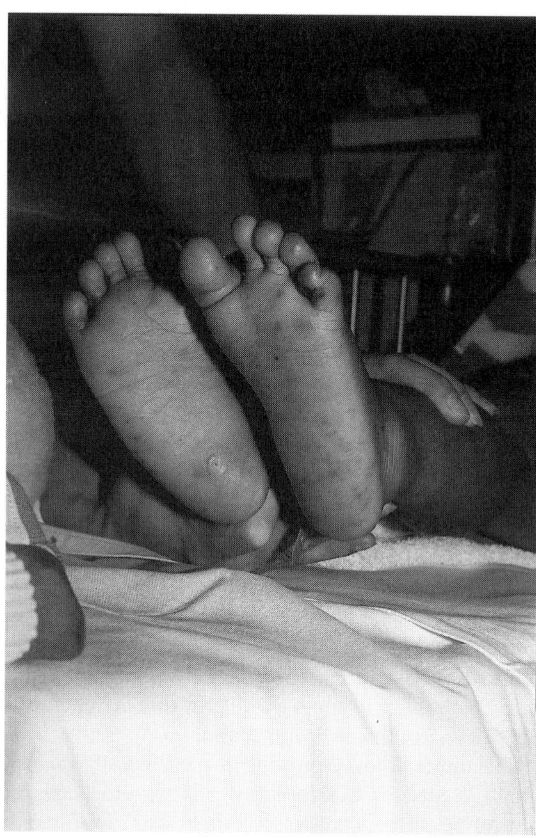

Fig. 2.1.2 Infective endocarditis. Necrotic embolic lesions due to emboli (Janeway lesions).

emboli, while right-sided endocarditis may lead to small pulmonary emboli, which are often clinically inapparent. Frequent clinical features include a new or changing heart murmur, the non-specific symptoms noted above, new or worsening congestive heart failure, petechiae, splinter haemorrhages and spleno-megaly. Classic immune-mediated, peripheral manifestations of IE such as Osler nodes, Janeway lesions and Roth spots are quite rare in children as compared to adults with IE. As with all other infectious diseases, the manifestations of IE in the neonate tend to be more subtle; often fever is not present. Long-standing IE is frequently characterized by evidence of immune activation, with immune complex formation and deposition and hyperglobulinaemia that can manifest clinically as vasculitis and/or glomerulonephritis. Neurological symptoms may develop early or late in IE, related to vasculitis, emboli or an associated brain abscess.

Laboratory features

The most important laboratory test for IE is, of course, the blood culture. Patients with IE typically have continuous shedding of low numbers of bacteria into the bloodstream. Because the most common bacterial causes of IE are also frequent contaminants of blood cultures, optimal aseptic technique and obtaining several sets of blood cultures prior to initiation of antibiotic therapy greatly enhance interpretation of results. Problems associated with blood cultures relate to the patient who has received antibiotics prior to obtaining the culture, with resultant false negative culture results, and to the patient suspected to have IE but who has repeated negative blood cultures in the absence of prior antibiotic therapy. The latter comprise the approximately 3–5% of patients in any series of IE who are considered to have 'culture-negative' endocarditis, often confirmed later at surgery or autopsy. Blood cultures are positive in only about 50% of patients with fungal endocarditis. Another important cause of 'culture-negative' endocarditis is infection with nutritionally deficient viridans streptococci (*Streptococcus defectivus*) that grow only on supplemented agar or adjacent to other bacteria. Three sets of blood cultures obtained over a 24 h period enable diagnosis of about 97% of cases of IE.

Other laboratory tests are less specific for IE. Acute-phase reactants are usually elevated, and rheumatoid factor is positive in about 50% of patients, particularly those with longer duration of symptoms. Most IE patients at diagnosis have mild–moderate anaemia (normochromic, normocytic) and some degree of leucocytosis. Haematuria is often present, reflecting immune complex-mediated nephritis.

Echocardiography is very useful for detecting the presence of vegetations, which can be visualized in more than half of patients. Trans-oesophageal echocardiography is substantially more sensitive than trans-thoracic echocardiography for detecting vegetations in adults and probably in children as well.

Prevention

Despite a lack of controlled clinical trials that demonstrate feasibility, it is recommended to attempt to prevent IE when at-risk patients undergo procedures that are associated with bacteraemia. This practice is based primarily upon extensive animal model data that demonstrate the efficacy of antibiotics given prior to bacteraemia in the prevention of IE. Clearly, prevention of all bacteraemic events is not possible, and IE may develop despite appropriate administration of prophylactic antibiotics. At-risk children should receive prophylaxis as recommended by the American Heart Association or by the British Working Party when undergoing a dental or surgical procedure likely to be associated with bacteraemia. Those at risk (Table 2.1.2) include patients with previous history of

Table 2.1.2   Cardiac conditions for which endocarditis prophylaxis is or is not recommended

Prophylaxis recommended
Prosthetic cardiac valves, including bioprosthetic and homograft valves
Previous bacterial endocarditis, even in the absence of heart disease
Surgically constructed systemic–pulmonary shunts
Most congenital cardiac malformations
Rheumatic and other acquired valvular dysfunction, even after valve surgery
Hypertrophic cardiomyopathy
Mitral valve prolapse with valvular regurgitation

Prophylaxis not recommended
Isolated secundum atrial septal defect
Surgical repair without residua beyond 6 months of:
    secundum atrial septal defect
    ventricular septal defect
    patent ductus arteriosus
Previous coronary artery bypass surgery
Mitral valve prolapse without valvular regurgitation
Physiological, functional or innocent heart murmurs
Previous Kawasaki disease without valvular dysfunction
Previous rheumatic fever without valvular dysfunction
Cardiac pacemakers and implanted defibrillators

Recommendations of the American Heart Association.[4]

IE, almost all forms of congenital or acquired heart lesions (except secundum atrial septal defect or coronary artery disease), and those who are postcardiac surgery (except secundum atrial defect repaired without a patch or patent ductus). Patients considered to be at particularly high risk for IE are those with prosthetic valves and those with surgically constructed systemic–pulmonary shunts; parenteral rather than oral prophylaxis may afford a higher level of protection for these high-risk patients, but this is somewhat controversial. Maintenance of optimal oral hygiene and dental care is also important in prevention of IE, and it is advisable for needed dental procedures to be performed prior to cardiac surgery, when possible, to minimize risk of prosthetic IE.

Common errors in antibiotic prophylaxis for IE include initiating antibiotics too long before the procedure, thus selecting resistant mucosal flora; continuing prophylaxis longer than 12 h after the procedure; using low-dose oral therapy, leading to inadequate serum concentrations; and failure to use prophylaxis for non-extraction dental procedures that are likely to result in gingival bleeding. Prophylaxis for gastrointestinal or genitourinary procedures likely to result in bacteraemia includes coverage for enterococcal organisms.

Treatment

Children with suspected or proven IE are best managed jointly by paediatric infectious diseases and paediatric cardiology specialists, and dental evaluation is generally indicated. General principles that guide management of IE include (1) parenteral administration of antibiotic therapy because of the high serum antibiotic concentrations achieved, (2) use of bactericidal antibiotics because of the lack of inflammatory cells within cardiac vegetations, (3) prolonged antibiotic therapy because of the high failure rates often associated with short courses, and (4) use of synergistic drug combinations when applicable (as in enterococcal endocarditis). It is generally desirable to monitor the peak serum bactericidal titre achieved using the patient's own microorganism; a titre $\geq 1:8$ is reassuring, but the poor standardization of these assays may make interpretation difficult. Patients with IE require close follow-up, including occasional blood cultures during the first several months after completion of therapy, since most relapses occur during this period. Except in the rare patient with acute fulminant (usually staphylococcal) endocarditis in whom prompt initiation of therapy is necessary, it is highly desirable to establish a bacteriological diagnosis prior to starting therapy, i.e. to withhold therapy until the laboratory reports positive blood cultures.

The role of cardiovascular surgical intervention in IE is highly individualized and determined by the site of infection and by the clinical course, including the haemodynamic status of the patient. General indications for surgical intervention include recurrent emboli or a single large embolus (especially from the left side of the heart), progressive cardiac failure despite therapy, significant valvar obstruction, and persistent bacteraemia for at least 10–14 days despite appropriate therapy. Early surgical replacement of an infected prosthetic valve or other device may reduce the high mortality associated with prosthetic endocarditis. Surgery should not be delayed specifically because the antibiotic course has not been completed. Successful management of fungal endocarditis almost always requires surgical resection of the lesion.

The most common organisms causing IE are the highly penicillin-sensitive streptococci, defined as those with minimal inhibitory concentrations (MICs) of penicillin $\leq 0.1\ \mu g/ml$. These include most viridans streptococci, *Streptococcus bovis*, and group A streptococci. Very high cure rates are associated with several regimens: 4 weeks of penicillin G or ceftriaxone alone, 4 weeks of penicillin with gentamicin for the first 2 weeks, or 2 weeks of penicillin with gentamicin. Two weeks of penicillin alone is not recommended because of unacceptable relapse rates. Recent studies have used 2 weeks of ceftriaxone with an aminoglycoside. Two-week regimens are not recommended for patients with complications such as extracardiac infection or intracardiac abscesses. For penicillin-allergic patients who cannot be desensitized, intravenous vancomycin or a first-generation cephalosporin for 4 weeks is effective.

Viridans streptococci with penicillin MIC values > 0.1 μg/ml and < 0.5 μg/ml, as well as nutritionally deficient streptococci, are best treated with 4 weeks of penicillin combined with gentamicin for the first 2 weeks, because of the readily demonstrable synergy between these agents for these organisms. For penicillin-allergic patients who cannot be desensitized, 4 weeks of vancomycin with or without gentamicin is appropriate. Fortunately, enterococcal endocarditis is rare in children, as this is a difficult infection to treat. Combination penicillin and aminoglycoside therapy for 4–6 weeks is necessary, with vancomycin and gentamicin for 4–6 weeks in penicillin-allergic patients. When high-level aminoglycoside resistance (MIC > 2000 μg/ml) is present, one can predict lack of synergy between penicillin and the aminoglycoside.

Therapy of methicillin-sensitive staphylococcal endocarditis in the absence of prosthetic material consists of a penicillinase-resistant penicillin (nafcillin, oxacillin or flucloxacillin) or a first-generation cephalosporin (cephalothin or cefazolin) for 4–6 weeks. Some favour adjunctive therapy with an aminoglycoside, at least for the initial 3–5 days. Rifampin/rifampicin (which can never be used as sole therapy because resistance will likely emerge) is often added to the therapy of patients who appear to be responding slowly to therapy. Those who are allergic to penicillin agents or who are infected with a methicillin-resistant staphylococcus should be treated with 4–6 weeks of vancomycin. When staphylococcal infections occur on prosthetic material, an additional 2 weeks of therapy is generally indicated.

Therapy for Gram-negative IE must be tailored to the specific agent. The HACEK organisms most often are treated successfully with ampicillin plus gentamicin or with ceftriaxone for 3–4 weeks (6 weeks with prosthetic material). Fungal endocarditis is particularly difficult to treat and is associated with high mortality, with most patients requiring surgery, as noted above. Diagnosis is difficult because candidaemia does not necessarily indicate the presence of IE, while endocarditis due to other fungi is rarely associated with positive blood cultures and is most often diagnosed at surgery or autopsy. Echocardiography is usually very helpful because fungal endocarditis is often manifested by large, bulky vegetations. Almost all patients require at least 6 weeks of amphotericin B intravenously with surgical extirpation. The role of adjunctive therapy with other antifungal agents remains unclear. Surgery is best performed after 1–2 weeks of medical therapy, if the patient's haemodynamic status permits.

Therapy for culture-negative endocarditis generally consists of nafcillin, oxacillin or flucloxacillin for 6 weeks, combined with an aminoglycoside for the initial 2 weeks (if the patient has responded well to treatment). Vancomycin should be used instead of a semi-synthetic penicillin for penicillin-allergic patients or those with prosthetic valves or other material.

MYOCARDITIS

Myocarditis is defined pathologically as infiltration of the myocardium by inflammatory cells. The spectrum of presentation and the prognosis in childhood vary according to age and immunocompetence, with neonates usually affected most severely.

Epidemiology

Coxsackie B virus and other enteroviruses such as echoviruses, as well as adenovirus and influenza virus, are the leading identifiable causes of childhood myocarditis. The list of infective causes is extensive (Table 2.1.3), and postinfectious causes, such as rheumatic fever, and radiation, chemical or drug injury to the myocardium, also should be considered. Acute Coxsackie B virus infection has a high incidence of myocardial involvement during the first year of life, lower incidence during later childhood, and a relative increase in incidence in adolescence. About 50% of neonatal myocarditis is caused by Coxsackie B. Myocarditis may account for up to 20% of non-accidental childhood sudden, unexpected death occurrences and may be present asymptomatically in some patients with viral infections.

Pathogenesis

Myocardial damage may be the result of various mechanisms. *Corynebacterium diphtheriae* produces a circulating toxin that is myocytotoxic. Immunological mechanisms are responsible for the formation of the endomyocardial Aschoff nodule and for myocarditis in acute rheumatic fever. An adjacent inflammatory process, or vasculitic endothelial damage as in cytomegalovirus myocarditis, may cause indirect myocardial injury. Enteroviruses may cause direct damage to myocytes, a major factor in neonatal myocarditis. However, several days after the onset of disease, immunologically mediated damage may become more important.

Clinical features

Neonates may present with lethargy, irritability, anorexia, temperature instability and tachycardia, which may progress rapidly to overt features of cardiogenic shock, with poor peripheral perfusion, cyanosis, hypotension, cardiomegaly, hepatomegaly and respiratory distress. Older patients are usually less severely

Table 2.1.3   Selected infectious causes of myopericarditis

Viruses	**Chlamydias**
Coxsackie A, B	*Chlamydia psittaci*
Echo	
Influenza A, B	**Protozoa**
Adeno	*Trypanosoma cruzii*
Mumps	*Entamoeba histolytica*
Rubella	*Toxoplasma gondii*
Varicella zoster	
Epstein–Barr	**Metazoa**
Cytomegalovirus	*Trichinella spiralis*
Polio	
Rubeola	**Miscellaneous**
	Kawasaki disease
Spirochaetes	Malignancy
Borrelia burgdorferi	
	Bacteria
Fungi	*Staphylococcus aureus*
Aspergillus fumigatus	Streptococcal species, e.g. *S. pneumoniae* and *S. pyogenes*
Candida albicans	*Haemophilus influenzae*
	Neisseria meningitidis
Mycoplasmas	Enteric Gram-negative bacilli including *Salmonella typhi*
Mycoplasma pneumoniae	*Corynebacterium diphtheriae*
	Legionella pneumophilia

affected. A history of preceding upper respiratory tract symptoms or diarrhoea is common. Adolescents may complain of chest pain from accompanying pericarditis or palpitations. In an infant who presents with respiratory distress, important clinical clues to the diagnosis of myocarditis may be tachycardia out of proportion to the degree of fever, or poor perfusion with diminished pulses and skin pallor, sometimes with progression to severe cardiac decompensation.

Laboratory substantiation of the diagnosis includes ECG changes, which may include non-specific ST segment and T wave abnormalities and arrhythmias, raised serum levels of troponin T or the MB fraction of creatinine kinase, and echocardiographic quantification of reduced systolic function. Magnetic resonance imaging of myocardium and indium-111 anti-myosin antibody imaging are newer diagnostic modalities. Endomyocardial biopsy is usually not indicated in the acute phase of the disease but may become more frequently utilized to obtain tissue for in situ molecular techniques such as the polymerase chain reaction, as advances in anti-enteroviral therapy require a specific aetiological diagnosis. Stool, respiratory and blood cultures for viruses and other pathogens, and acute and convalescent serological investigations should be employed for establishing an aetiological diagnosis. Serological studies are limited by the very large number of enterovirus serotypes.

Treatment

Supportive management is the cornerstone of therapy in the majority of cases, because no effective anti-enteroviral agent is available. When a treatable aetiological agent is verified, for example a rickettsial infection, specific management should be instituted. Excessive exercise should be avoided during other viral infections in which asymptomatic myocardial involvement may be present. Immunosuppressive therapy should be avoided, as both corticosteroids and non-steroidal anti-inflammatory agents generally are thought to have a deleterious effect during acute myocarditis. Recent reports suggest a possible benefit of high-dose intravenous gammaglobulin. Most cases recover completely; however, when chronic cardiomyopathy results, patients may become candidates for cardiac transplantation.

PERICARDITIS

Acute pericarditis (inflammation of the pericardium) occurs in all age groups and may be overlooked by the practitioner. Although most cases are silent, severe haemodynamic compromise and even death may result.

Epidemiology

Idiopathic and viral causes of pericarditis predominate (see Table 2.1.3). Many cases considered idiopathic are probably the result of viral infections. Enteroviruses predominate, with Coxsackievirus the most common cause of myopericarditis and epidemic pleurodynia (Bornholm disease). A relapsing course that extends months or years may complicate viral pericarditis. Acute purulent pericarditis still occurs in childhood, although usually not as a primary disease, since in about 85% of cases another site of bacterial infection is identifiable. *Staphylococcus aureus* is the most common bacterial pathogen; many other bacteria including *Haemophilus influenzae* type b may also cause pericarditis Fig. 2.1.3.

The spectrum of causative agents in immunocompromised patients differs: the human immunodeficiency virus may cause pericardial disease, but *Mycobacterium tuberculosis* and opportunistic pathogens such as fungi occur relatively more frequently. Advances in medical technology have been associated with an increase in non-infectious causes of pericardial disease.

Pathogenesis

Viruses reach the pericardium via the haematogenous route, and sequelae are rare, except for recurrent disease, which is often immunologically mediated. Bacteria commonly gain access to the pericardial space haematogenously or via spread from a contiguous focus.

Alternatively, the infection may originate from a focus within the heart, such as endocarditis, or by direct inoculation as with surgery. In tuberculosis, spread may also occur from affected lymph nodes adjacent to the pericardium. The pericardium reacts to acute injury by exuding fluid, fibrin and cells in various combinations, resulting in a pericardial effusion. Accumulation of substantial amounts of pericardial fluid usually occurs in bacterial infections and may lead to tamponade. Organization with adhesions, obliteration of the pericardial space, and calcification may develop and result in constrictive pericarditis, which occurs in up to 50% of tuberculous cases.

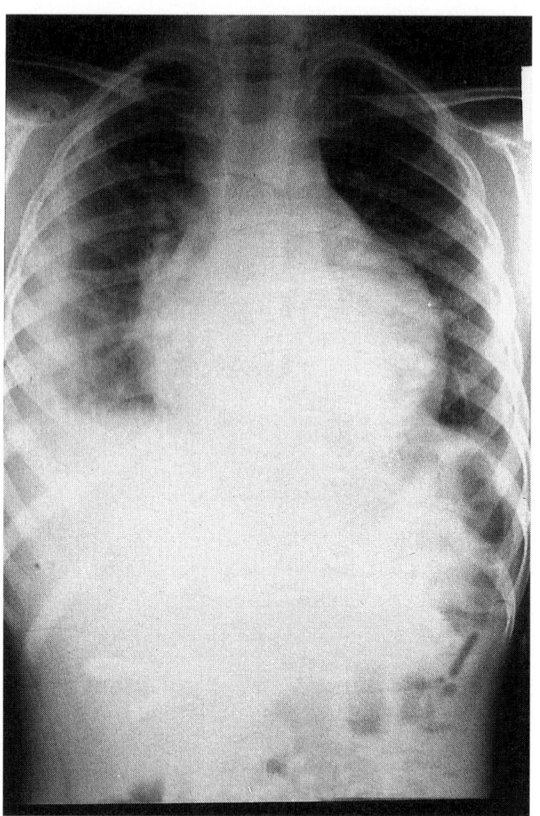

Fig. 2.1.3 Purulent pericarditis. Boy aged 4 years with right-sided empyema and enlarged globular heart shadow, due to *Haemophilus influenzae* type b.

Clinical features

Presentation varies according to aetiology. Patients with viral pericarditis commonly have chest pain; fever may be present, as well as a prodromal flu-like illness. Bacterial infections are associated with a more 'toxic' appearing patient, while the onset of tuberculous pericarditis is most often insidious.

Physical findings may include the classic three-component pericardial friction rub, which is infrequently present. When a large pericardial effusion is present, cardiac dullness on percussion may extend beyond the apical pulse, which may be poorly palpable. Heart sounds are usually muffled. Signs of tamponade (progressive reduction of ventricular diastolic filling, with increased systemic and pulmonary venous pressures) include palpable pulsus paradoxus, poor cardiac output resulting in systolic hypotension, hepatomegaly, elevated jugular venous pressure and signs of pulmonary oedema.

Diagnosis is assisted by ECG changes such as ST segment elevation and PR segment depression, reflecting subepicardial inflammation and injury. Chest radiograph may demonstrate an increased cardiac silhouette, but echocardiography is more reliable for diagnosis of a pericardial effusion. Although cardiac tamponade or constriction is a clinical diagnosis, two-dimensional echocardiography may display typical changes. Should an effusion be present, pericardiocentesis for microbiological and cytological analysis of the fluid is usually indicated. In cases in which the aetiological diagnosis is not obvious, pericardial biopsy should be considered. Other cultures and serological investigations should be employed in an attempt to reach an aetiological diagnosis.

Therapy

Myocarditis is often also present in cases of viral pericarditis, and the treatment is the same. Pain may be treated with salicylates. Bacterial pericarditis must be managed both with adequate pericardial fluid drainage (usually placement of a pericardial window) and appropriate parenteral antibiotics. Steroid management is important as adjunctive therapy for reducing the incidence of pericardial constriction in tuberculous pericarditis. Steroids are not indicated in acute pericarditis of other aetiology, and should be reserved for cases of persistent or recurrent disease, or possibly for managing enlarging effusions, for which patients should be monitored during the acute phase of the disease. Long-term follow-up is necessary to detect possible pericardial constriction, which may require surgical removal of the pericardium.

BIBLIOGRAPHY

1 Bayliss R, Clarke C, Oakley C M et al. The microbiology and pathogenesis of infective endocarditis. Br Heart J 1983; 50: 513–519.
2 Bisno A L. Group A streptococcal infections and acute rheumatic fever. N Engl J Med 1991; 325: 783–793.
3 Bisno A L, Dismukes W E, Durack D T et al. Antimicrobial treatment of infective endocarditis due to viridans streptococci, enterococci, and staphylococci. JAMA 1989; 261: 1471–1477.
4 Dajani A S, Bisno A L, Chung K J et al. Prevention of bacterial endocarditis: recommendations by the American Heart Association. JAMA 1990; 264: 2919–2922.
5 Denny F W. A 45-year perspective on the streptococcus and rheumatic fever. Clin Infect Dis 1994; 19: 1110–1122.
6 Drucker N A, Colan S D, Lewis B et al. γ-Globulin treatment of acute myocarditis in the pediatric population. Circulation 1994; 89: 252–257.
7 Durack D T. Prevention of infective endocarditis. N Engl J Med 1995; 322: 38–44.
8 Friedman R A, Duff D F. Myocarditis. In: Feigin R D, Cherry J D, eds. Textbook of pediatric infectious diseases, 3rd edn. Philadelphia: Saunders, 1992: pp 357–375.
9 Pinsky W W, Friedman R A, Jubelirer D P, Nihill M R. Infectious pericarditis. In: Feigin R D, Cherry J D, eds. Textbook of pediatric infectious diseases, 3rd edn. Philadelphia: Saunders, 1992: pp 377–386.
10 Savoia M C, Oxman M N. Myocarditis and pericarditis. In: Mandell G L, Bennett J E, Dolin R, eds. Mandell, Douglas and Bennett's Principles and practice of infectious diseases, 4th edn. New York: Wiley, 1995: pp 799–808.

11 Simmons N A. Recommendations for endocarditis prophylaxis. J Antimicrob Chemother 1993; 31: 437–438.
12 Special writing group of the committee on rheumatic fever, endocarditis, and Kawasaki disease of the council on cardiovascular disease in the young. American Heart Association: Guidelines for the diagnosis of rheumatic fever: Jones criteria, updated 1992. Circulation 1993; 87: 302–307.
13 Taranta A, Markowitz M, eds. Rheumatic fever, 2nd edn. Boston: Kluwer, 1989.
14 Veasy L G, Wiedmeier S E, Orsmond G S et al. Resurgence of acute rheumatic fever in the intermountain area of the U.S. N Engl J Med 1987; 316: 421–427.

CHAPTER 3

GASTRO-INTESTINAL TRACT

3.1 Infectious diarrhoea and vomiting

INTRODUCTION

Improvements in prevention and treatment have resulted in the displacement of acute diarrhoea by respiratory tract infections as the leading cause of mortality in childhood. In developed countries, mortality from diarrhoea is rare, but gastrointestinal infections are frequently encountered. Such improvements in mortality have had less impact on the morbidity of infectious diarrhoea. Persistent diarrhoea, which may complicate infectious diarrhoea, is a continuing problem. Specific therapy for persistent diarrhoea is generally lacking, and it remains a cause of malnutrition and death. The term 'gastroenteritis' to describe infectious diarrhoea and vomiting is falling from favour because there is little evidence for gastric involvement and, in the viral diarrhoeas, inflammation of the gut (enteritis) is not a prominent pathological feature.

EPIDEMIOLOGY

In the UK each general practitioner will see, on average, 18 children per year with diarrhoea and vomiting.[1] Gastrointestinal infections account for approximately 10% of admissions to general paediatric units.[2] In a study from Western Australia, intestinal infections were the cause of admission to hospital for 12% of Aboriginal and 5% of non-Aboriginal children.[3]

Risk factors for infectious diarrhoea include poor socioeconomic status and bottle-feeding.[4] Poor nutrition predisposes to prolonged episodes of diarrhoea, rather than increased attack rates.[5] Human breast milk contains a number of protective factors, including leucocytes, immunoglobulin, non-immunoglobulin and antiviral factors. Among the non-immunoglobulin protective factors are lactoferrin, which conjugates iron required by bacteria,[6] and analogues of the receptors to which bacteria and their toxins bind, which inhibit binding to the intestinal mucosa.[7] The stomach is an important defence barrier because the majority of ingested microorganisms, with the exception of *Candida*, are killed by gastric acid. It is not understood why the infectious dose of *Campylobacter* is as low as 500 organisms and *Shigella* 10 organisms, whereas *Vibrio cholerae* requires many more viable organisms to infect humans.[8] Nevertheless, hypochlorhydria is a risk factor for intestinal infection, and studies are in progress to determine whether infection of the stomach in infancy by *Helicobacter pylori* causes transient hypochlorhydria and a 'window of opportunity' for intestinal colonization by enteropathogens.[9] The second-line mechanical defence mechanism is small intestinal motility. The word 'jejunum' means 'empty', thereby testifying to the effectiveness of peristalsis, which rapidly conveys bacteria that survive the gastric acid barrier to the distal bowel. This defence mechanism can be overcome by bacteria which can adhere to the brush border of the jejunal mucosa, and may be impaired by antimotility drugs. The normal small intestinal flora improves the 'colonization resistance' of the intestinal tract; this effect can be perturbed by the use of antibiotics.[8]

There are over 500 000 000 children under 5 years of age in the Third World who have more than 1 500 000 000 episodes of diarrhoea annually. It is estimated that approximately 3 million children die each year from diarrhoeal diseases.[10] Potential infectious agents are isolated in up to 80% of episodes of acute diarrhoea, confirming the infective nature of the disease. Important diarrhoeal pathogens are listed in Table 3.1.1. This list is expanding with the description of pathogens such as enterotoxigenic *Bacteroides fragilis*[11] and a cyanobacterium or coccidian variously labelled 'cyanobacteria-like or coccidia-like body' (CLB) and now called *Cylospora cayetanensis*.[12]

In humans, both in developed and developing countries, and in all mammalian species examined, rotavirus is a leading cause of diarrhoea.[13] It causes a brief but severe illness, during the cooler months of the year, when it can account for up to 80% of admissions to hospital with acute diarrhoea. Excretion of rotavirus in the newborn period is often asymptomatic and protects against subsequent infection. Adenovirus shows less seasonal variation and is responsible for 5–10% of childhood diarrhoea.[14] It has become notorious for causing lethal diarrhoea in bone marrow recipients.[15] Epidemiological studies have confirmed the role of astrovirus in day care settings.[16] Small round structured viruses (SRSV) were previously named after the place of first isolation (e.g. Norwalk, Hawaii, Ditchling and Parramatta) or foodstuff (e.g. cockle). Each type is antigenically distinct and hence repeated attacks can occur throughout life; family outbreaks are common. Droplet spread occurs via vomitus containing the virus. The name of the illness associated with this group of viruses, viz. 'winter vomiting disease', attests to their seasonality. The epidemiological importance of SRSV may be underestimated as they cannot be cultured and diagnosis depends on electron microscopy of vomitus or stool.

Vibrio cholerae is one of three species of bacteria with the capacity to cause

Table 3.1.1   Diarrhoeal pathogens of epidemiological importance

---

Viruses
Rotavirus
Adenovirus
Astrovirus
Small round structured viruses

Non-invasive bacteria
Vibrio cholerae
Enterotoxigenic *Escherichia coli*
Enteropathogenic *E. coli*
Enteroaggregative *E. coli*
Diffusely adhering *E. coli*
Clostridium difficile

Invasive bacteria
Shigella
Enteroinvasive *E. coli*
Salmonella
Campylobacter
Yersinia

Protozoa
Entamoeba histolytica
Cryptosporidium parvum
Giardia duodenalis

---

pandemics (the others being *Shigella dysenteriae* 1 and *Yersinia pestis*). *V. cholerae* has two biotypes (classical and El Tor) and two serotypes (Inaba and Ogawa). A new antigenic type of *V. cholerae* O139, to which pre-existing immunity is non-protective, threatens to produce the eighth pandemic.[17] The organism is waterborne and probably occupies a marine environment between pandemics. Enterotoxigenic *Escherichia coli* is an important cause of diarrhoea in children in developing countries. Adults living in developed countries do not encounter this group of pathogens until they travel to the Third World; hence they are a major cause of travellers' (or emporiatic) diarrhoea, which affects as many as 11 million people annually.[18] Enteropathogenic *E. coli* is the leading cause of diarrhoea in children in South America.[19] Enteroaggregative *E. coli* is a novel group of enteropathogens with an epidemiological link with chronic diarrhoea.[20–22] A specific subgroup of enteropathogenic *E. coli* are termed enterohaemorrhagic *E. coli* because they cause an illness termed 'haemorrhagic colitis' in which the stools, although often watery, may resemble pure blood. These pathogens resemble enteropathogenic *E. coli* in their localized destructive interaction with the brush border of the intestinal tract. They differ from enteropathogenic *E. coli* which colonize the entire gastrointestinal tract by preferentially colonizing the colon.[23] They also differ by virtue of their ability to produce a cytotoxin resembling the toxin of *Shigella dysenteriae* 1 called Shiga-like toxin in the USA and Verocytotoxin (VT) in the UK.[24] The name Vero refers to the green monkey kidney cell line used to assay cytotoxic activity. Two types of VT (1 and 2) have been described. The most prevalent enterohaemorrhagic *E. coli* strains produce lipopolysaccharide of serogroup O157 and flagellae of serotype H7. This serotype is now the commonest cause of acute renal failure in developed countries.[24] These *E. coli* and also *Shigella dysenteriae* 1 cause the haemolytic uraemic syndrome in which the capillaries of the glomeruli and other organs become occluded with fibrin thrombi. The platelet count is low due to consumption of platelets in the thrombi. The threads of fibrin in the capillaries cleave passing red cells. This process is referred to as microangiopathic haemolytic anaemia.[25]

The epidemiological data implicating *E. coli* which adhere diffusely to tissue culture cells (enteroadhesive *E. coli*) as a cause of diarrhoea are controversial, with equal numbers of studies of acute diarrhoea either linking the excretion of these *E. coli* with symptoms or failing to find an association.[26]

With the exception of enterohaemorrhagic *E. coli* these species of enteric pathogens cause watery diarrhoea. The invasive bacteria also cause watery diarrhoea, but have the capacity to cause bloody diarrhoea or dysentery. The genus *Shigella* has four species: *S. dysenteriae*, *S. flexneri*, *S. boydii* and *S. sonnei*. *S. dysenteriae* 1 is confined to developing countries, where it causes the most severe disease with substantial mortality, due to complications such as haemolytic uraemic syndrome (HUS).[25] *S. flexneri* and *S. boydii* cause illnesses of intermediate and variable severity, while *S. sonnei* is associated with mild illness. Increasing utilization of day care for children has resulted in a resurgence of this organism in the UK to levels previously experienced in the 1950s.[27] Shigellae are restricted in species specificity to primates.[28] They are extremely infectious, with as few as 10 organisms capable of inducing the infection.[28]

Enteroinvasive *E. coli* are closely related to shigellae and testify to the repertoire of this species in causing diarrhoea by a wide variety of mechanisms. They account for 11% of bloody diarrhoea in Thai children.[29] Salmonellae are divided into more than 1500 species on the basis of antigenic differences. *Salmonella typhi* and *S. paratyphi* A and B are restricted to the human host and can cause typhoid, or enteric fever. Non-typhoid salmonellae, which cause acute diarrhoea, colonize the gut of many animal species, including man.[30] Certain phage types of

S. enteritidis cause widespread infection: PT4 in Europe, and PT6 and PT13a in the USA.[31] *Campylobacter* is the commonest bacterial cause of infectious diarrhoea in the UK, causing diarrhoea most often in young adults. Isolation rates are 300 per 100 000 in the UK and USA in children and 100–1000 times higher in developing countries.[32] Chickens and domestic pets are important reservoirs. Eating pork is a risk factor for *Yersinia pseudotuberculosis* and *Y. enterocolitica* infection.[33] *Entamoeba histolytica* is a global cause of infectious colitis, and hepatic abscesses.[34] Cysts of *Cryptosporidium parvum* and *Giardia duodenalis* (*G. lamblia*) can contaminate domestic water supplies.[35] Contact with farm animals, which can occur in city farms in urban settings, is a risk factor for *Cryptosporidium*.

DIAGNOSIS

Stool examination is indicated in the immunodeficient host, for infection control during epidemics, and for bloody diarrhoea, persistent diarrhoea and when diarrhoea follows foreign travel, since the latter three circumstances may be indications for treatment with a specific antibiotic. Routine urine culture is worthwhile, providing a clean sample is obtained, since urinary tract infection can present with vomiting and/or diarrhoea. Blood and cerebrospinal fluid (CSF) cultures may also be required if the child is seriously ill, since systemic sepsis may present with symptoms such as diarrhoea and vomiting.[36]

It is generally impossible to make a clinical aetiological diagnosis. In children older than 6 months who present in the cooler months with severe watery diarrhoea and fever, preceded by vomiting and upper respiratory tract infection, rotavirus is the most likely cause. Experienced staff can diagnose rotavirus on the basis of the particular odour of the stool, with reasonable sensitivity and specificity.[37] The presence of blood, pus and mucus points to one of the invasive bacteria listed in Table 3.1.1. Tests for the presence of leucocytes in stool are becoming available, based on measurement of stable white cell markers such as lactoferrin and calprotectin.[38] *Campylobacter* is notorious for producing flu-like symptoms and severe abdominal pain masquerading as an acute abdomen.[39] Diarrhoeagenic bacteria (especially enteropathogenic *E. coli*, enteroaggregative *E. coli* and *Salmonella*) and parasites are associated with persistent diarrhoea.[20] Entero-aggregative *E. coli* can cause simultaneous infection of the urinary tract and gut. The diarrhoea associated with enterohaemorrhagic *E. coli* may be virtually pure blood (haemorrhagic colitis). Enterohaemorrhagic *E. coli* and *Shigella dysenteriae* 1 can cause disseminated intravascular coagulation. The intravascular strands of fibrin cleave passing red cells and block glomeruli, thus producing HUS.

Examination of stool by electron microscopy can be used to demonstrate viral particles. When electron microscopy is unavailable, enzyme-linked immunosorbent assay (ELISA) can be used to detect rotavirus and the two serogroups of adenovirus (40 and 41) associated with diarrhoea. ELISA assays are also available to detect the production of exterotoxins by *V. cholerae* and enterotoxigenic *E. coli*. Enteropathogenic *E. coli*, diffusely adhering *E. coli* and enteroaggregative *E. coli* are diagnosed by observing the specific adhesion pattern to HEp-2 cells shown by these organisms. Enteropathogenic *E. coli* form micro-colonies resembling bunches of grapes on HEp-2 cells (localized adhesion). Enteroaggregative *E. coli* adhere in clumps and in chains resembling stacked bricks.[40] The adhesion process of enteropathogenic *E. coli* results in destruction (effacement) of microvilli, and formation of cup-like projections of cell membrane (pedestals) which partially invest the bacteria. The resulting perturbation of the cell skeleton, with condensation of actin underlying the pedestals, can be visualized by staining the actin with fluorescent labelled phalloidin.[41] Enteroaggregative *E. coli* do not perturb the cell skeleton. Strains of diffusely adhering *E. coli* have been described which cause changes in the cytoskeleton; it is possible that these are more pathogenic than those which adhere without damaging the cell.

Molecular diagnosis based on DNA hybridization assays have been available since the early 1980s but laboratories have been slow to introduce them. Increasingly, molecular techniques such as genomic fingerprinting, hybridization with DNA probes or the polymerase chain reaction (PCR) are being employed to identify such organisms as diarrhoeagenic *E. coli*, and shigellae.[42]

Presumptive identification of *Campylobacter* can be made by microscopy of Gram-stained stool samples; the organisms resemble seagulls' wings. Identification of amoebae also requires careful examination of fresh stool samples; pathogenic *Entamoeba histolytica* characteristically contain ingested erythrocytes.[34] Cryptosporidial cysts are demonstrated by modified Ziehl Nielsen stain of stool.[43] Cysts of *Giardia duodenalis* are seen in fresh stool and trophozoites in duodenal fluid; parasites may also be diagnosed on electron microscopy of jejunal biopsies.

The differential diagnosis of acute diarrhoea and/or vomiting is outlined in Table 3.1.2. Infections elsewhere than in the gastrointestinal tract may present with vomiting. Urinary cultures may be positive in infants with diarrhoea and vomiting. The *E. coli* isolated may demonstrate the enteroadhesive aggregative phenotype and be capable of causing urinary and gastrointestinal tract infection. Features which suggest an underlying surgical problem include a subacute presentation with vomiting (especially bile-stained), gross abdominal distension

Table 3.1.2 Differential diagnosis of acute diarrhoea and/or vomiting

Infectious diarrhoea

Ingestion of preformed toxin
  Staphylococcal food poisoning
  Scombrotoxin

Systemic infections
  Septicaemia
  Urinary tract infection
  Meningitis
  Respiratory tract infections

Surgical conditions
  Appendicitis
  Intussusception
  Pyloric stenosis
  Hirschsprung disease

Metabolic problems
  Diabetic ketoacidosis
  Congenital adrenal insufficiency
  Renal failure

Others
  Coeliac disease
  Cows' milk protein intolerance
  Chronic inflammatory bowel disease
  Immunodeficiencies
  Selective inborn errors of absorption
  Enterocolitis
  Poisoning

and/or tenderness, bloody stools and, in very low birth weight babies, redness or oedema of the abdominal wall due to necrotizing enterocolitis.[36]

ASSESSMENT OF SEVERITY

The most important consequence of acute diarrhoea is dehydration (Table 3.1.3). The severity of diarrhoea can be underestimated when there is enteropooling of secretions (so-called 'cholera sicca' or dry cholera) or when watery diarrhoea is mistaken for urine. Fever leading to febrile convulsions may be a consequence of invasive diarrhoea but also of viral diarrhoea or other infections and is noticeably absent in bloody diarrhoea due to enterohaemorrhagic E. coli.

Assessment of dehydration by clinical examination is more difficult in malnourished children. Loss of the periorbital fat causes enophthalmos simulating dehydration. Conversely dehydration in those with obesity or hypernatraemic dehydration may be underestimated because of maintenance of tissue turgor. Dehydration is graded as mild when there is a history of excess fluid loss (i.e. diarrhoea and/or vomiting) but no clinical signs of dehydration. This indicates that less than 5% of body weight has been lost as fluid. When signs of dehydration (sunken fontanelle, suppression of tear and saliva production, sunken eyes, loss of tissue turgor, peripheral cyanosis and rapid pulse) are present, between 5% and 10% of body weight has been lost as fluid depending on the severity of the signs. When shock occurs and the radial pulse is impalpable, then more than 10% of fluid has been lost as water.

Weighing the child is a useful objective measure of dehydration if a reliable, recent weight is available. If the history is longer than a few days, some of the weight loss will be due to loss of tissue as well as water. Serial weighing is also important to monitor therapy. If the weight is still low after rehydration, one of the chronic disorders listed in Table 3.1.2 may be present.

Biochemical assessment is not necessary for mild dehydration. In moderate or severe dehydration, the identification of hypernatraemia will change the rate at which oral rehydration therapy is administered (see below). If the child is critically dehydrated, the first priority is to obtain intravenous (or, failing this, intraosseous) access.

Table 3.1.3   Assessment of normonatraemic dehydration

Body weight lost (%)	Severity	Clinical state	Signs/symptoms
< 5	Mild	Not unwell	Thirst
5–10	Moderate	Apathetic Unwell	Dry mucous membranes, sunken eyes, sunken fontanelle
10–15	Severe	Shocked	Peripheral circulatory failure, peripheral vasoconstriction, hypotension, tachycardia
> 15	Critical	Moribund	Severely shocked

TREATMENT

The mainstay is oral rehydration therapy (ORT), which is effective in over 90% of moderately dehydrated patients.[44] The effectiveness of this form of treatment is based on the presence of hexose and amino acid carriers in the brush border of the jejunum, which require the simultaneous presence of sodium in the intestinal lumen to function effectively. The linked, active translocation of solute and sodium across the brush border is followed by the passive movement of water. ORT is the treatment of choice in hypernatraemic dehydration because convulsions occurring during treatment, which are a sign of cerebral overhydration, are less likely if oral rather than intravenous therapy is given.

Clinical trials indicate that the optimum sodium concentration for oral rehydration salt (ORS) solution is 60–75 mmol/l. The potassium concentration in ORS solution (20 mmol/l) is often insufficient to replace the substantial amounts of potassium lost in acute diarrhoea although the resulting deficiency rarely produces clinical symptoms. The correction of the sodium deficit assists in potassium conservation by preventing excretion of potassium in the urine in exchange for sodium in response to aldosterone. The glucose concentration should be no more than 100 mmol/l, as higher concentrations may not be tolerated, especially in viral diarrhoea. The ability to absorb glucose is limited and secondary monosaccharide intolerance will occur if excess carbohydrate is given. Replacement of glucose in ORS by cooked starch results in improved efficacy in cholera-like diarrhoea, but not in less severe diarrhoea.[45] The inclusion of citrate as a base precursor results in more rapid correction of acidosis but may be unnecessary except for cholera-like diarrhoea.

Children who are < 5% dehydrated should be encouraged to drink extra fluid. This approach is preferred to the administration of home-made solutions of sugar and salt; the opportunities for incorrect and potentially dangerous formulations are ever present. Those who are 5–10% dehydrated require 50–100 ml/kg ORS solution over 6–8 h to replace their fluid deficits. Basic fluid requirement can be provided by encouraging the child to drink water, or fruit juice diluted 1 : 3 with water, while continuing losses are replaced with either 50–100 ml/kg per day of ORS solution or by 5–10 ml/kg per loose stool, depending on severity. The child should be reassessed after 6–8 h, and if the child's state of rehydration has not improved (as judged by decreased clinical signs of dehydration and increased weight) then rehydration should be continued by the intravenous route. In hypernatraemic dehydration (serum sodium > 150 mmol/l) the same volumes of ORS solutions are given over 12–16 h rather than 6–8 h. The hyperglycaemia which accompanies hypernatraemia corrects spontaneously.

The majority of children will be fully rehydrated by this regimen and can resume a normal diet. Careful balance studies have failed to show any benefit from graded reintroduction of diet. Breast-fed babies should be encouraged to suckle throughout.[46]

Those in whom hydration has improved but residual signs of dehydration persist should receive continuing replacement of their deficits with ORS solution. Those with severe dehydration should receive intravenous rehydration with 150 mmol/l NaCl (normal saline 20 ml/kg over 20 min) followed by 75 mmol/l NaCl + 2.5% dextrose (half normal saline, 100 ml/kg over 4–6 h) with added potassium. Fluid may be administered to shocked children into the medullary cavity of the tibia by bone marrow biopsy needle if venepuncture fails. Continuing losses should be provided as for oral rehydration with 75 mmol/l NaCl + 2.5% dextrose and maintenance fluid and sodium requirements with 30 mmol/l NaCl + 4% dextrose (fifth normal saline). Alternatively, once the circulation is re-established, further rehydration therapy can be administered orally.

Dehydrated patients should have regular recording of blood pressure, weight, and output of stool, vomitus and urine. The occurrence of oliguria (< 1 ml/kg per hour) is an indicator of continuing dehydration or acute renal failure. In dehydration, the urine : plasma creatinine ratio is > 1.1 and the urine : plasma urea ratio is > 7. Elevation of plasma urea is no guide as values > 50 mmol/l occur in dehydration. If still oliguric after 8 h of rehydration therapy, frusemide (1 mg/kg) is given intravenously. If this does not produce a diuresis, or the urine quality, based on the above ratios of urine and plasma urea and creatinine, is inadequate then renal failure is present. Fluid is restricted to 80 ml/kg per 24 h for the first day without added potassium, then 30–40 ml/kg per 24 h + volume of the previous 24 h urinary output is administered. If the serum potassium concentration rises to 7.5 mmol/l, emergency treatment with intravenous calcium gluconate (0.5 ml/kg of 10% solution) is required, given over several minutes with ECG control. The presence of haematuria or a palpable renal mass suggests renal vein thrombosis, which can be confirmed by ultrasound. If polyuria persists after recovery then medullary necrosis may have occurred. The presence of anaemia and thrombocytopenia suggests that the oliguria is due to HUS secondary to enterohaemorrhagic *E. coli*. Administration of fresh frozen plasma (but not administration of antibiotics) has been shown to be beneficial.[47]

Hypokalaemia causes bradycardia and hypotension during rehydration. The ECG shows flattened T waves, U waves and a prolonged Q–T interval. Correction should be under ECG control. Hyperkalaemia produces tall T waves, flattened P waves and widening of the QRS complex. Replacement fluid should not contain more than 80 mmol/l of potassium because of the limited rate at which potassium can be transported into cells.

Other indications for intravenous rehydration are shown in Table 3.1.4. Severe diarrhoea indicates a rate of greater than 10 ml/kg per 24 h. The use of a nasogastric infusion of ORS solution may permit oral rehydration in spite of severe diarrhoea and vomiting. Ileus can complicate acute diarrhoea and will prevent successful oral rehydration. Coma is another contraindication, to avoid vomiting and aspiration. Children with appendicitis or intussusception may present with diarrhoea and vomiting; hence those with a distended or tender abdomen need intravenous therapy. In the vast majority of children, oral rehydration is the safest, simplest and most cost-effective method, with the added bonus of involving parents in the care of their sick child.

Antidiarrhoeal or antiemetic drugs are not indicated in the management of acute diarrhoea in childhood. The limited indications for antibiotics are shown in Table 3.1.5 and dosages of recommended agents in Table 3.1.6. They are seldom required, as the aetiology of acute diarrhoea and vomiting is so often viral, and most bacterial infections are self-limiting. When used they are often given empirically because rapid diagnostic methods are rarely available.[48] Specific recommendations are difficult in the presence of increasing resistance to antimicrobials, especially in shigellosis. Nevertheless, in severe shigellosis antibiotics decrease mortality. Whilst fluoroquinolones are recommended for adults, these antibiotics are not licensed for use in the UK for children because of the theoretical potential to damage growing bone cartilage. It seems unlikely that this complication will be seen after 1–3 days therapy yet children are thus deprived of these useful drugs. Travellers' diarrhoea is bacterial in origin in over 80% and duration is significantly shortened by antibiotics. *Campylobacter* is always resistant to trimethoprim. Erythromycin causes rapid elimination of the pathogen, and

Table 3.1.4   Indications for intravenous rehydration

Severe dehydration
Severe diarrhoea and vomiting
Ileus
Coma
Diagnostic doubt

Table 3.1.5   Indications for antibiotic therapy in diarrhoeal diseases

	Antibiotic	
Indication	Adults	Children
Severe shigellosis	Trimethoprim	Trimethoprim
Severe salmonellosis	Ciprofloxacin	Cefotaxime
Campylobacteriosis	Erythromycin	Erythromycin
Yersiniosis	Trimethoprim	Trimethoprim
Clostridium difficile	Vancomycin	Vancomycin
Cholera	Tetracycline	Furazolidone
Severe travellers' diarrhoea	Ciprofloxacin	Trimethoprim + erythromycin
Amoebiasis	Metronidazole + diiodohydroxyquin	Metronidazole + diiodohydroxyquin
Giardiasis	Tinidazole	Furazolidone

Modified from DuPont.[48]

Table 3.1.6   Dosage of antibiotic therapy in diarrhoeal diseases

	Dose			
Antibiotic	Adults	Children[a]	Total doses per day	Duration (days)
Trimethoprim	160 mg	10 mg/kg per day	2	3 (14 for severe salmonellosis)
Ciprofloxacin	300 mg	No	2	1–3 (14 for severe salmonellosis)
Erythromycin	250 mg	40 mg/kg per day	4	5
Vancomycin	125–250 mg	40 mg/kg per day	4	7–10
Tetracycline	500 mg	No	4	3
Furazolidone	100 mg	8 mg/kg per day	4	5 (3 for cholera; 10 for giardiasis)
Metronidazole	750 mg	30–50 mg/kg per day	3	5–10
Diiodohydroxyquin	650 mg	40 mg/kg per day	3	21
Tinidazole	2 g	No	1	1

Modified from DuPont.[48]
[a] Total daily dose.

generally shortens the illness. Antibiotics will also decrease the profound fluid and electrolyte loss in cholera. Salmonellae can cause extraintestinal infections which are an indication for antibiotics. Antibiotics should not be withheld in severe salmonella colitis because of concerns about development of antibiotic resistance. Furazolidone is recommended for giardiasis because there is a paediatric preparation available. Metronidazole has the advantage of activity against amoebiasis and overgrowth of the small intestine by bacteria. Severely ill infants with diarrhoea and vomiting should be given broad-spectrum systemic antibiotics in case there is associated sepsis.

Persistent diarrhoea is an important complication of infectious diarrhoea.[49] When diarrhoea persists for longer than 14 days, malnutrition is likely to occur, and, now that deaths from dehydration can be effectively prevented, there are clusters of diarrhoeal mortality in children with persistent symptoms, accounting for a third or more of all deaths from diarrhoea. The syndrome is due to an interaction of host and infecting agent. The complication is more likely in immunocompromised hosts such as young infants and children with defective cell-mediated immunity. Pre-existing malnutrition is also a risk factor. Infection with bacteria and protozoa rather than viruses is also a risk factor. Treatment strategies are being developed, based on modular diets consisting of protein (chicken or soy), carbohydrate (rice or glucose), fat (vegetable oil), vitamins and minerals.[50]

PREVENTION

Various measures to prevent diarrhoea have been assessed by Feachem et al.[51] Highly cost-effective measures include encouragement of breast-feeding and handwashing. Breast milk intake does not decrease during episodes of diarrhoea; breast-feeding decreases stool losses during acute diarrhoea, and prevents persistent diarrhoea. Measles immunization, a highly cost-effective measure in its own right, will prevent the diarrhoeal diseases which occur during convalescence when the child is temporarily immunosuppressed.[52] Supplementation with vitamin A has not been universally successful in preventing diarrhoea.[53] Zinc supplementation and general improvement in nutrition may be effective in decreasing duration of diarrhoea.[54] Provision of clean water is less cost-effective because of the high cost involved for every life saved; quantity of water available seems more important than quality.

The prospects for preventing diarrhoea by active immunization are improving. An effective live attenuated rotavirus vaccine should be available in the near future.[55]

REFERENCES

1 Orme R L'E, Piller G J. A report of a colloquium on health services in Britain and France, University of Exeter. Liverpool: Children's Research International, 1994.
2 MacFaul R, Glass E, Jones S. Appropriateness of paediatric admission. Arch Dis Child 1994; 71: 50–58.
3 Read A W, Gibbins J, Stanley F J, Morich P. Hospital admissions before the age of 2 years in Western Australia. Arch Dis Child 1994; 70: 205–210.
4 Savage F. Breast-feeding in the 1990s. Int Child Health 1992; 3: 29–33.
5 Baqui A, Sack R, Black R, Chowdhury H, Yunus M, Siddique A. Cell-mediated immune deficiency and malnutrition are independent risk factors for persistent diarrhea in Bangladeshi children. Am J Clin Nutr 1993; 58: 543–548.
6 Sánchez L, Calvo M, Brock J H. Biological role of lactoferrin. Arch Dis Child 1992; 67: 657–661.
7 Patton S. Detection of large fragments of the human milk mucin MUC-1 in feces of breast-fed infants. J Pediatr Gastroenterol Nutr 1994; 18: 225–230.
8 Sarkar S A, Gyr K. Non-immunological defence mechanisms of the gut. Gut 1992; 33: 987–993.
9 Walker-Smith J A. Malnutrition and infection. Trans R Soc Trop Med Hyg 1993; 87 (Suppl 3): 13–15.
10 WHO. Programme for control of diarrhoeal diseases Ninth Programme Report 1992–1993. Geneva: World Health Organization, 1994; WHO/CDD/94.46.
11 Sack R B, Myers L L, Almeido-Hill J et al. Enterotoxigenic Bacteroides fragilis: epidemiologic studies of its role as a human diarrhoeal pathogen. J Diarrhoeal Dis Res 1992; 10: 4–9.
12 Butcher A R, Lumb R, Coulter E, Nielsen D J. Coccidian/cyanobacterium-like body associated diarrhea in an Australian traveller returning from overseas. Pathology 1994; 26: 59–61.
13 Elliott E J. Viral diarrhoeas in childhood. Br Med J 1992; 305: 1111–1112.
14 Kotloff K L, Losonsky G A, Morris J G, Wasserman S S, Singh-Naz N, Levine M M. Enteric adenovirus infection and childhood diarrhea: an epidemiologic study in three clinical settings. Pediatrics 1989; 84: 219–225.
15 Troussard X, Bauduer F, Gallet E et al. Virus recovery from stools of patients undergoing bone marrow transplantation. Bone Marrow Transplant 1993; 12: 573–576.
16 Mitchell D K, Van R, Morrow A L, Monroe S S, Glass R I, Pickering L K. Outbreaks of astrovirus gastroenteritis in day care centers. J Pediatr 1993; 123: 725–732
17 Albert M J, Ansaruzzaman M, Bardhan P K et al. Large epidemic of cholera-like disease in Bangladesh caused by Vibrio cholerae O139 synonym Bengal. Lancet 1993; 342: 387–390.
18 Farthing M J. Travellers' diarrhoea. Gut 1994; 35: 1–4.
19 Gomes T A T, Blake P A, Trabulsi L R. Prevalence of Escherichia coli strains with

localized, diffuse, and aggregative adherence to HeLa cells in infants with diarrhea and matched controls. J Clin Microbiol 1989; 27: 266–269.

20 Bhan M K, Khoshoo V, Sommerfelt H, Raj P, Sazawal S, Srivastava R. Enteroaggregative Escherichia coli and Salmonella associated with nondysenteric persistent diarrhea. Pediatr Infect Dis J 1989; 8: 499–502.

21 Haider K, Faruque S M, Shahid N S et al. Enteroaggregative Escherichia coli infections in Bangladeshi children: clinical and microbiological features. J Diarrhoeal Dis Res 1991; 9: 318–322.

22. Cravioto A, Tello A, Navarro A et al. Association of Escherichia coli HEp-2 adherence patterns with type and duration of diarrhoea. Lancet 1991; 337: 262–264.

23 Tzipori S, Gibson R, Montanoaro J. Nature and distribution of mucosal lesions associated with enteropathogenic and enterohemorrhagic Escherichia coli in piglets and the role of plasmid-mediated factors. Infect Immun 1991; 57: 1142–1150.

24 Thomas A, Chart H, Cheasty T, Smith H R, Frost J A, Rowe B. Vero cytotoxin-producing Escherichia coli, particularly serogroup O157, associated with human infections in the United Kingdom: 1989–91. Epidemiol Infect 1993; 110: 591–600.

25 De Silva D G H, Mendis L N, Sheron N et al. Concentrations of Interleukin-6 and tumour necrosis factor in serum and stools of children with Shigella dysenteriae 1 infection. Gut 1993; 34: 194–198.

26 Candy D C A. Gastrointestinal infections in children. Curr Opin Gastroenterol 1995; 11: in press.

27 Anonymous. Dysentery due to Shigella infection. Commun Dis Rep CDR Weekly 1992; 2: 69.

28 Levine M M. Bacillary dysentery: mechanisms and treatment. Med Clin North Am 1982; 66: 623–638.

29 Taylor D N, Bodhidatta L, Echeverria P. Epidemiologic aspects of shigellosis and other causes of dysentery in Thailand. Rev Infect Dis 1991; 13 (Suppl 4): S226–230.

30 Candy D C A, Stephen J. Salmonella. In: Farthing M, Keusch G, eds. Enteric infection: mechanisms, manifestations and management. London: Chapman & Hall, 1989: pp 289–298.

31 Rampling A. Salmonella enteritidis five years on. Lancet 1993; 342: 317–318.

32 Savarino S J, Bourgeois A L. Epidemiology of diarrhoeal diseases in developed countries. Trans R Soc Trop Med Hyg 1993; 87 (Suppl 3): 7–11.

33 Doyle M P. Pathogenic Escherichia coli, Yersinia enterocolitica and Vibrio parahaemolyticus. Lancet 1990; 336: 1111–1115.

34 Weinke T, Friedrich J B, Hopp P, Janitschke K. Prevalence and clinical importance of Entamoeba histolytica in two high-risk groups: travelers returning from the tropics and male homosexuals. J Infect Dis 1990; 161: 1029–1031.

35 Gray S F, Rouse A R. Giardiasis: a cause of travellers' diarrhoea. Commun Dis Rep CDR Review 1992; 2.

36 Tripp J H, Candy D C A. Acute diarrhoea and vomiting: gastroenteritis. In: Tripp J H, Candy D C A, eds. Manual of paediatric gastroenterology and nutrition, 2nd edn. Oxford: Butterworth-Heinemann, 1992: pp 25–35.

37 Poulton J, Tarlow M J. Diagnosis of rotavirus gastroenteritis by smell. Arch Dis Child 1987; 62: 851–852.

38 Cantey J. Escherichia coli diarrhea. Gastroenterol Clin North Am 1993; 22: 609–622.

39 Kapperud G, Lassen J, Ostroff S M, Aasen S. Clinical features of sporadic Campylobacter infections in Norway. Scand J Infect Dis 1992; 24: 741–749.

40 Brook M G, Smith H R, Bannister B A et al. Prospective study of verocytotoxin-producing, enteroaggregative and diffusely adherent Escherichia coli in different diarrhoeal states. Epidemiol Infect 1994; 112: 63–67.

41 Knutton S, Baldwin T, Williams P H, McNeish A S. Actin accumulation at sites of bacterial adhesion to tissue culture cells: basis of a new diagnostic test for enteropathogenic and enterohemorrhagic Escherichia coli. Infect Immun 1989; 57: 1290–1298.

42 Islam D, Lindberg A A. Detection of Shigella dysenteriae type 1 and Shigella flexneri in feces by immunomagnetic isolation and polymerase chain reaction. J Clin Microbiol 1992; 30: 2801–2906.

43 Public Health Laboratory Service Study Group. Cryptosporidiosis in England and Wales: prevalence and clinical and epidemiological features. Br Med J 1990; 300: 774–777.

44 World Health Organization. A manual for the treatment of diarrhoea. WHO/CDD/Ser 80.2/Rev 2, 1990.

45 Gore S M, Fontaine O, Pierce N F. Impact of rice based oral rehydration solution on

stool output and duration of diarrhoea: metanalysis of 13 clinical trials. Br Med J 1992; 304: 287–304.

46 Brown K H, Lake A. Appropriate use of human and non-human milk for the dietary management of children with diarrhoea. J Diarrhoeal Dis Res 1991; 9: 168–185.

47 Loirat C, Sonsino, E, Hinglais N et al. Treatment of the childhood haemolytic uraemic syndrome with plasma: a multicentre randomized clinical trial. Paediatr Nephrol 1988; 2: 279–285.

48 DuPont H L. Diarrhoeal disease: current concepts and future challenges. Antimicrobial therapy and prophylaxis. Trans R Soc Trop Med Hygiene 1993; Suppl 3: 31–34.

49 Gracey M. Persistent childhood diarrhoea: patterns, pathogenesis and prevention. J Gastroenterol Hepatol 1993; 8: 259–266.

50 Booth I W, Candy D C A. Practical problems in protracted diarrhoea. J Trop Paediatr 1987; 33: 69–74.

51 Feachem R G, Hogan R C, Merson M H. Diarrhoeal disease control: reviews of potential interventions. Bull World Health Org 1983; 61: 637–640.

52 Sarker S A, Wahed M A, Rahaman M M, Alam A N, Islam A, Jahan F. Persistent protein losing enteropathy in post measles diarrhoea. Arch Dis Child 1986; 61: 739–743.

53 Stansfield S K, Muller P L, Lerebours G, Augustin A. Vitamin A supplementation and increased prevalence of childhood diarrhoea and acute respiratory infection. Lancet 1993; 342: 578–582.

54 Behrens R H. Diarrhoeal disease: current concepts and future challenges: the impact of oral rehydration and other therapies on the management of acute diarrhoea. Trans R Soc Trop Med Hyg 1993; Suppl 3: 35–38.

55 Vesikari T. Clinical trials of live oral rotavirus vaccines: the Finnish experience. Vaccine 1993; 11: 255–261.

3.2   Hepatitis

VIRAL HEPATITIS

Introduction

Infectious jaundice has been recognized as a clinical entity for centuries, but it is only during the lifetime of doctors still practising that clear recognition has been made of its aetiology and mode of transmission. The viral aetiology of 'serum hepatitis' was recognized in the 1940s, and epidemiological observations soon differentiated two forms of hepatitis: a long incubation period illness that was primarily transmitted parenterally, and a shorter incubation illness spread more readily. These two distinct infections are now known as hepatitis B and hepatitis A respectively. A variety of other infectious agents have since been shown to cause hepatitis, but less commonly than hepatitis A or B. These have been designated hepatitis C, D and E.[1] In addition, other viruses including the herpesvirus group can also cause liver disease and will be discussed.

Hepatitis A

Epidemiology

Hepatitis A infection is present worldwide, and is the commonest viral hepatitis in man. It is particularly prevalent in children, especially in areas of low socioeconomic status and poor hygiene. This is clearly associated with differences in faecal–oral transmission of the virus. In recent years the epidemiology of the virus has changed — as countries have developed improved levels of hygiene the overall incidence of infection worldwide has decreased, with a greater proportion of infections occurring in older individuals and primary infection in infants and children becoming less common.[2] Since symptoms in hepatitis A increase with increasing age, this epidemiological change is accompanied by a greater proportion of symptomatic infections.

Hepatitis A is caused by infection with a small RNA virus of the picornavirus family. It can infect man and a few other primates. It is quite stable to heat, acids and detergents, making it relatively resistant to disinfection. It can, however, be destroyed by boiling for a few minutes or by exposure to ultraviolet light.

Spread occurs particularly between children in the same household, especially in situations where there is overcrowding and poor sanitation. Epidemics have occurred from unhygienic food-handling by individuals excreting the virus, and particularly from shellfish harvested from contaminated waters, since many filter feeders concentrate viruses and other pathogens as they filter the water. Hepatitis A virus (HAV) can survive in contaminated seawater for a month or more. Transmission virtually never occurs by blood transfusion, except in neonates. Infection with hepatitis A is thought to confer immunity for life. Second attacks rarely if ever occur (but see under 'Relapse' below).

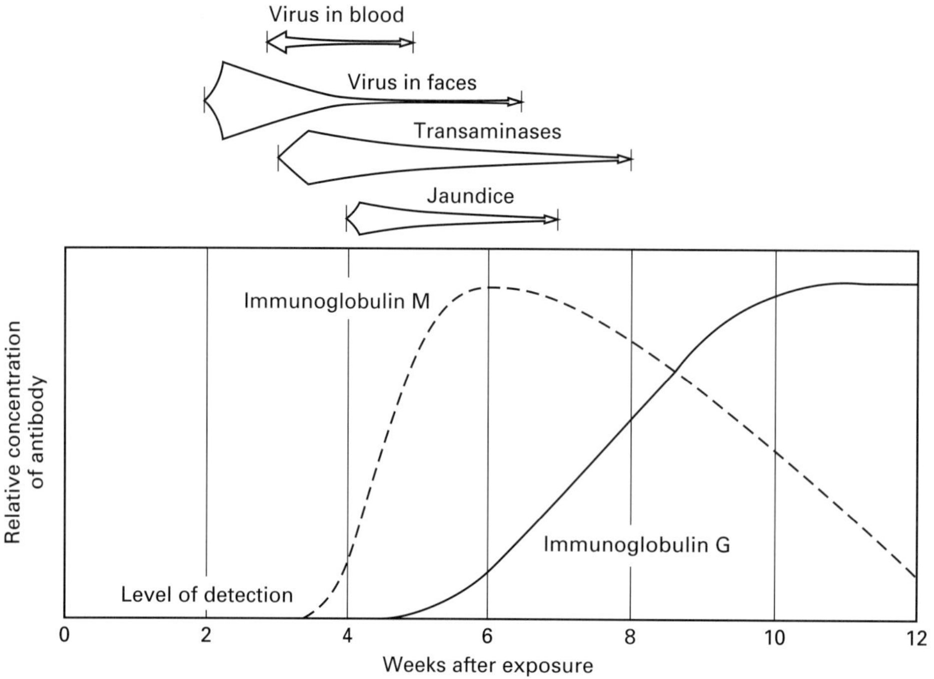

Fig. 3.2.1   Immunological and biological events associated with viral hepatitis A. (From Hollinger & Dienstag[12].)

Pathogenesis

Although it has long been thought that the cellular damage in hepatitis A was due to the direct action of the virus, work in recent years suggests that virus-specific CD8-positive T cells are important in the production of the liver damage and in the clearance of virus-infected cells from the liver.

Clinical features

The incubation period of hepatitis A is usually about 4 weeks, but can vary between 2 and 7 weeks. The illness is usually heralded by a non-specific prodrome characterized by tiredness, anorexia, vomiting and abdominal pain. Low-grade fever is also often present. The prodrome usually starts a week or so before jaundice, pruritus and dark urine are noted. It is this period that is associated with the highest excretion of virus in the stools. The appearance of jaundice marks a decrease in the degree of viral shedding, which usually stops within 2 weeks of the appearance of dark urine. Patients' faeces are infectious for up to 3 weeks before and 1 week after the onset of the jaundice.

Neither chronic liver disease nor a carrier state is recognized in association with hepatitis A.

Neonatal infection. Neonates can be infected with hepatitis A by transfusion from a donor in the prodromal phase of the illness or from a mother who can transmit the virus to the neonate during labour or delivery. Surprisingly, neonates infected in this way seldom show any clinical or biochemical features of hepatitis, although they excrete the virus in the stool and may infect other individuals.

Complications

Relapse. This is unusual but well recognized, particularly in adults. A second rise in aminotransferases occurs 8–12 weeks after the initial illness, and histological changes may persist for a year or more.

Fulminant hepatitis. Occasional patients (about 0.1% of symptomatic children) develop fulminant hepatitis. This can be diagnosed by the development of encephalopathy and by impairment of clotting. A good index of prognosis is the degree of prolongation of the prothrombin time after vitamin K. An international normalized prothrombin ratio (INR) of 1.6 or more should be an indication for transfer to a specialized liver unit — preferably one with facilities for liver transplantation. An INR of 4 or more is generally considered an indication for the child to be put onto the transplant list.[3]

Diagnosis

Hepatitis A is diagnosed by the appearance of specific IgM antibodies in the blood. These are present at or shortly after the clinical onset of the disease, and remain detectable for only about 3 months. IgG antibody is present for years after infection, and is good evidence of immunity.

Prevention

Passive immunization. Immune serum globulin is available for close contacts, particularly adult contacts of childhood cases, who are likely to be more severely affected than the index case. Travellers to endemic areas can be given prophylactic injections of immunoglobulin which last 4–6 months.

Active immunization. Hepatitis A vaccine prepared from an attenuated, formalin-inactivated strain of the virus ('Havrix', SmithKline Beecham) is available (although not yet licensed in Britain) and should be used where possible in preference to passive immunization.[4,5]. The vaccine is given as a three-dose regime, and probably affords long-lasting protection. It appears safe, and produces a high degree of protection (>90%) in clinical studies (see Ch. 18).[6]

Hepatitis B

Historical

Hepatitis B accounts for the vast majority of infections originally described as 'serum hepatitis' in the 1940s and 1950s. In the 1960s an antigen was first detected in the blood of Australian aborigines; this was initially thought to be an anthropological marker, and was called 'Australia antigen'. It soon became evident that this antigen was related to hepatitis B (serum hepatitis) infection, and it was renamed 'hepatitis-associated antigen' (HAA). Neither of these two names is now in use, and the currently agreed name for the antigen (now recognized to be the surface coat of the virus) is the hepatitis B surface antigen (HB_sAg).

The hepatitis B virus is a DNA virus which belongs to the hepadna group of viruses. Other members of this family produce hepatitis in ducks, in woodchuck and in ground squirrel, but the hepatitis B virus is thought to only infect man.

The virus consists of an outer protein coat, the hepatitis B surface antigen, and a viral core (see Fig. 3.2.2). The latter includes a core protein (hepatitis B core antigen, HB_cAg), another core antigen called e antigen associated with viral infectivity, and viral DNA and DNA polymerase. The whole virus particle seen under the electron microscope is known as a 'Dane' particle, after the virologist who first described it. The outer protein coat of the virus (HB_sAg), which is in itself non-infectious, is vastly over-produced both in infection and in the carrier state, and can be synthesized independently of the whole virus particle. Thus detection of the viral coat in blood does not necessarily indicate that the individual is infectious.

Epidemiology

The prevalence of the virus and the hepatitis B carrier state vary dramatically in

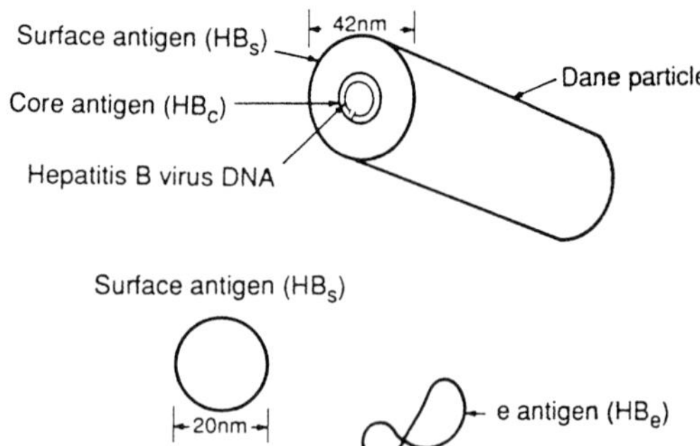

Fig. 3.2.2 Diagrammatic representation of electron microscopic appearance of hepatitis B virus.

different parts of the world. In Britain it is less than 1% of the population; similar low rates exist in other northern European countries, and in North America. Carriage rate is much higher in southern Europe, in Southeast Asia and in many areas of the developing world. There is evidence that this variation in carriage rate is not merely a reflection of social and environmental factors, but is also affected by the genetic background of the ethnic groups concerned. Both hepatocellular carcinoma and chronic hepatitis are clearly linked epidemiologically with hepatitis B infection, and areas with a high carriage rate also have a high rate of these diseases. It has been estimated that more than 25% of carrier infants will die from liver disease in adult life.

Modes of transmission

Parenteral and sexual routes are important methods of transmission worldwide, but in children the primary reason for hepatitis B carriage is vertical transmission of the virus from the mother to her child. This is particularly true in Southeast

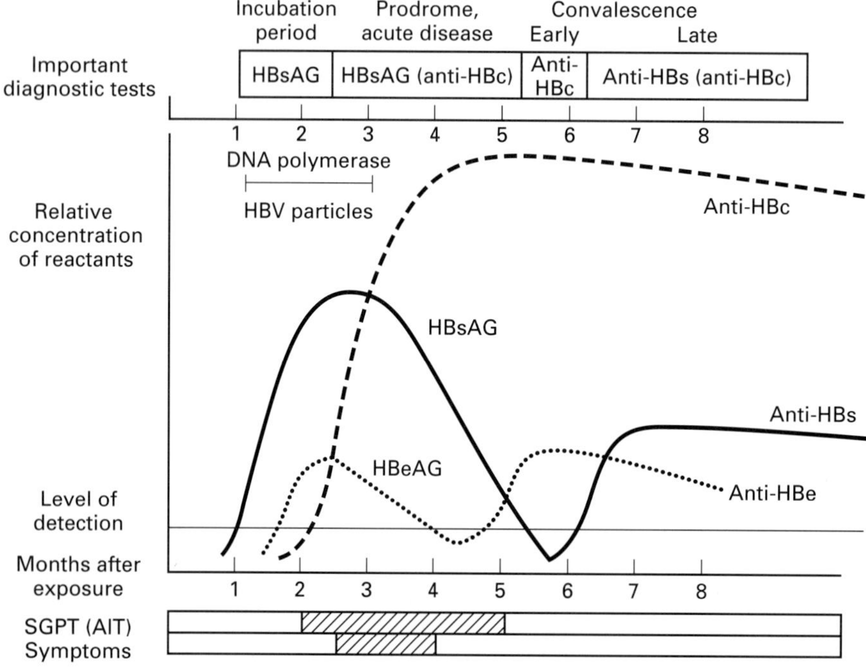

Fig. 3.2.3 Immunological events associated with hepatitis B (From Hollinger & Dienstag[12]).

Asia. However, in Africa horizontal transmission from one sibling to another is the most important mode of transmission and may result from sores and bed-bugs.[7] Exposure to infected blood or blood products accounts for an appreciable number of cases in Western countries with a low incidence of hepatitis B otherwise.

Diagnosis of hepatitis B

Interpretation of serological data. Because of the variety of viral antigens and associated antibodies, the interpretation of hepatitis B serology is sometimes confusing (Fig. 3.2.3).

Surface antigen (HB$_s$Ag). The presence of the surface coat of the virus in the blood indicates either current infection or the over-production of the surface protein typical of the carrier state. Surface antigen is also present in the blood in the incubation period of the illness for several weeks before symptoms develop.

Antibody to surface antigen (Anti-HB$_s$). Individuals with antibody to surface antigen are immune from hepatitis B. Antibody can be the result either of previous natural infection or of immunization.

Core antigen. The presence of core antigen (HB$_c$Ag) indicates whole virus particles in the blood stream, i.e. current infection.

Core antibody (Anti-HB$_c$). Antibody to core is only present in patients who have been infected in the past. Vaccine does not contain any of the virus apart from the outer protein coat, and vaccination will not, therefore, lead to production of core antibody.

IgM anti-core (IgM-anti-HB$_c$). This is present in acute or convalescent hepatitis, but also in carriers with chronic or progressive liver disease.

e antigen (HB$_e$Ag). e antigen is part of the viral core. Its presence in the blood correlates closely with the presence of complete viral particles (Dane particles), and with the presence of viral DNA polymerase. It is therefore used clinically as a marker of viral infectivity and of viral replication. It is not present in the blood in the absence of HB$_s$Ag.

e antibody (Anti-HB$_e$). This indicates progression towards elimination of the virus, either in acute infection or in the carrier state. e antibody can be found in the blood in normal convalescence, but is also present in patients who are carriers, and are in the process of eliminating the virus (this progression, when it occurs, is usually spread over several years).

HBV DNA. The presence of viral DNA in the blood is the 'gold standard' for viral replication. It can be interpreted in the same way as the presence of e antigen, but is more sensitive.

Mutants of the hepatitis B virus

A variety of mutants have been described; two are of particular clinical importance:

1. A mutation in the precore region of the viral DNA leads to a pathogenic virus which can cause fulminant hepatitis in infants of anti-HB$_e$ carrier mothers, i.e. mothers who otherwise would be considered of low infectivity. This phenomenon is rare but well recognized, and is an important reason for

immunizing infants born to 'low-infectivity' anti-HB_e-positive carrier mothers (see below).

2. A mutation in the DNA coding for hepatitis B surface antigen itself can lead to the production of an altered virus which is resistant to the effect of anti-HB_s antibodies. Immunization will therefore not protect individuals against infection with this mutant.

Pathogenesis

During the acute phase of the illness, and even during the prodromal period, circulating immune complexes are detectable, and arthralgia, fever and vasculitis may occur. Cell damage during the acute phase follows expression of viral antigen on the hepatocyte surface, with consequent cell lysis mediated by cytotoxic T cells. In chronic hepatitis B infection a reduced capacity to synthesize α- and β-interferons leads to reduced expression of HLA class I receptors on the hepatocyte surface. This means that these cells will express smaller amounts of viral antigen, and will therefore not be recognized or lysed effectively by cytotoxic T cells, resulting in prolonged infection. Other pathogenetic mechanisms also occur, but this is possibly the best understood, and the rationale for α-interferon treatment in chronic hepatitis B infection.

Clinical features of hepatitis B infection

Neonates. Only a tiny proportion of neonates infected from carrier mothers get significant acute disease, but approximately 90% go on to be chronic carriers of the virus. Boys are more likely to become chronic carriers than girls. Occasional neonates (1 : 1000 or less) born to anti-HB_e-positive mothers will get fulminant hepatitis;[8] many of these will only survive with liver transplantation (see mutant viruses above).

Hepatitis B in pregnancy. Infants infected from mothers who contract hepatitis B in the last trimester of pregnancy are at risk of serious disease, and should be protected at birth with both active and passive immunization.

Older children — acute infection. The incubation period is typically 3 months, but can be anything from 2 to 6 months. Many (about three-quarters) of children with hepatitis B are anicteric. The prodrome, which may last a week or more, is non-specific, but nausea, anorexia, abdominal pain and mild fever are prominent features. The icteric phase lasts 1–2 weeks in most children. Appetite usually returns before the jaundice clears completely. A small proportion of patients (0.1–0.5%) go on to have fulminant hepatitis. Premonitory features include a rising bilirubin and (particularly) a prolonged prothrombin index. As for hepatitis A infection, an INR > 1.6 after vitamin K should give rise to major concern; and an INR ≥ 4 is an indication for urgent transplantation. The derangement of clotting is probably a better indication of the degree of liver damage than the level of encephalopathy.

Older children — chronic infection

Chronic hepatitis B infection varies in severity from asymptomatic carriage of the virus, only detectable on virological testing, to severe liver disease which can be life-threatening. There is a very clear geographical and ethnic divide between areas of the world where a high rate of hepatitis B carriage exists (e.g. Southeast Asia, West Africa), and those areas where the carriage rate is low (Western Europe and North America). In the former, hepatitis B infection is the commonest cause of chronic liver disease in childhood, and the incidence of hepatocellular carcinoma (a largely hepatitis B-related disease) is high. In areas where the carriage rate is low, hepatitis B is an uncommon cause of chronic liver disease in childhood, and hepatocellular carcinoma is not a major problem.

Breast-feeding

Although HBV DNA and the HBV virus can be excreted in breast milk, infants of carrier mothers are at little if any extra risk by being breast-fed. They should, nevertheless, be immunized against hepatitis B as early as possible in life. In developing countries with a high infant mortality, the risks of bottle-feeding clearly outweigh any potential infection from breast milk.

Treatment

α-interferon has some effect in reducing the viral load. Approximately 30% respond to treatment, some HB_eAg-positive carriers converting to HB_eAg negativity, and others eradicating the virus altogether.[9] Response may be enhanced by associated treatment with steroids.

Treatment is parenteral, and needs to be continued for many months. The administration of α-interferon is often associated with significant side-effects, primarily of fever and influenza-like symptoms. At our present state of knowledge it should probably be considered only for those patients with severe chronic disease.

Immunization

The current vaccine consists of the outer protein coat of the virus (the HB_sAg), and is prepared using molecular techniques in yeast cells. The earlier vaccine, which was prepared from plasma donated by HB_sAg-positive carriers, is no longer used. Infants of carrier mothers are best protected by a 'belt and braces' approach using vaccine and specific anti-HBV immunoglobulin. In situations where this is not economically possible (e.g. in developing countries), vaccine alone is used. A policy of universal neonatal immunization against hepatitis B appears to offer 90+% protection against the disease (see Ch. 18).

Hepatitis C

In recent years, a further virus in addition to hepatitis B has been identified which produces a parenterally transmitted illness. This was first identified epidemiologically as a cause of post-transfusion hepatitis in patients who had no evidence of hepatitis A or B. By sophisticated molecular biological techniques, almost all the viral genome has now been cloned and sequenced, although the virus has not yet been seen under the electron microscope or grown in cell culture. Hepatitis C virus (HCV) is an RNA virus distantly related to the flaviviruses, but sufficiently different to be put in a different family.

Pathogenesis

As with other hepatitis viruses, the liver injury is probably largely immunological, the result of the host immune response rather than direct viral damage to the liver cell.

Clinical features

Hepatitis C appears to be parenterally acquired in many instances, although some cases are sporadic. When acquired parenterally, it has a mean incubation period of 8 weeks, but this can vary within wide limits.

Clinical features are similar to other forms of viral hepatitis. The illness is usually milder than hepatitis B, and the aminotransferase levels usually lower.

Characteristic features of the illness include:

- a high likelihood of chronic disease (about 50% of patients), with aminotransferase levels abnormal for 6 months or longer.
- a relapsing and remitting course with recurrent relapses over many months.
- the production of chronic active hepatitis or chronic persistent hepatitis.
- the existence of a carrier state like hepatitis B.
- an increased incidence of hepatocellular carcinoma in patients (but hepatitis B remains a much more important risk factor for hepatocellular carcinoma).

Modes of transmission

Most hepatitis C is transmitted parenterally, in association with blood and blood products. HCV RNA has not been detected in the milk of hepatitis C carrier mothers, and therefore breast-feeding can be encouraged in these mothers.

Unlike hepatitis B, vertical transmission is not a major problem with hepatitis C. Studies with antibodies and with polymerase chain reaction (PCR) detection of viral nucleic acid have shown that vertical transmission does occur, but that it is almost always trivial, producing a slight elevation of aminotransferases at most. Affected infants usually appear to develop antibody and become immune, rather than becoming chronic carriers as is the norm with hepatitis B infection. HIV infection in the mother appears to increase the likelihood of vertical transmission of coincident hepatitis C.

Diagnosis

It is not possible to differentiate one form of viral hepatitis from another reliably on clinical grounds.[10] Diagnosis of hepatitis C depends on detection of antibody to specific viral antigens, or detection of viral nucleic acid by PCR. The original 'first generation' enzyme-linked immunosorbent assay (ELISA) test for antibody to viral antigen was of low sensitivity and often does not become positive for many months after infection. It also yielded false positives on occasion, especially in patients with autoimmune hepatitis. Further assays have since been introduced — a second-generation ELISA and recombinant immunoblot assays (RIBA) — but insufficient information exists at present to assess them adequately or to compare them with PCR techniques, which are still primarily a research technique.

Treatment

Like hepatitis B, hepatitis C may respond to treatment with α-interferon,[11] with some children becoming seronegative (up to 40% of adult hepatitis C carriers respond to interferon therapy). As with hepatitis B, treatment needs to continue for many months, and there is no guarantee of success. It should probably be reserved for those with significant or rapidly progressive liver disease.

Hepatitis D

Hepatitis D is also known as delta agent. It is a defective virus which has no outer coat, and which uses the hepatitis B surface antigen for this purpose. It is therefore only transmitted with hepatitis B, and has no independent existence. Individuals who are positive for hepatitis D as well as hepatitis B have a more severe clinical illness, with a more rapid progression to chronic liver disease.

Superinfection in a patient already infected with hepatitis B causes an exacerbation of clinical illness. The diagnosis can be made by detecting hepatitis D antibodies in the blood (IgM in the case of acute infection, IgG in patients previously affected). Hepatitis D occurs much more commonly in some parts of the world than others. In Britain it is a particular problem in intravenous drug abusers. There is no specific treatment.

Hepatitis E

This virus, which has caused waterborne epidemics of hepatitis similar to hepatitis A, is spread by the faecal–oral route. It has, as yet, been little studied, but appears to cause relatively mild disease in children, although pregnant mothers appear to be at high risk of fulminant liver failure from the disease. There is no specific treatment, and chronic disease does not occur.

Recent evidence suggests that hepatitis E can be vertically transmitted and can cause appreciable disease in affected infants.

Hepatitis F, G and H

These have been described in experimental studies, or from histological and epidemiological evidence, but currently are not of clinical importance.

Neonatal hepatitis

This term is used to encompass all children with evidence of significant liver damage in the neonatal period. It is usual to exclude children with evidence of bile duct obstruction, i.e. those with biliary atresia. Neonatal hepatitis should be looked on as a syndrome rather than a single disease. Infective causes include cytomegalovirus, toxoplasmosis, herpes simplex virus infection and rubella, as well as hepatitis B. It should be stressed, however, that metabolic disease such as α_1-antitrypsin deficiency, galactosaemia or tyrosinosis can produce a very similar clinical picture both clinically and histologically. Hepatitis viruses are an unusual cause of neonatal hepatitis in Britain — the disease is much more likely to be metabolic in aetiology.

OTHER ORGANISMS CAUSING HEPATITIS

Cytomegalovirus, Epstein–Barr virus, toxoplasmosis enteroviruses and herpes simplex virus infections can all affect the liver, and should be considered in any unusual hepatitis when serology for conventional hepatitis viruses is negative. In addition, Weil's disease can also be associated with liver involvement. In the immunocompromised, liver damage can be caused by many pathogens; varicella is particularly important and varicella hepatitis may present without any significant generalized rash.

Infection may trigger haemolysis in patients with glucose 6-phosphate dehydrogenase deficiency, and this can be associated with slight elevation of the aminotransferases. The levels, however, will never approach those found in true hepatitis, but will only be marginally above the normal range.

Occasionally a patient with Wilson's disease will present with an acute or even fulminating illness which can be indistinguishable from viral hepatitis, and should be considered in all appropriate cases. Wilson's disease does not occur until the liver has accumulated enough copper to cause damage; it does not need to be considered in children below school age, and does not usually occur until adolescence.

REFERENCES

1 Ramos-Soriano A G, Schwartz K B. Recent advances in the hepatitides, Gastroenterol Clin North Am 1994; 23: 753–767.
2 Innis B L, Snitbhan R, Hoke C H, Munindhorn W, Laorakpongse T. The declining transmission of hepatitis A in Thailand. J Infect Dis 1991; 34: 191–193.
3 Bhaduri B, Lau J Y N, Heaton N et al. Acute hepatic failure in childhood: aetiology, prognostic indicators, and role of orthotopic liver transplantation (OLT). Hepatology 1992; 16: 516–520.
4 Boughton C R. Hepatitis A vaccine. Med J Aust 1991; 155: 508–509.
5 Werzberger A, Mensch B, Kuter B et al. A controlled trial of a formalin inactivated hepatitis A vaccine in healthy children. N Engl J Med 1992; 327: 453–457.
6 Innis B L, Snitbhan R, Kunasol P et al. Protection against hepatitis A by an inactivated vaccine. JAMA 1994; 271: 1328–1334.
7 Vall Mayans M, Hall A J, Inskip H M et al. Risk factors for transmission of hepatitis B virus to Gambian children. Lancet 1990; 336: 1107–1109.
8 Beath S V, Boxall E H, Watson R M, Tarlow M J, Kelly D A. Fulminant hepatitis B in infants born to anti-HBe hepatitis B carrier mothers. Br Med J 1992; 304: 1169–1170
9 Perrillo R P. Antiviral therapy of chronic hepatitis B: past, present and future. J Hepatol 1993; 17 (Suppl 3): S56–63.
10 Gregorio G V, Mieli-Vergani G, Mowat A P. Viral hepatitis. Arch Dis Child 1994; 70: 343–348.
11 A-Kader H H, Balistreri W F. Hepatitis C virus: implications to pediatric practice. Pediatr Infect Dis J 1993; 12: 853–867.
12 Hollinger F B, Dienstag J L. Manual of clinical microbiology, 4th edn. American Society for Microbiology, 1985.

3.3   Liver abscess

BACKGROUND

Liver abscess is rare in children, and is often diagnosed late because it has not been considered. There are two main types of liver abscess: pyogenic and amoebic. These will be considered separately although they have many similar features.

PYOGENIC LIVER ABSCESS

Most cases of liver abscess in children occur in immunosuppressed or immuno-deficient individuals. Chronic granulomatous disease is a particular predisposing factor. Diabetes and sickle cell anaemia also predispose to infection here as elsewhere.

In most cases in which a source can be found systemic bacteraemia is followed by localization of the organism in the liver. Other well-recognized pathogenic mechanisms include direct spread from neighbouring infection (e.g. in association with cholecystitis, cholangitis or pancreatitis), following portal pyaemia (from appendicitis, omphalitis or inflammatory bowel disease), or following blunt or penetrating abdominal trauma.

Microbiology

Important aetiological agents include *Staphylococcus aureus* (commonest), Gram-negative bacteria such as *Escherichia coli*, and anaerobes. The latter have been particularly highlighted as of importance in recent years.[1] Relevant anaerobes include *Peptostreptococcus* species, *Bacteroides fragilis* and *Fusobacterium* species.

Staphylococci are most likely to be associated with septicaemic spread, enteric organisms with abdominal disease such as appendicitis, and anaerobes as mixed infections in a variety of conditions. Several reported cases have been associated with *Fusobacterium necrophorum* infection.

Clinical features

Clinical features are often relatively non-specific, and the clinician must therefore have a high index of suspicion. Fever, nausea, vomiting, anorexia, weakness and malaise are typical but do not help to localize the infection.

Features to be looked for include hepatomegaly (present in most patients), tenderness in the right upper quadrant and localized rigidity and guarding.

Laboratory investigations are generally unhelpful. Liver function tests may be normal, and if raised aminotransferases are present, they are more likely to reflect associated cholangitis or other liver disease than to be due to the abscess. Most patients have anaemia and leucocytosis, but these again are non-specific. Blood cultures are usually sterile.

Investigations

The important investigations are radiological. Chest X-ray is often particularly helpful. An elevated right hemidiaphragm, a small pleural effusion, or right lower lobe atelectasis may be important clues to the diagnosis. Computed tomographic (CT) scanning provides the most sensitive probe for liver abscess, and can detect lesions as small as 1 cm in diameter. Ultrasound is, however, a more practical first investigation for most paediatricians, as it is also sensitive, does not involve radiation exposure, and is readily available in most units.[2,3]

Treatment

Liver abscesses should be treated either by open surgery or by percutaneous needling and/or drainage together with antibiotic therapy. Most undiagnosed and untreated patients die.

Abscess drainage is usually performed as an open procedure, but percutaneous catheter drainage has been widely performed in adults, although paediatric experience is limited.[4] Liver abscesses should always be cultured both aerobically and anaerobically. Fungi are better identified histologically, and if they are suspected it is important to arrange with the pathologist for special stains to be used.

Antibiotic treatment

Appropriate antibiotics depend on the likely source of the organisms. Many patients will have more than one organism present in the abscess. If anaerobes are known or suspected to be present, metronidazole, clindamycin, or a penicillin together with a β-lactamase inhibitor should be used. Third-generation cephalosporins and aminoglycosides are active against enteric organisms, and flucloxacillin or clindamycin are effective antistaphylococcal agents. Antibiotic treatment should continue for at least 4 weeks, or for longer if the child is being managed without surgical drainage of the abscess.

Chronic granulomatous disease

This disorder of neutrophil function predisposes to infections with catalase-positive organisms such as *Staphylococcus aureus*, and to fungal infections with *Candida* and *Aspergillus* species. Up to 40% of patients with chronic granulomatous disease get hepatic abscesses.

Fungal abscess

Fungal liver abscesses are the exclusive province of the immunocompromised, particularly leukaemics on prolonged parenteral feeding regimes, and patients with chronic granulomatous disease. Antifungal treatment with amphotericin (preferably liposomal) and other antifungals may need to be prolonged, and interferon γ may be of value in chronic granulomatous disease.[5]

AMOEBIC LIVER ABSCESS

Up to 10% of children with amoebiasis develop amoebic liver abscesses.

Clinical features

As in pyogenic liver abscess, non-specific features predominate. However, hepatomegaly is usual, and high fever with liver tenderness is the most common presentation.[6]

Most children do not give a history of preceding dysentery, and this together with the non-specific clinical features mean that the clinician needs to have a high index of suspicion in all febrile children from an endemic area in whom an alternative diagnosis is not apparent. Liver function tests are not usually abnormal. Jaundice is unusual.

Detection of amoebiasis

If the child is from or has recently visited an endemic area, evidence of amoebic infection should be sought. Cysts of *Entamoeba histolytica* are seldom present in the stools, and failure to detect them should not rule out the diagnosis. Serological studies can be very helpful, and are much more likely to be positive in patients with invasive amoebiasis than in disease localized to the colon.

Investigations

As well as the investigations detailed above, chest X-ray may be very helpful, and abdominal ultrasound or CT scanning should be performed as for suspected pyogenic liver abscess.

Management

The most important complication of amoebic liver abscess is rupture of the abscess into the abdomen or chest, with associated shock and a high mortality. Most patients are managed with a long-term amoebicide (metronidazole is usually the drug of choice); the abscess can be drained by percutaneous needle aspiration under ultrasound control. Treatment is continued for several weeks in a dose of 50 mg/kg per day, and the abscess or abscesses followed by repeated abdominal ultrasound.

Prognosis

When the diagnosis is promptly made and appropriate treatment instituted, the outlook is usually good. No patients died of a series of 24 children reported from Karachi over a 5-year period.[6] Once abscesses rupture, however, the mortality rises dramatically.

REFERENCES

1 Brook I, Fraizer E H. Role of anaerobic bacteria in liver abscesses in children. Pediatr Infect Dis J 1993; 12: 743–747.
2 Newlin N, Silver T M, Stuck K J, Sandler M A. Ultrasonic features of pyogenic liver abscess. Radiology 1981; 139: 155–159.
3 Laurin S, Kaude J V. Diagnosis of liver–spleen abscesses in children: with emphasis on ultrasound for the initial and follow-up examinations. Pediatr Radiology 1984; 14: 198–204.
4 Piniero-Carrero V M, Andres J M. Morbidity and mortality in children with pyogenic liver abscess. Am J Dis Child 1989; 143: 1424–1427.
5 Hague R A, Eastham E J, Lee R E, Cant A J. Resolution of hepatic abscess after interferon gamma in chronic granulomatous disease. Arch Dis Child 1993; 69: 443–445.
6 Nazir Z, Moazam F. Amebic liver abscess in children. Pediatr Infect Dis J 1993; 12: 929–932.

3.4 Cholecystitis

BACKGROUND

Acute cholecystitis in infants and children is unusual but not rare; when it occurs in children it is often not diagnosed for months or years because it has not been considered as a possibility. Gall-bladder disease is usually considered to be the realm of the adult physician rather than the paediatrician.

Cholecystitis, or inflammation of the gall-bladder, is seldom primarily of infectious origin, although the inflamed gall-bladder with impaired drainage will very readily become secondarily infected. Most cases of cholecystitis are associated with predisposing factors. The commonest of these are gallstones: cholelithiasis. Cholecystitis is usually divided into calculous and non-calculous disease, depending on whether or not coincident gallstones are present.

CALCULOUS CHOLECYSTITIS

In infants and children pigment stones are the commonest biochemical variety; they are composed primarily of calcium bilirubinate and occur in situations where bilirubin excretion in the bile is increased, particularly in congenital haemolytic anaemias. Because of the calcium they contain, they are usually radio-opaque.

In older children and adolescents, cholesterol stones are commoner; these are radiolucent, and therefore are better detected by ultrasound than by X-ray.

Mixed stones, also radio-opaque, may occur in adolescents and older children.

ACALCULOUS CHOLECYSTITIS

In the absence of gallstones, gall-bladder infection can occur as a primary event, particularly with *Salmonella typhi*,[1] but also with β-haemolytic streptococci, *Staphylococcus epidermidis* and leptospirosis.

In other patients, stasis or obstruction of the gall-bladder is a necessary prerequisite for infection. This therefore may occur in association with dehydration, surgery, intravenous feeding or other similar factors. Treatment with high-dose ceftriaxone, which produces biliary sludge, has also been associated with acute cholecystitis.[2] In the tropics, parasitic obstruction to the gall-bladder with *Ascaris* or with other worms may occur. *Fasciola* infection has also been reported as a cause of cholecystitis.

Clinical features

The clinical features in children are similar to those in adults. Unlike adults, however, there is an equal sex incidence of cholecystitis in childhood. The most characteristic feature is severe abdominal pain. This is usually localized to the right upper quadrant or to the epigastrium. In a minority of cases, the pain is less well localized, or may be referred to the peri-umbilical region. As in adults, pain in the right shoulder due to diaphragmatic irritation is not uncommon.

Fever is generally present, although it is usually only moderate. Rigors are unusual. Only a minority of children will be jaundiced. Many give a history of recurrent attacks of similar pain.

Clinical examination reveals abdominal tenderness and guarding, almost always in the right upper quadrant; in a small number of patients a tender mass may be felt in the region of the gall-bladder.

Investigations

Ultrasound is the investigation of choice,[3,4] although pigment stones in young children are often visible on straight X-ray. Not only will ultrasound detect gall-stones of any sort, but thickening of the gall-bladder wall can also be found. This is a very useful sign of cholecystitis, although not totally specific for it. If ultrasound is inconclusive, a technetium scan using HIDA or one of its analogues may be useful. Non-filling of the gall-bladder is suggestive of obstruction to the cystic duct, usually by a gallstone. Oral cholecystography can also be performed if the child is not jaundiced.

Other tests

Blood picture usually shows a mild leucocytosis with a left shift, and liver function tests are generally normal or only mildly disturbed apart from an elevated bilirubin in up to half the cases. Marked abnormalities of liver function are more consistent with hepatitis than with cholecystitis.

Evidence of sepsis, with fever, rigors and leucocytosis, should lead to blood cultures, and bile should be cultured both aerobically and anaerobically if any can be obtained at the time of surgery or other invasive procedure.

Management

Since obstruction is usually the primary cause of acute cholecystitis, its treatment is surgical. The inflammation is usually due to chemical damage by retained bile salts, and in most cases infection is only a secondary feature. Cholecystectomy is usually the procedure of choice, but in children who are too sick for this, cholecystotomy is a satisfactory alternative, although it is usually necessary to remove the gall-bladder later as an elective procedure in these children.

Microbiology and antibiotic treatment

In most cases surgical removal or drainage of the gall-bladder is sufficient, and antibiotics are not indicated. More prolonged illness than usual (pain for more than 3–4 days) is, however, almost always associated with secondary bacterial infection and should be treated with an antibiotic. Antibiotics should also be used if clinical features of sepsis, with high fever and rigors are present. It is important to use an antibiotic that is excreted in bile such as ampicillin or a cephalosporin. Some organisms such as *Salmonella typhi* grow well in bile; most pathogens, such as pneumococci and *Streptococcus pyogenes*, are very unhappy in such an environment. Most infections of the gall-bladder and biliary tree are with bile resistant organisms: coliforms, *Enterococcus faecalis*, and anaerobes such as clostridia and anaerobic streptococci.[5] Antibiotics which are effective against these organisms and which attain adequate concentrations in bile include co-trimoxazole and the cephalosporins. If aminoglycosides are used they should be combined with a penicillin because of their low activity against streptococci. Ampicillin is no longer a first-line drug in this situation, since increasing numbers of coliforms are now resistant. In general, cephalosporins are to be preferred to aminoglycosides because of their lower toxicity. However, ceftriaxone should not be used because its tendency to produce biliary sludging might only exacerbate any obstructive element to the illness. In those patients who have had previous biliary tract surgery, anaerobes are important and metronidazole together with mezlocillin or piperacillin might then be used.

COMPLICATIONS

Perforation of the gall-bladder

This is the commonest complication of acute cholecystitis. Perforation can lead to a bile peritonitis, which is associated with severe shock and has a high mortality (30% or more). This infected cavity can be walled off as an abscess, or can perforate into the gut to form a choledochoenteric fistula. All of these need surgical management.

Acute cholangitis

This ascending infection of the biliary tree is diagnosed because of increasing signs of sepsis in the patient with cholecystitis. There is almost always an associated ileus and more marked jaundice and abnormalities of liver function occur than are found in uncomplicated disease. Cholangitis should alert the paediatrician to the possibility of a structural abnormality of the biliary tree. The following are the most important.

Biliary atresia

Following a Kasai procedure or similar porto-enterostomy for biliary atresia the biliary tree outside the liver is entirely removed, and a Roux-en-Y loop of jejunum linked with the porta hepatis. This procedure allows gut bacteria direct access to the liver, and is frequently followed by recurrent episodes of ascending cholangitis, each of which causes further damage to the already impaired organ. Long-term prophylactic antibiotic treatment is usually recommended for these children, in whom the clinical features of cholangitis may be relatively mild or non-specific.

Unexplained fever or jaundice in a child who has had a Kasai operation should therefore be assumed to be due to cholangitis until some alternative explanation is found, and should be treated vigorously with antibiotics.

Caroli's syndrome (congenital ectasia of the bile ducts)

Caroli's syndrome is a rare abnormality of the bile ducts characterized clinically by recurrent episodes of cholangitis with jaundice. The abnormal and dilated bile ducts may sometimes be detectable on ultrasonography, but in many cases CT scanning will more readily detect them. This situation, too, will need to be treated vigorously with antibiotics, and should be managed in conjunction with a hepatology service.

Choledochal cyst

Choledochal cysts classically present with the clinical triad of jaundice, an abdominal mass and abdominal pain. In infancy, however, the presentation is rarely typical; the commonest type is a saccular or fusiform dilatation of the bile duct. This can readily get infected, probably because of relatively stagnant bile within the cyst. Operative or percutaneous cholangiography provide the 'gold standard' for the diagnosis, but many cases can be detected by ultrasound or CT scanning. All children with 'ascending cholangitis' without apparent cause should be assumed to have an anatomical abnormality of the bile ducts until proven otherwise.

Congenital hepatic fibrosis

This genetic disorder, inherited as an autosomal recessive, usually presents with hepatic enlargement and portal hypertension. It probably forms part of the same spectrum of disorders as Caroli's disease, and may present in early life with cholangitis. Splenomegaly is usual, and liver function is generally normal despite the hepatomegaly and hepatic fibrosis.

Cholecystitis in the neonate

Several reports over the last decade have defined cholecystitis in the newborn.[6,7] This is usually associated with concurrent systemic illness and with a mass in the right upper quadrant of the abdomen. With the increasing trend for preterm neonates to be treated with long-term parenteral nutrition, this is becoming recognized as a cause of cholecystitis in the neonate. As in cases diagnosed in older children, primary treatment is surgical, although adjunct antibiotic therapy is indicated.

REFERENCES

1 Yulevich A, Cohen Z, Maor E, Bryk T, Mares A J. Acute acalculous cholecystitis caused by Salmonella typhi in a six year old child. Eur J Paediatr Surg 1992; 2: 301–303.
2 Jacobs R F. Ceftriaxone associated cholecystitis. Pediatr Infect Dis J 1988; 7: 434–436.
3 Mirvis S E, Vainwright J R, Nelson A W et al. The diagnosis of acute acalculous cholecystitits: a comparison of sonography, scintigraphy and CT. Am J Roentgenol 1986; 147: 1171–1175.
4 Pedersen J H, Hancke S, Christensen B et al. Ultrasonography, 99mTc-DIDA cholescintigraphy, and infusion tomography in the diagnosis of acute cholecystitis. Scand J Gastroenterol 1982; 17: 77–80.
5 Marne C, Pallares R, Martin R, Sitges Serra A. Gangrenous cholecystitis and acute cholangitis associated with anaerobic bacteria in bile. Eur J Clin Microbiol 1986; 5: 35–39.
6 Ziv Y, Feigenberg Z, Dintsman M. Acute inflammation and distension of the gall bladder in infancy. Aust Paediatr J 1987; 23: 53–54.
7 Traynelis V C, Hrabovsky E E. Acalculous cholecystitis in a neonate. Am J Dis Child 1985; 139: 893–895.

Renal

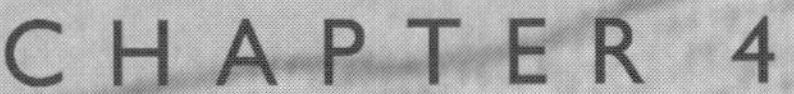

4.1. Urinary tract infection

4.2. Glomerulonephritis

J. Craig   J. Knight

4.1   Urinary tract infection

Urinary tract infection (UTI) is one of the commonest bacterial infections of children. The condition presents unique problems of urine collection, diagnosis and investigation that often make management difficult. The principles of management should include prompt diagnosis with the commencement of effective therapy, and the prevention of renal damage. The purpose of this review is to provide the paediatric physician with guidelines so that these principles can be pursued more readily.

DEFINITIONS

UTI is defined as the presence of significant numbers of viable bacteria in the urine. Children who present with UTI may be symptomatic or asymptomatic. The latter condition is also called covert, latent or screening bacteriuria; as the name implies, children with this diagnosis present with an intercurrent illness or take part in a screening programme and are found to have a significant bacteriuria. UTI can also be classified according to whether there is an associated renal tract abnormality such as urinary obstruction, urolithiasis, or a neuropathic bladder, in which case the UTI can be termed 'complicated'. If no abnormality is present the UTI can be regarded as 'uncomplicated'. UTI can also be divided into lower tract involvement only (cystitis), or ascending infection with involvement of the renal parenchyma (acute pyelonephritis). Infections can either be the first or recurrent. The latter includes the same organism (true recurrence) or a different organism (reinfection). These terms, though in widespread use, have limited clinical usefulness. The exceptions are pyelonephritis, which is complicated by permanent renal damage in some children, and covert bacteriuria, which generally does not require specific treatment.

Chronic atrophic pyelonephritis is a term used to describe a characteristic intravenous pyelogram appearance (clubbed calyces, contraction of the associated papilla and a defect in the renal cortical outline), and/or a chronic inflammatory reaction in the renal parenchyma on histological examination, and/or chronic renal infection. Reflux nephropathy is a term which denotes the association between vesicoureteric reflux and renal parenchymal abnormality.[1] Often reflux nephropathy and chronic atrophic pyelonephritis are used interchangeably.

DIAGNOSTIC METHODS

The diagnosis of UTI can only be made on the demonstration of significant bacteriuria. Adjunctive tests such as pyuria, abnormal urinalysis, elevated antibody titres, impaired concentrating ability, raised plasma urea and electrolytes, and the various forms of renal imaging available may assist in localizing the infection or prompting early diagnosis, but should not be used for routine diagnostic purposes. Counts of $10^8/l$ ($10^5/ml$) or more of a single pathogen in a fresh, uncentrifuged, voided, mid-stream specimen are generally regarded as diagnostic of UTI. Lower counts and/or the presence of two organisms can also be significant. Repeated urine cultures increase the likelihood of a correct diagnosis being made.

Any growth on a suprapubic bladder tap specimen or a urethral catheter specimen is also usually accepted as significant.[2]

Collection and transport of urine samples

Few techniques in clinical medicine can be as simple but as frustrating as the collection of an uncontaminated urine sample in a young child. In the older child who is able to void on request, the collection of an uncontaminated, voided mid-stream sample should present few difficulties, provided that the parent is instructed, in detail, on the method required. Unfortunately it is often left to the poorly instructed parent, and/or the most junior member of the medical or nursing team, to ensure that the sample is obtained appropriately. This often results in poorly obtained specimens, contamination of the urine with skin and mucosal organisms, with potentially misleading culture results, and leads to over- or under-treatment of the child. As urine samples collected after antibiotics have been commenced are non-diagnostic, it is the attending clinician's responsibility to ensure that a suitable urine sample has been obtained before antibiotics have been prescribed. Because the diagnosis of UTI carries with it particular implications for renal tract investigation, which are time consuming, invasive and unpleasant, the clinician needs to be sure that the possibility of contamination has been excluded, before treatment has commenced. The parent should be instructed to clean the urethral meatus/preputial fold with water and to 'catch' the middle specimen of urine while the child voids in an uninterrupted manner. Cleansing of the area with antiseptic may reduce the colony count and is therefore not recommended.

If the young child cannot void on request, a suprapubic bladder tap or a urethral catheter sample is required before treatment of a suspected UTI can be initiated. Of the two techniques the suprapubic bladder tap is preferable because of the lower frequency of contamination and iatrogenic UTI. If performed immediately following a failed bladder tap, urethral catheterization is usually successful. An adhesive plastic bag is often used to collect urine for infants. The advantage of this technique is the ease with which a sample of urine is obtained. Because of the unacceptably high number of contaminated samples, bags should not be used for the diagnosis of UTI unless all other techniques have failed.

Because of the exponential increase in the urinary colony count at room temperature, the specimen should be sent to the laboratory immediately after collection. If this is not possible, the sample can be stored at 4°C for a short period without significant alteration in the bacterial count.

Urine culture

Most laboratories process the urine in a semi-quantitative manner. For example, a wire loop, calibrated to deliver a standard volume of 1 µl, can be immersed into the urine and then used to inoculate media. The colony count can be read directly from the plate 24–48 h after inoculation. To determine the sensitivities of the isolate, most laboratories use diffusion tests. These tests use standardized filter paper disks which have been impregnated with a fixed amount of antibiotic. The isolate is seeded onto the surface of an agar plate and the disks are added. At 24 h the zones of inhibition, corresponding to the degree of susceptibility of the isolate to the antibiotic, are recorded.

Other diagnostic methods

White blood cells in the urine (pyuria) indicate inflammation of the urogenital tract that may be due to urinary tract infection. Pyuria is best quantified using a sample of uncentrifuged urine placed into a counting chamber and viewed through a microscope. Normal urinary white cell values for boys are $< 10 \times 10^6/l$, and for girls $< 50 \times 10^6/l$. Pyuria can be estimated by dipstick urinalysis testing using a leucocyte esterase test strip. Nitrites are produced in the urine by certain bacteria, and they can be detected by a test strip impregnated with nitrate.

Bacteria are frequently visible on wet mount microscopy and/or detected by Gram stain of uncentrifuged urine. Like the detection of pyuria, the presence of bacteria on microscopic examination of the urine enables the clinician to suspect the diagnosis and treat early, especially in the unwell child while the results of urine culture are awaited. Because of a significant false positive and false negative rate compared with the gold standard (urine culture) children who are suspected of having UTI should have their urine cultured in all instances, regardless of the urinalysis or urine white cell count.

EPIDEMIOLOGY

The incidence of symptomatic UTI in children under 11 years of age is estimated to be 2% for boys and 7% for girls.[3] Infancy is the age of greatest predisposition, particularly for boys. After infancy, girls more frequently present with a symptomatic infection (Fig. 4.1.1). UTI recurrence is more common in girls, with up to 50% developing at least one further infection.[4] The incidence of asymptomatic bacteriuria is similar to symptomatic infection.[5]

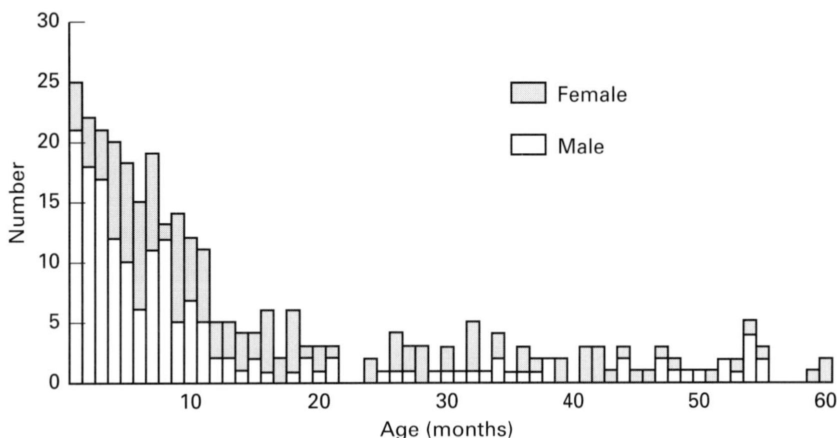

Fig. 4.1.1 Age of first-time symptomatic UTI by gender.

CLINICAL FEATURES

The clinical features of UTI are mainly due to the systemic effects of infection, and local effects on detrusor stability and urethral mucosal irritation. In children under 2 years of age the clinical features are generally non-specific and include fever, anorexia, vomiting, diarrhoea and lethargy. After 2 years of age symptoms referrable to the urinary tract such as frequency, dysuria, abdominal pain and urinary incontinence are more common, but not invariable. It is inappropriate for a non-specific febrile illness to be diagnosed as 'viral' in origin unless the urine culture is known to be sterile. A characteristic presentation, which is particularly worrying to parents, is the older boy who presents with macroscopic haematuria. While other causes of macroscopic haematuria should be considered such as glomerulonephritis, UTI is most commonly the correct diagnosis.

BACTERIAL AETIOLOGY

Most urinary pathogens are commensal bowel flora and gain access to the urinary tract via the urethra. *Escherichia coli* is the predominant pathogen in children, with over 80% of all UTIs caused by this organism. *Klebsiella* and *E. faecalis* are most frequently pathogens in infants. *Proteus* is a common isolate in older boys, and *Staphylococcus saprophyticus* in pubertal girls. In children with an associated renal tract abnormality, infection due to *Pseudomonas, Staphylococcus epidermidis, Corynebacterium* spp. and *Candida* spp. can occur, although *E. coli* remains the predominant invader (Fig. 4.1.2). Infection due to one of these unusual isolates should alert the clinician to the probability of a predisposing functional and/or anatomical renal tract abnormality.

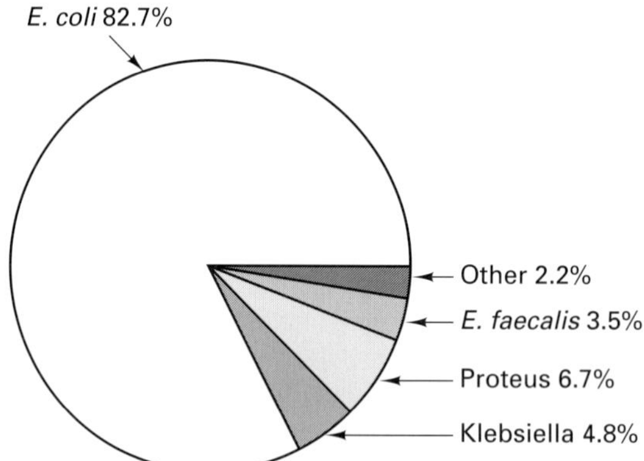

Fig. 4.1.2 Causative organisms in 304 consecutive urinary tract infections in preschool children.

ACUTE MANAGEMENT

Principles of acute management should include clinical examination to ascertain the presence of urinary obstruction and/or dehydration, early commencement of appropriate antimicrobials, and specific treatment of dehydration and electrolyte disorders.

Children who present with a symptomatic UTI should be examined with special reference to the state of hydration including blood pressure, the back, the external genitalia and the abdomen. A thorough lower limb neurological examination should be performed. If an abnormality is detected, an early renal tract ultrasound should be performed to rule out associated urinary obstruction.

The cause of dehydration in children who present with a urinary tract infection is two-fold. First, UTI frequently results in salt and water loss due to vomiting and diarrhoea which is not adequately replaced due to concomitant anorexia. Secondly, if renal parenchymal infection occurs, renal tubular salt and water wasting results in further predisposition to dehydration. This renal tubular dysfunction is particularly marked in infants under 3 months of age who have immature renal tubular function. The characteristic presentation in these children is a pattern of electrolyte abnormality which mimics congenital adrenal hyperplasia with hyponatraemic, hypochloraemic and hyperkalaemic dehydration with metabolic acidosis.[6] As the salt loss is generally of the order of 70 mmol/l of Na, the appropriate empiric fluid therapy should consist of a solution with at least this concentation of sodium (e.g., half-normal saline). Generally blood for urea and electrolytes should be drawn from any child who requires inpatient care, and urine should be sent not only for microscopy and culture, but also for an estimation of Na concentration and osmolality to assist with the rational administration of fluid therapy.

There are no data concerning the relative efficacies of intravenous versus oral antimicrobial administration. Indications for inpatient treatment with intravenous antibiotics should probably include clinical failure of oral administration, UTI in children under 3 months of age (who absorb oral antibiotics erratically), dehydration, electrolyte abnormalities, or a clinically severe illness. Empiric therapy should be based on the antibiotic sensitivities of the local urinary tract isolates (Fig. 4.1.3).

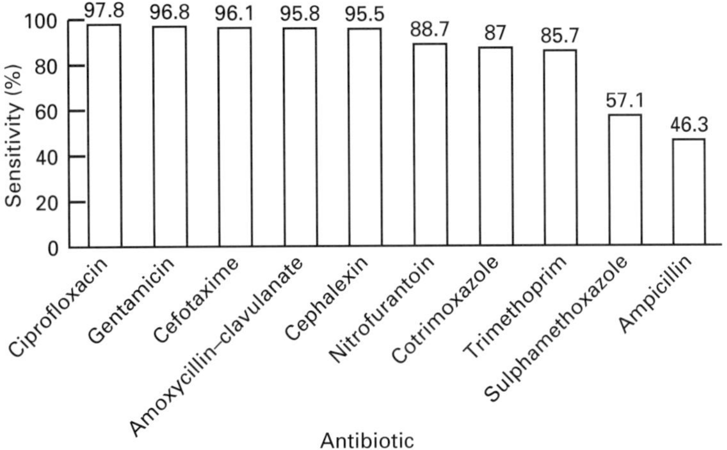

Fig. 4.1.3 Antibiotic sensitivity of isolates in 304 consecutive urine infections in children under 5 years of age.

If oral therapy is appropriate, trimethoprim alone or as co-trimoxazole (4 mg/kg per day of trimethoprim and 20 mg/kg per day of sulphamethoxazole given in two divided doses), and cephalexin (25 mg/kg per day given in three divided doses) are the agents generally regarded as the first-line antimicrobials. Amoxycillin–clavulanate (50 mg/kg per day in three divided doses) and nitrofurantoin (5 mg/kg per day in four divided doses) demonstrate similar in vitro efficacy but are more likely to cause gastrointestinal side effects. Because over 50% of all urinary pathogens are β-lactamase producing, amoxycillin/ampicillin is inappropriate as empiric therapy. Gentamicin (7.5 mg/kg per day in three divided doses) or a third-generation cephalosporin such as cefotaxime (100 mg/kg per day in three divided doses) are appropriate empiric antimicrobials for intravenous therapy. The addition of ampicillin (100 mg/kg per day in three divided doses) confers coverage against *E. faecalis* and should probably also be given to children under 3 months of age until the isolate has been identified. In all cases, once the in vitro susceptibility of the isolate has been performed, the antibiotic can be changed to a suitable and potentially less toxic alternative.

There are insufficient data in children to support the use of single-dose oral treatment. Antimicrobials should be given for 7–10 days. The decision to cease intravenous antibiotics and commence oral therapy is a clinical one, and is based on fever defervescence and an improvement in the general condition of the child.

All children should have a follow-up urine culture after the cessation of the antibiotic course. Antimicrobial administration need not be ceased before the urine specimen is collected. Persistent bacteriuria is a rarity (3%), and is usually a reinfection.[4] Treatment should be determined by the antibiotic susceptibility of the isolate.

Failure of treatment

It is imperative to distinguish between bacteriological and clinical failure. The latter is more common, and occurs when children who receive oral antimicrobials have persistent gastrointestinal upset and/or fever. It can be difficult to differentiate whether the persistent gastrointestinal disturbance is due to the antibiotic or the infection, although persistent fever often indicates that the UTI is causal. A repeat urine culture of these children is usually sterile and a period of intravenous antibiotics results in 'cure'. Clinical failure with persistent fever for more than 48–72 h should also suggest concomitant urinary obstruction and is an indication for an urgent renal tract ultrasound. Persistent bacteriuria is usually due to the administration of an antimicrobial agent to which the isolate is not susceptible. Renal calculi or impaired glomerular filtration that result in subtherapeutic levels of antibiotic in the affected renal tract can also cause persistent bacteriuria.

These conditions can be determined by examination of the urinary pathogen antibiogram, blood creatinine, renal ultrasonography and a plain abdominal X-ray.

PATHOGENESIS

The characteristic sex and age distribution of UTI in childhood strongly suggests that UTI is not due to faecal soiling and the relative shortness of the female urethra. There is also no evidence that bubble bath, poor hygiene or swimming predispose to UTI. Constipation and bladder instability may play a role, especially in the group of children who have recurrent UTI. Incomplete bladder emptying is probably important in those children with significant renal tract abnormality. These conditions include ureterocele, posterior urethral valves, pelvi-ureteric or vesicoureteric junction obstruction, primary megaureter, large bladder diverticuli, renal calculi and neuropathic bladder associated with sacral agenesis or meningomyelocele. Vesicoureteric reflux (VUR) is proposed as a predisposing factor for UTI because of the association between VUR and UTI in all series of children who present with a symptomatic UTI. The frequency of VUR in these children is almost invariably 20–30%. This figure is compared with the rate of VUR in 'normal' children (which varies from 0–60%,[7,8] but is often regarded as < 1%), and it is concluded that this confirms that VUR causes UTI. This is, at best, weak epidemiological evidence. The antegrade flow of refluxing urine into the bladder, once micturition has ceased, is the postulated mechanism. To date, apart from children with obstructive renal tract abnormality, these 'host factors' do not adequately explain why some children get UTI. Recently, from prospective cohort studies of children with antenatal renal tract dilatation who are found to have VUR on postnatal investigation, evidence has emerged that abnormal renal parenchyma (congenital renal hypo/dysplasia) may predispose to UTI, rather than the causal link being in the reverse direction as is commonly asserted.[9] There are clearly, as yet unknown, generalized and local host defence factors, which vary with age and sex, and predispose some children to UTI.

In contrast the various properties of the organism which predispose to UTI are better elucidated.[10] This is particularly true for *E. coli*, where a number of virulence factors have been identified. These virulence factors are certain O-antigens (cell wall), K-antigens (polysaccharide component of the capsule), and H- or flagellar antigens. The lipid component of the O-antigen, lipid A, is released after cell lysis. In the animal model this has been shown to reduce ureteric peristalsis so that the pathogen may gain access to the upper tract. Some mannose-resistant (MR) fimbriae adhere to the glycolipid determinant of blood group P and have been designated P fimbriae. P receptors are also present on uroepithelium, and have been implicated in animal studies and in children in the pathogenesis of acute pyelonephritis.[11]

It is widely held that colonization of the intestine and periurethra area must proceed before UTI can occur. Ascent of the pathogen into the bladder is followed by rapid multiplication, overwhelming of the host defences and, in some, continued ascent to the upper tracts. Bacteraemia occurs in 10% of children under 6 months old who present with a symptomatic UTI. This has been used to support the theory that infection in young infants is blood-borne, although the evidence is scanty.

INVESTIGATION

Few areas in paediatrics are as controversial as the mode and timing of the investigation of a child who presents with a symptomatic UTI. It has been held for over 20 years that the investigation of a child with a UTI is mandatory. This view stems from the observed association of severe permanent renal parenchymal damage with UTI and VUR.[1] The discovery of children with a predisposing renal tract abnormality (chiefly VUR) by the screening of children who present with a UTI, and the commencement of chemoprophylaxis, is clearly an attractive preventive strategy for the development of additional renal damage. Unfortunately this is unproven. Generally, however, investigation of a child with a UTI, to detect a 'predisposing abnormality' and to determine the severity of the infection, is standard clinical practice. A number of imaging modalities and their relative advantages and disadvantages are given in the following sections.

Renal tract ultrasound

The examination of the renal tract by real-time B-mode ultrasound is widely available, safe, painless and is almost universally acceptable to parents. It provides reasonable information on kidney, ureteric and bladder anatomy and does not require exposure to radiation. However, it is unreliable in the detection of VUR, acute and permanent renal parenchymal abnormality and renal calculi, and can provide no information on renal function. Renal ultrasonography is very operator dependent, and where possible should only be performed by an experienced paediatric sonographer. The major role of ultrasound is the detection of significant pelvic and/or ureteric dilatation which may indicate obstruction, and the detection of major renal parenchymal damage.

Intravenous pyelogram (IVP)

The IVP was, until recently, the gold standard investigation for renal parenchymal damage and urinary obstruction. It is widely available and provides good visualization of the anatomy of the renal parenchyma, collecting system and bladder. It has also been used extensively in prospective cohort studies so that the outcome of children with various grades of IVP-defined renal 'scarring' can be predicted with reasonable accuracy. Renal growth can also be reliably measured. However, the IVP is invasive, involves radiation exposure, and requires significant bowel preparation. Despite bowel preparation, the renal outlines are often obscured by overlying bowel gas. Anaphylactic reactions and nephrotoxicity can complicate the injection of the iodinated contrast. Because the IVP requires adequate glomerular function before the anatomy can be determined, it is seldom useful in children under 6 weeks of age. A lag time of up to 2 years has been reported before 'scarring' is visible. Information on function is not provided, and the IVP is less sensitive than the DMSA scan for both acute and chronic renal parenchymal damage.[12] The major role of the IVP is the confirmation of renal tract obstruction and the detection of renal parenchymal damage where nuclear imaging facilities are not available.

[99m]Tc-labelled dimercaptosuccinic acid (DMSA) scan

The DMSA is a relatively new radionuclide scan. DMSA is administered intravenously and scintiscans are taken after the renal tubular cells have been given sufficient time to take up the isotope. Any disorder of proximal renal tubular function related to the amino acid reabsorptive function will result in an area of photon deficiency. This may be due to acute or chronic tubular damage or due to a generalized tubular abnormality such as nephropathic cystinosis. Differential function of each of the renal units can also be obtained by measuring the functional tubular mass. The DMSA is generally accepted as the 'gold standard' for renal parenchymal abnormality, both for acute pyelonephritis and 'reflux nephropathy' (Fig. 4.1.4). However, it is not widely available, is invasive, provides no information on the collecting system anatomy, and involves exposure of the kidney to radiation. Perhaps most importantly the long-term clinical correlation with an abnormal DMSA scan is not available and the detection of small parenchymal defects, which are most unlikely to cause clinically significant impairment in renal function, probably results in unnecessary doctor–patient–parent anxiety.

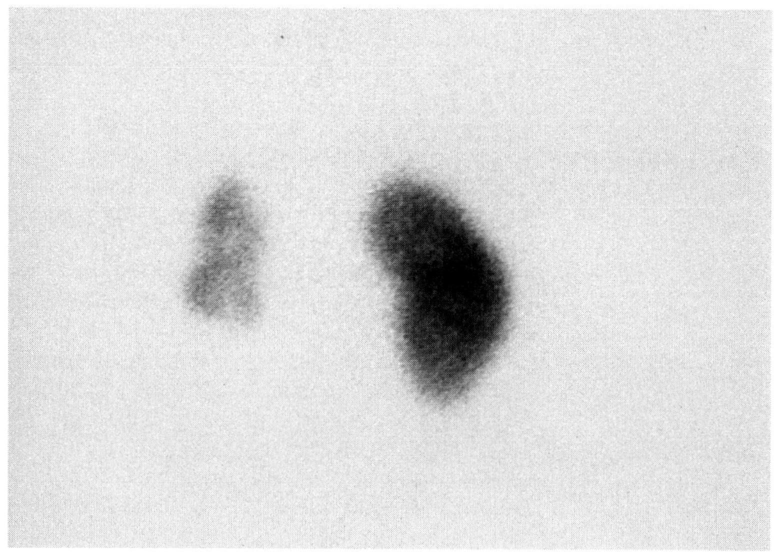

Fig. 4.1.4 A DMSA scan, which demonstrates diffuse renal parenchymal abnormality of the left kidney (NB: scintiscan taken from behind).

Currently DMSA scans are widely used to accurately determine the state of the renal parenchyma.

Micturating cystourethrogram (MCU)

Both the radiological and radionuclide MCU are used to detect VUR. The latter results in a significantly lower radiation dose, but does not provide as much information on urethral or bladder anatomy, and precise grading of the VUR cannot be performed.[5] Most data on the natural history of VUR is also based upon the radiological MCU. Generally the radioisotope MCU (usually ^{99m}Tc-labelled colloidal sulphur) is restricted to girls (because posterior urethral valves do not occur in females), or in the follow-up of children with known VUR. Indirect MCUs are advocated by some because they do not require bladder catheterization, but they are significantly less sensitive than 'direct' MCUs, and are generally not recommended. The MCU is the most invasive of all renal tract investigations and is the test that is most disliked by doctors, parents and patients. It provides no information on the state of the renal parenchyma, but is required if the presence of VUR needs to be determined. It should be understood that VUR is an active process and the presence and grade of VUR at one point in time does not give a complete picture of what may be occurring at other times or during a UTI. VUR can be graded, and the grading system used by the International Reflux Study is given in Fig. 4.1.5.[13] Higher grades of reflux and intrarenal reflux are particularly associated with parenchymal abnormality (Fig. 4.1.6).

Other investigations

A plain abdominal X-ray should be performed to exclude renal calculi, unless the MCU has included a baseline plain film. Radioisotope scans (e.g., diethylamine triamine pentaacetic acid or DTPA) with saline loading and frusemide diuresis are used to diagnose renal tract obstruction when renal tract dilatation is detected by ultrasonography.

Recommendations

Unfortunately, definitive recommendations for the mode and timing of renal tract investigations for a child who presents with a UTI cannot be given as the most clinically relevant questions concerning risk factors for long-term adverse outcome and UTI recurrence have not, as yet, been answered. If the detection of VUR is required then the MCU should be performed; if obstruction or gross renal parenchymal damage is the most important question then a renal ultrasound scan should be performed; and if the accurate detection of renal parenchymal damage is required then a DMSA scan should be the investigation of choice. Usually recommendations are made using these three imaging methods depending on the age of the child. For children over 5 years of age a renal ultrasound and plain abdominal X-ray are almost universally recommended as the minimum investigations. Because infancy is generally regarded as the period of greatest risk for

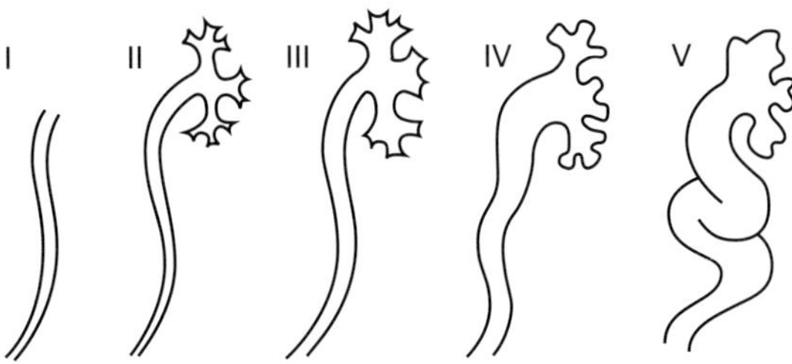

Fig. 4.1.5 Grades of VUR according to the International Reflux Trial.

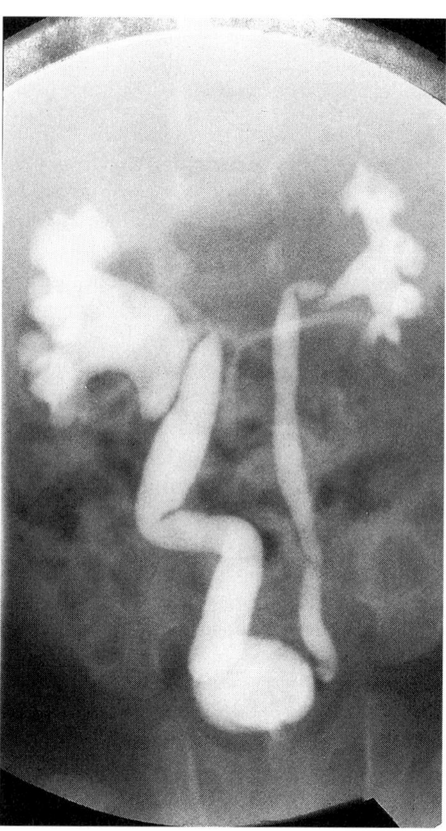

Fig. 4.1.6 Grade V VUR on the right and grade II on the left.

acute pyelonephritis and renal scarring, and additional renal damage in a previously normal renal tract is unusual after 5 years of age, more investigations are performed for the preschool age child. A renal ultrasound, MCU and DMSA scan (performed at least 3 months after the symptomatic infection to allow time for most of the acute changes to resolve) is the current mode of investigation, which will detect almost all abnormalites. Some authorities limit the MCU to infants only, others to children under 2 years of age. Prospective cohort and randomized controlled studies are currently being undertaken which will result in a more rational rather than traditional approach to this important aspect of management.

FOLLOW-UP

Chemoprophylaxis

The administration of low-dose antibiotic therapy has been shown to reduce the frequency of recurrent infection. This is recommended for the following indications:

1. After a symptomatic UTI until renal tract investigations have been carried out.
2. If renal tract investigations have demonstrated VUR, particularly dilating VUR, children are usually placed on long-term chemoprophylaxis until either the reflux is shown to have resolved by a repeat MCU or until the child reaches an age when additional renal damage is most unlikely to occur (4–5 years for a child with normal upper tracts and 7 years for a child with renal damage).

3. For children with demonstrable renal tract obstruction who are awaiting surgery.
4. There are a group of children who have frequent symptomatic recurrences despite normal renal tracts. For these children the problems and risks of long-term chemoprophylaxis are outweighed by the morbidity associated with UTI recurrence; 6–12 month periods of chemoprophylaxis, followed by a trial off chemoprophylaxis, is usually advised.

Surgical referral

Referral to a paediatric urologist should be considered in the following situations:

1. Nephrolithiasis.
2. Renal tract obstruction.
3. Breakthrough UTI in the presence of vesicoureteric reflux.

CIRCUMCISION AND UTI

In 1982 Ginsburg and McCracken published a series of 100 children who presented with a UTI within the first year of life; 62 children were boys, and of these only three were circumcised.[14] They concluded that an intact foreskin may predispose infant boys to UTI. To date a number of cross-sectional analytical, retrospective cohort, case–control and ecological studies have been published and have concluded in a similar manner. The following is an attempt to summarize the data, critically appraise the literature and provide some guidelines for the clinical application of the data.

Cross-sectional analytical studies

These include the original study of Ginsburg and McCracken and other published case series of infants and children with UTI. At best they provide very weak evidence, and conclusions on whether circumcision prevents UTI should not be drawn from studies with this methodology.

Case–control studies

Two relevant case–control studies have been published. The first was published by Herzog in 1989.[15] The study subjects were infant boys who presented to Boston Children's Hospital with an acute illness and who had a urine sample obtained. Cases were defined as those with significant bacteriuria, and controls those infant boys without bacteriuria. Of the 36 cases, no boy had been circumcised. This compared with the 76 control subjects, of whom 52 had been circumcised. The second study was published in 1992 and examined the incidence of symptomatic UTI in a group of men who attended an STD clinic.[16] A case was defined as a man with a positive urine culture, and the controls were those men who had a negative urine culture. Of the 26 cases, 18 were circumcised. Of the 52 controls, 46 were circumcised. The odds ratio for UTI in uncircumcised men was 3.4 (95% CI 1.0–11.2), with a p-value of 0.04. Both studies are at best weak evidence that circumcision prevents UTI. Both studies are hospital-based studies rather than the preferable population-based design. A major difficulty with the first study was the exclusion of 99 of the originally eligible 211 in a non-blinded fashion. The second study was also non-blinded and the criterion of UTI occurring in adult men who are attending an STD clinic can be questioned.

Cohort studies

The retrospective cohort studies of Wiswell and colleagues provide the strongest evidence that circumcision is protective.[17] A number of papers have been published on a very large cohort of newborn boys who were born in army hospitals and were subsequently admitted during the first year of life with a UTI. The odds ratio for UTI in uncircumcised male infants is 9.3 (95% CI 7.4–11.8). The magnitude of the odds ratio make confounding an unlikely reason to explain this result. Selection bias and differential misclassification remain unanswered criticisms. It is unclear how many servicemen 'drop out' of the service in any given year and whether this is more likely to occur in families who tend to be circumcised or uncircumcised. Every study is again non-blinded, but perhaps more importantly only infant boys who were hospitalized and had a bladder puncture or catheter-proven UTI were included. It is unclear how many boys had a UTI and were not admitted, or only had a voided urine sample to confirm the presence of infection. It is conceivable that more circumcised boys were treated as outpatients or did not have a urine sample taken by an invasive technique because the clinician thought that it was less likely that contamination would occur if a voided urine sample was taken in an uncircumcised male infant. No attempt at exploring this potential for bias has been made in any of the papers.

Before/after and ecological studies

Here Wiswell and colleagues attempt to correlate the falling rates of circumcision with the rising incidence of UTI in the same cohort of infant boys born in army hospitals.[18] This study design is also weak for questions of causality and detailed analysis of the data suggest that more factors are operative than the changing incidence of circumcision. It has also been suggested that the different gender ratios reflect the different rates of circumcision in different countries.[19] This also is unconvincing.

Proposed mechanism of action

It has been demonstrated that the degree of periurethral colonization by uropathogenic organisms is higher in uncircumcised than circumcised males, and adherence of these organisms seems enhanced by the presence of non-keratinized mucosa such as occurs on the prepuce.[20] This then is the putative mechanism by which a non-circumcised state predisposes to UTI.

Summary and clinical applications

Despite the difficulties with each of the studies, the general uniformity of the direction and magnitude of the apparent protective effect of circumcision for UTI makes it likely that this observed effect is 'true'. Proponents of routine newborn circumcision argue that the available evidence supports this practice as a public health measure. Before this can be advocated three difficulties must be countered. First, the surgical complication rate of circumcision is between 0.2% and 4.0%. Local infection and haemorrhage are the most common complications, but bacteraemia, meningitis, necrotizing fasciitis, scrotal abscess, phimosis, skin bridge, concealed penis, urethrocutaneous fistula, penile necrosis, meatitis, meatal stenosis, chordee, inclusion cysts, lymphoedema, bivalve penis, anaesthetic complications, gastric and bladder rupture, acute renal failure and death have all been reported. Second, it can be estimated that if the odds ratio for non-circumcision is 10.0, and the incidence for UTI in the first year of life for an uncircumcised male is 1%, one would need to circumcise 1000 male infants to prevent nine UTIs. During this time between two and 40 infants would have sustained significant complications from the procedure. Third, the short- and long-term morbidity and mortality of UTI in children are not of sufficient proven magnitude to warrant a putative prophylactic routine procedure such as circumcision. Certainly UTI causes an unpleasant acute illness in some children but the associated mortality is now less than 1%. Whether acute UTI causes renal damage of sufficient severity to cause hypertension and chronic renal failure, and which can be prevented by circumcision is unproven. On current data there seems insufficient evidence to support routine circumcision of the newborn as a public health measure to prevent UTI and possible long-term renal sequelae.

Circumcision may benefit the small group of boys who develop recurrent UTIs despite chemoprophylaxis, and for whom no additional form of therapy is available. There is no randomized controlled trial to support this practice, but there is some anecdotal evidence in favour.

REFERENCES

1 Bailey R R. The relationship of vesico-ureteric reflux to urinary tract infection and chronic pyelonephritis: reflux nephropathy. Clin Nephrol 1973; 1: 132–141.
2 Report of a working group of the research unit, Royal College of Physicians. Guidelines for the management of acute urinary tract infection in childhood. J R Coll Physicians Lond 1991; 25: 36–42.
3 Hellström A, Hanson E, Hansson S, Hjälmås K, Jodal U. Association between urinary symptoms at 7 years old and previous urinary tract infection. Arch Dis Child 1991; 66: 232–234.
4 Winberg J, Andersen H J, Bergstrom T, Jacobsen B, Larson H, Lincoln K. Epidemiology of symptomatic urinary tract infection in childhood. Acta Paediatr Scand 1974; 252 (suppl): 1–20.
5 Wettergren B, Hellström M, Stokland E, Jodal U. Six-year follow up of infants with screening bacteriuria. Br Med J 1990; 301: 845–848.
6 Melzi M L, Guez S, Sersale G et al. Acute pyelonephritis as a cause of hyponatraemia/ hyperkalaemia in young infants with urinary tract malformations. Pediatr Infect Dis J 1995; 14: 56–59.
7 Kjellberg S R, Ericsson N O, Rudhe U. The lower urinary tract in childhood. Chicago: Yearbook, 1957.
8 Kollermann M W, Ludwig H. Uber den vesico-ureteralen Reflux beim normalen Kind im Sauglings und Kleinkinderalter. Z Kinderheilk 1967; 100: 185–191.
9 Burge D M, Griffiths M D, Malone P S, Atwell J D. Fetal vesicoureteric reflux: outcome following conservative postnatal management. J Urol 1992; 148: 1743–1745.
10 Hanson L Å, Ahlstedt S, Jodal U et al. The host–parasite relationship in urinary tract infections. Kidney Int 1975; 8: S28–34.
11 Initiation of clinical pyelonephritis: the role of p-fimbriae-mediated bacterial adhesion. Contr Nephrol 1984; 39: 252–272.
12 Goldraich N P, Ramos O L, Goldraich I H. Urography versus DMSA scan in children with vesicoureteric reflux. Pediatr Nephrol 1989; 3: 1–5.
13 International Reflux Committee. Medical versus surgical treatment of primary vesicoureteric reflux. Pediatrics 1981; 67: 392.
14 Ginsberg C M, McCracken G H Jr. Urinary tract infections in young infants. Pediatrics 1982; 69: 409–412.
15 Herzog L W. Urinary tract infections and circumcision. Am J Dis Child 1989; 143: 248–250.
16 Spach D H, Stapelton A E, Stamm W E. Lack of circumcision increases the risk of urinary tract infection in young men. JAMA 1992; 267: 679–681.
17 Wiswell T E, Roscelli J B. Corroborative evidence for the decreased incidence of urinary tract infections in circumcised male infants. Pediatrics 1986; 78: 96–99.
18 Wiswell T E, Enzenauer R W, Holton M E et al. Declining frequency of circumcision: implications for changes in the absolute incidence and male to female sex ratio of urinary tract infections in early infancy. Pediatrics 1987; 79: 338–343.
19 Winberg J, Bollgren I, Gothefors L, Herthelius M, Tullus K. The prepuce: a mistake of nature? Lancet 1989; i: 598–599.
20 Fussell E N, Kaack M B, Cherry R, Roberts J A. Adherence of bacteria to human foreskins. J Urol 1988; 140: 997–1001.
21 Kaplan G W. Complications of circumcision. Urol Clin North Am 1983; 10: 543–549.

4.2 Glomerulonephritis

INTRODUCTION

Bacterial infection is the most common cause of acute glomerulonephritis in the world. Post-streptococcal glomerulonephritis is probably the best-recognized and most studied form of infection-associated nephritis, and will be considered here in some detail. The practical principles of management apply equally across the broad clinical spectrum of autoimmune, glomerulo-interstitial inflammatory reactions to infectious processes (Table 4.2.1).

EPIDEMIOLOGY

The incidence of infection-associated glomerulonephritis has fallen dramatically since the turn of the century. The fall antecedes the discovery of antibiotics and is often said to relate to improvements in general standards of hygiene. Glomerulonephritis is still very common, however, in poor countries[1-3] and in disadvantaged minorities living in wealthy countries.[4] The syndrome may occur at any age but is most common between the ages of 2 and 12 years. Symptomatic disease is twice as common in males as in females. There is a substantial incidence of subclinical disease, detectable by urinalysis surveys of children with sore throats. One prospective study showed that one in 26 non-streptococcal upper respiratory infections resulted in subclinical glomerulonephritis.[5]

In Japan, where the standard of living is high, annual screening has shown that 0.5–0.9% of children have blood or protein in their urine. The abnormality was attributed to recent glomerulonephritis in about 5% of children detected.[6] In Australian Aboriginal children, in contrast, the incidence of recent glomerulonephritis is as high as 8.9% of all school-age children.[3]

PATHOGENESIS AND PATHOLOGY

Certain strains of streptococci are particularly nephritogenic (M-types 1, 2, 4, 12, 18, 25, 49, 55, 57 and 60).[7] Antigens have been isolated from nephritogenic strains, and are demonstrable in the glomerulus in acute disease. At the same time, the alternate pathway of complement is activated and glomerular deposition of C3 and of the membrane attack complex (C5b-9) are demonstrable immunohistochemically. Platelets aggregate in glomerular capillary loops; the balance between fibrinolysis and coagulation becomes perturbed, procoagulant factor is excreted and extensive fibrin deposition ensues.

Table 4.2.1   Infectious diseases associated with postinfectious glomerulonephritis

The formal proof that an organism has caused postinfectious glomerulonephritis is made by demonstrating the presence of the infectious agent, or subunits thereof, in the glomerulus (or the presence of antibodies specific for the organism). This strict standard of proof is rarely achieved, if only because renal biopsy is rarely used in the management of postinfectious glomerulonephritis.

The list which follows is based on more relaxed criteria — case reports or series in which the antecedent infection seemed clinically likely to have provoked the renal disease.

Upper respiratory infection	Group A β-haemolytic *Streptococcus* (especially M serotypes 1, 3, 4, 12, 25, 49)
	Adenovirus
Skin infection	Group A β-haemolytic *Streptococcus* (especially M serotypes 2, 49, 55, 57, 60)
	Corynebacterium
	Propionibacterium
	Streptococcus pneumoniae
Lower respiratory infection	*Streptococcus pneumoniae*
	Mycoplasma
	Influenza A
	Adenovirus
Bacterial endocarditis	*Staphylococcus aureus*
	Streptococcus viridans
Shunt nephritis	*Staphylococcus aureus*
	Staphylococcus epidermidis
	Streptococcus viridans
Meningitis	*Neisseria meningitidis*
Visceral abscesses	*Staphylococcus aureus*
	Escherichia coli
	Pseudomonas aeruginosa
	Proteus mirabilis
	Klebsiella sp.
	Clostridium perfringens
	Atypical mycobacteria
Acute systemic infections	Epstein–Barr virus
	Cytomegalovirus
	Measles
	Mumps
	Varicella
	Rubella
	Coxsackievirus
	Echoviruses
	Rocky Mountain spotted fever
	Ross River virus
	Cat-scratch fever
Chronic systemic infections	Syphilis
	Leprosy
	Yersiniosis
	Brucellosis
	Leptospirosis
	Hepatitis B
	HIV
	Trichinosis
	Malaria (*Plasmodium falciparum* and *Plasmodium malariae*)
	Schistosomiasis (*Schistosoma haematobium* and *Schistosoma mansoni*)
	Toxoplasmosis
	Filariasis
	Rickettsiae
	Fungi (*Candida albicans* and *Coccidioides immitis*)

Cell-mediated immunity also plays a role in the pathogenesis of infection-associated glomerulonephritis: the renal interstitium is invaded by T lymphocytes, macrophages and neutrophils.

CLINICAL FEATURES

In developing countries, the initiating infection is typically a streptococcal impetigo. In developed countries, streptococcal pharyngitis predominates. The acute nephritic syndrome typically commences 1–2 weeks after throat infection and 3–4 weeks after skin infection.

The most common reasons for seeking medical attention are oedema (particularly periorbital oedema) or macroscopic haematuria — the urine is typically smoky brown in colour and described as resembling Coca-Cola or black tea. Bright red urine is more usual in IgA nephropathy than in postinfectious glomerulonephritis. On questioning there may be a history of oliguria, tiredness, poor appetite and general malaise. There may have been recent sore throat or skin infection.

The physical examination often reveals pitting oedema of the ankles or the sacrum, a blood pressure above the 95th percentile for age, and blood and protein in the urine on dipstick testing. In more severe cases, tachypnoea and crackles at the bases of the lung fields may betray the presence of pulmonary oedema.

DIAGNOSIS

The diagnosis of an acute nephritis can be made definitively by the examination of a spun sediment of fresh urine under the microscope. Ten millilitres of urine are centrifuged for 10 min at 3000 rpm, the supernatant poured off and the sediment resuspended by tapping the base of the test tube gently. A drop of the resultant fluid is placed on a microscope slide under a cover slip and examined under high power. The presence of red cell casts confirms the haematuria as glomerular. Casts break up rapidly in alkaline or concentrated urine, so this is a task which should be performed by the clinician, not by a laboratory technician. Copious white cells are also often seen in the urinary sediment in an early acute nephritis, and the unwary will be tempted to misdiagnose bacterial infection of the kidney.

It is traditional to confirm the diagnosis of post-streptococcal glomerulonephritis by demonstrating low C3 and normal C4 concentrations in the serum, together with evidence of high-titre antibodies to at least one of the common streptococcal surface antigens, streptolysin O or DNase B. However, even in Western teaching hospitals these results can take 7–10 days to return from the lab, and are therefore of little use in immediate clinical decision making. Of far more importance are the serum electrolytes (sodium, bicarbonate, potassium, calcium and phosphate), albumin, urea, creatinine and a full blood count. While the serum creatinine may not be higher than the upper limit of normal for an adult male (120 µmol/l), the use of the height/creatinine formula (glomerular filtration rate = 48 × height in centimetres ÷ serum creatinine in µmol/l)[8] will often reveal that the child has lost 30–50% of glomerular filtration rate. Serum potassium must always be checked but is seldom dangerously elevated. There will often be evidence of phosphate retention and accompanying hypocalcaemia. The serum albumin should be measured so that the importance of the hypocalcaemia can be assessed, and to avoid missing a mixed nephritic/nephrotic picture. The blood count will often show a mild normocytic, normochromic anaemia due to the temporary suppression of erythropoietin production. As the most important differential diagnosis in younger children is the haemolytic uraemic syndrome, the clinician should ascertain that platelets are plentiful and that there is no red cell fragmentation on the blood film.

TREATMENT

There is no specific treatment for nephritis. In post-streptococcal disease, the process proceeds to a benign outcome in virtually all cases over a period of weeks. In other infections the nephritis may continue until the underlying infection is treated or resolves. In the case of malaria and schistosomiasis, however, renal failure can result even when the infection itself is eliminated. In general, then, treatment is aimed at maintaining homeostasis until the kidneys recover.

If the blood pressure and serum creatinine are within the normal range at presentation, the child can be managed as an outpatient. It is useful to ask the parent to weigh the child daily and to bring him or her for review if the weight increases by more than half a kilogram — a sure sign of increasing fluid retention.

If the blood pressure is high, or renal impairment is present, hospital admission must be considered. While glomerular filtration rate may be reduced by as much as 30–50%, filtration seldom ceases entirely, so frusemide will be effective, although larger than usual doses must be used. The typical child with acute nephritis, puffy eyes and mild to moderate hypertension will produce a satisfying diuresis in response to an oral dose of frusemide, 5 mg/kg. The dose can be repeated every 12 h until the blood pressure has normalized and the oedema has gone. Twice-daily measurement of weight can be useful in judging when to back off on the diuretic regimen.

If the blood pressure is greater than 150 mmHg systolic, or 100 mmHg diastolic at presentation, an antihypertensive should also be used as a short-term measure until the frusemide has had a chance to work. A single dose of a calcium channel blocker such as nifedipine will lower the blood pressure safely and effectively for 4–6 h by vasodilatation, and if adequate diuretic has been given it should not be necessary to repeat the dose. Attention should be paid to the formulation of the drug: for example, nifedipine comes both in rapid-onset, liquid-filled 10 mg capsules and in sustained-release tablets. The former should be used. The dose is approximately 1 mg for each year of life, so that a 5-year-old would receive 5 mg, a 10-year-old 10 mg. Sublingual administration is difficult for small children, and unnecessary — uptake is just as rapid from the stomach.

Strict bed rest was used in the past, but is completely without value. Similarly, severe fluid restriction is an unnecessarily harsh measure, as fluid status can be controlled by adjusting the dose of diuretic. It is reasonable to limit access to high-salt junk foods like potato crisps, but the child should eat a normal diet.

PREVENTION

Improvements in general hygiene and living conditions are said to be the reason for the decrease in the incidence of infection-associated glomerulonephritis in recent decades, and it seems clear that as the standard of living improves in the poorer countries of the world, this problem will diminish in scope and severity. Where specific immunization is available for the underlying infection (for example, hepatitis B), this will clearly prevent the associated glomerulonephritis as well.

However, for the common postinfectious glomerulonephritis, no specific preventative measure has been identified. In particular, there is no evidence that the liberal use of oral antibiotics for sore throats or other upper respiratory symptoms can be justified on the grounds of the prevention of glomerulonephritis.

PROGNOSIS

The overwhelming majority of children with postinfectious glomerulonephritis due to streptococcal infection suffer mild disease and make a complete recovery.[9] It is usual to confirm that activation of the humoral immune system has largely ceased by repeating the measurement of the serum complement levels — they should have returned to normal by 6–8 weeks after the initial episode of glomerulonephritis. Prolonged hypocomplementaemia suggests the presence of chronic glomerulonephritis (such as mesangiocapillary glomerulonephritis type II) and is an indication for renal biopsy. It is important to recognize that while the complement levels should return to normal relatively rapidly, urinary sediment abnormalities on dipstick testing can persist for up to 12 months after the acute episode, and will sometimes become more florid if the child develops another sore throat. This slow resolution should be expected, and does not in itself throw doubt on the original diagnosis or constitute an indication for biopsy, as long as the child is well and has normal blood pressure and renal function.

The prognosis for glomerulonephritis due to other infectious agents depends on the prognosis of the primary infection.

Very occasionally, a child with postinfectious glomerulonephritis will develop a rapidly progressive crescentic glomerulonephritis and acute renal failure. In this circumstance, referral to a specialized paediatric nephrology service for renal biopsy, dialysis and consideration of empiric immunosuppressive therapy is appropriate.

REFERENCES

1 Elzouki A Y, Amin F, Jaiswal O P. Prevalence and pattern of renal disease in eastern Libya. Arch Dis Child 1983; 58: 106–109.
2 Tewodros W, Muhe L, Daniel E, Schalen C, Kronvall G. A one year study of streptococcal infections and their complications among Ethiopian children. Epidemiol Infect 1992; 109: 211–215.
3 Markowitz M. Streptococcal disease in developing countries. Pediatr Infect Dis J 1991; 10: S11–S14.
4 Van Buynder P G, Gaggin J A, Martin D, Pugsley D, Mathews J D. Streptococcal infection and renal disease markers in Australian aboriginal children. Med J Aust 1992; 156: 537–540.
5 Smith M C, Cooke J H, Zimmerman D M et al. Asymptomatic glomerulonephritis after nonstreptococcal upper respiratory infections. Ann Intern Med 1979; 91: 697–702.
6 Murakami M, Yamamoto H, Ueda Y, Murakami K, Yamauchi K. Urinary screening of elementary and junior high-school children over a 13 year period in Tokyo. Pediatr Nephrol 1991; 5: 50–53.
7 Colman G, Tanna A, Efstratiou A, Gaworzewska E T. The serotypes of Streptococcus pyogenes present in Britain during 1980–1990 and their association with disease. J Med Microbiol 1993; 39: 165–178.
8 Schwartz G J, Haycock G B, Edelman C M Jr, Spitzer A. A simple estimate of glomerular filtration rate in children derived from body length and plasma creatinine. Paediatrics 1976; 58: 259–263.
9 Perlman L, Herdman R C, Kleiman H, Vernier R L. Post streptococcal glomerulonephritis: a ten year follow-up of an epidemic. JAMA 1965; 194: 175–182.

CHAPTER 5

GENITAL TRACT

5.1. Vulvovaginitis

5.2. Sexually transmitted diseases and sexual abuse

5.1 Vulvovaginitis

INTRODUCTION

Vulvovaginitis in children is usually a benign condition. It has been reported as the most common gynaecological symptom in adult women.[1] The term vulvovaginitis is used to describe all inflammatory conditions involving the vulva and vagina in children, as both are usually involved and when occurring separately are difficult to differentiate. It is characterized by the complaint of discomfort or soreness in the vulval region. Itch and dysuria may be noted.

EPIDEMIOLOGY

The neonatal girl frequently has a small amount of white mucoid vaginal discharge. This is due to shedding of vaginal mucosa, hypertrophied by the action of maternal oestrogens. Gradually cellular activity decreases, the quiescent state of infancy and childhood is established and the vaginal pH rises to 6.5–7.5. From 3 months of age until puberty vaginal discharge is unusual.

Vulvovaginitis occurs most commonly between 2 and 7 years of age.[2] The normal flora of the prepubertal vagina includes lactobacilli, diphtheroids, *Staphylococcus epidermidis* and Gram-negative enteric organisms (mainly *Escherichia coli*).

The vulval area of the child is vulnerable to irritants and minor infection due to the relatively thin vaginal mucosa, and lack of labial fat pad. Common irritants are non-absorbent underwear, wet swimming costumes, perfumed and highly detergent soaps and threadworm.

Specific infections are caused by a variety of organisms. *Streptococcus* (*S. pyogenes* (Fig. 5.1.1), *S. pneumoniae*), *Haemophilus influenzae*, *Staphylococcus aureus* and enteric pathogens are most commonly isolated.[3]

Vulvovaginitis is an uncommon presentation of sexual abuse, but in these circumstances infection with *Neisseria gonorrhoeae*, *Chlamydia trachomatis* and herpes simplex virus may be found.[4]

Vulvovaginitis may be associated with the presence of a foreign body, anatomical abnormalities of the lower urinary tract, skin disease (e.g. psoriasis) and various acute systemic illnesses, e.g. measles, varicella, mononucleosis and Kawasaki disease.

Threadworms (*Enterobius vermicularis*) are found in at least 10% of affected children. The irritation is the result of nocturnal migration of the parasite into the vagina.[2,5] Urinary tract infection is found in a small proportion of these children but many who have dysuria have sterile urine.[7]

CLINICAL FEATURES

Intermittent complaint of a sore bottom is the most common presentation. Inter-

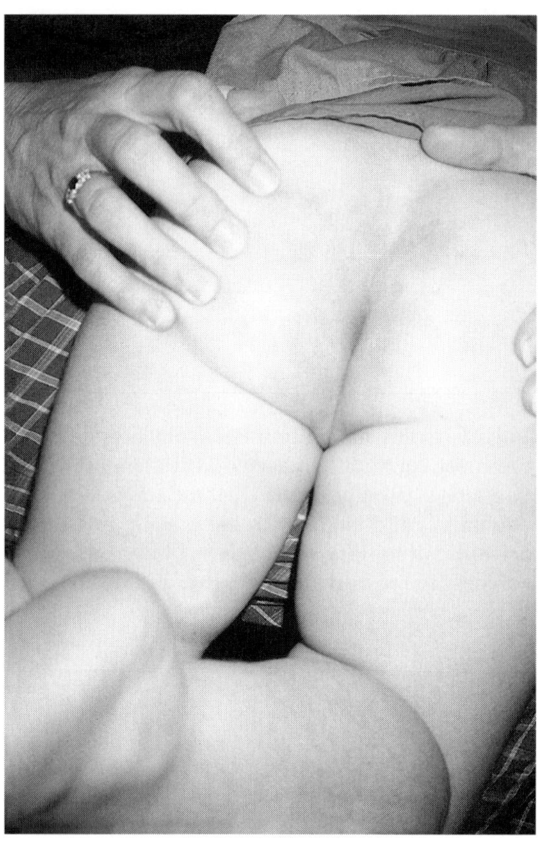

Fig. 5.1.1 Group A streptococcal vulvovaginitis with perianal cellulitis. See also colour plate.

mittent dysuria is common but may only be discovered on specific interrogation. In contrast, dysuria in a child with a urine infection is usually severe and persistent.

Nocturnal itch is suggestive of threadworm infestation. Vaginal discharge is uncommon although a small amount of white to yellowish staining of the child's pants may be noted. The discharge does not have an offensive odour.

The vulva and labia are red and a little oedematous. The surface is tender but bleeding is not a feature. If the symptom has been present for many weeks there may be some fusion of the labia minora.

When major underlying pathological processes are present there may be offensive discharge, which may be copious, purulent and blood-stained.

Ulcerated lesions are suggestive of primary genital herpes simplex virus infection (Fig. 5.1.2).

DIAGNOSIS

Non-specific vulvovaginitis is diagnosed on the basis of the history and a non-invasive, non-instrumental examination of the vulva. The examination of the vulva is satisfactorily performed with the child supine with legs abducted. A simple explanation of what the examination involves must be given to the child and her permission obtained. A swab of an obvious discharge can easily be obtained. No attempt should be made to separate fused labia.

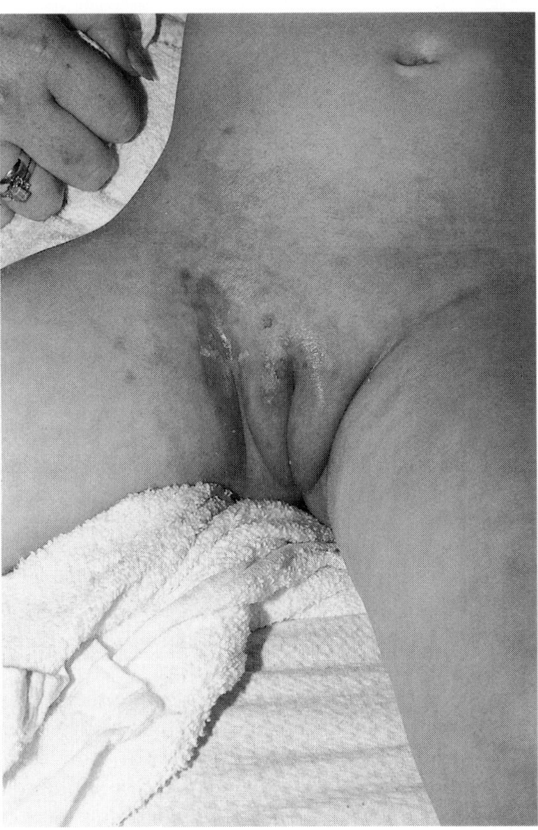

Fig. 5.1.2 Primary herpes simplex virus vulvovaginitis. Note ulcerated lesions. See also colour plate.

A urine culture should be obtained if dysuria is a prominent symptom.

If nocturnal itching is a feature the threadworms can usually be seen by the parents when the child wakes with the symptom. The vulva is examined with a torch with the child's thighs abducted, the room lights being dimmed. The worms are easily seen on the reddened vulva and in the vagina. They are white, about 1 cm long and 0.5 mm in diameter and are mobile.

A more detailed examination is necessary if the symptoms are recurrent, a copious or malodorous discharge is present, if bleeding is present or if there is a history of sexual abuse. Under these circumstances vaginal swabs using a saline-moistened calcium alginate swab may be collected or vaginal contents cultured by inserting a catheter within a larger catheter slowly into the vagina, injecting 1–2 ml of 0.9% saline and withdrawing this into a syringe via the inner catheter.[6]

If a more detailed physical examination is indicated it should be conducted by someone experienced in the area and general anaesthesia may be required. If urgent examination of the vagina is required, a view of the vagina and cervix may be obtained in a proportion of prepubertal girls by examination in the knee–chest position. The buttocks are held apart and as the child takes a deep breath the vagina usually becomes visible.

MANAGEMENT

Non-specific vulvovaginitis

For acute symptoms the child may sit in a basin of warm water (about 5 litres) to which about 5 g (1 teaspoon) of sodium bicarbonate or one small crystal of potassium permanganate (to make the water just visibly pink) has been added. The child sits in the water for 5–10 min gently irrigating her perineum. It is usually easy to obtain the child's cooperation as relief is prompt. This may be done once or twice a day until the symptoms resolve.

The child should wear only cotton underwear and should not use perfumed highly detergent soaps or bubble baths. The child must change out of a wet swimming costume as soon as possible after leaving the water. Unless the child's toileting habits are clearly unhygienic it is not helpful to change the normal practices of the family.

If nocturnal itching occurs, an attempt should be made to demonstrate the presence of threadworms but, as they are ubiquitous, if the symptoms persist mebendazole 100 mg should be given and repeated a week later. If this is a major factor, recurrences are common.

Labial agglutination

Application of 0.01% dienoestrol cream twice daily to the area of fusion usually leads to spontaneous lysis within 7–10 days. Application of petroleum jelly twice daily should continue for a month to prevent recurrence.

Recurrent vulvovaginitis

The problem has a tendency to recur during the first 5–6 years of childhood in spite of attention to the avoidance of irritants, and repeated symptomatic treatment may be necessary.

A review of the history may reveal more obvious urinary symptoms, localized abdominal pain, bowel symptoms, or purulent offensive discharge. These features would lead to specific investigation or more detailed physical examination. In the event that a pathogenic organism was cultured, a course of antibiotics as indicated by the culture and sensitivity pattern should be given. Primary or secondary emotional problems may occur.

Prevention

Girls should wear cotton underwear, change out of wet swimming costumes as soon as possible after leaving the water and avoid perfumed, highly detergent soaps including bubble baths. If these principles were followed, the incidence of non-specific vulvovaginitis would be reduced.

REFERENCES

1 Hatch K D. Vulvar and vaginal disorders. Curr Opin Obstet Gynecol 1992; 4: 904–906.
2 Pierce A M, Hart C A. Vulvovaginitis: causes and management. Arch Dis Child 1992; 67: 509–512.
3 Emans S J, Goldstein D P. Pediatric and adolescent gynecology, 3rd edn. Boston: Little Brown & Co, 1990.
4 Lowy G. Sexually transmitted diseases in childhood. Pediatr Dermatol 1992; 9: 329–333.
5 Aruda M M. Vulvovaginitis in the prepubertal child. Nurs Pract Forum 1992; 3: 149–151.
6 Vandeven A M, Emans S J. Vulvovaginitis in the child and adolescent. Pediatr Rev 1993; 14: 141–147.
7 Heale W F, Weldon A P, Henistone A A. Reflux nephropathy: presentation of urinary infection in childhood. Med J Aust 1973; 1: 1138–1140.

N. E. MacDonald   P. R. Gully

5.2 Sexually transmitted diseases and sexual abuse

INTRODUCTION

Sexually transmitted diseases (STD) encompass a broad group of microbial agents which in adults are spread primarily by sexual contact. These infections may be transmitted to children or non-sexually active adolescents through sexual abuse by oral–genital, genital–genital, and anogenital contact. Unlike the situation in adults and adolescents, in children the presence of an STD may be the first indication that abuse has occurred. Thus, detection of an STD in a child warrants consideration for evaluation for sexual abuse.[1] Similarly, an evaluation for STD is recommended as part of the workup for selected children who may have been sexually abused.[1,2] One must bear in mind that even for adolescents in whom STD are primarily acquired through consensual sexual relationships, they are also at risk for transmission through sexual abuse and assault.

Great care must be taken in the diagnosis and management of a child with an STD. Misidentification of organisms such as *Neisseria gonorrhoeae* can result in inappropriate child abuse investigations. Furthermore, one must try to distinguish whether the organism was sexually transmitted or acquired through non-sexual means.

NON-SEXUAL ROUTES OF TRANSMISSION OF MAJOR STD ORGANISMS

Non-sexual transmission of STD occurs most frequently from an infected woman to her child in utero or at the time of delivery. STDs which may be acquired in utero include syphilis, human immunodeficiency virus infection, and herpes simplex virus infection. STDs transmitted during delivery include gonorrhoea, chlamydia, herpes, hepatitis B and human papillomavirus infections. Non-sexual, non-perinatal transmission of most STD via fomites, autoinoculation and close physical contact are thought to be unusual.[3]

The probability that child sexual abuse rather than persistence of perinatal organisms has caused an infection varies with the STD pathogen and the age of the child. While *N. gonorrhoeae* can be acquired perinatally, asymptomatic infection has not been shown to persist beyond the neonatal period. Furthermore, transmission via fomites is distinctly unusual. Thus identification of *N. gonorrhoeae* from an oral or rectal/genital site in a child greater than 1 month of age and particularly over 6 months of age is highly suggestive of sexual transmission. In contrast, *Chlamydia trachomatis* infection acquired perinatally has been shown to persist for up to 2 years.[4] Thus some experts have suggested that *C. trachomatis* isolation from the rectum or genital tract of children greater than 6 months of age merits consideration for evaluation for sexual abuse,[5] while others have suggested evaluation only if over 2 years of age.[4]

For genital and perianal warts, the time after birth at which onset of lesions can no longer be attributed to perinatal infection is unknown. However, a comparison of data on transmission of human genital papillomavirus disease in adults and children strongly suggests that anal–genital HPV diseases of children that appear after infancy are usually acquired through abusive sexual contact, not by transmission by fomites or autoinoculation.[6]

While *Trichomonas vaginalis* infection of the nasopharynx and vagina can be acquired perinatally, the prepubertal vagina which lacks glycogen and has a relatively high pH does not provide a favourable environment for long-term persistence of the infection. Unfortunately, there are no reported studies that confirm or deny the role of non-sexual transmission beyond the neonatal period. However, trichomonad infections in children are so uncommon that the possibility of easy spread by fomites seems unlikely. Thus, non-neonatal cases of trichomoniasis in a prepubertal child have a high probability of sexual transmission and a low probability of accidental transmission via fomites.

The pattern for herpesvirus infection is not as clear. Perinatal acquisition of HSV II is well established with onset of symptoms in the first month of life. However, HSV II can be transmitted by autoinoculation from oral lesions to the genitalia.[7] Fomites probably do not play a major role in acquisition of genital HSV since transmission requires direct contact of viable virus with either a mucous membrane or an abraded skin surface. Thus isolation of HSV from a primary genital lesion in a prepubertal child beyond 3 months of age should raise the suspicion of sexual abuse but alternative routes such as autoinoculation must also be considered.

Bacterial vaginosis (non-specific vaginitis) is a polymicrobial vaginal infection that appears to be more prevalent in adolescents and adults diagnosed with STD. While bacterial vaginosis has been reported more often in sexually abused children than in non-abused children,[8] the possibility remains that non-sexual transmission may occur.[9] Similarly, most studies of *Gardnerella vaginalis* in children show that this organism is more commonly found in children who have been sexually abused but can be found in a small proportion of children with no history of abuse.[10,11]

EPIDEMIOLOGY

The prevalence of STD among abused children is relatively low (Table 5.2.1) and varies considerably from centre to centre, country to country, and reflects the referral bias of the study populations as well as the incidence and prevalence of STD in the population within which the children live.[10,12–18] Between 0 and 10% of the abused children studied were infected with *N. gonorrhoeae*, with as many as 44% of infected children having asymptomatic disease.[18] Chlamydial infections have been documented in 0.7–17% of abused children. Of importance, in a study of over 1300 children evaluated for possible sexual abuse in North Carolina, less than half of the girls with culture-proven vaginal *Chlamydia* had a discharge on presentation or within the previous 6 months by history.[12]

Other STDs have been identified in sexually abused children but the numbers tested are much smaller, making it harder to draw conclusions. *Trichomonas vaginalis* has been identified in 2–16% of sexually abused children and bacterial vaginosis in 7–26%.[8,12,13] Rectal and/or genital warts have been found in 0.6–1.8% of cases.[13,18] The risk of acquiring syphilis appears to be quite low[12,19] except in the studies from South Africa.[14,17] Case reports suggest that HIV may be acquired during sexual abuse[20,21] but the degree of risk is unknown. None of the 288 girls

Table 5.2.1 Prevalence of STD in recent surveys of children evaluated for sexual abuse

Reference	No. tested	Ages (years)	STD	% Positive
Ingram et al (1992)[12] (USA)	1538	1–12	GC	2.8
			CT	1.2
			HPV	1.8
			S	0.1
			HSV	0.1
	141		TV	2.1
	99		BV	7
Gardner (1992)[10] (Australia)	209	2.1–14.9	GC	1
			CT	0.7
			HSV	0.5
			GV	7.2
Yordan & Yordan (1992)[13] (USA)	288 all female	0.4–18	GC	1.7
			CT	6.6
			HSV	0.3
			HPV	3.8
			TV	1.0
DeVilliers et al (1992)[14] (S. Africa)	152	<3 – >16	GC	1.3
			CT	0.7
			TV	0.7
			S	1.9
Fuster & Neinstein (1987)[15] (USA)	50	1–12.5	CT	17
			GC	0
Walker et al (1988)[16] (Canada)	381	0.5–15	GC	1.0
			CT	0.8
Jaffe & Roux (1988)[17] (S. Africa)	88	–	GC	10
			S	9
Dejong (1986)[18] (USA)	532	0.5–13	GC	4.7
			HPV	0.6
			HSV	0.2
			BV	0.5

Key: GC, gonorrhea; CT, *Chlamydia* infection; HPV, human papillomavirus infection; S, syphilis; HSV, herpes simplex virus infection; TV, trichomoniasis; BV, bacterial vaginosis.

referred to a sexual abuse clinic in Connecticut between 1988 and 1992 were shown to have HIV infection.[13]

A survey of 2143 medical, public health, social service and legal/judicial professionals involved in child abuse programmes across Canada and the USA detected 28 children with abuse-related HIV from an estimated total of 5622 HIV antibody tests performed during 113 198 sexual abuse assessments.[22]

CLINICAL EVALUATION

Evaluation for STD should be carried out on all children who have been sexually abused in a manner in which transmission of an STD is possible, i.e. genital–genital, oral–genital or rectal–genital contact. Since obtaining a complete history is difficult, especially from young or poorly verbal children, and asymptomatic infection may occur, the decision to evaluate the child for STDs must be made on an individual basis. Situations involving a high risk for STDs and a strong indication for testing include the following: (1) suspected offenders known to have an STD or be at high risk, e.g. multiple sexual partners, i.e. more than one partner per year, or past history of an STD; (2) the child or adolescent has

Table 5.2.2   Symptoms or signs of STD in children/adolescents[a]

	Symptoms	Signs
Urethritis	Urethral discharge Burning on urination Irritation in the distal urethra or meatus Unwillingness to void Enuresis Vague lower abdominal pain	Urethral discharge Meatal inflammation (infrequent) Unexplained pyuria in an adolescent male
Cervicitis: adolescents	Vaginal discharge Lower abdominal pain of recent onset Intermenstrual, postcoital or prolonged abnormal vaginal bleeding Deep dyspareunia	Purulent or mucopurulent cervical discharge Induced mucosal bleeding on taking first endocervical swab[b] If ectopy present, oedema and erythema in the area of ectopy
PID: adolescents	Low abdominal pain of recent onset Metrorrhagia, intermenstrual or postcoital vaginal bleeding Deep dyspareunia Vaginal discharge that is not readily explained	Cervical motion tenderness Adnexal tenderness on bimanual examination with or without a mass Cervicitis: ~30% Fever (<40% cases)
Prepubertal vulvovaginitis	Vaginal discharge Perineal irritation	Vaginal discharge
Postpubertal vaginitis (a) Candidiasis (b) Trichomoniasis	Itch External dysuria Painful, itchy, foul-smelling discharge,	Mild to moderate erythema, oedema of vagina and introital region discharge: clumpy and adherent Vaginal erythema and discharge ranging from white to frothy green
(c) Bacterial vaginosis	Grey to white vaginal discharge plus amine (fishy) smell	Grey to white adherent vaginal discharge plus amine (fishy) smell
Genital warts	Warty growth May be asymptomatic or may cause bleeding, pruritus or discharge	Warty growths on anogenital and/or mucous membrane In adolescent female, may involve cervix
Genital ulcers (a) HSV	Genital pain Painful ulcers Fever, malaise	Ulcer; often multiple ↑ Inguinal lymph node non-fluctuant, tender
(b) Primary syphilis	Painless ulcer	Papule → chancre Indurated with serous exudate Usually single ulcer Smooth margin and base
(c) Chancroid[c]	Painful ulcers Painful swollen regional lymph nodes	Usually two or more ulcers Indurated, ragged, undermined Irregular margin Swollen, painful regional lymph node with oedema, erythema overlying skin
Epididymitis	Painful unilateral scrotal swelling	Unilateral scrotal swelling or tenderness — unusual in prepubertal boys

[a] STD may be asymptomatic.
[b] Less reliable if areas of ectopy.
[c] Unusual infection in developed countries.

symptoms or signs of an STD (Table 5.2.2); (3) the prevalence of STD is high in the community.[23]

INTERVIEW AND EXAMINATION

In order to minimize the stress to the child or adolescent, a person supportive

Table 5.2.3   Points of emphasis in STD/sexual abuse interview

General
Non-judgmental
Terminology that child understands
Avoid leading questions

Past history
Perinatal history
  Maternal STD
  Perinatal STD/symptoms
Previous accidents, injuries, burns, ingestion
Developmental history
Past STD
Behaviour changes/school problems

Social and family history
Family structure; residential care; day care; other caregivers
Family medical history including
  STD, sexual or physical abuse, substance abuse
Family stress: financial, social

Table 5.2.4   Points of emphasis in STD/sexual abuse physical examination

Complete physical examination
Include:
  Growth parameters
  Sexual development (Tanner scale)
Examine for evidence of physical abuse and neglect as well as sexual abuse

Directed examination
Examine:
  Vaginal area, buttocks, rectum, penis for signs of trauma/infection, e.g. erythema,
  discharge, abrasions/tears, scarring, inflammation, presence of warts, ulcers
  Mouth, breasts

to the patient should be present during the interview and examination. The
history should be thorough and careful, with particular attention to the details
of the abuse (Table 5.2.3).

The physical examination (Table 5.2.4) needs to be carried out in a relaxed
atmosphere in order to minimize the child's or adolescent's stress. Each step needs
to be explained in advance and reassurance given. If the child is unable to
cooperate due to age and/or anxiety, then examination under anaesthesia may
be helpful. The oral, anal and genital areas should be carefully inspected for
signs of trauma or infection. If assault has been very recent (within hours), then
re-evaluation 24–48 h later may allow detection of bruising or other injuries that
take time to become evident. The examiner should confirm the historical events
during the physical examination by asking the patient to indicate areas where
touched or areas where pain is experienced. While a patulous sphincter in a
child should be regarded with suspicion, this alone is not adequate evidence for
confirmation of sexual abuse since a patulous anus can be seen in children with
chronic faecal retention and in those with neurological abnormalities involving
the sacral area.

SPECIMEN COLLECTION AND LABORATORY DIAGNOSIS

The suggested procedures for evaluation for STD in sexually abused children
and adolescents are shown in Table 5.2.5. To minimize upset to the child, appro-

Table 5.2.5 Specimen collection and laboratory diagnosis for STD in the evaluation of sexually abused children/adolescents

Site	Procedure
Pharynx	*N. gonorrhoeae* culture[a]
Rectum	*N. gonorrhoeae* culture[a] *C. trachomatis* culture[b] HSV culture[c]
Urethra (males) — see text	*N. gonorrhoeae* culture[a] *C. trachomatis* culture[b] HSV culture[c]
Urine in males	Examine for *T. vaginalis*[d] Examine for *C. trachomatis* if test available[e]

Vagina in prepubertal females[f] — see text	*N. gonorrhoeae* culture[a]
	C. trachomatis culture[b]
	Gram stain of smear, saline wet mount and 10% KOH preparation for:
	  T. vaginalis[d]
	  Clue cells and amine odour
	  pH — not useful if prepubertal
	  Yeast
	HSV culture[c]

Cervix in postpubertal females[f]	*N. gonorrhoeae* culture[a] *C. trachomatis* culture[b] Gram stain of smear HSV culture[c]

Vagina in postpubertal females[g]	Gram stain of smear, saline wet mount and 10% KOH preparation for:
	  T. vaginalis[d]
	  Clue cells and amine odour
	  pH — not useful if prepubertal[h]
	  Yeast

Genital ulcers	HSV culture *Haemophilus ducreyi* culture[i] Serology for *Treponema pallidum*[j] and at 6 weeks
Genital warts	Clinical evaluation Consider biopsy and histological confirmation
Serological samples	Syphilis[k] HIV[l] HBV[m] Frozen sample to be saved

[a] Due to medical–legal issues, culture of *N. gonorrhoeae* is the preferred method of diagnosis.

[b] Due to medical–legal issues, culture of *C. trachomatis* is the preferred method of diagnosis.

[c] Cultures for HSV if inflammation present.

[d] Culture if available is more sensitive for the detection of *T. vaginalis* than wet mount.

[e] Centrifuged first-void urine (20 ml) may yield equal positivity rates to swabs for *C. trachomatis* when collected from a symptomatic male.

[f] The prepubertal counterpart to cervicitis is vaginitis. A speculum examination is rarely indicated in a prepubertal child (see text).

[g] Collection of vaginal swabs from adolescents is usually done as part of the speculum examination. If present, pooled vaginal secretions are collected; if not, the vaginal wall in the posterior fornix is swabbed.

[h] Vaginal pH is not thought to be a useful marker for bacterial vaginosis in the prepubertal girl because of a lack of known standards.

[i] To ensure optimal processing of specimens for *H. ducreyi*, the laboratory should be contacted before the specimen is collected.

[j] Dark-field examination of fluid from ulcer base is helpful but the test is not widely available.

[k] Testing for syphilis is optional depending upon the circumstances of abuse and the prevalence of syphilis in the community. In the case of acute assault, the test is repeated 6 weeks later.

[l] Testing for HIV is optional depending upon the circumstances of abuse and the prevalence of HIV in the community. In the case of acute assault, the test is repeated 12–24 weeks later.

[m] Testing for hepatitis B is optional depending upon the circumstances of the abuse, the prevalence of hepatitis B in the community, and whether the child is fully immunized against hepatitis B. In the case of acute assault, a repeat test should be performed 6–12 weeks following the initial test. If the assailant is known to be HB$_s$Ag positive, hepatitis B immune globulin and hepatitis B vaccine should be given if the child is not immunized.

priate specimens should be obtained during a single visit. If the suspected sexual abuse occurred within 72 h of the initial assessment, microbiological testing should be deferred for 3–10 days since false negatives can occur if tested too early. In cases of chronic abuse or when the incident has occurred >72 h earlier, specimens should be obtained at the time of physical examination.

For prepubertal girls, a speculum examination is not necessary since the prepubertal counterpart to cervicitis is vaginitis. Vaginal specimens can be taken without a speculum in a relaxed child. As long as the hymenal ring is not touched, there is little or no sensation with collection of swab specimens. Vaginal specimens may be obtained through aspiration of vaginal contents with a sterile eyedropper or with a moistened dacron swab. A speculum examination is rarely required in a prepubertal child and anaesthesia should be considered if full cervical and vaginal visualization is necessary. Collecting an intraurethral specimen in a prepubertal boy is often difficult and painful due to the small diameter of the urethra. For practical rather than scientific reasons, a meatal rather than an intraurethral specimen may be obtained using a thin swab on a flexible wire shaft. The swab can be rotated in the meatal opening rather than introduced further into the urethra.

In postpubescent females, a speculum examination with cervical specimen collection is indicated but must be done in a gentle reassuring manner so there will be a minimum sense of being reassaulted. Similarly, for postpubescent males, intraurethral specimens should be collected.

Due to the legal consequences surrounding child sexual abuse, cultures for both *N. gonorrhoeae* and *C. trachomatis* are the optimal diagnostic tests for children being screened for STDs. Confirmation of identification of an isolate as *N. gonorrhoeae* using biochemical and enzyme–substrate or serological assays is imperative to avoid inappropriate child abuse investigations.[24] Non-culture tests are less reliable in children due to the higher probability of false positive results as a result of the low prevalence of these organisms in children. Thus, these results must be interpreted with caution as an indicator of possible STD and as an indication for treatment. For example, diagnostic tests for *C. trachomatis* using either monoclonal antibodies in direct immunofluorescent stains or enzyme-linked immunosorbent assays are not sufficiently sensitive or specific in low-risk populations such as children to be acceptable.[25,26] However, if culture tests for *N. gonorrhoeae* or *C. trachomatis* are unavailable or impractical, then referring the child to a regional centre or cautious interpretation of non-culture results are options to consider. If available, vaginal secretions should be cultured for *T. vaginalis* since this is more sensitive than wet mount examination.[27] All STD agents isolated from a victim of child sexual abuse should be stored at –70°C for possible future studies. Further investigations such as serotyping of *N. gonorrhoeae* by a reference laboratory should be considered.

TREATMENT

Management of children and adolescents who have been sexually abused must include psychological and social support for the patient as well as other affected family members. With respect to STDs, prophylactic antibiotics are not usually indicated for children when sexual abuse is suspected, due to the low infection rate and the low risk of complications in prepubertal children. Very few cases of pelvic inflammatory disease or peritonitis in prepubertal girls or epididymitis in prepubertal boys have been documented. Treatment should be considered if the child or adolescent, on initial examination, has clinical signs of infection, the

Table 5.2.6   Synopsis of treatment regimens for selected STD in adolescents and children

	Adolescents	Children
Uncomplicated gonococcal infection	Ceftriaxone 125 mg i.m. in a single dose or Cefixime 400 mg p.o. in a single dose *plus* doxycycline or azithromycin[a]	Ceftriaxone 125 mg i.m. or cefixime 16 mg/kg (max 400 mg) p.o. in a single dose *plus* erythromycin[a]
Chlamydial infection	Doxycycline 100 mg p.o, b.i.d. for 7 days or azithromycin 1 g p.o. in a single dose	Erythromycin 50 mg/kg per day p.o. in four divided doses for 10–14 days
Bacterial vaginosis	If asymptomatic, treatment is unnecessary. If symptomatic, metronidazole 500 mg p.o. b.i.d. for 7 days or metronidazole 2 g p.o. in a single dose	Metronidazole 15–20 mg/kg per day p.o. in three divided doses for 7 days (max. 250 mg per dose)
Trichomonas vaginalis	Metronidazole 2 g p.o. in a single dose	Metronidazole 15–20 mg/kg per day in three divided doses p.o. for 7 days (max. 250 mg per dose)

[a] To ensure effective treatment against possible co-infection with *C. trachomatis*.

assailant is known to be infected, or the child or adolescent is likely to be lost to follow-up. Otherwise, STD treatment can be deferred until the agent is identified. A synopsis of treatment regimens recommended for the common STDs is given in Table 5.2.6.[1,23]

If an STD is diagnosed, contact tracing of sexual contacts should be carried out and other children or adolescents at risk of abuse, e.g. siblings, household contacts and close social contacts, need to be assessed. Follow-up cultures for 'test of cure' is important if an STD is found and treated. For gonorrhea, trichomoniasis and bacterial vaginosis, this should occur approximately 4–7 days after completion of therapy, and 3–4 weeks after completion of therapy for *C. trachomatis*. Follow-up treatment for the prepubertal child or adolescent with syphilis is similar to that of adult patients.[1,23]

REFERENCES

1 Canada Communicable Disease Report. Canadian guidelines for the prevention, diagnosis, management and treatment of sexually transmitted diseases in neonates, children, and adults. Gully P, Bowie W R, MacDonald N E, eds. Health and Welfare Canada, 1992.
2 Report of the Committee on Infectious Diseases. American Academy of Pediatrics, 1994.
3 Schwarcz S K, Whittington W L. Sexual assault and sexually transmitted diseases: detection and management in adults and children. Rev Infect Dis 1990; 12 (suppl 6): S682–S690.
4 Oriel J D. Chronic Chlamydia trachomatis infections in infants. In: Chlamydial infection: Proceedings of the sixth international symposium, 1986.
5 Hammerschlag M R, Doraiswamy B, Alexander E R, Cox P, Price W, Gleyzer A. Are rectogenital chlamydia infections a marker of sexual abuse in children? Pediatr Infect Dis 1984; 3: 100–104.
6 Gutman L T, Herman-Giddens M E, Phelps W C. Transmission of human genital papillomavirus disease: comparison of data from adults and children. Pediatrics 1993; 91: 31–38.
7 Nahmias A J, Dowdle W R, Naib Z M, Josey W E, Luce C F. Genital infection with herpesvirus hominis types 1 and 2 in children. Pediatrics 1968; 42: 659–666.
8 Hammerschlag M R, Cummings M, Doraiswamy B, Cox P, McCormack W M. Nonspecific vaginitis following sexual abuse in children. Pediatrics 1985; 75: 1028–1031.
9 Bump R C, Buesching W J. Bacterial vaginosis in virginal and sexually active adolescent females: evidence against exclusive sexual transmission. Am J Obstet Gynecol 1988; 158: 935–939.
10 Gardner J J. Comparison of the vaginal flora in sexually abused and nonabused girls. J Pediatr 1992; 120: 872–877.

11 Bartley D L, Morgan L, Rimsza M E. Gardnerella vaginalis in prepubertal girls. Am J Dis Child 1987; 141: 1014–1017.

12 Ingram D L, Everett V D, Lyna P R, White S T, Rockwell L A. Epidemiology of adult sexually transmitted disease agents in children being evaluated for sexual abuse. Pediatr Infect Dis J 1992; 11: 945–950.

13 Yordan E E, Yordan R A. Sexually transmitted diseases and human immunodeficiency virus screening in a population of sexually abused girls. Adolesc Pediatr Gynecol 1992; 5: 187–191.

14 de Villiers F P R, Prentice M A, Bergh A M, Miller S D. Sexually transmitted disease surveillance in a child abuse clinic. S Afr Med J 1992; 81: 84–86.

15 Fuster C D, Neinstein L S. Vaginal Chlamydia trachomatis prevalence in sexually abused prepubertal girls. Pediatrics 1987; 79: 235–238.

16 Walker F E, Doherty J A, Jessamine A G. STD testing of suspected sexually abused children at a pediatric hospital. Can Dis Week Rep 1988; 14-44: 201–204.

17 Jaffe A M, Roux P. Sexual abuse of children: a hospital-based study. S Afr Med J 1988; 74: 65–67.

18 De Jong A R. Sexually transmitted diseases in sexually abused children. Sex Trans Dis 1986; 13: 123–126.

19 Lande M R, Richardson A C, White K C. The role of syphilis serology in the evaluation of suspected sexual abuse. Pediatr Infect Dis J 1992; 11: 125–127.

20 Gutman L T, St Claire K K, Weedy C, Herman-Giddens M E, Lane B A, Neimeyer J G, McKinney R E. Human immunodeficiency virus transmission by child sexual abuse. Am J Dis Child 1991; 145: 137–141.

21 Siegel R, Christie C, Myers M, Duma E, Green L. Incest and Pneumocystis carinii pneumonia in a twelve year old girl: a case for early human immunodeficiency virus testing in sexually abused children. Pediatr Infect Dis J 1992; 11: 681–682.

22 Gellert G A, Durfee M J, Berkowitz C D, Higgins K V, Tubiolo V C. Situational and sociodemographic characteristics of children infected with human immunodeficiency virus from pediatric sexual abuse. Pediatrics 1993; 91: 39–44.

23 Centers for Disease Control and Prevention. 1993 sexually transmitted diseases treatment guidelines. MMWR 1993; 42 (RR-14): 1–102.

24 Whittington W L, Rice R J, Biddle J W, Knapp J S. Incorrect identification of Neisseria gonorrhoeae from infants and children. Pediatr Infect Dis J 1988; 7: 3–10.

25 Hammerschlag M R, Rettig P J, Shields M E. False positive results with the use of chlamydial antigen detection tests in the evaluation of suspected sexual abuse in children. Pediatr Infect Dis J 1988; 7: 11–14.

26 Porder K, Sanchez N, Roblin P M, McHugh M, Hammerschlag M R. Lack of specificity of Chlamydiazyme[R] for detection of vaginal chlamydial infection in prepubertal girls. Pediatr Infect Dis J 1989; 8: 358–360.

27 Kreiger J N, Tam M R, Stevens C E et al. Diagnosis of trichomoniasis: comparison of conventional wet mount examination with cytologic studies, cultures, and monoclonal antibody staining of direct specimens. JAMA 1988; 259: 1223–1227.

NEUROLOGICAL

M. A. Herbert   E. R. Moxon

6.1   Meningitis: bacterial, viral, tuberculous, fungal, recurrent meningitis and parameningeal focus

INTRODUCTION

Infections of the central nervous system include meningitis (bacterial and aseptic), parameningeal foci and parenchymatous infections (encephalitis and cerebral abscess). Meningitis and parameningeal foci are the subject of this chapter. Encephalitis, cerebral abscess, shunt infections and subdural empyema are dealt with in Chapters 6.3–6.5.

Meningitis is inflammation of the meninges, predominantly the pia-arachnoid, and of the cerebrospinal fluid (CSF) in the subarachnoid space. Viral meningitis is the most common form, but has much less of an impact than bacterial meningitis which causes several hundred thousand deaths per year worldwide and leaves many survivors severely neurologically handicapped. Acute bacterial meningitis (ABM) most frequently affects children less than 2 years old — an age at which infection may be particularly devastating as it coincides with the 'critical period' of postnatal brain development. This potentially catastrophic illness makes major demands on hospital and community resources. Tuberculous meningitis (TBM), which will be considered separately from ABM, accounts for 30–60% of all bacterial meningitis in Africa and Asia, and contributes substantially to these populations' total burden of morbidity and mortality. TBM is rare in Europe, North America and Australia, but the few cases generate disproportionate costs as hospital stays may be prolonged.

EPIDEMIOLOGY OF ACUTE BACTERIAL MENINGITIS

The three organisms of greatest public health importance are *Neisseria meningitidis*, *Streptococcus pneumoniae* and *Haemophilus influenzae* (Fig. 6.1.1). Although other bacteria do cause ABM, their individual contribution is relatively small, at least in immunocompetent hosts. The neonatal period, in which meningitis is most commonly caused by group B streptococci, *Escherichia coli* or *Listeria monocytogenes*, is a period of relatively high risk, but neonatal cases add only a small percentage to total childhood meningitis.

The risks of developing meningitis vary with age and geographical location, and are summarized in Table 6.1.1.

The three major pathogens of ABM have several common features. Transmission is by the respiratory route, with intimate, usually sustained contact being necessary for acquisition. The optimal host-pathogen relationship is carriage of the organism as a commensal. In a small percentage of children, this relationship breaks down, bacteria breach the nasopharyngeal mucosa and cause invasive disease. Attack rates are highest among the poor, in large families, where overcrowding is manifest, and in closed populations such as school dormitories

Table 6.1.1   Geographical and age-related risk of acquiring meningitis

Meningitis type	Relative risk per year			Case-fatality rate
Bacterial meningitis	1:12 500	All ages	Overall rate	10%
Developed world[1–6]	1:1200	<1 year	*H. influenzae*	3–6%
	1:6000	1–4 years	*N. meningitidis*	3–13%
	1:36 000	5–9 years	*S. pneumoniae*	9–26%
	1:60 000	10–14 years		
Bacterial meningitis	1:900	Africa — meningitis belt		22%
Other continents[7,8]	1:2600	Africa — the rest		45%
	1:2200	South America		33%
	1:3–10 000	Asia (<5 years)		
Aseptic meningitis	1:450–900	<1 year		0%
	1:5000	1–4 years		
	1:20 000	5+ years		
Tuberculous meningitis[9,10]	1:500 000	UK/Australia		20–30%
	1:10 000	China		
	1:350	India (<35 years)		

Asian figures: D. Leboulleux, personal communication.

(notably for meningococcal spread) and day care centres. Breast feeding may be protective, and passive smoking is a risk factor. Disease incidence shows seasonal variation, which differs with geographical location. Meningococcal meningitis in the UK, for example, has a peak incidence in winter, and is temporally linked with some viral upper respiratory tract infections; whereas in Africa, meningococcal epidemics start in the middle of the dry season and subside with the rains.

Certain socioeconomically marginalized groups in developed countries acquire more meningitis, such as Eskimos, Navajo and Apache Indians, and Aborigines. In a 1987–1991 meningococcal epidemic in central Australia, the Aboriginal population (all ages) had an attack rate of 1 in 625 persons/year, compared with 1 in 25 000 for the rest of the population.[11] The cause for the enhanced risk is obscure, but may relate to economic status, crowding, earlier acquisition, density of nasopharyngeal colonization and genetic predisposition. One in twenty-four children with sickle cell disease will develop pneumococcal meningitis by 4 years old.

The major neonatal and childhood pathogens of ABM, Group B streptococcus, *E. coli*, *S. pneumoniae*, *N. meningitidis* and *H. influenzae* are all encapsulated, with the exception of *L. monocytogenes* which has no capsule. In defending against invasion by capsulate bacteria, the major host clearance mechanisms include serum antibody to the capsule, complement and mononuclear/macrophage phagocytosis. Defects of any of these, such as terminal complement deficiencies, hypogammaglobulinaemia, sickle cell disease, splenectomy, malignancy and HIV, predispose to more frequent and severe infections.

The three major organisms of childhood meningitis are dissimilar in that *N. meningitidis* has a capacity to cause large scale epidemics, particularly group A and to a lesser extent group C, whereas *S. pneumoniae* and *H. influenzae* generate only sporadic cases. Group B and C meningococci usually cause only small outbreaks, or may be transiently hyperendemic. *N. meningitidis* group B can be hyperendemic for many years, such as in Norway. A summary of some individual characteristics of the three major meningeal pathogens is given in Table 6.1.2.

The availability of *H. influenzae* type b conjugate vaccine has dramatically reduced the incidence of *H. influenzae* invasive disease in many countries in Europe, in North America and in Australia.[1] The efficacy of the vaccine (>98% in the UK) indicates that a 50% reduction in all ABM is now a realistic possibility,

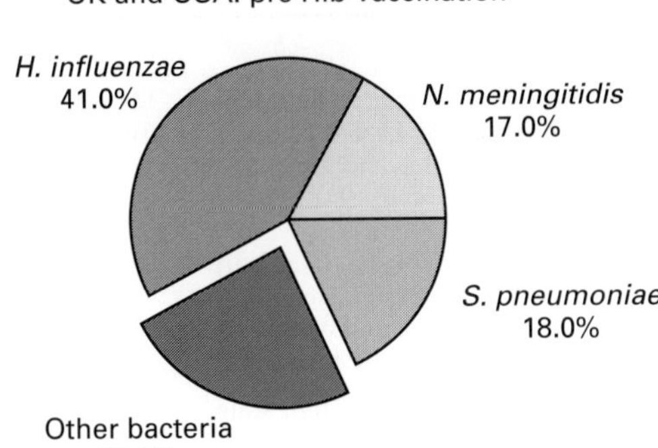

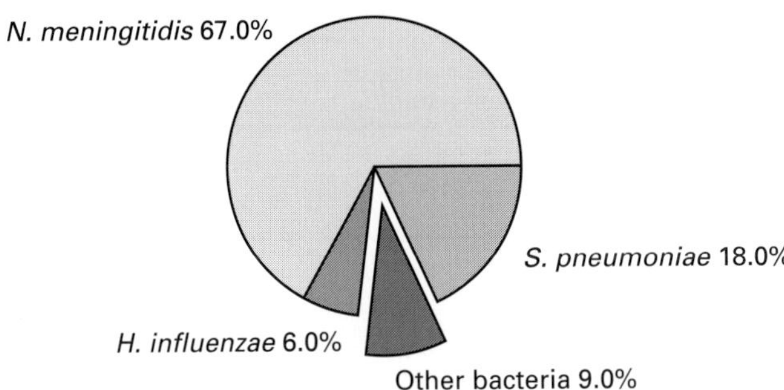

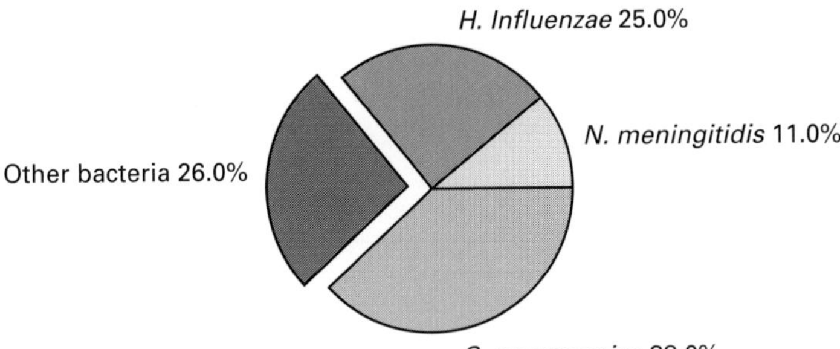

Fig. 6.1.1   The contribution of three pathogens to acute bacterial meningitis.

although substantial economic and logistical problems remain in making Hib conjugate vaccines available through the Expanded Programme of Immunization.

Pathogenesis and pathophysiology

The mechanisms underlying entry of microbes into the central nervous system, the induction of inflammation and the ensuing tissue injury vary depending on the particular biological attributes of the organisms, e.g. tropism, extracellular or intracellular replication, and virulence factors. In bacterial meningitis, there are usually four steps: (i) colonization of the nasopharynx, (ii) invasion and blood stream survival, (iii) meningeal entry and (iv) multiplication in the pia-arachnoid/ CSF.[2,14] However, other mechanisms must be considered (e.g. direct implantation

Table 6.1.2 Features of the three main pathogens of ABM

	N. meningitidis[12]	*S. pneumoniae*[13]	*H. influenzae*[2]
Capsular type	Serogroups A, B, C, D, E29, W-135, X, Y, Z B is responsible for 60–75% of disease, and C for 25–40% in developed nations. Groups A + C cause most disease in the tropics.	The 7 serotypes associated with most meningitis are: Developing world 14, 6, 5, 1, 19, 9 and 23; Developed world 14, 6, 19, 18, 9, 23 and 4 Types 6, 14, 19 and 23 are notable in that they cause much disease, are poorly immunogenic, and are most associated with antibiotic resistance.	Six serotypes: a–f Type b causes most disease worldwide
Carriage	5–10%, but much higher if child has a viral respiratory infection.	20–40% of children. A different stain colonizes 25% of the population per year, and invasion tends to occur within a month of new carriage.	60–90% of children carry non-capsulate strains, and 2–5% capsulate.
Peak attack rates	Most meningitis develops at age <2 years, especially infants aged 3–5 months. A second peak occurs in adolescence.	50% of invasive disease happens in the first year of life, a further 30% up to 2 years and 5–10% up to 3 years. It then continues to be a cause of meningitis throughout adult life.	Peak disease is at 7–14 months, with almost all meningitis afflicting those <5 years.

Table 6.1.3 Mechanisms of microbial entry into the CNS

Bacterial meningitis	Nasopharyngeal colonization and bloodstream spread Direct entry via skull fracture Neurosurgical procedures, including VP shunts Defects of craniospinal axis (congenital dermal sinuses and meningomyelocele)
Viral meningitis	Retro-axonal spread along peripheral nerves (herpes simplex, varicella zoster virus, Epstein-Barr virus) Via blood after replication in the respiratory tract (measles, mumps) Multiplication in intestinal tract and local lymph nodes before blood spread (polio and enteroviruses) Arthropod borne, subcutaneous, lymph nodes, vascular endothelial and macrophage replication, and then spread to the CNS after viraemia[a] (arboviruses)
Parameningeal foci	Spread from adjacent sites (sinusitis, otitis, vertebral or skull osteomyelitis, spondylitis, and dental abscess) Metastatic spread from a distant focus of infection A consequence of poorly treated meningitis

[a] Viraemia is a feature of most viral infections, yet only a few viruses can invade and replicate within the CNS.

following accidental trauma or neurosurgery). Table 6.1.3 summarizes possible mechanisms of CNS entry by different pathogens. Despite the proximity of the nasopharyngeal mucosa to the cribriform plate and the contiguous route afforded by the olfactory nerves, few microbes reach the CNS by this route. Notable exceptions include herpes simplex virus and the necrotizing invasion of the cribriform plate by *Naegleria agglomerans*, a fresh water amoeba.

In the early stages of infection, the CSF is immunologically isolated by the effect of tight junctions which characterize the endothelial cells of the blood brain barrier, and by the absence of specific immunological clearance mechanisms; bacteria can initially multiply relatively unchallenged. As the bacterial density of the CSF exceeds a threshold, inflammatory cells breach the blood brain barrier and enter the CSF. Cytokines have a central role in the induction of this inflammation. In meningococcal meningitis, for instance, TNF, IL-1, IL-6 and IL-8 are often raised, in CSF as well as blood. TNF released in response to bacterial components, such as lipopolysaccharide, may induce or up-regulate IL-1, IL-6 and

IL-8 which appear to arise in coordinated sequence. The expression of selectins on neutrophils, and integrins or ICAM-1 on the cells of the blood brain barrier, is regulated by cytokines. Antibodies that inhibit cytokines are able to block specific components of inflammation, for instance, the interaction of neutrophil CD18 with endothelial ICAM-1 can be inhibited by anti-CD18 antibodies, and leucocyte migration into the CNS is prevented.[15]

Irrespective of the mechanisms of transfection to the CNS, the pathophysiological consequences depend upon both the location and number of organisms and the cytotoxic properties of the infecting microbes. Neurological damage is a consequence of direct bacterial cytotoxicity, indirect injurious agents (intense inflammation, diffusion of 'toxins', ischaemia, vasculitis, oedema) and systemic effects (shock, cerebral hypoperfusion, convulsion and impairment of ventilation in severely ill patients).

Hypoperfusion is a consequence of raised intracranial pressure, primarily from cerebral oedema, and loss of cerebral vascular autoregulation, during which brain perfusion is reliant solely on the maintenance of systemic blood pressure. The aetiology of cerebral oedema can be any of the following:

Vasogenic	Leakage of the blood brain barrier secondary to endothelial cell damage. The oedema is composed of a plasma filtrate.
Cytotoxic	Cell membrane alterations lead to intracellular fluid loss.
Interstitial	Increased CSF collection between cells because of obstructive hydrocephalus.

Clinical manifestations and pathophysiological relationship

Eighty-five percent of children with meningitis have fever, vomiting, and severe headache. The majority have pyrexia for 1–4 days, about 13% for 5–9 days, 13% for >10 days, and 16% have a recurrence after 24 hours of normal temperature.[3] Infants, in contrast to older children, have an immature inflammatory cytokine response, and consequently, less frequently exhibit fever. Recurrent or prolonged fever is most commonly associated with another focus of infection (e.g. arthritis or pneumonia), with hospital acquired coincidental infection, thrombophlebitis, subdural effusions or drug fever.[3]

Severe headache is characteristic of meningeal irritation, but as with pyrexia, is usually a less reliable sign in the younger child. Positive Brudzinski and Kernig tests are elicited in around a third of children, whereas back pain and nuchal rigidity occur more commonly; all reflect inflammation of nerve roots of the spinal canal and adjacent sensory nerves. The most comfortable position for the patient, an extended neck but flexed hips and knees, minimises tension on the nerves arising from the spinal cord. A positive Brudzinski sign is involuntary muscular contraction causing flexion of the legs, when the neck is passively flexed by the examining physician. Kernig sign is elicited when there is back pain with extension of the leg which stretches the sciatic nerve. Infants under 1 year old may rarely develop neck stiffness in the very late stages.

Raised intracranial pressure is evident as headache, and in those aged less than 18 months, as a bulging fontanelle. Inadequate and disturbed cerebral perfusion, deranged cerebral metabolism and the inadequate clearance of anaerobic metabolic products, all contribute to the encephalopathy of meningitis, which typically manifests as lethargy, irritability, reduced consciousness or coma. Inappropriate release of ADH is a common accompaniment of the cerebral dysfunction, and the degree and duration of the hyponatraemia correlates with a worse outcome.

Petechiae occur in 50% or more of children with meningococcal meningitis, which has a worse prognosis if shock complicates the meningitis. Petechiae should be sought carefully, including on the buccal mucosa and conjunctiva. The rash may initially be urticarial or maculopapular, before becoming purpuric. Rarely, petechiae are a feature of overwhelming Haemophilus and pneumococcal meningitis, especially in a child who has had a splenectomy. An unusual sign is tache cerebrale, a non-specific sign of inflammation: stroking the skin with a blunt instrument produces a raised red streak.

Thirty percent of children have fits, 20% at presentation, and a further 10% within 72 hours. Early onset fits are of no great prognostic value. Focal and late onset fits (>72 hours) may reflect sequelae and are worrying signs associated with abnormal neurology at follow up. Ataxia can occasionally be the presenting feature, thought to be a result of labyrinthitis. Ten to 20% of children have cranial nerve palsies (mainly III, IV, VI or VII), or other focal signs (hemiparesis, quadriparesis and visual field defects) on admission; these may reflect either localized brain injury or elevated intracranial pressure. Patients who die do so of overwhelming sepsis or from pressure changes within the brain.

Table 6.1.4 outlines clinical features by age, and Table 6.1.5 lists the signs of prognostic relevance.[2,5,16]

Lumbar puncture

The rationale for performing a lumbar puncture (LP) is to make a definitive diagnosis of meningitis upon which a confident treatment plan can be based. By confirming meningitis, doubts and anxieties over many other possible central nervous system differential diagnoses can be alleviated. Some indications for undertaking an LP that may be considered useful are outlined in Table 6.1.6.

There is no routine need for a repeat LP of a child being treated for ABM unless there is doubt about clinical improvement at 48–72 hours, but it may be particularly helpful in Gram-negative, tuberculous and neonatal meningitis, and where antibiotic resistant organisms are identified.[16]

Table 6.1.4 Clinical signs

Preterm neonate	Exceedingly subtle signs Can mimic respiratory distress syndrome
Neonate	Non-specific, with few signs referable to the CNS Bulging fontanelle Fits (in up to 40%) Temperature instability (fever in only 50%) Irritable ± high-pitched cry Lethargic Poor feeding, vomiting, distended abdomen Tachypnoea, apnoea and cyanosis
Infants (1–18 months)	Fever Irritability alternating with lethargy Vomiting Cries in pain when moved Bulging fontanelle Fits (approx. 20% at presentation)
Child (>18 months old)	Fever (in 60% or more) Vomiting Nuchal rigidity Cerebral dysfunction – confusion, delirium, lethargy and coma Kernig sign Brudzinski sign

Table 6.1.5 Poor prognostic features in acute bacterial meningitis

Indicators of increased bacterial load	Delay in presentation and initiation of therapy
	High bacterial density in CSF by Gram stain
Inadequate or overwhelmed host inflammatory response	Younger age (neonates especially, and <1 year)
	Delayed sterilization of CSF
	Leucopenia
Systemic hypotension and shock	Petechiae (suggests meningococcal pathogen, and likelihood of septic shock with meningitis)
	Poor peripheral perfusion
	Hypotension is a late sign
Signs suggesting severe meningitis	Impaired consciousness and coma
	Hyponatraemia: degree and duration
	Deranged clotting functions
	Thrombocytopenia
Focal brain insults, or coning impending	Focal neurological signs before the start of treatment
	Focal fits (more likely to herald neurological sequelae)
	Late fits, after first 72 h of treatment
Complications	Subdural empyema

Table 6.1.6 Indications for lumbar puncture

Any child should be considered for LP if they have fever without a focus
Less than 3 months old and fever, for instance >38°C
3 months to 2 years old, lethargy and pyrexia, for instance >39°C
Infants <12 months old with a febrile fit (whether there is a focus of infection or not)
A febrile convulsion at <18 months old if no focus for infection (and a low threshold for LP even where there is a focus)
Meningeal irritation guides the need for LP in children older than 2 years
The adage 'If you think of doing an LP, do it' applies more strongly, the younger the child

Risks of lumbar puncture

Several complications have been attributed to performing an LP. They may be relatively minor and transient, such as post LP headache, diplopia and temporary squint, or they may be more severe, as in the herniation syndromes leading to coning (tonsillar compression). The issue of whether coning is caused by LP, or whether it is merely a reflection of the severity of the meningitis and coincides with LP, is controversial, but it is likely that removal of CSF is a predisposing factor.

All children with meningitis have raised intracranial pressure. Herniation begins when the raised pressure is directed caudally, so that the subarachnoid space is compressed at the cisterna magna. Obstructing CSF flow between the cranial vault and the lower pressure spinal cord encourages the brain to shift with compression of the brain stem. Coning can follow meningitis alone, can follow a sudden rise in intracranial pressure after a convulsion, and occur after an LP. A few children cone immediately after LP, but usually there is a delay of around 8–12 hours. The amount of CSF sampled at the time of the LP is less important than the continued leakage of CSF through the dural puncture. When there is a widely open fontanelle, the brain can expand without caudal obstruction of CSF, and herniation is extremely unlikely; it is our personal practice though to defer LP in babies with the same criteria as we would defer LP in older children. Cord compression is a rare sequel similar to coning, and is due to constriction of the anterior spinal artery by the cerebellar tonsils. It may cause upper spinal cord ischaemia and quadriplegia.

Other causes for raised pressure, such as acute hydrocephalus, cerebral oedema, abscess, subdural haematoma, bleeding from an AV malformation and posterior fossa tumours, are much more likely than meningitis to be associated with herniation after LP. These conditions frequently produce papilloedema, compared

Table 6.1.7   Signs which contraindicate lumbar puncture

Clinical signs	Reason for delaying LP
Papilloedema; or Focal neurological signs	Suggests an alternative diagnosis or excessively raised intracranial pressure
Coma (Glasgow Coma Score <8); or Recent fit (within 30 m); or Prolonged fits (>30 m duration)	Excessively raised intracranial pressure
Hypertension with bradycardia; or Irregular or slow respiration; or Fixed dilated pupils; or Decorticate or decerebrate posturing	Impending cerebral herniation (coning)
Septic shock (especially <1 y)	Risk of cardiorespiratory compromise during procedure
Skin infection at LP site Bleeding diathesis	Risk of introducing infection Risk of bleeding

with less than 1% of patients with early ABM; papilloedema should therefore alert to an alternate diagnosis in which an LP is hazardous. Reasons for deferring LP are summarised in Table 6.1.7.

In general, the risks of LP are very small, there are clear benefits to confirming or ruling out a diagnosis of meningitis, and the patients in whom it should not be done, or in whom it should be deferred can be readily identified on clinical criteria.

Role of CT scan

The primary role of a CT scan is to exclude other pathology. Its urgency is dictated by the severity of signs, and rate of decline of the child. A CT scan may also give some information on early herniation (i.e. ventricular system displacement, sulcal effacement). A normal CT scan does not exclude the later occurrence of herniation, as in 18–36% of children who die from coning, there is a normal CT finding prior to death.[17] Thus, if the CT scan is normal but clinical signs contraindicate doing an LP, then antibiotics should be given and the LP delayed. If there is doubt about the diagnosis, or concern that complications have ensued, obtain a CT scan. One strategy for when to undertake LP and CT scan is given in Fig. 6.1.2.[17,18]

Interpreting LP findings

Interpretation of CSF results is mostly uncomplicated, but can sometimes be an exacting task. Several studies have defined the range of CSF normality and the changes that occur with various forms of meningitis.[19,20]

CSF white cell count

Outside the neonatal period, a white cell count (WCC) greater than $5 \times 10^9/l$ raises doubt about meningitis, and over $10 \times 10^9/l$ is considered abnormal. The occurrence of fits at any age does not appreciably alter the WCC. The CSF absolute neutrophil count (ANC) is $\geq 1 \times 10^9/l$ in 99% of babies and children with meningitis. Conversely, CSF from 95% of non-infected children has an absolute neutrophil count (ANC) $<1 \times 10^9/l$, but $1 \times 10^9/l$ is considered allowable by some physicians if all other CSF parameters are normal; although even $1 \times 10^9/l$ neutrophils raises concern.

CSF GLUCOSE

A common evaluation of CSF glucose is through comparison with that in plasma,

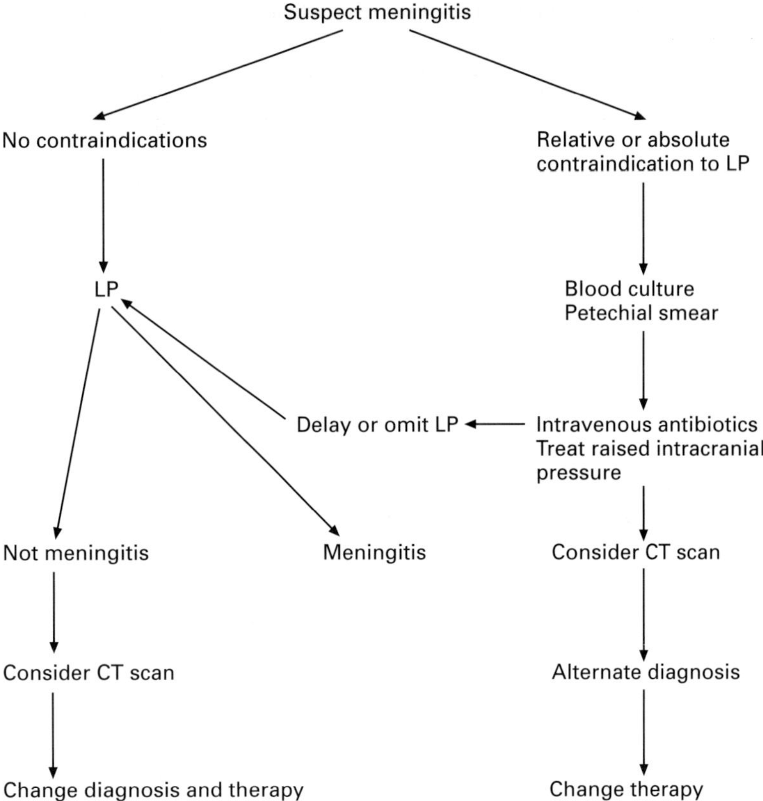

Fig. 6.1.2 Decision tree: when to do an LP, or request a CT scan.

and a ratio of ≥ 0.6 (CSF : blood levels) is considered normal, whereas ≤ 0.4 has a specificity of detecting ABM of 98% and a sensitivity of 80%. A ratio of 0.35 to 0.5 can be seen in viral meningitis.[3] A raised plasma glucose, such as occurring with stress around the time of an LP, is transmitted to the CSF slowly, over a few hours. The CSF : blood glucose ratio can thus be erroneously depressed; measurement of an absolute CSF glucose value is considered by some clinicians to be a better indicator of true hypoglycorrhachia. In several childhood series, the normal range for CSF glucose was 2.5–3.6 mmol/l,[3] whereas the mean CSF glucose in ABM ranged from 1.1 to 1.6 mmol/l; and in one such study, a CSF glucose of <2.2 mmol/l was found in 81% of children with ABM.[19]

GRAM STAINING OF CSF

The Gram stain appearance may give a clue to the pathogen. Many factors such as differential uptake of stain, the presence of fragmented bacteria, and inexperience in detecting artifacts may lead to errors; initial therapy should therefore not be based solely upon Gram stain findings.

BLOODY TAP

About 14% of neonatal lumbar punctures result in bloody CSF, and another

14% provide inadequate CSF for full investigations. One leucocyte per 700 erythrocytes is permitted by some, but such calculations prove to be of limited usefulness, many clinicians err on the side of caution and assume that the WCC would be the same if the LP were not blood contaminated. Blood in the CSF raises the protein content 0.01 g/l for each 1000 erythrocytes per ml.[3] The normal range for CSF protein is 0.2–0.45 g/l.[3,19] Protein is raised in the CSF of 60% of school-aged children with ABM, and almost all preschool children. The mean CSF protein in ABM ranges from 1.3–3.0 g/l.[19]

OVERLAP BETWEEN NORMAL AND MENINGITIC CSF

If the diagnosis is unclear from a first LP, a repeat at around 6 hours may clarify the interpretation.

Outside infancy, a CSF WCC >1000 × 10^9/l, and predominantly neutrophils, for instance >60% of the total WCC, is likely to be due to bacterial meningitis. A WCC of 10–500 × 10^9/l and predominantly lymphocytes probably reflects viral meningitis, although the possibility of TBM, partially treated ABM or of a parameningeal focus should be considered.

Despite these differences, raised CSF parameters in almost all young children are often treated as bacterial meningitis until CSF cultures are sterile at 48 hours. Viral meningitis may occasionally have a WCC >1000 × 10^9/l, and early onset viral infection may show a predominance of neutrophils in CSF. In older patients, clinicians are often able to be more discriminating between viral meningitis and ABM, and each of the following findings on its own correlates with 99% certainty of bacterial (as distinct from viral) meningitis: CSF glucose <1.9 mmol/l, CSF : blood glucose ratio <0.23, protein >2.2 g/l, WCC >2000 × 10^9/l, ANC >1180 × 10^9/l.[19]

Occasionally, in pneumococcal or meningococcal meningitis, children may have no CSF pleocytosis. This is especially likely in young infants who have immature chemotaxis of inflammatory cells, but in this situation there is often raised protein and depressed CSF glucose. In older children, CSF may be obtained in the early phases of meningitis when the bacterial load is increasing, but has not reached the threshold for inflammation. Where meningitis exists without CSF pleocytosis in the older child, the protein and glucose levels are usually also normal, bacteria are of low density and are either not visible on Gram staining, or are easily missed.

PCR AND ANTIGEN TESTING

The PCR is being evaluated for identification of many meningitic pathogens, including enteroviruses, bacteria and tuberculosis. Although still under investigation, it is likely to be a highly sensitive and specific tool.[21] Antigen tests to identify *S. pneumoniae*, *N. meningitidis*, *H. influenzae* type b, *E. coli* and type III group B streptococcus are available using enzyme linked immunosorbent assay (ELISA), latex agglutination tests or countercurrent immunoelectrophoresis. The speed and ease of performance are greatest with the latter two tests, whereas ELISA is the most sensitive and specific. Antigen-based assays are beneficial in confirming ABM where the clinical and CSF examinations leave little doubt over the diagnosis but where the exact organism is unknown, for example when culture is negative because of prior antibiotic treatment, but where the CSF WCC, glucose and protein clearly indicate ABM. High false negative test results, false positives due to cross reacting antigens, and less sensitivity when the bacterial load is low, make these assays less useful when they are needed most, in making an early diagnosis of ABM when the CSF findings are equivocal. The sensitivity of latex agglutination in CSF can be as low as 50%.[22]

The diagnosis of *N. meningitidis* may also be made through Gram staining of a petechial smear, and in fulminant episodes of sepsis, by staining of the buffy coat of blood.

ANTIMICROBIAL TREATMENT

Antibiotic therapy should not be delayed if bacterial meningitis is suspected. Initial treatment should cover expected organisms for the age group until culture and sensitivity results are available at around 48 h.[2,7,23,24]

Infants aged between 1–3 months, tend to be in one of two groups: previously healthy babies at home, or preterm infants who remain on a neonatal unit. The latter group are exposed to nosocomial infections, and are treated the same as neonates. For a term baby at home, the pathogens are most likely to be one of the 3 main community acquired childhood bacterial causes, but could also be late onset *L. monocytogenes*, group B streptococcus, or more rarely *E. coli* or enterococcus; cefotaxime with ampicillin is the most appropriate treatment.

Since the development of widespread *H. influenzae* resistance to ampicillin and the rarer chloramphenicol resistance, third generation cephalosporins, cefotaxime or ceftriaxone, have become the main therapy for children older than 3 months. *S. pneumoniae* resistance is also increasing. Only 2–3% of *S. pneumoniae* are resistant to penicillin in the UK, but over 40% in some European countries, such as Hungary and Spain.

Treatment is normally for 7 days for *N. meningitidis*, and for 7–10 days for *S. pneumoniae* or *H. influenzae* meningitis. Dosages are given in Table 6.1.8.

FLUID BALANCE

Antidiuretic hormone is secreted inappropriately during meningitis.[26,27] The resultant hyponatraemia can worsen cerebral oedema. Maintenance fluids are therefore usually given at two-thirds normal requirements. Patients in shock or those dehydrated and with poor perfusion require cautious administration of colloid. It is often a difficult balance to correct hypovolaemia and yet not exacerbate cerebral oedema through water overload. Plasma urea, and plasma and urine electrolytes and osmolarities should be measured at least daily. The duration and degree of hyponatraemia correlates with fits and abnormal neurological examination at 1 month.

Table 6.1.8 Dosages of commonly administered antibiotics

Ampicillin	50 mg/kg per dose 12-hourly (1st week of life), 6-hourly (2–4 weeks), 3-hourly (4+ weeks)
Benzylpenicillin	60 mg/kg per dose 12-hourly (1st week), 6-hourly (2–4 weeks), 4-hourly thereafter
Cefotaxime	50 mg/kg per dose 12-hourly (if preterm), 8-hourly (1st week), 6-hourly (2–4 weeks), 4-hourly (4+ weeks)
Ceftriaxone	50–75 mg/kg per dose daily (1st week), 12-hourly (2+ weeks)
Chloramphenicol	25 mg/kg per dose 8-hourly (not to be used in neonates). Toxicity (grey syndrome) develops in infants with levels >20 mg/l, and in older children with levels >200 mg/l. Levels are also important when an infant is changed to oral therapy, where serum concentrations are especially unpredictable, making it difficult to achieve adequate therapeutic levels

GENERAL MEASURES

Any child with shock requires admission to an intensive care unit, and full supportive management, including central venous pressure monitoring and inotrope infusions. Neonates especially, but also older children, may need ventilation depending on degree of shock, hypoxia and coma. Clotting studies and platelets are measured for evidence of disseminated intravascular coagulation.

ANTIMICROBIAL PROPHYLAXIS

Rifampicin is given to contacts of *N. meningitidis* and *H. influenzae* type b meningitis, but not of *S. pneumoniae*.[28] Alternative drugs that can eradicate nasopharyngeal carriage are ceftriaxone and ciprofloxacin. There is no role for protective chemotherapy during an outbreak, as it does not prevent disease in those incubating the infection, it encourages resistance development, and it confuses the clinical presentation.

DEXAMETHASONE THERAPY

The rationale behind the use of steroids in meningitis is a belief that it is the host inflammatory reaction, rather than the bacteria, which causes most harm, and this has been most convincingly demonstrated in *H. influenzae* type b meningitis. Steroids given with, or prior to (at least 15 minutes before) the first dose of antibiotics, are considered to dampen the inflammatory response to microbial cell wall components associated with bacterial lysis, such as endotoxin. The arguments for and against currently using dexamethasone (DXM) are:

Arguments in favour of steroids

1. Experimental models, in which *H. influenzae* is the pathogen, support the concept of steroids dampening inflammation; *S. pneumoniae* has also been used in a few studies.[29] There is less CSF inflammation when steroids are given, and lower CSF pleocytosis and cytokine activity, and elevated glucose.
2. Although many controlled trials of DXM in human subjects have given equivocal results, some appear to show outstanding benefit (i.e. reduction in sensorineural hearing loss from 15 to 3%), and meta-analyses of selected trials in one review showed a statistically significant benefit from steroids.[29,30]
3. There is a theoretical likelihood of the same mechanisms of neuronal damage and deafness in *S. pneumoniae* and *N. meningitidis* meningitis as in *H. influenzae* meningitis. Coupled with higher neurological sequelae in pneumococcal meningitis, it is reasonably likely that steroids will be of benefit.
4. There is no delay in clearance of bacteria from CSF when steroids are administered.

Against steroids

1. Since the introduction of Hib-conjugate vaccines, the incidence of *H. influenzae* meningitis has rapidly declined and it may soon disappear in developed countries. The vast majority of patients in trials of DXM had infection with *H. influenzae*; the results of these studies may therefore not now be applicable to meningitis.
2. *S. pneumoniae* release exotoxins (i.e. pneumolysin) in addition to

Table 6.1.9   Who should receive prophylaxis?

H. influenzae type b	All family, if one member is <4 years, and has not had Hib conjugate vaccine[a]
	Unvaccinated children <2 years in a nursery if contact is for >25 h per week[b]
	Staff of a nursery if more than 2 cases in 60 days[b]
N. meningitidis	All household and 'kissing' contacts
	Preschool groups: all contacts
	Primary + secondary schools, and colleges: only for those whose exposure is similar to household contacts, i.e. shared dormitory, and for 'kissing' contacts

[a] 'Vaccinated' is defined as ≥2 vaccines if ≤13 months old, and ≥1 vaccine if ≥13 months old.
[b] There is no unifying agreement on the need to provide prophylaxis to staff and children in nurseries. These are two suggestions, but consider consulting with local public health teams for individual area policies.

proinflammatory cellular components such as lipoteichoic acid. Exotoxins may cause direct neuronal damage, whereas steroids can only suppress inflammation. The relative contribution of each of these deleterious factors, and hence of the role of steroids, is therefore unknown.

3. In meningococcal meningitis, hearing loss may have an alternate aetiology, such as hypovolaemia associated with septic shock. The use of steroids for meningococcal septicaemia may be harmful, and DXM is therefore not advocated in meningitic patients with purpura and hypotension.

4. Many trials that show a benefit from steroids have had higher than usual sequelae rates. Inadequate antibiotics (i.e. cefuroxime), late presentations of patients or less than optimal supportive care (for example in developing countries, Egypt and Costa Rica), may have contributed to these higher rates. Benefits from steroids may be greater where sequelae are common, and marginal in developed countries, where cefotaxime/ceftriaxone are used and supportive facilities are optimal.[31]

5. There have been only 2 clinical trials that advocate DXM in pneumococcal meningitis (a subgroup of patients in an Egyptian trial, and a small retrospective analysis from Dallas).

6. DXM is not of proven benefit in neonatal meningitis.

7. Side effects of steroids such as gastrointestinal bleeding must always be considered: this occurs in up to 2% of patients.

Opinion remains divided on whether DXM should be given for ABM,[31,32] and the importance of the time of administration. The usual dose is 0.15 mg/kg/dose 6 hourly. A two-day regimen (0.4 mg/kg/dose 12 hourly) has also been used, but experience with it is limited.

ISOLATION PROCEDURES

Handwashing must be observed between all patients. In general, no isolation procedures are required for organisms that are usually commensals. Table 6.1.10 provides a guide to the isolation procedures for the conventional pathogens.[33]

Recurrent meningitis   Recurrent bacterial meningitis results from fractures of the skull (base and temporal bone), ventriculo-peritoneal shunts and other neurosurgical procedures, and congenital defects of the craniospinal axis, such as a dermoid sinus or meningomyelocele. Rhinorrhoea or otorrhea may accompany skull fracture or CSF fistula. The bacteria implicated are those that constitute the flora of the nasopharynx, sinuses and skin: *S. pneumoniae*, *H. influenzae/parainfluenzae*, Gram

Table 6.1.10   Isolation measures

Organism	Isolation strategy	Gown + gloves
N. meningitidis	Respiratory isolation, until given 24 h of rifampicin (or other 'carriage-eliminating' antimicrobial)	No
S. pneumoniae	Respiratory isolation until 24 h of antimicrobial therapy has elapsed	No
H. influenzae type b	Respiratory isolation until given 24 h of rifampicin	No
Group B streptococcus	No isolation necessary, unless nursery outbreak	No
Salmonella meningitis	Isolation, or cohorting of ill/colonized patients	Yes
Herpes simplex	Contact isolation for neonates, and for older children with florid skin lesions, but not for isolated CNS infection	Yes
Enteroviruses	Isolation for duration of stay. Enteric precautions, especially diligent handwashing following nappy changing	Yes
Tuberculous meningitis	Infants and children rarely require isolation, unless frequent coughing with open pulmonary TB	No

negative bacilli (*E. coli*, Pseudomonas spp.), anaerobes, Staphylococcus spp., Streptococcus spp. and Corynebacterium spp.

Mollaret's meningitis is benign, recurrent, aseptic meningitis of unknown aetiology. It occurs sporadically and presents at greater than 5 years old. Symptoms are the same as in acute bacterial meningitis, including neck rigidity, fits and coma. Complete spontaneous recovery follows within a few days. Cerebrospinal fluid has <3000 × 10^9/l leucocytes, predominantly lymphocytes, macrophages and large endothelial (Mollaret) cells, CSF protein is increased and glucose decreased.

Syndromic causes of recurrent meningitis are Behcet's disease, Vogt-Koyanagi-Harada syndrome and Iceland disease. Behcet's does occasionally occur in older children, and is the triad of mucous membrane ulceration, uveitis and meningo-encephalitis. The CSF shows a raised protein and pleocytosis. Filamentous virus-like particles may be implicated. Vogt-Koyanagi-Harada syndrome is a triad of acute eye involvement (field defects, blindness or uveitis) with meningo-encephalitis and skin features (vitiligo, alopecia or poliosis). Twenty percent arise in those under 20 years old, and 80% in adults. There is some speculation over a chronic viral aetiology. Iceland disease is a benign myalgic encephalomyelitis that has seasonal epidemics. CSF is usually normal, and recovery complete. A viral aetiology is assumed.

PARAMENINGEAL FOCI OF INFECTION

Purulent focal infections in the CNS are:[34,35]

Cerebral abscess (Chapter 6.3)
Cranial subdural empyema (Chapter 6.3)
Cerebral epidural abscess
Spinal abscess (spinal epidural abscess, subdural empyema and intermedullary spinal abscess)
Intervertebral disc infection
Osteomyelitis of the skull/vertebral purulent abscess
Cold abscess of vertebrae

Parameningeal focal infections are life threatening and may leave severe neurological sequelae. They form a group of differential diagnoses of meningitis, often with similar presentations or with CSF changes that might mislead to a diagnosis of meningitis. Delayed recognition of a spinal or cerebral abscess can have tragic consequences. The commonest causative organisms are *S. aureus*, anaerobes, Gram negative bacilli, *H. influenzae* and *S. pneumoniae*.

Epidural abscess

Cerebral epidural abscess has the same aetiology, pathogenesis and bacteriology as subdural empyema. It occurs as a direct extension of osteomyelitis, sinusitis, otitis media, mastoiditis or dental abscess, with extension of infection to the epidural space. Surgical procedures (neurosurgical, dental, otologic) or skull fractures may also introduce infection. Symptoms are mild and insidious, with local pain and tenderness, headache, low grade fever and minimal or no neurological deficits. Cerebral epidural abscess is a leading cause of dural sinus thrombosis, which may then lead on to benign intracranial hypertension (which despite its name can cause optic nerve atrophy). The erythrocyte sedimentation rate is >100 mm/h, and LP shows increased or normal pressure. The CSF is usually normal, but may show a 'parameningeal reaction' with moderate pleocytosis, raised protein, and low glucose. CT scan can make the diagnosis, but false negative scans occur in up to 30% of post-neurosurgical infections, and enhanced CT or MRI is better. Treatment demands antibiotics and surgery if the abscess has a mass effect (craniotomy/craniectomy rather than burr hole drainage). Occasionally conservative management is successful with antibiotics alone. Extension of infection from the epidural space to the subdural space, producing a subdural empyema, causes rapid neurological deterioration.

Spinal abscess

Spinal abscesses are mostly epidural; spinal subdural empyema and intramedullary spinal abscesses are inordinately rare in children. Infection is the result of metastatic spread via the veins of Batson's plexus, or results from direct extension of spondylitis, lung or perinephric abscess. Congenital dermal sinuses may also predispose. Spinal abscesses occur mostly in the thoracic and lumbar regions. The onset is acute and symptoms advance rapidly, even in hours, to paraplegia. Well-defined backache and tenderness progress to spinal root signs and widespread sharp pain. Once sensory deficits appear, paraplegia is imminent. Initially there is leg weakness, then gait difficulty, sphincteric loss and finally paraplegia. Loss of sphincter control and leg weakness are poor prognostic signs, and by the time paraplegia is recognized, the chance of recovery is small. CSF shows a parameningeal reaction. Culture and Gram stain of CSF will be negative unless the spinal needle passes through the abscess. Diagnosis is most accurate with CT or MRI, but when these investigations give equivocal results, myelography and contrast CT are necessary. Early identification and decompressive laminectomy and irrigation are essential for a good outcome. Achieving this aim though is unfortunately unusual.

Disc infections

Intervertebral disc infections are more frequent in children than in adults; and present with fever, malaise, localized back or abdominal pain, and refusal to walk. X-rays may show narrowing of disc space and demineralization of adjacent vertebrae. Treatment is with antibiotics. Surgery is not necessary unless infection extends to become a spinal abscess.

Cold abscess

Cold abscesses of vertebrae are due to tuberculosis. They are exceptionally uncommon in Europe and Australia since the decline in TB, but do still occur in developing countries. Pott's paraplegia is spinal cord compression from vertebral collapse. X-rays may show a paravertebral abscess and bony lesions. Treatment involves orthopaedic surgery and antituberculous therapy.

ASEPTIC MENINGITIS

Aseptic meningitis is historically defined as a syndrome of a typically lymphocytic meningitis which broadly covers all meningitis aetiologies other than acute bacterial meningitis.

Enteroviruses are the commonest cause of this syndrome, accounting for approximately 85% of all cases of aseptic meningitis. The differential diagnosis is long and includes: other viruses, partially treated ABM, TBM, rickettsial and spirochaetal agents, fungi, protozoa and helminths (toxoplasmosis, cysticercosis, malaria and amoebiasis), and non-infectious causes. CSF pleocytosis also occurs with subarachnoid haemorrhages, chemical irritation (as in spinal anaesthesia) ventriculoperitoneal shunts for hydrocephalus, vasculitis (e.g. Kawasaki disease, SLE), CNS tumours and CNS leukaemia.

A more helpful classification is subdivision of meningitis into ABM, viral, TBM, fungal, other microbial agents and non-infectious causes. The CSF characteristics of some of these groups are as outlined in Table 6.1.11.

Some of the commoner viruses are as follows:[2]

Enteroviruses

In temperate climates the incidence of enteroviral meningitis is greatest in summer and autumn, whereas in tropical regions there is equal year round incidence. Spread is mostly faecal-oral, and infants and young children are predominantly affected. Immunodeficiency predisposes. Coxsackie B2 and B5, and echoviruses 4, 6, 9, 11, 16 and 30 are the commonest causing meningitis.

Mumps

Ten to thirty per cent of infections in a non-immunized population will manifest meningitis if mumps infection is acquired. It is a benign and self-limiting meningitis. Mumps is transmitted by respiratory spread and the incidence is highest in children aged 5–9 years. In the developed world, immunization protects the majority from mumps.

Table 6.1.11   Differentiating meningitis on CSF findings[3,19]

	CSF pleocytosis ($\times 10^9$/l)	Gram stain/antigen test/culture	Protein (g/l)	Glucose (mmol/l)
Normal	0–5 lymphocytes	Negative	0.2–0.45	2.5–3.6
Bacterial	100–2000, mostly neutrophils	Positive	1.3–3.0	1.1–1.6
Viral	10–500 lymphocytes	Negative	0.5–1.0	Slightly low to normal
TBM	60–280 lymphocytes and neutrophils and up to 4000 cells	Acid-fast bacilli positive	1.0–6.0	Low
Recurrent (Mollaret's)	<3000 lymphocytes, macrophages, Mollaret's cells	Negative	0.5–1.0	Low

Herpesviruses

These include varicella zoster, herpes simplex virus 1 and 2, Epstein-Barr virus, human herpes viruses 6 and 7, and cytomegalovirus.

Meningitis is self-limiting and benign, whereas encephalitis is life threatening, hence it is vital to differentiate the conditions. Encephalitis is part of fulminant septicaemia in the neonate, whereas in childhood, presentation can be distinctly either meningitis or encephalitis. HSV can be recurrent (Mollaret's meningitis also associated with EBV). CMV is notable for causing meningitis in the immuno-compromised host.

Acyclovir is the treatment of choice for HSV meningitis ($500\,mg/m^2/dose$ 8 hourly intravenously). Early empiric administration is vital, especially if encephalitis, rather than meningitis, is suspected.

Lymphocytic choriomeningitis virus

This is a murine virus which can be transmitted to man, notably laboratory workers. Human–human transmission does not occur.

Human immunodeficiency virus

Five to ten percent have an acute meningo-encephalitis during or after the early mononucleosis-like syndrome of HIV infection.

Adenovirus

Cases are usually sporadic, but may occasionally be epidemic. Serotype 7 is most associated with meningitis; serotypes 1, 6 and 12 less so.

Polio

The natural history is of a minor illness occurring over 1–3 days. In 1–5% of patients, a 2–5 day symptom-free period precedes a major illness, with a meningitic stage heralding acute flaccid paralysis in 0.1–2%.

Arboviruses

These are viruses spread by insect vectors, with most cases occurring in warm months and in temporate climates. Children are more likely to manifest meningitis than adults.

NON-VIRAL CAUSES OF ASEPTIC MENINGITIS

Two important and relatively common forms are worth mention, *Mycoplasma pneumoniae* and Leptospirosis.

Mycoplasma

Aseptic meningitis is one of many extra-pulmonary complications of *Mycoplasma pneumoniae* infection.[36] CNS manifestations occur in 1:1000 infections, encephalitis is more common than meningitis, and when meningitis is present encephalitis often coexists. Sixty per cent have normal CSF, and 40% have a pleocytosis with up to $230 \times 10^9/l$ leucocytes. CSF protein varies from 0.2 to 1.6 g/l. Children are affected usually from 3 years old upwards, and meningitis may be the lone manifestation without pneumonia. Identification of *M. pneumoniae* can be with the non-specific finding of positive cold agglutinins, and the more specific complement fixation test. The organism is fastidious and culture is not usually undertaken.

Leptospirosis

Leptospira organisms are excreted by many wild and domestic animals. Leptospirosis is acquired by humans through contact with urine of an infected animal, either directly or through contaminated pools, puddles and streams. Leptospirosis is an abrupt onset, biphasic illness with a 7–12-day incubation period.[37] The first 'blood-borne' phase lasts 4–7 days and is mild and flu-like. There is a gap of 1–2 days, and then the most severe features may appear during a second, 'immune phase', which lasts 4–30 days. Antibody develops during this second phase and organisms are usually cleared from CSF and blood; aprupt onset of headache and fever may herald aseptic meningitis. The headache is intense, unremitting and throbbing, frontal or bitemporal and may be associated with retrobulbar pain. Benzylpenicillin or ampicillin most effectively ameliorate symptoms if started in the first phase of illness, but do seem to have a role in reducing sequelae even if started late in the second phase. Treatment is recommended in any hospitalized patient for 5–7 days.

TUBERCULOUS MENINGITIS

Tuberculous meningitis (TBM) is three times more common in children (6 months to 6 years) than in adults. Mycobacterium tuberculosis usually enters the body via the lungs or gastrointestinal tract. Dissemination to regional lymph nodes is followed by blood stream spread to other organs (i.e. apex of the lungs and the central nervous system). Meningitis occurs much later than haematogenous dispersal, and it is likely that it results from rupture of a caseous tuberculous focus into the CSF. Approximately 50% of all children with TBM have a prior history of TB.[9,10]

Pathology of TBM

At post mortem, a thick grey diffuse exudate often involves the meninges, especially around the basal cisterns and the spinal cord. The exudate microscopically contains lymphocytes, plasma cells, epithelioid cells and large amounts of fibrin. Hydrocephalus may result from occlusion of the basal cisterns and IVth ventricle outflow aqueducts. Phlebitis leads to infarcts, often accompanied by haemorrhage. Blood vessels may become hard and woody.

Clinical

There is a prodrome of malaise, anorexia, fatigue, fever (typically less than 39°C), myalgia and headache over 2–8 weeks. Infants have irritability, drowsiness, poor feeding and abdominal pain. The headache gradually worsens until it becomes continuous. Increasing irritability can progress to nausea, vomiting, confusion, fits and occasionally psychosis. Fifteen to 30% of children have cranial nerve palsies on admission. Papilloedema is frequent, and choroid tubercles may be seen on fundoscopy in 10%.

Hemiparesis and a variety of movement disorders are seen, usually a consequence of vasculitis. Involuntary movements occur more frequently in children than adults and include chorea, hemiballismus, athetosis, cerebellar ataxia and myoclonus.

Chest X-ray changes are seen in 50–90% of children with TBM (adults only 25–50%). CT scan of the head may show thickening of the meninges, hydrocephalus, infarction, oedema (periventricular predominantly), and mass lesions (tuberculoma, TB abscess). Tuberculin testing is positive in 85–90% of children with TBM (40–65% of adults). Some children may have a normal CXR and tuberculin test and yet have TBM. Early morning gastric aspirates for culture and Ziehl-Nielsen/Kinyoun staining are necessary if aseptic meningitis exists and TBM is suspected.

LP in TBM

Fifty per cent have raised opening CSF pressure. There is not the same risk of herniation following LP in TBM as in acute suppurative bacterial meningitis, despite the frequent presence of papilloedema. The median CSF WCC is 60–$280 \times 10^9/l$, but may be normal or massively raised ($>4000 \times 10^9/l$). A high CSF protein is the rule (1–2 g/l), and glucose is low. Acid fast bacilli are seen in up to 25% of CSF samples, and TB is cultured in 25–70%. Culture takes from two to several weeks to become positive. Preliminary reports of PCR for detection of mycobacterial DNA indicate sensitivities and specificities for this test of greater than 90%.

TBM and HIV

HIV increases the risk of a person contracting TBM, but HIV does not alter the mode of presentation, response to therapy, nor prognosis for the TBM.

Treatment of TBM

First line drugs are isoniazid, rifampicin, pyrazinamide, ethambutol and streptomycin. Dosages are given in Table 6.1.12.

There is reasonable evidence to support the adjunctive use of steroids in treating TBM.

Prognosis

Despite treatment, the mortality from TBM is 20–30%. Poor prognostic indicators are advanced stage, young children, very high CSF protein and markedly low CSF glucose. Clinical improvement usually occurs within 2 weeks of therapy commencing. There may be a transient worsening at the start, a form of Jarisch-Herxheimer reaction. Resolution of fever often takes weeks. Abnormalities of glucose, protein and pleocytosis in CSF persist for months. Late deterioration at 2–18 months can be due to swelling of a residual tuberculoma and is steroid responsive.

Twenty-five per cent of child survivors have long-term sequelae: cognitive, fits, hemiparesis, ataxia, persistent CNS palsies and optic atrophy.

Table 6.1.12   Treatment

Isoniazid	Hepatotoxicity, peripheral neuropathy (when not given with pyridoxine), altered mental state and hypersensitivity	5–10 mg/kg per day, up to 15 mg/kg per day if not used with rifampicin
Rifampicin	Vomiting, orange discoloration of tears and urine, staining of contact lenses, hepatitis, thrombocytopenia, 'flu-like' illness, and renders the contraceptive pill ineffective	10–20 mg/kg per day (maximum 600 mg per day)
Pyrazinamide	Hepatotoxicity, cochlear damage (correlates with total accumulated dose). Generally well tolerated by children	20–35 mg/kg per day. Use only for 4–8 weeks (maximum 12)
Ethambutol	1% get optic neuritis, therefore only use in older children in whom ophthalmic examination can reliably be made (visual acuity and colour perception)	15–25 mg/kg per day. Tuberculostatic at 15 mg/kg per day and tuberculocidal at 25 mg/kg per day. Optic neuritis occurs at higher doses
Streptomycin	Ototoxicity and vestibular disorders	

FUNGAL MENINGITIS

Fungal meningitis is rare in immunocompetent children, but is an important differential diagnosis in the febrile neutropenic or transplant patient, and in very low birth weight neonates. Candida and Aspergillus spp. are the main pathogens in children with oncological conditions, and Cryptococcus in AIDS and immune suppressive disorders.

REFERENCES

1 Adams W G, Deaver K A, Cochi S L et al. Decline in childhood Haemophilus influenzae type b (Hib) disease in the Hib vaccine era. JAMA 1993; 269: 221–226.
2 Tunkel A R, Scheld W M. In: Mandell G L, Bennett J E, Dolin R (eds) Mandell, Douglas and Bennett's Principles and practice of infectious diseases, vol 1. 4th edn. Edinburgh, Churchill Livingstone 1995; pp 831–865.
3 Feigin R D, McCracken G H, Klein J O. Diagnosis and management of meningitis. Pediatr Infect Dis J 1992; 11: 785–814.
4 Carter P E, Barclay S M, Galloway W H, Cole G F. Changes in bacterial meningitis. Arch Dis Child 1990; 65: 495–498.
5 Baraff L J, Lee S I, Schringer D L. Outcomes of bacterial meningitis in children: a meta-analysis. Pediatr Infect Dis J 1993; 12: 389–394.
6 Synott M B, Morse D L, Hall S M. Neonatal meningitis in England and Wales: a review of routine national data. Arch Dis Child 1994; 71: F75–F80.
7 Greenwood B M. The epidemiology of acute bacterial meningitis in tropical Africa. In: Williams J D and Burnie J (eds). Bacterial meningitis. London, The Beecham Colloquia. 1987; Academic Press pp 61–91.
8 Noah N D. Epidemiology of bacterial meningitis: UK and USA. In: WIlliams J D, Bumie J (eds). Bacterial meningitis. 1987; London, The Beecham Colloquia. Academic Press pp 93–115.
9 Berger J R. Tuberculous meningitis. Curr Opin Neurol 1994; 7: 191–200.
10 Teoh R, Humphries M. Tuberculous meningitis. In: Infections of the Central Nervous System. Lambert H P (ed). 1991; Kass Handbook of Infectious Diseases. Philadelphia, Decker pp 189–206.
11 Patel M S, Merianos A, Hanna J N, Vartto K, Tait P, Morey F, Jayathissa S. Epidemic meningococcal meningitis in central Australia. Med J Aust 1993; 158: 336–340.
12 Broome C V. The carrier state: Neisseria meningitidis. J Antimicrob Chemother 1986; 18: s25–34.
13 Gray B M, Dillon H C. Natural history of pneumococcal infections. Pediatr Infect Dis J 1989; 8: s23–25.
14 Tunkel A R, Scheld W M. Pathogenesis and pathophysiology of bacterial meningitis. Annu Rev Med 1993; 44: 103–120.
15 Brandtzaeg P. Pathogenesis of meningococcal infections. In: Cartwright K (ed). Meningococcal disease. 1995; Chichester, Wiley pp 71–114.
16 Lebel M H 1992 Adverse outcome of bacterial meningitis due to delayed sterilisation of cerebrospinal fluid. In: Schonfeld H, Helwig H (eds) Bacterial meningitis. Antibiot Chemother. Basel Karger, vol 45, pp 226–238.
17 Rennick G, Shann F, de Campo J. Cerebral herniation during bacterial meningitis in children. BMJ 1993; 306: 953–955.
18 Mellor D H. The place of computed tomography and lumbar puncture in suspected bacterial meningitis. Arch Dis Child 1992; 67: 1417–1419.
19 Bonadio W A. The cerebrospinal fluid: physiologic aspects and alterations associated with bacterial meningitis. Pediatr Infect Dis J 1992; 11: 423–432.
20 Spanos A, Harrell F E, Durack D T. Differential of acute meningitis — an analysis of predictive value of initial observations. JAMA 1989; 262: 2700–2707.
21 Ni H, Knight A I, Cartwright K, Palmer W H, McFadden J 1992 Polymerase chain reaction for diagnosis of meningococcal meningitis. Lancet 340: 1432–1434.
22 Hill R B, Adams S, Gunn B A, Eberly B J. The effects of nonclassic pediatric bacterial pathogens on the usefulness of the Directigen latex agglutination test. Am J Clin Pathol 1994; 101: 729–732.
23 Klein J O. Antimicrobial treatment and prevention of meningitis. Pediatric Annals 1994; 23: 76–81.

24 Booy R, Kroll S. Bacterial meningitis in children. Curr Opin Pediatr 1994; 6: 29–35.

25 Shann F, Duncan A, Butt W, Henning R, South M, Tibballs J. Drug doses. 1994 Intensive care unit, Royal Children's Hospital, Parkville, Victoria 3052, Australia. 8th edn. Collective Pty Ltd, Australia.

26 Nathavitharana K A, Tarlow M J. Current trends in the management of bacterial meningitis. Br J Hosp Med 1993; 50: 402–407.

27 Brown L W, Feigin R D. Bacterial meningitis: fluid balance and therapy. Pediatr Ann 1994; 23: 93–98.

28 American Academy of Paediatrics. Haemophilus influenzae infections, and meningococcal infections. In: Peter G (ed) 1994 Red Book: Report of the Committee on Infectious Diseases. 23rd edn. Illinois: American Academy of Paediatrics; 1994: 203–216 and 323–326.

29 Bhatt S M, Cabellos C, Nadol J B, Halpin C, Lauretano A, Xu W Z, Tuomanen E. The impact of dexamethasone on hearing loss in experimental pneumococcal meningitis. Paediatr Infect Dis J 1995; 14: 93–96.

30 Kennedy W A, Hoyt M J, McCracken G H. The role of corticosteroid therapy in children with pneumococcal meningitis. Am J Dis Child 1991; 145: 1374–1378.

31 Schaad U B, Lips U, Gnehm H E, Blumberg A, Heinzer I, Wedgwood J for the Swiss Meningitis Study Group. Dexamethasone therapy for bacterial meningitis in children. Lancet 1993; 342: 457–461.

32 The Meningitis Working Party of the British Paediatric Immunology and Infectious Diseases Group. Should we use dexamethasone in meningitis? Arch Dis Child 1991; 67: 1398–1401.

33 American Academy of Paediatrics. Section 2, infection control for hospitalised children, isolation precautions. In: Peter G (ed) 1994 Red Book: Report of the Committee on Infectious Diseases. 23rd edn. Illinois: American Academy of Paediatrics; 1994: 93–101.

34 Carmel P W. Purulent focal infections. In: Rudolph A M (Ed). Rudolph's Textbook of Pediatrics. 19th edition. California, Appleton and Lange; 1991; pp 1843–1849.

35 Greenlee J E. Epidural abscess. In: Mandell G L, Bennett J E, Dolin R (eds) Mandell, Douglas and Bennett's Principles and practice of infectious diseases, vol 1. 4th edn. New York, Churchill Livingstone 1995; pp 901–906.

36 Koskiniemi M. CNS manifestations associated with Mycoplasma pneumoniae infections: summary of cases at the University of Helsinki and review. Clin Infect Dis 1993; 17: s52–57.

37 Farrar W E. Leptospira species (leptospirosis). In: Mandell G L, Bennett J E, Dolin R (eds). Mandell, Douglas and Bennett's Principles and Practice of infectious diseases, vol 2. 4th edn. New York, Churchill Livingstone 1995; pp 2137–2141.

D. W. Webb   C. R. Kennedy

6.2   Acute viral meningitis, encephalitis and parainfectious encephalopathy

INTRODUCTION

In this chapter we discuss acute viral meningitis and encephalitis and childhood postinfectious encephalopathies. For an account of 'chronic' viral infections of the central nervous system (CNS), including neurological manifestations of human immunodeficiency virus and a more detailed account of CNS complications of virus infections in general, the reader is referred to texts dealing exclusively with these topics.[1,2]

Several principles are important by way of introduction to viral infection of the CNS:

1. A particular clinical picture is seldom specific to a single virus.
2. Most CNS viral infections are uncommon complications of common systemic viral infections.
3. The syndromes of aseptic meningitis and encephalitis form a continuum caused by the same viruses, although some viruses are more likely to cause meningitis and others to cause encephalitis.
4. Although the term 'encephalitis' is strictly speaking a histological one, the diagnosis, with the exception of herpes simplex encephalitis, has usually been a clinical one, and accordingly imprecise.

CLINICAL FEATURES

Viral infection of the CNS, if confined to the meninges, may be clinically manifest as one or more of headache, lethargy, photophobia, abdominal pain, vomiting, fever (not invariable) and meningism. In the young infant there may just be fever and irritability, with less than 10% having signs of meningeal irritation.[3] If infection spreads to the parenchyma of the brain (encephalitis), in addition to the above symptoms, depression in the state of consciousness, seizures, focal neurological deficits and raised intracranial pressure may be present separately or together and are not specific to the infecting agent.

DIAGNOSIS

A careful history, with an appreciation of the significance of geographical and seasonal factors, and a thorough general and neurological examination, may provide important clues as to the causal agent of viral CNS infection. A high diagnostic yield from investigations is possible provided that appropriate specimens are obtained and correctly processed. The proportion of positive findings from both viral culture and serology falls progressively after the first week of the illness, so that early investigation is crucial.[4] Identification of the virus helps rationalize treatment and improve prediction of outcome.[5,6]

Appropriate specimens to seek a viral cause of infection (Table 6.2.1) should be transported to the laboratory immediately, or on melting ice if there is any delay. If storage is necessary this should be at 4°C and for as short a time as possible. Viruses are most likely to be cultured from respiratory specimens taken within 3–4 days of the onset of symptoms.[7] Stool culture has a higher yield than rectal swabs.[8,9]

Because viruses may be carried asymptomatically in the throat or stool an associated high serum level of specific IgM or a four-fold rise in IgG titre is needed to establish recent viral infection.[8,10] The proportion of CNS viral infections in which cause could be established would be greatly increased if antibodies against the relevant group of viruses were sought in appropriate paired sera using existing methods.

The IgG index is a measure of intrathecal IgG synthesis by comparing cerebrospinal fluid to serum ratios of total IgG and albumin. It is a useful index of CNS viral infection.[11] It should be interpreted with caution if there is evidence of an abnormality of the blood–brain barrier (raised CSF : serum albumin ratio). An elevated IgG index and the presence of oligoclonal bands provide support for intrathecal IgG synthesis but cannot be used to confirm that a neurological illness is attributable to a specific virus.

The virus-specific IgG ratio compares the CSF to serum ratio of specific antiviral IgG with that of total IgG and can be used to identify infection by a specific virus in the CNS.[10,12] If the fraction of specific antiviral IgG in the CSF exceeds that in the serum by more than a factor of two then intrathecal synthesis of antibody against that virus is very probable.[13] The IgG index and virus-specific IgG ratio are only likely to be helpful if measured on convalescent samples, which are often difficult to obtain.

Table 6.2.1   Investigation of a child with a presumed viral infection of the CNS

Specimens for viral culture	Transport
Blood	EDTA/heparinized sample
Respiratory secretions	Viral transport medium
Throat swab	Viral transport medium
Stool sample	Sterile container
Urine	Sterile container
CSF	Sterile container

Serology
Paired specific serum IgG (and where available IgM) concentrations at presentation, 2 and 6 weeks later

CSF IgG index — 6 weeks after presentation

$$\frac{\text{CSF total IgG conc.}}{\text{Serum total IgG conc.}} \times \frac{\text{Serum albumin conc.}}{\text{CSF albumin conc.}}$$

CSF specific IgG ratio — 6 weeks after presentation

$$\frac{\text{CSF specific antiviral IgG conc.}}{\text{Serum specific antiviral IgG conc.}} \times \frac{\text{Serum total IgG conc.}}{\text{CSF total IgG conc.}}$$

CSF Oligoclonal bands — 6 weeks after onset of CNS illness

Antigen detection — at presentation
CSF viral specific monoclonal antibodies
CSF viral amplification (PCR)

Table 6.2.2   Causes of viral meningoencephalitis in childhood. The viruses are listed under their most common clinical presentation.

Family	Commonest clinical presentation	
	Aseptic meningitis	**Encephalitis**

Picornavirus	Enteroviruses
	   Coxsackie B1–B6
	   Echovirus 1–30
	   Coxsackie A1–A24
	   Enterovirus 68–72
	   Poliovirus 1–3	

Herpes virus		Herpes simplex 1 Herpes simplex 2 Cytomegalovirus Varicella
	Herpes virus 6	Epstein-Barr
Paramyxovirus	Mumps	Measles RSV Parainfluenza
Orthomyxovirus		Influenza
Rubivirus		Rubella
Adenovirus		Serotype 7
Arena virus	LCM virus	Lassa fever
Rhabdovirus		Rabies
Arbovirus		see Table 6.2.6

Key: RSV, respiratory syncytial virus;
   LCM, lymphocytic choriomeningitis virus.

The polymerase chain reaction (PCR) technique enables the amplification of nucleic acid sequences in 8–10 h and is likely to be the way forward in providing accurate and early evidence of CNS viral infection.[14–17] The major causes of acute viral meningitis and encephalitis in childhood are listed in Table 6.2.2 and discussed below.

The presence of interferon in the CSF, although only moderately sensitive, is highly specific for viral CNS infection.[10] Its measurement can be a useful adjunct to diagnosis in the acute phase, although the test is not widely available.

VIRAL MENINGITIS

Viral meningitis, by definition, is infection confined to the meninges, choroid plexus and ependyma and is considered a defined clinical entity because of the similarities in presentation, course and benign outcome caused by a wide variety of viral agents. However, potentially lethal and treatable infections of the CNS can initially present as aseptic meningitis, so the first important task is to exclude more serious infection and in particular bacterial meningitis (perhaps partially treated), tuberculous meningitis, bacterial endocarditis, parameningeal foci of infection and Lyme disease (Table 6.2.3).

The major point of departure in assessment of a child suspected of having viral meningitis is examination of the cerebrospinal fluid (CSF). In most cases the typical CSF profile is of a total white cell count of less than $500/mm^3$ ($500 \times 10^6/l$) with a lymphocyte predominance, a protein concentration of less than 100 mg/dl

Table 6.2.3   Other causes of aseptic meningitis in children

Infective

Bacterial	Partially treated bacterial meningitis
	Bacterial endocarditis
Mycobacteria	Tuberculosis
Spirochaetes	*Borrelia burgdorferi* (Lyme disease)
Fungi	*Cryptococcus neoformans*
Parasites	*Toxoplasma, Naegleria* or *Hartmanella*
Rickettsiae	*Rickettsia ricketsii* (Rocky Mountain spotted fever)

Brain abscess
Parameningeal infection
Septic embolism

Non-infective
Leptomeningeal malignancy
Vasculitis
Sarcoidosis
Kawasaki disease

Table 6.2.4   Recent CSF profiles identified in bacterial and viral meningitis[15,44]

CSF profile	Features with 99% certainty of bacterial infection (422 cases)	Profile seen in >90% of cases of viral meningitis (277 children)
WCC	>2000 × 10³/ml	<1000 × 10³/ml
PMN	>1180 × 10³/ml	
CSF protein	>220 mg/dl (2.2 g/litre)	<17 mg/dl (0.17 g/litre)
CSF glucose	<1.9 mmol/litre	>2.0 mmol/litre
CSF/blood glucose	<0.23	>0.4

Key: WCC, white cell count; PMN, neutrophil count.

(1 g/litre) and a normal glucose level. Notable exceptions to this pattern are (1) the predominance of polymorphs at presentation in 40% of enteroviral infections of the CNS[18] (a conversion to lymphocyte predominance generally occurs within 24 h although this is not invariable) and (2) the low CSF glucose and moderately raised protein sometimes seen in infections with herpes simplex, mumps and lymphocytic choriomeningitis virus infections. It is also worth remembering that CSF white cell counts of less than 250/mm³ are seen in 21% and an initial lymphocyte predominance in 15% of all cases of bacterial meningitis.[19,20] Recent surveys of meningitis have reported CSF profiles in bacterial and viral CNS infection (Table 6.2.4).[8,19]

A low CSF white cell count with a lymphocyte predominance is also seen in tuberculous meningitis but CSF protein levels are usually considerably raised (often 1.0–3.0 g/litre) and CSF glucose is modestly low (less than 50% serum concentration).[21] A similar profile is seen with Lyme disease, although the CSF glucose is generally normal.[22]

VIRAL ENCEPHALITIS

Acute encephalopathies of viral or unknown origin occur most commonly in the first decade of life, with a peak incidence of 1–2/1000 in the first 6 months.[23] The diagnosis of viral encephalitis is supported by a mild lymphocellular pleocytosis in the CSF (absent in up to 50% of cases), mild elevation of protein and normal glucose. Electroencephalographic (EEG) abnormalities are seldom

Table 6.2.5 Causes of acute encephalopathy in childhood

1. Intracranial infection
   See Table 6.2.3
2. Parainfectious insult
   Acute disseminated encephalomyelitis
   Acute haemorrhagic leucoencephalitis
   Reye's syndrome
   Haemorrhagic shock encephalopathy
   Septicaemia (Gram-negative, staphylococcal)
3. Trauma
4. Hypoxic ischaemic injury
5. Fluid, electrolyte, glucose and acid–base disorders
6. Endogenous toxins
   Organ failure (kidney, liver)
   Inherited metabolic disorders
7. Exogenous toxins
   Drugs, poisoning
8. Status epilepticus
9. Hypothermia and hyperthermia
10. Mass lesion or CSF obstruction
11. Vascular
    Cerebrovascular accident
    Vasculitis
    Hypertension

specific, with background slowing or epileptiform discharges that may be diffuse or focal. Cranial computed tomography (CT) is often normal or may show diffuse or focal low attenuation (oedema) which is non-specific. Magnetic resonance imaging (MRI) is more sensitive.[24]

Immediate goals in the management of presumed viral encephalitis should be to give intravenous acyclovir promptly (even in the absence of focal features to suggest herpes virus infection); to detect other treatable causes of an acute encephalopathy (Table 6.2.5); and to protect the child's brain against further insult. Maintenance of cerebral perfusion and supportive care are of crucial importance in encephalitis, as the pathological process often appears to be temporary or reversible to the extent that a deficit that appears very severe at the height of the illness may be followed by an excellent recovery. Supportive measures of vital importance include seizure control, temperature control, attention to airway and circulation, maintenance of electrolyte balance (in the knowledge that inappropriate antidiuretic hormone secretion is common) and nutritional support.

Raised intracranial pressure and decreased cerebral perfusion pressure (the difference between systolic blood pressure and intracranial pressure) are associated with a higher mortality in Reye's syndrome, near drowning and CNS infections in childhood.[25–27] Decreased cerebral perfusion pressure distinguishes non-survivors from survivors of CNS infection much more clearly than raised intracranial pressure, thus emphasizing the importance of maintaining or if necessary increasing systemic arterial pressure.[25] Maintenance of cerebral perfusion pressure seems a logical goal of treatment, although direct evidence that such intervention improves the prognosis in CNS infections in general, or in viral infections in particular, is sparse.

VIRUSES CAUSING ACUTE CENTRAL NERVOUS SYSTEM INFECTION

Non-polio enteroviruses

From the late neonatal period and throughout childhood most cases of aseptic meningitis are now caused by non-polio enteroviruses (Coxsackie A and B and echoviruses). These have a worldwide distribution and accounted for over 90% of viral isolates in recent surveys of early childhood and late neonatal aseptic meningitis.[8,28–30] More than 90% of cases were due to Coxsackie B and echovirus infection.[8] They account for about 5% of all cases of viral encephalitis in the USA, although the figure rises to 25% of cases during epidemics.[31]

Enteroviral infection has a marked seasonal variation, with 80% in the Northern hemisphere occurring in the months July to October.[8] Orofaecal spread and respiratory droplet are the usual routes of transmission. Incubation periods are variable, averaging from 5 to 10 days. Infection becomes established in the pharynx and gastrointestinal tract, sometimes with related prodromal symptoms. In addition to gastroenteritis and respiratory tract disease, conjunctivitis, ex-anthematous illness, myopathy, myocarditis/pericarditis, hepatitis, herpangina and hand, foot and mouth disease can also occur. However, the majority of infected individuals have subclinical disease.

The frequency with which enteroviral illness is complicated by CNS infection is age dependent. Those at highest risk appear to be young infants, and aseptic meningitis is diagnosed in almost half of enterovirus-infected infants younger than 3 months who undergo lumbar puncture for evaluation of a fever.[32] The yield of CSF culture for enterovirus isolation is about 35%.[8] Cultures of pharyngeal, urine and stool specimens can increase the overall yield to 60%, but in an immunocompetent patient should only be interpreted as evidence of infection with appropriate serology. Serological confirmation can be laborious because of the large number of serotypes, but it is possible to look for neutralizing anti-bodies to an isolated virus or less specifically at IgM antibodies against groups of viruses (e.g. Coxsackie). Detection of viral nucleic acid using PCR has been shown to be sensitive and specific for the diagnosis of enteroviral meningitis.[14] This technique also permits identification of Coxsackie A viruses, which have previously required animal inoculation to be detected reliably.

Non-polio enteroviral CNS infection is usually a self-limiting disease with a good outcome,[33] although infants may suffer neurological sequelae and neonatal disease can be particularly severe.[34] There is no specific treatment.

Children with agammaglobulinaemia are at risk of chronic CNS enteroviral infection. Intravenous and/or intrathecal immunoglobulin therapy may provide some clinical benefit.[35]

Polioviruses

The introduction of polio and mumps vaccines has dramatically reduced the inci-dence of these organisms as causes of aseptic meningitis in effectively vaccinated populations.[36] Unvaccinated individuals remain at risk as do large populations in the developing world. More than 90% of natural polio virus infections are asymptomatic or produce only mild symptoms. Aseptic meningitis occurs in 4–8% of cases, and paralytic disease in 1%.[36] Live attenuated oral polio vaccine (OPV) has caused a small number of vaccine-related infections.[37] The risk of vaccine-associated disease is approximately 1 case per 2.6 million doses of OPV distributed, and is seen in young, often immunodeficient, children or their adult, unimmunized contacts. Cases of vaccine-related disease are indistinguishable clinically from natural disease.

Mumps virus

In the prevaccine period mumps was the second most common cause of viral meningitis. Cases of vaccine-related mumps meningitis have been reported,[38–40] although the incidence was greatest by far with the Urabe strain. Mumps infec-tion occurs most commonly in late winter and spring and there is a 6–18-day incubation period. Fifty per cent of those with mumps parotitis have CSF pleocytosis. Symptomatic CNS disease occurs in 1–10% and usually follows the onset of parotitis by several days to weeks.[36] Males are three times more likely to develop neurological complications.[41] Meningitis is the only manifestation of infection in 50% and may precede the parotitis.[42] Other clinical clues in these cases include orchitis, oophoritis and pancreatitis, while the serum amylase may be raised. Mumps virus can be isolated from the CSF and infection can also be confirmed serologically. Serious sequelae are reported to occur in 1/6000 cases of mumps meningitis and residual, unilateral deafness in less than 1/30 000.[43] Neurological sequelae of mumps encephalitis occur in up to 25% of patients and include cortical blindness, cerebellar ataxia, myelitis, aqueduct stenosis and sensorineural deafness.[44] A chronic relapsing encephalitis has also been reported.[45]

Herpes simplex virus 1

Herpes simplex virus type 1 (HSV-1) can occasionally cause aseptic meningitis but more commonly causes a focal encephalitis (HSE). This has a 70% mortality if untreated and less than 10% of survivors return to normal function. HSE has an annual incidence of approximately 1/250 000 with no seasonal variation.[47,48] Onset may be insidious or rapid and there is usually a high fever (39–40°C). This is followed by behaviour change and, in 65%, focal seizures of temporal lobe origin. The classical signs of HSE are focal neurological deficits localized to the temporal or frontal lobes (hemiparesis, paraesthesiae, aphasia) with a depressed level of consciousness. However, the presence of focal neurological signs is not invariable, nor is it specific to HSE.[48] A history of mucocutaneous herpes is no more common in children with HSE than other causes of viral encephalitis.[48]

EEG findings include slowing and spike and slow wave epileptiform activity localized to the temporal lobe. These appearances have a sensitivity of 84% and a specificity of 33% for HSE.[48] CT shows focal abnormality in only 60%. Virus is isolated from the CSF in less than 5% of cases. Since the majority of patients are seropositive prior to their illness, seroconversion is not usually helpful except in very young children. Anti-HSV-1 titres in CSF are useful and rise 20-fold in 40% of proven cases between 5 and 10 days and in 90% in those with symptoms for more than 2 weeks.[49] Measurement of HSV-1-specific IgM in the CSF can provide an accurate diagnosis within 4–10 days.[50] Antigen detection using a monoclonal antibody to HSV-1 is sensitive by the second week but only detects 62% in the first week.[51] PCR has been used to confirm HSE,[52] but a negative PCR does not totally exclude the diagnosis.

The natural history of HSE has been shown to be improved by specific antiviral treatment. Outcome is related to the level of consciousness at the start of therapy, so that treatment with acyclovir should not be delayed.[53] Mortality from HSV-1 falls from 70% to 28% in acyclovir-treated patients and to 8% for those in whom treatment is started within 4 days of neurological symptoms.[54] In a follow-up study 38% were normal or had mild impairment, 9% had moderate sequelae and 53% died or had severe impairment.[54] Relapse or secondary deterioration in appropriately treated HSE has been reported and chorea is often a prominent feature if this occurs.[55] This may be due to a postinfectious neuroallergic process and immunomodulation therapy may be appropriate.

Herpes simplex virus 2

The incidence of neonatal HSV infection is estimated to be 1/3000–1/5000 deliveries in the USA, with 70% being due to HSV-2 and 30% to HSV-1.[48]

Neonatal CNS infection with HSV-1 infection has a better prognosis than with HSV-2.[54] Neonatal HSV infection generally follows primary maternal genital HSV, though rarely it can follow recurrent maternal disease. In less than 25% of cases of neonatal HSV infection is there a history of any maternal genital lesion. Neonatal HSV encephalitis may present de novo, usually in the second to third week of life with a median age of 11 days. However, untreated localized HSV infection (skin, eye, mouth) has a greater than 80% risk of progressing to disseminated infection, including CNS, if untreated. In possible neonatal HSV encephalitis, a history of maternal genital lesions should be sought, and the baby examined for skin lesions, keratoconjunctivitis, oral lesions, pneumonitis and hepatitis. However, all may be absent. The CSF protein is often raised (500–1000 mg/dl) and the yield of viral culture from CSF is high. Early treatment with acyclovir decreases the incidence of disseminated disease and reduces the overall mortality from 80% to 19%.

Other herpes viruses

Varicella zoster, cytomegalovirus and Epstein–Barr virus (EBV) can all cause aseptic meningitis. The incidence is highest in the immunocompromised host, who is also predisposed to more severe infection and meningoencephalitis. Systemic but not neurological infection with human herpesvirus type 6 (which causes roseola infantum) has been documented in children with seizures, acute encephalopathy and transverse myelitis.

Varicella zoster primary infection leads to chickenpox. Neurological complications occur in 1/1000 chickenpox infections and in half they consist of a self-limiting cerebellitis with ataxia, which has an excellent prognosis. Meningoencephalitis can also occur, and both classically start 4–8 days after the onset of the rash but may also precede it.[56] Other sequelae of varicella infection include Guillain–Barré syndrome, myelitis, cranial neuropathies and optic neuritis. There is uncontrolled evidence for efficacy of acyclovir in herpes zoster-associated meningoencephalitis in the immunosuppressed.[57]

EBV is known to cause aseptic meningitis, encephalitis, cerebellar ataxia, Bell's palsy, Guillain–Barré syndrome, transverse myelitis, and the rare post-EBV psychosis with altered perception, the so-called 'looking glass' syndrome. Neurological symptoms usually appear 1–3 weeks after the onset of infectious mononucleosis, although children in particular may have no prodromal illness. Prognosis is excellent.

Measles

Measles infection is commonly associated with asymptomatic EEG and CSF abnormalities. Acute encephalitis is reported to occur in about 1/1000 cases.[1] This typically occurs in a child recovering from measles infection with a fading exanthem, who then deteriorates with a high fever, altered consciousness and, frequently, focal or generalized seizures.[58] It has a waxing and waning course and can involve involuntary movement disorders, hallucinations, hypotonia or spasticity. Occasionally myelitis, cerebellar ataxia or optic neuritis is a feature. Neurological sequelae are seen in 23–35% and include epilepsy, hemiplegia, mental retardation and behaviour problems.[59] CSF and EEG findings are not of prognostic value. Neurological sequelae of measles vaccination have an incidence of 1.79 per million, approximately equal to the background incidence of viral encephalitis.[60] Subacute sclerosing panencephalitis is a rare but devastating complication in which measles virus acts as a slow virus, usually presenting at 6–10 years of age as a chronic progressive dementia with convulsions. It occurs with an incidence of 1/1 000 000 cases of wild-type measles infection, is more likely to occur in infants who have measles before 1 year of age, and can be prevented by measles immunization.

Adenovirus

Adenovirus infections in childhood generally cause respiratory infections, fever or conjunctivitis, or are asymptomatic. CNS complications are generally confined to the immunosuppressed and to children with severe respiratory or generalized disease. They are the cause of less than 5% of all cases of meningoencephalitis in the USA and this complication has been particularly associated with serotype 7.[61]

Rubella

Rubella encephalitis is said to complicate rubella infection in 1/20 000 cases.[1] Focal neurology is rare and survivors generally recover rapidly with few sequelae. Congenital rubella panencephalitis and chronic progressive rubella panencephalitis, which mimics SSPE, are two quite distinct neurological complications.

Rare causes of childhood encephalitis

Arenaviruses

Lymphocytic choriomeningitis has a natural reservoir in the field mouse and hamster, and virus is transmitted to humans by contact with infected rodents or their excreta.[36] It can be acquired by aerosol, direct contact or the bite of an infected animal. The peak incidence is in late autumn and early winter. The incubation period is 1–3 weeks and infection begins with an influenza-like illness, with approximately 15% of patients developing signs of meningitis. Diagnosis is by viral culture or serology. Meningitis is usually self-limiting although occasionally protracted. Lassa fever virus is a cause of meningoencephalitis and haemorrhagic fever which is initially acquired from rats but can be spread from man to man.[1] It has been reported to respond to ribavirin therapy.[46]

Arboviruses

Arboviruses represent the most frequent cause of epidemic encephalitis in the USA,[36] with more than 400 varieties (Table 6.2.6). They are arthropod-borne, and usually transmitted to man from a bird or mammal pool, with a peak incidence in the July to October months. A tick-borne disease (louping ill) which can cause cerebellar ataxia and encephalitis is the only arboviral illness recognized in the UK.[62]

Japanese B encephalitis is probably the commonest of these infections world-

Table 6.2.6 The more common arboviral infections with their vector and distribution

Arboviruses	Vector	Distribution of disease
Bunyavirus		
Rift Valley	Sandfly	Africa, Egypt
California	Mosquito	USA — north and mid-west
Togaviruses		
Western equine	Mosquito	USA — west of Mississippi
Eastern equine	Mosquito	USA — Atlantic and Gulf coasts
St Louis	Mosquito	USA — nation-wide
Venezuelan equine	Mosquito	USA — Florida, southwest Central and South America
Japanese B	Mosquito	Japan, Korea, China, Taiwan, Singapore, Malaysia, Indonesia, Thailand, Burma, Nepal, India
Murray Valley	Mosquito	Australia
Colorado fever	Tick	USA — Rocky Mountains
Eastern	Tick	Eastern Russia
Central European	Tick	Central Europe
Louping ill	Tick	Northern UK

wide, causing 10 000 cases and 1000 deaths per annum in China alone.[63] A recent survey from India identified Japanese B infection in 23% of children with acute unexplained encephalopathy.[64] Involvement of the basal ganglia is common in childhood. Eastern equine encephalitis is the most sinister variety of the North American arboviruses and is associated with a high incidence of infection in children. Outbreaks characteristically occur at the end of wet summers.[31] The other North American arboviruses that cause CNS infection all produce similar non-descript encephalitis which resolves without residua in the majority of cases. Australian arboviruses associated with encephalitis include Australian encephalitis (previous Murray Valley encephalitis) and Barmah Forest viruses.

Rabies

Rabies is one of the world's deadliest infections, and kills 25 000 people in India each year.[65] Cases originating from domestic animal bites are a rarity in North America and Europe and the most common animal reservoirs are now the skunk, fox, racoon, coyote and insectivorous bat.[54] Airborne infection has been reported. Nearly half of all cases occur in children. The incubation period is usually 1–3 months, though may be up to several years, and is related to the extent of innervation of the bitten area and to age (being shorter in children). The prodrome consists of paraesthesiae at the site of the bite, headache, malaise, anorexia and meningism. Two to 10 days later there is onset of seizures, delirium and periods of hyperexcitability which may be stimulus-sensitive. Painful laryngospasm induced by attempting to drink (hydrophobia) is common and a minority manifest as ascending paralysis with areflexia. Diagnosis is often difficult. Virus can be detected by fluorescent antibody stains of corneal or skin sections. Serology may also be helpful. Postexposure management involves administration of antiserum (rabies immunoglobulin) and immunization, ideally with the newer tissue culture vaccines, which are expensive but have less serious neuroparalytic complications than cheaper neurotissue vaccines.[65,66]

POSTINFECTIOUS ENCEPHALOMYELITIS

This is characterized by an initial latent phase between the acute illness and the onset of neurological symptoms and is thought to be an immunologically mediated disease initiated by the viral pathogen. It is sometimes associated with widespread changes in white matter and referred to as acute disseminated encephalomyelitis (ADEM). There is also a more fulminant variant known as acute haemorrhagic leukoencephalitis whose pathophysiology may be similar.

Table 6.2.7   Antiviral encephalitis therapy

Herpes simplex virus and varicella	
Acyclovir	500 mg/m² or 10 mg/kg 8-hourly, i.v. for 10–14 days
Vidarabine	15–30 mg/kg per day
	i.v. over 12 h for 10–14 days
Cytomegalovirus	
Ganciclovir	5 mg/kg 12-hourly
	i.v. for 14–21 days
Influenza A	
Amantadine	2 mg/kg 12-hourly, orally for 5–7 days
Postinfectious encephalomyelitis	
Prednisolone	2 mg/kg daily orally for 5 days

Measles is the commonest identified infection associated with ADEM but it has also been reported with varicella and influenza infection and rarely after HSE. There is anecdotal evidence that steroids have been of benefit.[67]

Prognosis

Determining a specific cause of encephalitis is helpful in improving the accuracy of prognosis by placing this into three broad categories: (1) high mortality (30–100%) — Eastern equine encephalitis, Japanese B encephalitis and rabies; (2) moderate mortality rates (10–30%) — measles, rubella, adenovirus and herpes simplex virus encephalitis treated with acyclovir; and (3) low (less than 10% mortality) — enteroviruses, mumps and chickenpox.

Clinical features are helpful in predicting the outcome for the significant proportion of children with viral encephalitis for whom no virus is identified and in whom the concern is really whether neurological sequelae are likely. In a prospective study, several clinical criteria predicted a poor outcome based on neurological examination, developmental quotients and behaviour assessment at 8 months follow-up (Table 6.2.8).[4]

Table 6.2.8 Factors which may be used to predict a poor outcome in childhood encephalitis[4]

(a) Age — less than 3 years at presentation
(b) Coma Score — less than 9/15 on modified Glasgow Coma Scale
(c) Brain stem responses — abnormal oculocephalic responses
(d) Blood–brain barrier — high CSF : serum albumin ratios
(e) Evidence of CNS infection — positive serology + either isolation of virus from the CSF, raised CSF interferon or high IgG-specific ratios

REYE'S SYNDROME

Reye's syndrome is a childhood illness characterized by an onset with profuse vomiting and a deteriorating level of consciousness in the setting of hypoglycaemia and deranged liver function.[68] Diagnosis is based on the finding of elevated serum hepatic transaminases and/or blood ammonia (greater than three times the upper normal limit), but normal bilirubin and is confirmed by liver histology, which shows diffuse intense microvesicular panlobular fatty change. Coagulopathy and cerebral oedema are universal features.

The incidence is 1–6 cases per million children under 16 years and appears to be falling.[69] In most children it is a biphasic illness following an apparently innocuous viral infection (varicella, adenovirus, influenza A and B viruses). An association with prior ingestion of therapeutic doses of salicylates has been supported in case control studies.[70]

Reye's syndrome is a diagnosis of exclusion. An inherited metabolic disease should be considered in all children who present with a Reye-like illness as a growing number of inherited metabolic defects (Table 6.2.9) have been found to be associated with the syndrome.[69,71] This is particularly important in a young child (under 3 years) with a previous personal or family history of unexplained neurological illness or in whom the attack is atypical with no viral prodrome. First-line tests should include blood glucose, acid–base status, urinary ketones and plasma ammonia. If Reye's syndrome is suspected, the clinical chemistry laboratory should be asked to deep-freeze and store any surplus plasma or urine already collected and note the time and date of all specimens. Ideally blood should be taken before any intravenous glucose is given.

Table 6.2.9 Metabolic disorders that may present as a Reye-like syndrome are listed with their supporting biochemical markers and the appropriate diagnostic tests

Disorder and biochemistry	Diagnostic tests
Fatty acid oxidation disorder (including carnitine deficiency)	
No fasting ketonuria	Urinary organic acids
Abnormal plasma carnitine	Fibroblast/tissue enzymes
	DNA studies
Urea cycle disorders	
Respiratory alkalosis	Plasma and urinary amino acids
No hypoglycaemia	Urinary organic acids
	Tissue (liver) enzyme
	DNA studies
Organic acid disorders	
Metabolic acidosis	Urinary organic acids
Ketonuria	Fibroblast/tissue enzymes
Pyruvate metabolism	
Lactic acidosis	Plasma and urinary amino acids
	Tissue (liver/muscle) enzymes
	DNA studies
Carbohydrate metabolism	
Lactic acidosis	Plasma and urinary fructose
Hyperbilirubinaemia	Tissue (liver) enzyme

If the child is likely to die before definitive results are available it is necessary to perform more rigorous sampling either pre-mortem or as soon as possible after death. Details of appropriate samples and storage conditions have been published[69] and are summarized in Table 6.2.10. If no urine is available, a bladder stab should be considered and contaminated urine should be centrifuged to remove blood cells before freezing. Cardiac puncture may be necessary to obtain blood. Skin samples that are taken within 24 h post mortem are likely to be viable if not infected.

Children with Reye's syndrome should be managed in a paediatric intensive care unit. The aim is to re-establish normal homeostasis by correcting hypoglycaemia, dehydration, acidaemia and raised intracranial pressure, and to control seizures and fever. Evidence suggests that cerebral perfusion pressure should be maintained above 40 mmHg to ensure a satisfactory outcome.[72] In one study mortality was 12.5%, and 10% had sustained severe neurological sequelae. Poor outcome was associated with early onset of seizures, profound hypoglycaemia and coma.[73]

Table 6.2.10 Emergency sampling requirements for biochemical analysis in a child with Reye's syndrome

Urine	5–10 ml (plain bottle)	Store at –20°C
Plasma	5 ml (lithium heparin)	Store at –20°C
	1 ml (fluoride tube)	
Whole blood	5 ml (EDTA tube)	Store at –20°C
Skin	Must be sterile — 2 mm cube into transport medium or sterile isotonic saline	Straight to laboratory or store at +4°C Do not freeze
Tissues[a]	Needle biopsy (plastic tube)	Snap freeze (liquid nitrogen) store at –70°C
CSF	1 ml (plain bottle)	Store at –20°C

[a] Tissues: liver, heart and skeletal muscle.

HAEMORRHAGIC SHOCK ENCEPHALOPATHY SYNDROME

Haemorrhagic shock encephalopathy syndrome was first reported in 1983 by Levin and colleagues as an apparently new and devastating illness of young infants.[74] Although subsequent cases have been widely reported and the clinical presentation more clearly delineated the aetiopathogenesis remains obscure. A close similarity to the features of heatstroke has been noted.[75]

Most infants have onset between 3 and 4 months of age and there are no geographic clusters or secular trends.[76] In the typical case the infant is found comatose in the early morning after a mild prodromal illness with respiratory or gastrointestinal symptoms. A very high temperature is usual (over 40°C in 50%) and the infant is shocked, with profuse diarrhoea and abnormal respirations. Hepatomegaly and convulsions are a feature in two-thirds. The onset of bloody diarrhoea, sometimes accompanied by haematemesis or haemoptysis, heralds a severe disseminated intravascular coagulopathy. Investigations reveal a falling haemoglobin and platelet count, hypoglycaemia (75%), acidosis, hypernatremia (96%), and hepatic and renal dysfunction. Serum ammonia, CSF analysis and microbiological investigations are normal. The initial EEG shows prolonged runs of often rhythmic discharges which fluctuate in amount and amplitude with varying distribution and morphology — 'electrical storms'.[77] Cerebral oedema or areas of ischaemia have been reported on cranial imaging.[76,78] Cerebral atrophy is a late feature.

Mortality in the largest series was 46%.[76] Among those in deep coma and with refractory seizures, death usually ensues within 1–2 days. The majority of survivors are severely handicapped, although full recovery has been reported.[76] Treatment is supportive.

REFERENCES

1 Johnson R T. Viral infections of the nervous system. New York: Raven Press, 1982.
2 Boos J, Esiri M M. Viral encephalitis. Oxford: Blackwell 1986.
3 Rorabaugh M L, Berlin L, Heldrich F et al. Aseptic meningitis in infants younger than 2 years of age: acute illness and neurologic complications. Pediatria 1993; 92: 206–211.
4 Kennedy C R, Duffy S W, Smith R, Robinson R O. Clinical predictors of outcome in encephalitis. Arch Dis Child 1987; 62: 1156–1162.
5 Wilden S, Chonmaitree T. The importance of the virology laboratory in the diagnosis and management of viral meningitis. Am J Dis Child 1987; 141: 454–457.
6 Chonmaitree T, Menegus M A, Powell K R. The clinical relevance of 'CSF viral culture': a two year experience with aseptic meningitis in Rochester, NY. JAMA 1982; 247: 1843–1847.
7 Hurrell G D, Sturdy P M, Frood J D L, Gardner P S. Viruses in families. Lancet 1971; i: 769–774.
8 Berlin L, Rorabaugh M L, Heldrich F, Roberts K, Doran T, Modin J F. Aseptic meningitis in infants under 2 years of age: diagnosis and etiology. J Infect Dis 1993; 168: 888–892.
9 Mintz L, Drew W L. Relation of culture site to the recovery of non-polio enteroviruses. Am J Clin Pathol 1980; 74: 324–326.
10 Kennedy C R, Chrzanowska K, Robinson R O, Tyrrell D A J, Valman H B, Webster A D B. A major role for viruses in acute childhood encephalopathy. Lancet 1986; i: 989–991.
11 Stephenson J B P, King M D. Handbook of neurological investigations in children. London: Butterworth-Heinemann, 1989.
12 Skoldenberg B, Forsgren M, Alestig K et al. Acyclovir versus vidarabine in herpes simplex encephalitis: randomised multicentre study in consecutive Swedish patients. Lancet 1984; 1: 707–711.
13 Johnson R T, Griffin D E, Hirsch B L et al. Measles encephalomyelitis: clinical and immunological studies. N Engl J Med 1984; 310: 137–141.

14 Rotbart H A. Diagnosis of enterviral meningitis with the polymerase chain reaction. J Pediatr 1990; 117: 85–89.

15 Cohen B A, Rowley A H, Long C M. Herpes simplex type-2 in a patient with Mollaret's meningitis: demonstration by polymerase chain reaction. Ann Neurol 1994; 35: 112–116.

16 Shoji H, Honda Y, Murai I, Sato Y, Oizumi K, Hondo R. Detection of varicella zoster virus DNA by polymerase chain reaction in cerebrospinal fluid of patients with herpes-zoster meningitis. J Neurol 1992; 239: 69–70.

17 Imai S, Usai N, Suguira M et al. Epstein–Barr virus genomic sequences and specific antibodies in cerebrospinal fluid in children with neurologic complications of acute and reactivated EBV infections. J Med Virol 1993; 40: 278–282.

18 Feigin R D, Shackelford P G. Value of repeat lumbar puncture in the differential diagnosis of meningitis. N Engl J Med 1973; 289: 571–574.

19 Spanos A, Harrell F E, Durack D T. Differential diagnosis of acute meningitis. JAMA 1989; 262: 2700–2707.

20 Powers W J. Cerebrospinal fluid lymphocytosis in acute bacterial meningitis. Am J Med 1985; 79: 216–220.

21 Newton R W. Tuberculous meningitis. Arch Dis Child 1994; 70: 364–366.

22 Steere A C. Lyme disease. N Engl J Med 1989; 321: 586–596.

23 Wang D, Bortolussi R. Acute viral infection of the CNS in children: an eight year review. Can Med Assoc J 1981; 125: 585–589.

24 Schroth G Gawehn J, Thron A et al. Early diagnosis of herpes simplex encephalitis by MRI. Neurology 1987; 37: 179–183.

25 Goitein K, Tamir I. Cerebral perfusion pressure in central nervous system infections of infancy and childhood. J Pediatr 1983; 103: 40–43.

26 Mayer T, Walker M L. Emergency intracranial pressure monitoring in paediatrics. Clin Pediatr 1982; 21: 391–396.

27 Shaywitz B A, Rothstein P, Venes J. Monitoring and management of increased intracranial pressure in Reye's syndrome: results in 29 children. Pediatrics 1980; 66: 198.

28 Hristeva L, Booy R, Bowler I, Wilkinson A R. Prospective surveillance of neonatal meningitis. Arch Dis Child 1993; 69: 14–18.

29 McIntyre J P, Keen G A. Laboratory surveillance of viral meningitis by examination of cerebrospinal fluid in Cape Town, 1981–89. Epidemiol Infect 1993; 111: 357–371.

30 Shattuck K E, Chonmaitree T. The changing spectrum of neonatal meningitis over a fifteen year period. Clin Pediatr 1992; 31: 130–136.

31 Toltzis P. Viral encephalitis. Adv Pediatr Infect Dis 1991; 6: 111–136.

32 Dagan R, Jenista J A, Menegus M A. Association of clinical presentation, laboratory findings and virus serotypes with the presence of meningitis in hospitalized infants with enterovirus infection. J Pediatr 1988; 113: 975–978.

33 Wilfert C M, Thompson R J, Sunder T R, O'Quinn A, Zeller J, Blacharsh J. Longitudinal assessment of children with enteroviral meningits during the first three months of life. Pediatrics 1981; 67: 811–815.

34 Sells C J, Carpenter R L, Ray G C. Sequelae of central nervous system enterovirus infections. N Engl J Med 1975; 293: 1–4.

35 Erlendsson K, Swartz T, Dwyer J M. Successful reversal of echovirus encephalitis in X-linked hypogammoglobulinemia by intraventricular administration of immunoglobulin. N Engl J Med 1985; 312: 351–353.

36 Hammer S M, Connolly K J. Viral aseptic meningitis in the United States: clinical features, viral etiologies, and differential diagnosis. Curr Clin Top Infect Dis 1992; 12: 1–25.

37 Nkowane B M, Wassilak S C F, Orenstein W A, Bart K J, Schonberger L B, Hinman A R. Vaccine associated paralytic poliomyelitis: United States 1973 through 1984. JAMA 1987; 257: 1335–1340.

38 Gray J A, Burns S M. Mumps meningitis following measles, mumps and rubella immunisation. Lancet 1989; ii: 297.

39 Murray M W, Lewis M J. Mumps meningitis following measles mumps and rubella vaccination. Lancet 1989; ii: 677.

40 Cizman M, Mozetic M, Radescek-Rakar R et al. Aseptic meningitis after vaccination against measles and mumps. Pediatr Infect Dis J 1989; 8: 302–308.

41 Johnstone J A, Ross C A, Dunn M. Meningitis and encephalitis associated with mumps infection. Arch Dis Child 1972; 47: 647–651.

42 Levitt L P, Rich T A, Kinde S W et al. Central nervous system mumps: a review of 64 cases. Neurology 1970; 20: 829–834.

43 Russell R R, Donald J C. The neurologic complications of mumps. Br Med J 1958; 2: 27–30.

44 Koskiniemi M, Donner M, Pettay O. Clinical appearance and outcome in mumps encephalitis in children. Acta Paediatr Scand 1983; 72: 603–606.

45 Vaheri A, Julkenen I, Koskiniemi M. Chronic encephalomyelitis with specific increase in intrathecal mumps antibodies. Lancet 1982; ii: 685.

46 McCormick J B, King I J, Webb P A et al. Lassa fever: effective therapy with ribravarin. N Engl J Med 1986; 314: 20–26.

47 Corey L, Spear P G. Infections with herpes simplex viruses. N Engl J Med 1986; 314: 749–757.

48 Whitley R J. Herpes simplex virus infection of the central nervous system; encephalitis and neonatal herpes. Drugs 1991; 42: 406–427.

49 Nahmias A J, Whitley R J, Visintine A N et al. Herpes simplex virus encephalitis: laboratory evaluations and their diagnostic significance. J Infect Dis 1982; 145: 829–836.

50 Lakeman F D, Koga J, Whitley R J. Detection of antigen to herpes simplex virus in cerebrospinal fluid from patients with herpes simplex encephalitis. J Infect Dis 1987; 155: 1172–1178.

51 Hanada N, Kido S, Terashima M, Nishikawa K, Morishima T. Non-invasive method for early diagnosis of herpes simplex encephalitis. Arch Dis Child 1988; 63: 1470–1473.

52 Puchhammer-Stockl E, Popow-Kraupp T, Heinz F X, Mandl C, Kunz C. Establishment of PCR for the early diagnosis of herpes simplex encephalitis. J Med Virol 1990; 32: 77–82.

53 Whitley R J, Alford C A, Hirsch M S et al. Vidarabine versus acyclovir therapy in herpes simplex encephalitis. N Engl J Med 1986; 314: 144–149.

54 Whitley R J. Viral encephalitis. N Engl J Med 1990; 323: 242–250.

55 Pike M G, Kennedy C R K, Neville B G R, Levin M. Herpes simplex encephalitis with relapse. Arch Dis Child 1991; 66: 1242–1244.

56 Goldstern A S, Millichap J G, Miller R H. Cerebellar ataxia with pre-eruptive varicella. Am J Dis Child 1963; 106: 197–200.

57 Steele R W, Keeney R E, Bradsher R W et al. Treatment of varicella zoster meningoencephalitis with acyclovir: demonstration of virus in cerebrospinal fluid by electron microscopy. Am J Clin Pathol 1983; 80: 57–60.

58 LaBoccetta A C, Tornay A S. Measles encephalitis, report of 61 cases. Am J Dis Child 1964; 107: 247–255.

59 Boughton C R. Morbilli in Sydney. Part II. Neurological sequelae of morbilli. Med J Aust 1964; ii: 908–915.

60 White F. Measles vaccine associated encephalitis in Canada. Lancet 1983; ii: 613–614.

61 Simila S, Jouppila R, Salmi A, Pohjohnen R. Encephalomeningitis in children associated with adenovirus type 7 epidemic. Acta Paediatr Scand 1970; 59: 310–316.

62 Brewis F G, Neubauer C, Hurst E W. Another case of louping-ill in man. Lancet 1949; i: 689–691.

63 Kennedy C R. Acute viral infections excluding herpes simplex, rabies and HIV. In: Lambert H P, ed. Infections of the central nervous system. London: Edward Arnold, 1991.

64 Kumar R, Mathur A, Kumar A, Sethi G D, Sharma S. Virological investigations of acute encephalopathy in India. Arch Dis Child 1990; 65: 1227–1230.

65 Dutta J K, Dutta T K. Rabies in endemic countries. Br Med J 1994; 308: 488–489.

66 Seghal S, Bhatia R. Rabies: epidemiology, principles of control and treatment. New Delhi: National Institute of Commuinicable Diseases, 1992: p 4.

67 Pasternak J F, De Vivo D C, Prensky A L. Steroid responsive encephalomyelitis in childhood. Neurology 1980; 30: 481–486.

68 Reye R D K, Morgan G, Baral J. Encephalopathy and fatty degeneration of the viscera. Lancet 1963; ii: 749–752.

69 Green A, Hall S M. Investigation of metabolic disorders resembling Reye's syndrome. Arch Dis Child 1992; 67: 1313–1317.

70 Hall S M, Plaster P A, Glasgow J F T, Hancock P. Preadmission antipyretics in Reye's syndrome. Arch Dis Child 1988; 63: 857–866.

71 Robinson R O. Differential diagnosis of Reye's syndrome. Dev Med Child Neurol 1987; 29: 110–120.

72 Jenkins J G, Glasgow J F T, Black G W, Fannin T F, Hicks E M, Keilty S R et al. Reye's syndrome: assessment of intracranial monitoring. Br Med J 1987; 294: 337–338.

73 Glasgow J F T, Moore R. Reye's syndrome 30 years on. Br Med J 1993; 307: 950–951.

74 Levin M, Kay J D S, Gould J G et al. Haemorrhagic shock and encephalopathy: a new syndrome with a high mortality in young children. Lancet 1983; ii: 64–67.

75 Sofer S, Phillip P, Hershkowits J, Bennett H. Hemorrhagic shock and encephalopathy syndrome: its association with hyperthermia. Am J Dis Child 1986; 140: 1252–1254.

76 Bacon C J, Hall S M. Haemorrhagic shock encephalopathy syndrome in the British Isles. Arch Dis Child 1992; 67: 985–993.
77 Harden A, Boyd S G, Cole G, Levin M. EEG features and their evolution in the acute phase of haemorrhagic shock encephalopathy syndrome. Neuropediatrics 1991; 22: 194–197.
78 Vles J S H, de Vries L S, Wilms G, de Roo M, Casaer P J M. Computed cranial tomography, magnetic resonance imaging and single photon emission tomography in haemorrhagic shock encephalopathy syndrome: a report of three cases. Neuropediatrics 1992; 23: 24–27.

6.3   Brain abscess and subdural empyema

INTRODUCTION

The importance of these uncommon conditions, marked by intracranial collections of pus, is that while they are eminently treatable the consequences of delay in diagnosis can be catastrophic. Optimal management requires close cooperation between the paediatrician, radiologist, neurosurgeon, and microbiologist.

PREDISPOSING FACTORS, INCIDENCE AND EPIDEMIOLOGY

In children with normal immune systems, brain abscesses most commonly occur in those with chronic suppurative infections of the upper respiratory tract (URT) — in particular the sinuses, middle ear space and mastoid air cells — or with cyanotic congenital heart disease (CCHD). It is quite unusual for bacterial meningitis to be complicated by abscess formation, but this is an occasional finding in neonatal meningitis,[1] particularly where caused by Gram-negative enteric bacilli other than *Escherichia coli*. Children with profound defects in cell-mediated immunity such as occur in AIDS are also at risk of cerebral abscesses caused by the protozoal pathogen *Toxoplasma gondii*. Anyone is at risk of a brain abscess after penetrating brain injury, though there is small comfort to be gained from the observation that heat from high-velocity bullets tends to sterilize damaged tissues. About 13% of brain abscesses occur in the absence of any clear predisposing factor (Table 6.3.1).

In cases of subdural empyema, as in cases of brain abscess, there is an important association with chronic suppurative sinusitis, but in contrast another frequent association is with bacterial meningitis in early childhood.

Both diseases are rare. The incidence of brain abscess over all ages has been estimated at about 1/100 000,[2] and subdural empyema is substantially rarer. The

Table 6.3.1   Predisposing factors associated with brain abscess in six reported series

Reference	Wright et al[14]	Nestadt et al[15]	Fischer et al[16]	Jadavji et al[17]	Saez-Llorens et al[8]	Aebi et al[12]	Totals
Period of study	1946–65	1950–60	1945–80	1960–84	1960–88	1967–87	
Study size	30	35	94	74	101	28	362
Associated condition							
URT sepsis	14	21	24	17	31	8	115 (32%)
CCHD	4	4	47	18	14	13	100 (28%)
Trauma	–	3	5	7	11	–	26 (7%)
Meningitis	–	–	7	7	24	–	38 (10%)
Unknown	5	5	4	10	20	4	48 (13%)

In each series other possible predisposing conditions were identified in about 10% of cases. These included chronic pulmonary sepsis (bronchiectasis, cystic fibrosis), foci of chronic infection elsewhere, and extracardiac right-to-left shunts.

figures for brain abscess, however, bear closer inspection. The incidence varies considerably between populations, particularly in relation to the different predisposing conditions. It is relatively commoner where chronic URT infection is widely found, and in childhood occurs particularly in adolescents with chronic suppurative sinus or mastoid disease.[3] Where antibiotics are routinely used in childhood infections brain abscess is rarer and the great majority of cases are found in association with CCHD, though rarely before the age of 2 years. In a prospective study of 483 infants with CCHD, Piper et al[4] found an overall annual incidence of 0.45% but a year-on-year increasing age-specific incidence reaching a maximum of 1.75% at 12 years. In their first two decades, the risk of brain abscess in patients with Fallot's tetralogy — the commonest association with brain abscess — was a substantial 12.1%.

PATHOPHYSIOLOGY AND PATHOGENESIS

Pyogenic brain abscesses evolve from an initial stage of cerebritis to central liquefaction with formation of a surrounding capsule of vascular connective tissue. In the context of chronic suppurative URT infection, the initiating event is probably thrombophlebitis spreading from the extracranial focus via penetrating emissary veins to a venous sinus, leading to congestion and inflammation of underlying brain. Abscesses that occur are generally single and predictably located: frontal or occasionally temporal when related to paranasal sinusitis, temporal or sometimes cerebellar when associated with ear infections. In CCHD, the risk of brain abscess correlates with the degree of hypoxia.[5] These children are at risk of developing microscopic areas of brain infarction due to their severe hypoxaemia coupled with the increased viscosity of their polycythaemic blood, in particular when reduced flow in the microcirculation becomes critical during episodes of dehydration or cardiac dysfunction. Episodes of low-grade bacteraemia are common as right-to-left shunting of blood bypasses the filter of the pulmonary capillary bed, and seeding of such devitalized areas establishes foci of cerebritis. Abscesses, not surprisingly, are often multiple and may be anywhere, though they are most commonly found in the territory of the middle cerebral artery.

In contrast to the focal nature of the infection in brain abscess, in subdural empyema infection can spread widely over the surface of the brain in the potential space defined by the dura and arachnoid. These membranes are not firmly attached to each other so the potential space between them is extensive, bounded only in the midline by the falx cerebri and caudally by the tentorium cerebelli. Where associated with sinusitis, intracranial extension of inflammation again is thought to occur through emissary veins. In empyema complicating meningitis, the pathogenesis is of secondary infection of subdural effusion, a common association particularly of *Haemophilus* meningitis.

MICROBIOLOGY

Reports of the comparative frequency of isolation of different bacterial species from brain abscesses are hard to amalgamate as patient populations and the extent of microbiological investigation available are so variable. With careful and prolonged aerobic and anaerobic culture, organisms can nearly always be identified in aspirates of pus from brain abscesses.[6] Polymicrobial infections are not unusual. Streptococcal species are among the commonest organisms found, in particular *Streptococcus milleri*. Other anaerobic/microaerophilic streptococci,

Bacteroides spp. and *Fusobacteria* are also common in CCHD-associated brain abscesses, reflecting the origin of infecting organisms in the mouth and URT. Similar organisms are found in abscesses complicating chronic URT sepsis. *Proteus mirabilis* and other Gram-negative bacilli have been found in abscesses associated with an otitic focus, while streptococci and *Staphylococcus aureus* are commonly found in association with sinusitis. Brain abscesses occurring after head injury, not surprisingly, often contain *S. aureus* and other skin commensals. The unusual meningitis pathogen *Citrobacter diversus*[7] has a peculiar propensity to cause penetrating neonatal brain infection.[7]

Anaerobic streptococci, *Bacteroides* and *S. aureus* in pure and mixed culture are also found in subdural empyema associated with sinusitis. Meningitis-associated cases are usually caused by the meningeal pathogen.

CLINICAL PRESENTATION AND DIFFERENTIAL DIAGNOSIS

The classic presentation of brain abscess is with a triad of headache, fever and focal neurological deficit. Headache is of course difficult to establish in infants, and in a large retrospective study[8] the full set of these symptoms and signs was only reported in 28% of 101 children. Fever and vomiting are common initial complaints, associated before long with other signs of raised intracranial pressure such as alteration in behaviour or lethargy, and focal neurological signs (42% in the same series). Seizures are common (46% in the same series, 37% generalized). The tempo of the illness is often fairly slow, and symptoms may precede diagnosis by a long time: in the series cited[8] the mean was 13 days (range 3–120 days). Brain abscess should always be considered in the differential diagnosis of a febrile child with CCHD or chronic URT infection, and delays largely reflect a failure to consider the diagnosis where the presentation is with non-specific illness, aggravated by a lack of ready access to computed tomographic (CT) imaging of the brain. Cases may, however, occasionally present in a more fulminant fashion, when the outcome is worse both in terms of mortality and residual neurological damage in survivors.[9]

As the presentation is essentially that of an intracranial mass lesion, tumour is important in the differential diagnosis. Viral encephalitis (Ch. 6.2) can present with the same constellation of symptoms and signs. Meningitis generally presents more acutely, but there are important examples with an insidious onset, such as tuberculous meningitis and cryptococcal meningitis in the immuno-compromised.

Subdural empyema usually presents in a more rapid fashion. Typically, a child with sinusitis (not necessarily obvious),[10] develops signs of meningitis — fever, headache, vomiting, a stiff neck — rapidly progressing to focal neurological abnormality and often seizures. Signs of raised intracranial pressure are often prominent. Where subdural empyema occurs as a complication of meningitis, the presentation is of secondary fever and neurological deterioration, which may be dramatic.

INVESTIGATIONS

The risk of coning makes lumbar puncture absolutely contraindicated where brain abscess or subdural empyema is suspected. Where tomographic imaging of the brain — CT and now magnetic resonance (MR) scanning — is available, as is increasingly the case, less definitive investigations such as isotope scanning are

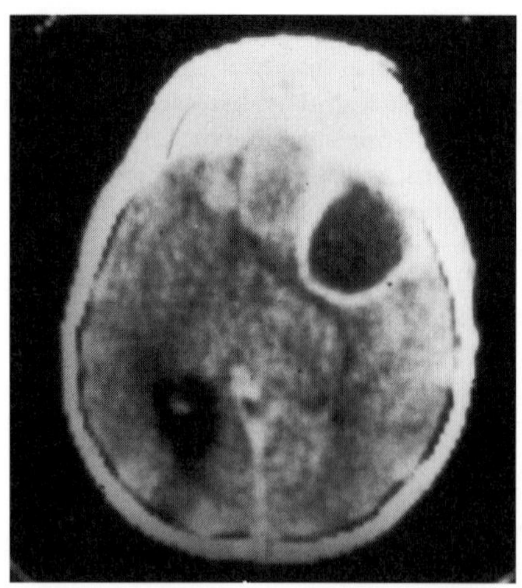

Fig. 6.3.1 Brain abscess. Contrast-enhanced CT scan image of the brain of a 4-year-old boy with cyanotic congenital heart disease. A ring-enhancing lesion is seen in the deep frontal white matter with surrounding oedema causing mid-line shift due to mass effect. On other cuts a second lesion was seen adjacent to this. Mixed aerobic and anaerobic flora were cultured from pus aspirated from the cavity.

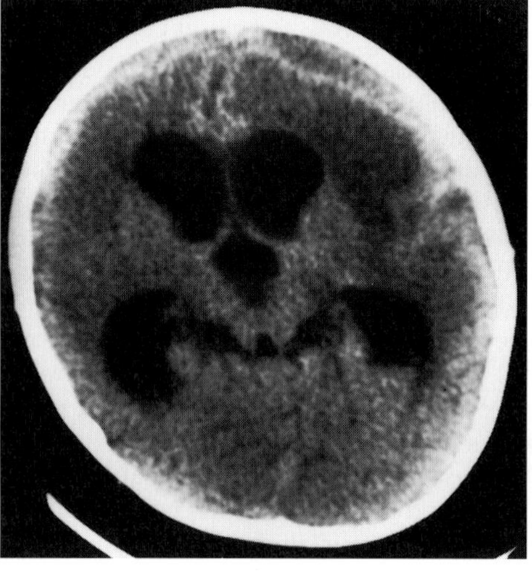

Fig. 6.3.2 Subdural empyema. Unenhanced CT scan image of the brain of an infant with *Haemophilus influenzae* meningitis. A cellular subdural effusion is shown tracking along the left frontal cerebral convexity, consistent with an empyema. The cerebral ventricles are markedly dilated and on other cuts there is layering of cellular debris in the CSF space at the posterior aspects of the occipital horns of the lateral ventricles. The deep white matter is of lower attenuation than normal due to marked cerebral oedema.

becoming outmoded as first-line investigations. Brain abscesses are characteristically seen on CT as mass lesions with surrounding oedema. Lesions 'ring-enhance' after injection of contrast medium, the highlighted vascular capsule suggesting that a mass lesion is an abscess rather than neoplasm (Fig. 6.3.1). In the clinical context in which it is sought, subdural empyema also has a characteristic appearance (Fig. 6.3.2).

TREATMENT

For adequate treatment of brain abscess, neurosurgical intervention is virtually always needed in addition to prolonged antibiotic therapy. It is unlikely that antibiotics alone can ever be sufficient once cavitation occurs, though there have been convincing successes where diagnosis has been early, in the cerebritis stage.[11] There is continuing controversy over the relative merits of stereotactic/CT-guided repeated aspiration of abscess cavities and their complete excision, though the former approach is the most widely used and the latter is considered by many to carry unacceptable postoperative morbidity of brain scarring and epilepsy.[12] Antibiotic choice is directed initially by the likely microorganisms involved, later modified by the results of culture. The traditional approach has been to give a long course (3–6 weeks) of parenteral penicillin, chloramphenicol and metronidazole, a combination which provides wide anaerobic and antistreptococcal cover with good brain penetration. An antibiotic with activity against staphylococci, e.g. flucloxacillin, is substituted for penicillin in cases associated with sinusitis or head trauma. The third generation cephalosporin ceftazidime, with broad Gram-negative and antipseudomonal cover, appears to penetrate intracranial pus well,[13] and has been substituted for penicillin/chloramphenicol in cases associated with meningitis or otitis, though there is little experience to guide the use of such drugs in this context. The place of intracavitary antibiotic therapy is not defined, and carries the risk of seizures resulting from the direct action of antibiotic on surrounding brain. In the acute phase of the illness, when cerebral oedema surrounding the abscess may cause life-threatening raised intracranial pressure, a brief course of steroids and the use of mannitol may be life-saving. The mainstay of management for subdural empyema has long been prompt neurosurgical intervention combined with appropriate antibiotics, selected on the same basis as described above, in high dosage.

OUTCOME AND COMPLICATIONS

Where prompt CT scanning has allowed more rapid diagnosis, the mortality from brain abscess is around 10%, with about 50% of survivors having significant long-term neurological deficits. Rupture of an abscess into the ventricular system is a particularly feared complication, with high mortality. The rarer, more aggressive, subdural empyema has a mortality rate of around 30% and substantial morbidity in terms of hydrocephalus, focal brain damage and epilepsy. Extensive cerebral thrombophlebitis and cerebral infarction are the dreaded complications in what remains a disease with a very gloomy prognosis.

REFERENCES

1 Sutton D L, Ouvrier R A. Cerebral abscess in the under 6 month age group. Arch Dis Child 1983; 58: 901–905.
2 Nicolosi A, Hauser W A, Beghi E, Kurland L T. Epidemiology of central nervous system infections in Olmstead County, Minnesota, 1950–1981. J Infect Dis 1986; 154: 399–408.
3 Rosenfeld E A, Rowley A H. Infectious intracranial complications of sinusitis, other than meningitis, in children: 12-year review. Clin Infect Dis 1994; 18: 750–754.
4 Piper C, Horstkotte D, Arendt G, Strauer B E. Brain abscess in children with cyanotic heart defects. Z Kardiol 1994; 83: 188–193.
5 Takeshita M, Kagawa M, Yonetani H, Izawa M, Yato S, Nakanishi T, Monma K. Risk factors for brain abscess in patients with congenital cyanotic heart disease. Neurol Med Chir Tokyo 1992; 32: 667–670.
6 de Louvois J, Gortvai P, Hurley R. Bacteriology of abscesses of the central nervous system: a multicentre prospective study. Br Med J 1977; 2: 981–984.
7 Renier D, Flandin C, Hirsch E, Hirsch J F. Brain abscesses in neonates. J Neurosurg 1988; 69: 877–882.
8 Saez-Llorens X J, Umana M A, Odio C M, McCracken G H Jr, Nelson J D. Brain abscess in infants and children. Pediatr Infect Dis J 1989; 8: 449–458.
9 Seydoux C, Francioli P. Bacterial brain abscesses: factors influencing mortality and sequelae. Clin Infect Dis 1992; 15: 394–401.
10 Skelton R, Maixner W, Isaacs D. Sinusitis-induced subdural empyema. Arch Dis Child 1992; 67: 1478–1480.

11 Berg B, Franklin G, Cuneo R, Boldrey E, Strimling B. Nonsurgical cure of brain abscess: early diagnosis and follow-up with computerized tomography. Ann Neurol 1978; 3: 474–478.

12 Aebi C, Kaufmann F, Schaad U B. Brain abscess in childhood: long-term experiences. Eur J Pediatr 1991; 150: 282–286.

13 Green H T, O'Donoghue M A T, Shaw M D M, Dowling C. Penetration of ceftazidime into intracranial abscess. J Antimicrob Chemother 1989; 24: 431–436.

14 Wright R L, Ballantine H T. Management of brain abscesses in children and adolescents. Am J Dis Child 1967; 114: 113–122.

15 Nestadt A, Lowry R B, Turner E. Diagnosis of brain abscess in infants and children. Lancet 1960; ii: 449–453.

16 Fischer E G, McLennan J E, Suzuki Y. Cerebral abscess in children. Am J Dis Child 1981; 135: 746–749.

17 Jadavji T, Humphreys R P, Prober C G. Brain abscesses in infants and children. Pediatr Infect Dis J 1985; 4: 394–398.

6.4 Shunt infections

INTRODUCTION

The treatment of many central nervous system (CNS) diseases involves gaining access to the cerebrospinal fluid (CSF) spaces. Indications for such access can be classified as diversion, drainage or monitoring. All of these involve prosthetic implants. These may be temporary or permanent. The usual reason is for continuous CSF diversion, or 'shunting' for the treatment of hydrocephalus. The risk of infection continues to be a major cause of morbidity and mortality for patients with CSF shunts.

EPIDEMIOLOGY

As patients who require CSF shunting usually require their shunt for life, and those with benign diseases will probably require several shunt revisions for non-infectious reasons, a distinction must be made between 'case infection rate' and 'operative infection rate'. The former refers to the infection rate per patient, and the latter refers to the infection rate per procedure. Even if the operative infection rate remained constant, the case infection rate increases as the patients grow older and require more revisions. In recent years the case infection rate has ranged from 10% to 40% and the operative infection rate ranges from 5% to 14%.[1-4] Two studies have reported a greater operative infection rate for shunt revisions.[2,3] Recently, there has been a decline in the operative infection rate. Factors which are implicated in this include: changes in materials used in shunt manufacture; changes in packaging and sterilization procedures; fewer pre-shunting invasive procedures (lumbar puncture, pneumoencephalography, ventricular tap); improvements in operating room facilities; surgical experience; preoperative patient preparation; and reduced duration of surgery.[5] There is an increased risk of infection in patients undergoing revision following treatment for shunt infection, with an operative incidence of 10–20%. In these, the same organism is cultured in 50% of cases.[1,6]

Shunt infections occur in a bimodal distribution from the time of shunt surgery; 70–80% present by 6 months postoperatively, with a second peak after 12 months.[4]

The most important of the host factors that determine the incidence of shunt infections is age: children <6 months old at surgery, and particularly neonates, are at increased risk.[3]

AETIOLOGY

Table 6.4.1 shows the most common organisms isolated from infected shunts.

Table 6.4.1 Causes of shunt infection

Organism	Infection rate (%)
Gram-positive	
Coagulase-negative staphylococci	45–70
Staphylococcus aureus	10–30
Streptococci	8–10
Diphtheroids	1–15
Gram-negative	
Escherichia coli	8–10
Klebsiella species	3–8
Pseudomonas/Proteus	2–8
Anaerobes	6
Mixed cultures	10–15

Adapted from reference 5.

Most infections are due to skin or bowel flora. There is no difference in the distribution of organisms associated with acute or delayed infections. There is also no obvious contribution from the position of the distal end of the shunt. The only identifiable association is when the distal end of a ventriculoperitoneal shunt has perforated a hollow viscus, resulting in infection by mixed Gram-negative species. Infection by organisms usually associated with bacterial meningitis (*Haemophilus influenzae, Neisseria meningitidis, Streptococcus pneumoniae*) only cause about 5% of shunt infections, although there is a suggestion that patients with shunts are more susceptible to these organisms.[6]

The initial step in shunt infection must be attachment of bacteria. Once bacteria have adhered to a catheter, they are not easily removed.

PATHOGENESIS

Four mechanisms have been postulated by which shunts become infected (Table 6.4.2).

Probably the most frequent cause of shunt infection is colonization at the time of surgery. This is suggested by the fact that most shunt infections occur within several weeks of surgery, and usually with skin organisms.[4]

Breakdown of surgical wounds or of skin overlying the shunt allows direct access of microbes to the shunt. Extension of tissue infections adjacent to the shunt are also included in this category.

Haematogenous seeding of shunts is probably uncommon. Shunts with their distal end in the venous system, e.g. ventriculo-atrial shunts, are at continuous risk of infection from bacteraemia. Transient or asymptomatic bacteraemia has not been definitely associated with shunt infection. It seems that sustained bacteremia, recent shunt surgery with the presence of devitalized tissue and haematoma is necessary.[7] Even then, shunt infection in these circumstances is rare.

There are several reports of *Haemophilus influenzae* shunt infections which

Table 6.4.2 Mechanisms of shunt infection

Colonization at the time of surgery
Wound or skin breakdown
Haematogenous seeding
Retrograde infection from the distal end of the shunt

occur late relative to surgery, have an extra-CNS source of infection, and usually positive blood cultures. These probably do not represent true shunt infection, but direct haematogenous CNS infection, with secondary shunt infection.[4,8]

Retrograde infection is usually associated with infections of externalized devices where organisms invade from the exit site.

CLINICAL FEATURES

Clinical presentation varies depending on the causative organism and the type of shunt. Symptoms are usually caused by shunt malfunction secondary to infection, and include headache, nausea, lethargy and deteriorating mental status. Fever and pain are not uniformly present. Signs are related to the site where the infection originated. Proximal infection may cause shunt malfunction or obstruction. As the shunt lies within the CSF space, infection results in meningitis or ventriculitis. With ventricular shunts, meningitis is rare as there is usually no communication between the ventricles and meninges. Distal infections usually have symptoms specific to the location of the end. Infected vascular shunts have associated bacteraemia. A complication of these is shunt nephritis which develops in about 4% of infected vascular shunts.[4] It is an immune complex-mediated disease, similar to that seen in bacterial endocarditis. Infected shunts that terminate in the pleural or peritoneal space will usually present with failure of CSF absorption. In the peritoneum, encystment of the catheter and loculation of pockets of CSF (CSF-oma) can occur. These may become large and palpable, particularly in infants. If more severe, peritonitis will be present.[9] Some shunt infections are insidious, causing few symptoms. There may only be low-grade, intermittent malaise or fever. This is commonly seen when patients have received repeated courses of antibiotics for intercurrent infections.

DIAGNOSIS

The main principle in diagnosing shunt infection is to have a high index of suspicion. Infection should be considered in any patient with a shunt who develops fever, although only rarely will the fever be secondary to shunt infection.

The diagnostic procedure of choice is direct culture of CSF from within or around the shunt. All other investigations, apart from blood cultures in the presence of a vascular shunt, are indirect pointers to shunt infection.[10]

Most implanted devices have an access reservoir which can be sampled. The only risk from sampling is introduction of infection. Any positive culture should be carefully evaluated. If the CSF is infected, a pleocytosis and variable biochemical changes may be found. In the majority of shunt infections culture of the tapped fluid is positive, even sometimes without a positive Gram stain, with a normal cell count and normal chemistry.[4,11] The culture may take several weeks to become positive, particularly in infections due to fastidious organisms, and the result may be confounded by prior antibiotic treatment.

In distal shunt infection without shunt dysfunction, the CSF may be completely normal. There may only be localized signs in the peritoneum, ranging from mild discomfort to peritonitis.

In all cases, correlation of the clinical features, laboratory findings and culture must be made. Because of the often insidious presentation of shunt infection, any positive culture should be taken seriously.

TREATMENT

There are no published well-conducted trials of any method of treating shunt infection. However, removal of the infected shunt is absolutely necessary for successful treatment.[3,4] Antibiotic therapy usually begins without positive bacteriological diagnosis. Coverage is selected for the most likely organisms. Most infections are due to staphylococci, therefore appropriate antistaphylococcal therapy is necessary. Gram-negative aerobes are also common, and may be suggested by a more severe clinical course. Culture results and sensitivity will subsequently allow treatment to be modified.

Vancomycin has been shown to be effective in staphylococcal shunt infections. Its efficacy is increased by adding rifampicin, which penetrates CSF well. Rifampicin is not used alone, as resistance rapidly develops.

For Gram-negative coverage, a third-generation cephalosporin such as ceftriaxone or ceftazidime penetrates inflamed meninges reasonably well. Aminoglycosides do not penetrate even inflamed meninges well, and their use should be restricted to Pseudomonas infection, where they are used in combination with an antipseudomonal penicillin or ceftazidime.[12]

Direct instillation of antibiotics into the CSF is achieved through a ventriculostomy or via a reservoir. The most commonly used intraventricular antibiotics are vancomycin and gentamicin, but detailed studies of efficacy and pharmacokinetics are not available, so dosage and frequency are empirical.

Treatment of an infected shunt should include parenteral antibiotic therapy, complete removal of the infected shunt at the beginning of treatment and placement of an external ventriculostomy, which can also be used for antibiotic instillation. This gives a cure rate of >90%. Duration of therapy is guided by the infecting organism, response to therapy and the duration of positive cultures. Usually 7–10 days of therapy following the last positive culture and removal of the infected device is sufficient. Shunt revision is usually carried out following 72 h of observation off antibiotics.[5]

PREVENTION/PROPHYLAXIS

There are no well-conducted studies showing a reduction in operative infection rate with any method of prophylaxis. However, most authorities would recommend fastidious skin preparation, minimal operative manipulation and the use of disinfectants such as Bacitracin; many neurosurgeons continue to use perioperative antistaphylococcal antibiotics despite lack of data that they reduce the operative infection rate.

CONCLUSION

Shunt infections remain a significant neurosurgical complication. Morbidity and mortality may be reduced by early detection and aggressive therapy. They are difficult to diagnose and treat, so prevention will offer the biggest advance in the reduction of morbidity.

REFERENCES

1 Ersahin Y, McLone D G, Storrs B B, Yogev R. Review of 3017 procedures for the management of hydrocephalus in children. Concepts Pediatr Neurosurg 1989; 9: 21–28.
2 George R, Leibrock L, Epstein M. Long-term analysis of cerebrospinal fluid shunt infections: a 25 year experience. J Neurosurg 1979; 51: 804–811.
3 Odio C, McCracken G H, Nelson J D. CSF shunt infections in pediatrics. Am J Dis Child 1984; 138: 1103–1108.
4 Schoenbaum S C, Gardner P, Shillito J. Infections of cerebrospinal fluid shunts: epidemiology, clinical manifestations, and therapy. J Infect Dis 1975; 131: 543–552.
5 Kaufman B A, McLone D G. Infections of cerebrospinal fluid shunts. In: Scheld W M, Whitley R J, Durack D T, eds. Infections of the central nervous system. New York: Raven Press, 1991: pp 561–585.
6 Meirovitch J, Kitae-Cohen Y, Keren G, Fiendler G, Rubenstein G. Cerebrospinal fluid shunt infections in children. Pediatr Infect Dis J 1987; 6: 921–924.
7 Shurtleff D B, Christie D, Foltz E L. Ventriculoauriculostomy-associated infection: a 12 year study. J Neurosurg 1971; 35: 686–694.
8 Lerman S J. *Haemophilus influenzae*: infections of cerebrospinal fluid shunts. J Neurosurg 1981; 54: 261–263.
9 James H E. Infections associated with cerebrospinal fluid prosthetic devices. In: Sugarman B, Young E J, eds. Infections associated with prosthetic devices. Chicago: CRC Press, 1984: pp 23–42.
10 Noetzel M J, Baker R P. Shunt fluid examination: risks and benefits in the evaluation of shunt malfunction and infection. J Neurosurg 1984; 61: 328–332.
11 Myers M G, Schoenbaum S C. Shunt fluid aspiration. Am J Dis Child 1975; 129: 220–222.
12 Everett E D, Strausbaugh L J. Antimicrobial agents and the central nervous system. Neurosurgery 1980; 6: 691–714.

I. Andrews   R. Ouvrier   P. Grattan-Smith

6.5 The child with paralysis or weakness

INTRODUCTION

The general approach to the diagnosis of weakness in childhood, based upon history, examination and investigations, is applicable to weakness and paralysis in children with ongoing or recent infection. The initial step is to identify the weakness and the accompanying features of the various neuromuscular diseases, and then the anatomical site of dysfunction producing the weakness. In the clinical context of a child with ongoing or recent infection, the aetiological diagnosis of that infection may facilitate diagnosis and institution of therapy for the neuromuscular dysfunction.

A careful history may elicit symptoms suggestive of specific patterns of weakness; for example, prominent and early bladder and bowel dysfunction suggest a spinal cord lesion such as epidural abscess; or new onset of nasal voice and nasal regurgitation, followed by distal weakness and sensory symptoms, suggest diphtheritic neuropathy. The tempo of the neuromuscular dysfunction, site of initial symptoms and subsequent progression, involvement of ocular, bulbar or respiratory musculature, and sphincter disturbance are important data in the diagnosis of the cause of weakness and in assessment of disease severity. Characterization of the temporal relationship of the onset of weakness to infection may help separate infectious and 'postinfectious' causes of weakness.

The neurological examination aims to localize the site of neuromuscular dysfunction. Weakness and paralysis may result from dysfunction at any level of the central nervous and neuromuscular systems. Clinical examination can usually localize the site of the lesion causing the weakness to the cerebral hemispheres, posterior fossa, spinal cord, anterior horn cell, peripheral nerve, neuromuscular junction or muscle (see Table 6.5.1). Correlation between the site of the lesion and the underlying or recent infection often reduces the list of diagnostic possibilities. For example, Guillain–Barré syndrome and transverse myelitis are common 'postinfectious' causes of weakness in childhood. Separation of these diagnoses is possible by physical examination (see Table 6.5.1) and localization of dysfunction to distinct parts of the neuromuscular system, the first to peripheral nerves and the second to the spinal cord.

Appropriate laboratory investigations, such as nerve conduction velocity studies, electromyography, muscle enzyme levels, cerebrospinal fluid (CSF) analysis, muscle biopsy, 'tensilon' test and specific investigations related to the precipitating infection, guided by the clinical features and diagnostic suspicions, may further localize the site of the dysfunction and occasionally suggest the underlying pathogenesis.

Similarly, this general approach to childhood weakness will provide an estimation of the severity of weakness, guidelines for supportive therapy and, in the

Table 6.5.1   Clinical examination features which aid in localization of CNS or neuromuscular dysfunction

Anatomical site of CNS or neuromuscular dysfunction	Typical clinical features
Cerebral hemisphere	Intellectual decline Seizures Visual field defect Hemiparesis, hemineglect, hyperreflexia, hypertonia, extensor plantar response Dystonia, chorea Diminished alertness Endocrine dysfunction Vomiting, headache
Posterior fossa	Diminished alertness Cranial nerve palsies Hemiparesis, hyperreflexia, hypertonia, extensor plantar response Ataxia, nystagmus, incoordination Vomiting, headache
Spine	Weakness below the lesion Bladder and bowel dysfunction Hyperreflexia, hypertonia, extensor plantar response Babinski reflex Loss of cutaneous abdominal reflexes Sensory loss below the lesion
Anterior horn cell	Proximal and distal weakness Hypotonia Hypo- or areflexia Fasciculations Wasting Preserved sensation
Peripheral nerve	Distal weakness[a] or weakness restricted to specific nerves Peripheral hypotonia or hypotonia restricted to specific nerves Hypo- or areflexia Wasting Glove and stocking sensory loss or sensory loss restricted to specific nerves
Neuromuscular junction	Proximal weakness Weakness of extraocular muscles Fatiguability Normal or reduced tone Normal or reduced reflexes Wasting (rarely) Preserved sensation
Muscle	Proximal weakness[b] Normal or reduced reflexes Normal or reduced tone Wasting Preserved sensation

[a] Although peripheral nerve disease typically produces distal weakness, some patients with Guillain–Barré syndome may develop proximal muscle weakness early in the disease course.

[b] Although muscle disease typically produces proximal weakness, some myopathies, such as myotonic dystrophy, have distal weakness as prominent features, and some such as congenital centronuclear myopathy or facioscapulohumeral muscular dystrophy have prominent facial weakness.

context of the infectious disease, characterization of disease pathogenesis may facilitate specific therapeutic measures.

Pre-existing neuromuscular disease

Acute infection and associated systemic dysfunction may exaggerate pre-existing neuromuscular disease. Examples include exacerbation of weakness and deterioration of function in chronic inflammatory demyelinating peripheral neuropathy, congenital and autoimmune myasthenia gravis, Duchenne dystrophy, other myopathies and the periodic paralyses, during or following infection. Even pre-existing central nervous system (CNS) dysfunction may be exacerbated by hypoxia or hyperglycaemia, which may accompany infection.

Specific infections associated with specific forms of neuromuscular disease

Polio, diphtheria, botulism and tick paralysis exhibit characteristic syndromes of weakness and paralysis (see below). Human immunodeficiency virus (HIV) infection has been associated with weakness due to neuromuscular dysfunction at multiple levels, including myositis, neuromuscular junction dysfunction, peripheral neuropathy, radiculitis and an amyotrophic lateral sclerosis-like illness. Lyme disease (due to *Borrelia burgdorferi* infection) may also produce weakness secondary to myositis, neuropathy (especially facial nerve palsy), radiculitis or myelopathy. Multiple infectious agents, including coxsackievirus, arboviruses, influenza virus, echovirus (in agammaglobulinaemic patients), Epstein–Barr virus, *Mycoplasma*, cat scratch disease and several parasitic infections may cause myositis, but generally weakness is not the major feature with these infections.

In addition, drugs used in the treatment of specific infections may also produce weakness. For example, zivodudine and DDT, used in the treatment of HIV infection, may produce weakness due to myopathy and neuropathy respectively, chloroquine used in the treatment of malaria may produce a painless myopathy, or aminoglycoside antibiotics may induce a myasthenic-like syndrome or exacerbate myasthenia gravis.

GUILLAIN–BARRÉ SYNDROME

Introduction

The Guillain–Barré syndrome (acute inflammatory demyelinating polyradiculoneuropathy, AIDP) is an acute inflammatory disorder of peripheral nerves and nerve roots characterized pathologically by lymphocyte and macrophage infiltration and by myelin destruction. It is thought to be an autoimmune disorder. Excellent reviews of the disorder have been published.[1,2] In addition numerous paediatric series have been reported which are reviewed by Ouvrier et al.[3]

The annual incidence of Guillain–Barré syndrome is about 1 : 100 000 of the population. The disease occurs at all ages and has been reported in the neonatal period and at 4 months of age. Very young cases should be suspected of having infantile botulism. There is no apparent sex predilection in the first two decades and no definite seasonal peak in the usual form of the disorder. In a more recently described variant of this disorder, which affects motor nerves predominantly, there is a peak in the summer months.[4]

Approximately half to two-thirds of patients are reported to have a prodromal illness within a 4-week period prior to the onset of AIDP. Most commonly, the illness affects the upper respiratory tract; a predominantly gastroenteritic infection is next most common. Recent attention has focused on *Campylobacter* infections. Certain specific infections have been implicated as definite (*Mycoplasma*, cytomegalovirus, Epstein–Barr virus, vaccinia, variola), probable (varicella zoster, measles, mumps, hepatitis A or B) or possible aetiological antecedents (rubella, influenza A and B, coxsackievirus and echovirus).[1] More recently, the HIV virus has been implicated. Only rarely is an organism cultured from the CSF.

Non-specific triggers, such as surgery or malignant disease, are exceptionally rare in children.

Clinical features

Weakness, particularly of the lower limbs, is the initial complaint in almost all patients. In the youngest patients, weakness may be interpreted as ataxia. The weakness is generalized in about 50% of patients, predominantly distal in about 30% and mainly proximal in about 20%.[3,5] This high rate of proximal involvement in childhood occasionally leads to misdiagnosis. The weakness, which is usually symmetrical, may ascend and progress in severity over several days to weeks. Fifty per cent of children have reached the nadir of their weakness by 1 week, 80% by 2 weeks and over 90% by 3 weeks. By arbitrary definition, all children with uncomplicated AIDP will have reached their maximum level of weakness by 4 weeks from onset. Cases in whom weakness progresses or relapses after 4 weeks are considered to have chronic progressive or relapsing inflammatory demyelinating polyradiculoneuropathy (CIDP). There is facial weakness, often asymmetrical, in 20–50% of children and some evidence of bulbar involvement in about one-quarter of patients. The oculomotor nerves (III, IV and VI) are involved in about 8–10% of children and total ophthalmoplegia may follow. The Miller–Fisher syndrome, in which weakness confined to the facial and extraocular muscles is associated with ataxia and hyporeflexia, has a frequency of 1% in children with AIDP.[6] Particular strains of *Campylobacter* have now been associated with the Miller–Fisher syndrome. Although ophthalmoplegia may be associated with a relatively benign course, some cases progress to severe paralysis with respiratory failure.[7]

The most serious complication of the weakness, that of respiratory involvement, is detectable in about half the patients. Mechanical ventilation is required in approximately 7–15% of cases. In the older child, monitoring of respiratory function is possible by regular estimation of vital capacity. In the very young child, this approach is not practical and careful clinical evaluation as well as monitoring of pulse, and of blood gases by transcutaneous measurement, may be essential to avoid unexpected collapse due to respiratory failure.

After reaching its maximum, weakness persists for several days but improvement is generally evident within 2 weeks of reaching plateau levels. Recovery, virtually complete in two-thirds of patients, then proceeds over a period of months.

In most cases, all deep tendon reflexes are eventually abolished, often early in the illness. Occasionally, the proximal reflexes may be retained and rarely, in otherwise typical cases, the reflexes may be preserved throughout the illness.[5] Extensor plantar responses are occasionally observed.

Pain and paraesthesiae were present in 63% of the Sydney cases at presentation. Objective sensory findings are infrequent at presentation but have been noted to develop in up to 65% of cases in some series. Position, vibration, pain and touch sensation are impaired in descending order of frequency.

Although common in children, autonomic dysfunction is less serious than in adults. Constipation is present in approximately 40% and urinary retention or incontinence in about 10% of cases. Urinary difficulties are transitory. Vasomotor disturbances such as bouts of excessive sweating with peripheral vasoconstriction are seen in up to 50% of children. Treatment of impending respiratory failure should be the first consideration when such vasomotor episodes occur. Hypertension, usually mild, is present in 10–30% of children and hypotension is occasionally encountered. Cardiac rhythm disturbances occurred in 32% of the cases in one study[5] but are uncommon in the authors' experience.

Papilloedema has been described in about 5% of cases in some series but observed only once by the authors. The papilloedema resolved after several weeks' treatment with acetazolamide. The syndrome of inappropriate antidiuretic hormone is seen in about 3% of cases.

Ancillary investigations

A rise in the level of CSF protein in the absence of a pleocytosis of more than 10 cells/mm³ is considered a hallmark of the disease. The CSF protein level may, however, be normal in 10–20% of children with otherwise typical Guillain–Barré syndrome. Lumbar puncture should be delayed until the second week of the illness, as the protein level is commonly normal during the first week. In approximately 10% of cases there is a CSF pleocytosis of more than 10 cells/mm³.

Clinical neurophysiology

The earliest abnormality in clinical neurophysiological studies is a drop in the amplitude of the evoked muscle action potential and conduction block. Most patients develop conduction block in one or more nerves during the first 2 weeks of the illness, usually after the first week. Marked slowing of nerve conduction (less than 40 m/s in the median and ulnar nerves; less than 30 m/s in the peroneal nerve) is characteristic. Most children with Guillain–Barré syndrome have definite abnormalities of nerve conduction. The nerve conduction disturbances are patchy, some nerves conducting normally while others demonstrate markedly reduced conduction velocities. The abnormalities have been correlated with segmental demyelination in peripheral nerves.

In the acute motor axonal neuropathy syndrome, sensory nerve conduction studies are normal but muscle compound action potential amplitudes are much reduced. F wave latencies are absent and there is only mild slowing of motor nerve conduction.

Pathological findings

The Guillain–Barré syndrome is a multifocal, non-infective, inflammatory process causing demyelination and sometimes axonal degeneration of peripheral nerves. There is swelling and cellular infiltration, by lymphocytes and macrophages, of the proximal nerve roots in particular but the entire peripheral nervous system may be affected. Sural nerve biopsy may show evidence of demyelination and inflammatory cell infiltration in routine transverse sections[8] but biopsies close to the motor end-plate and teased fibre preparations provide the most sensitive demonstration of such changes.

Pathogenesis

The current hypothesis is that a viral infection or other trigger exposes neuritogenic antigens on myelin which are normally sequestered. An autoimmune reaction which causes demyelination is thereby triggered. An alternative hypothesis is that the antecedent viral infection causes a fall in the normal population of suppressor T cells. As a result of this fall, there is a proliferation of T and B lymphocytes which recognize and commence to attack nervous system antigens.[9]

Diagnosis

In the young child with apparent ataxia, careful examination will usually reveal weakness and areflexia, enabling the exclusion of cerebellar disease as the primary cause of the clinical picture. However, in early or uncooperative patients, this distinction is not always easy.

The rapid onset of weakness carries a wide differential diagnosis. In the child under 1 year of age, infantile botulism is an important possibility. Preceding constipation, the presence of pupillary abnormalities and the results of ancillary investigations allow ready distinction.

In the older child, acute viral myositis occasionally causes weakness and even areflexia but the creatine kinase is elevated and CSF protein and nerve conduction studies are normal. The condition is usually short lived.

Spinal cord lesions such as tumours and inflammatory processes may cause confusion. Whenever a motor or sensory level is apparent, myelography or magnetic resonance imaging (MRI) examination should be considered.

Poliomyelitis and other paralytic conditions due to enteroviruses are usually distinguishable by the presence of fever, asymmetry of weakness, CSF findings and results of laboratory investigations.

When neuropathy is diagnosed, the possibility of acute or subacute toxic neuropathies may be raised. Porphyric neuropathy is very rare in childhood.

In endemic regions, tick-bite paralysis causes a picture closely resembling AIDP. The differentiation is discussed in the section on tick paralysis.

Prognosis

The mortality in most published series is about 5%, but in a French study and in the Sydney experience it was about 1%. Most deaths in childhood are due to preventable respiratory complications. Pulmonary emboli or fatal arrhythmias, major causes of death in adults, are rare in childhood.

Although the prognosis for survival is generally good, a significant proportion of children is left with residual disabilities. Seventeen of sixty-nine (25%) patients followed up in the Paris study had residual disabilities.[5] The commonest disabilities include footdrop, pes cavus and postural tremor. Persisting weakness of the hands is occasionally seen. Only a small percentage of those with residual disability at 1 year after the illness recover completely.

Treatment

Supportive, symptomatic treatment is the mainstay of therapy. In the early stages of the illness, the child should be closely observed in hospital, preferably in an intensive care unit. The latter is particularly important in the child under the age of 4 years where objective assessment of respiratory function is difficult. In the older child, regular measurement of vital capacity is performed. Ventilatory support should be considered if vital capacity falls below 30% of predicted values and instituted if there is evidence of respiratory insufficiency.

If respiratory therapy is required for more than 1 week, tracheostomy is recommended. Dysphagia or bulbar paresis may necessitate nasogastric or gastrostomy feeding.

Chest and limb physiotherapy are important to clear secretions and maintain limb mobility. Splints may be required to prevent foot- and wristdrop. Frequent turning of the patient is essential to avoid pressure areas.

ACTH therapy was found to shorten the duration of the illness in a small controlled study but a larger randomized trial of prednisolone in adults with AIDP led to the conclusion that steroid treatment was not beneficial. Steroids are not recommended for the routine treatment of the Guillain–Barré syndrome in childhood. A short course may be beneficial in relieving severe pain,[10] for which quinine and codeine are also reported to be effective.

Plasmapheresis has been shown to be effective in decreasing the severity and improving the outcome of AIDP in patients over 12 years of age.[11,12] Several uncontrolled paediatric series have shown apparent favourable outcomes with plasmapheresis. In the study of Epstein & Sladky,[13] in which the authors analysed their experience with plasmapheresis in nine children with Guillain–Barré syndrome compared with 14 similarly affected controls, the time to recover independent ambulation was significantly shorter in the treated patients. Similar results were noted in the study of Yoshioka et al[14] and Lamont & Sladky.[15]

Because of the technical difficulty with plasmapheresis in young children, the finding of an outcome equivalent to or better than that with plasmapheresis using intravenous gamma globulin originally demonstrated by Van Der Meche et al[16] assumed particular significance in childhood. Several uncontrolled studies of intravenous gamma globulin use in childhood have now been undertaken.[17,18] The advantages of gamma globulin infusions which are usually given in a dosage of 0.4 g/kg per day for five successive days are the ease of administration and relative freedom from side-effects. Currently children under the age of 10 who are deteriorating rapidly (for example those who become non-ambulant within the first 7 days or so, or those patients who appear to be approaching this degree of severity in the first few days of illness) are treated with intravenous gamma globulin. Older patients may receive plasmapheresis in similar circumstances. Most patients, however, are still treated without specific therapy.

DIPHTHERIA

Diphtheria is an acute infectious disease caused by *Corynebacterium diphtheriae*. It is now an extremely rare disease in regions with prophylactic immunization. Typically the pharynx is infected and covered by a white or grey membranous exudate and the patient is mildly febrile, anorexic and may complain of irritability, malaise and headache. The larynx, skin wounds or umbilicus may also be sites of infection. One or two weeks into the illness, the patient may develop cardiac involvement with circulatory failure, or arrhythmias, which may be severe. Most patients have resting tachycardia.[19]

Diphtheritic paralysis is a relatively common sequel of infection, occurring in about 20% of patients. Involvement of the nervous system follows a predictable pattern. Palatal paralysis, characterized by nasal speech, dysphagia and regurgitation (often through the nose), begins in the first week or two of the illness and progresses over the next few weeks, lasting about 7 weeks in total. In some cases respiratory embarrassment and aphonia occur due to diaphragmatic and laryngeal paralysis. During the fourth or fifth week of the illness, ocular accommodation due to weakness of ciliary muscle produces blurred vision. Extraocular muscle weakness may occasionally ensue over the next few weeks. Pupillary responses to light are preserved. In some cases these cranial nerve pareses resolve spontaneously without more widespread weakness, but in others a peripheral neuropathy develops between the fifth and eighth weeks. This sensorimotor neuropathy is characterized by peripheral weakness, hyporeflexia, alterations in all sensory modalities and sometimes muscle tenderness, which may progress and ascend over a few weeks to impair respiratory function, before slow, spontaneous resolution, in a manner akin to Guillain–Barré syndrome. Rarely, cerebral lesions are associated with diphtheria infection and may be embolic or infective in origin.[19] CSF may show elevated protein and a mild pleocytosis, which parallels disease severity. Peripheral nerve conduction velocities may remain normal in the first weeks of the illness, despite obvious weakness. Subsequently conduction velocities slow to 15–35 m/s for several months despite clinical resolution.

Pathophysiology

Clinical and experimental studies indicate that weakness associated with diphtheria is due to nerve injury by diphtheria toxin, a potent inhibitor of protein synthesis. Pathological examination reveals demyelination with preservation of axon continuity, concentrated in the nodose ganglion of the vagus nerve, the dorsal root ganglia, and adjacent regions of the dorsal, ventral and mixed spinal nerve roots. Inflammatory infiltrates are lacking. Localization of the pathology in animals experimentally injected with diphtheria toxin parallels regions of relatively permeable blood–nerve barrier. The toxin is predominantly transported by the bloodstream, but the early onset and severity of pharyngeal weakness with 'faucial' diphtheria and the local weakness associated with peripheral infective foci indicate a role for local diffusion of toxin.

Diagnosis

Diagnosis early in the course depends upon culture of the organism. Later in the course, the diagnosis of diphtheritic neuropathy depends upon the distinctive progression of weakness and associated clinical features, coupled with slowed motor and sensory nerve conduction velocities.

Treatment

Diphtheria can be prevented by immunization using diphtheria toxoid. If initiated within 2 days of the primary infection, diphtheria antitoxin significantly reduces the incidence and severity of cardiac and neurological complications,[19,20] but is of no benefit once the polyneuropathy begins. A dosage regime for antitoxin is outlined by Krugman et al.[20] Patients seen early in the disease and those seen late in the disease, from whom the bacilli can still be cultured from the site of infection, should be treated with penicillin or erythromycin. Bed rest and treatment of cardiac failure and arrhythmias are important in patients with myocarditis. Patients with severe pharyngeal paralysis may suffer aspiration, so gastric or duodenal feeding may be useful. Respiratory support may occasionally be required for respiratory failure secondary to neuropathy and myocarditis. With supportive therapy, spontaneous, complete resolution of the peripheral nerve disease associated with remyelination can be expected.

Exposed intimate contacts should have throat cultures and be treated with antibiotics if cultures are positive. Unimmunized contacts and contacts with unknown immunization histories should receive antibiotics and active immunization.[19]

POLIOMYELITIS

Introduction

Poliomyelitis is an infectious disease caused by polioviruses, a subset of the enterovirus family. This disease is now rare in countries where immunization against polio is common, but remains prevalent in the Third World. The vast majority of individuals infected with potentially pathogenic strains of poliovirus exhibit no symptoms or only a mild, non-paralytic, febrile illness with diarrhoea. Less than 1% of infected individuals develop paralytic poliomyelitis, which is likely secondary to host factors influencing predisposition to poliomyelitis.

Clinical features

Paralytic poliomyelitis has a biphasic clinical course.[21] The initial illness consists of a few days of fever, malaise, headache and gastrointestinal disturbance, and is associated with viraemia. This resolves spontaneously, but after 2–5 days meningoencephalomyelitic symptoms develop with fever, vomiting, headache, neck and back pain and occasionally delirium. CSF shows polymorphonuclear cells and lymphocytes initially, with predominantly lymphocytes and elevated protein in the second week. About half of these patients go on to develop paralysis, beginning within 5 days of the meningoencephalomyelitic phase and progressing over the next 1–3 days. Paralysis may be widespread or focal. The paralysis is often asymmetrical and involves large muscle groups more commonly than small muscle groups, which aids differentiation from Guillain–Barré syndrome. Exercise may exacerbate the weakness. Cranially and spinally innervated muscles may be affected. Bulbar weakness and respiratory failure (due to diaphragmatic and intercostal weakness) can be lethal.

Examination at this stage discloses evidence of anterior horn cell dysfunction, with flaccid paralysis, prominent fasciculations, absent or reduced reflexes and early onset of muscle wasting (see Table 6.5.1). Sensation is characteristically normal. Rarely more diffuse spinal cord dysfunction may also be apparent.[21] In mild cases recovery may begin within 1 week of paralysis, but usually begins 1–3 weeks after peak paralysis. The greater part of recovery is evident within the first months, but may continue for several years. Although partial recovery is expected, residual weakness of a proportion of affected muscles is typical.

A similar clinical disease may be seen after oral vaccination with live attenuated polio virus in about one in three million vaccinations. Although this unfortunate complication may occur in normal children, it is more likely in immunocompromised patients. Rare cases of poliomyelitis occurring in previously immunized children have been reported. Infections with other enteroviruses including coxsackieviruses and echoviruses may rarely produce a similar clinical picture.

Pathogenesis

The disease is caused by infection of anterior horn cells by bloodborne virus.[21] Anterior horn cells are destroyed and surrounded by inflammatory changes of microglial infiltrates and reactive astrocytosis.

Diagnosis

Diagnosis rests upon clinical features, seroconversion, and recovery of the virus from the oropharynx and stool, which is possible from 19 days prior to paralysis, to 3 months after paralysis.

Treatment

As there is no specific treatment of poliomyelitis, emphasis is placed on worldwide prophylaxis by immunization, using oral live attenuated virus vaccines (Sabin) or inactivated virus vaccines (Salk), which include all three types of poliovirus pathogenic in humans. Immunocompromised patients and close contacts of immunocompromised patients should be immunized with parenteral, inactivated virus (Salk vaccine). In affected individuals only supportive measures are available, including ventilatory support, gastric or duodenal feeding and physical therapy.

SPINAL EPIDURAL ABSCESS

Introduction

Spinal epidural abscess is a rare disease. It is, however, an important childhood infection (presenting with weakness), because of its potentially devastating consequences, but with effective treatment if diagnosed and treated quickly. Although most cases are secondary to bloodborne sepsis or surgery, epidural abscess has also been reported as a complication of a dermal sinus.

Clinical features

Fifty-seven childhood cases of spinal epidural abscess were reviewed by Rubin et al.[22] Older children are most commonly affected, but the disorder may occur in any age group. Onset is typically with fever and back pain, followed over hours to 2 weeks by spinal cord dysfunction, including paresis, sphincter dysfunction, and sensory loss below the level of the lesion, and radicular pain at the level of the lesion. A paraspinous mass is palpable in 16%.

Investigations

The white blood cell count is typically elevated and blood culture is positive in two-thirds. Plain radiographs of the spine are normal, but myelogram, computed tomography (CT) myelogram or MRI of the spine typically reveals the lesion. These procedures and surgical exploration localize the abscess to the posterior part of the epidural space in 86%, laterally in 7%, anteriorly in 2% and circumferentially in 2%. Lumbar puncture is dangerous because it may contaminate the subarachnoid space but, if performed, a large-bore needle may facilitate drainage of pus and determination of the organism. CSF, when collected, is normal in 25% and shows mild leucocytosis, low glucose or elevated protein in the remainder. *Staphylococcus aureus* is the most common causative organism, accounting for 79% of childhood cases, but other organisms and mixed cultures have been reported.

Differential diagnosis

This diagnosis should be considered particularly in patients suspected to have transverse myelitis and spinal cord infarction, and also in patients with 'discitis' and spinal osteomyelitis.

Treatment

Treatment involves immediate surgical decompression of the spinal cord and drainage of pus, often with open packing of the wound. Antibiotic therapy should be instigated quickly and include both anti-*Staphylococcus aureus* and broad-spectrum cover. With instigation of treatment prior to neurological dysfunction or with weakness, but not paralysis, 90% recovered completely. Of those treated after paralysis, one-third recovered, but the majority remained paralysed or died.

TICK PARALYSIS

Introduction

Tick paralysis is caused by a toxin secreted by engorging female ticks of various species, mainly *Ixodes* spp. in Australia and *Dermacentor* spp. in North America.

Clinical features

Symptomatic onset usually occurs 5–7 days after attachment. The first sign is often unsteadiness or weakness of the lower limbs. An ascending paralysis with subsequent loss of deep tendon reflexes follows, although in some cases the reflexes can be preserved. In severe cases ophthalmoplegia, facial and bulbar weakness and respiratory failure can occur. Young girls are particularly susceptible perhaps due to the tick escaping detection in their long hair. In North America, where tick paralysis is commonly caused by *Dermacentor andersoni* or *D. variabilis*, the presenting features are usually also those of ascending paralysis. There is, however, a major difference in the clinical course. Removal of the tick usually results in rapid improvement. In contrast, not only does *Ixodes holocyclus* cause more systemic disturbance but also continued deterioration for 24–48 h following the removal of the tick has been repeatedly demonstrated. This should always prompt a search for further undetected ticks but must be recognized as part of the natural history of *I. holocyclus* paralysis.

In some cases, the paralysis may be confined to one region, for example facial paralysis due to an engorged tick close to the parotid gland or brachial plexus palsy due to an axillary attachment of the tick.

Neurophysiology

Tick paralysis is thought to be due to the action of several neurotoxins produced in the salivary glands of the engorging tick. A protein neurotoxin called holocyclotin has been isolated from the salivary glands of *I. holocyclus*. Acetylcholine release is reduced at the motor end-plate possibly due to reduced calcium entry into nerve terminals or interference with presynaptic excitation–secretion coupling. This produces a decrease in number of miniature end-plate potentials which are, however, of normal size. The neurophysiological consequence of this is a reduced amplitude of the compound muscle action potential (CMAP) in nerve conduction studies. Some prolongation of distal motor latencies but normal motor and sensory nerve conduction velocities are also observed.

Treatment

The most important step in the treatment of tick paralysis is the discovery and then removal of the tick. Many methods of tick removal have been advocated, but it has been found that traditional methods such as the application of a lighted match, alcohol or petroleum jelly are not effective. It is recommended that the tick be grasped close to the skin with curved forceps and removed with steady pressure. It is possible that pyrethrin-containing aerosol sprays may be effective, but we are not aware of any controlled trials of this.

In most cases of human paralysis caused by *I. holocyclus*, respiration is not compromised and once the tick is removed recovery follows, although at times slowly, without specific treatment. Nevertheless, careful observation of respiratory and bulbar function as for the Guillain–Barré syndrome is indicated. Ventilation is sometimes indicated for impending or actual respiratory failure. Hyperimmune serum prepared from dogs is the usual treatment for paralysed animals. In humans it has been used sparingly and only in severely ill patients because of the risk of acute reactions and of serum sickness.

Conclusion

Although often occurring in the spring and summer, tick paralysis can present at any time of the year. It should be considered in any child presenting with an unsteady gait, ascending paralysis, ptosis, facial weakness or unreactive pupils. The tick must be removed carefully, but even when this is done there is often deterioration in the following 24–48 h and the child must be carefully observed over this period. Once the danger has passed the child may not return to normal for several weeks. Hyperimmune serum may have a role in seriously ill children, but acute allergy or serum sickness is a likely consequence.[24]

DERMATOMYOSITIS

Dermatomyositis is a relatively rare multisystem disease characterized mainly by a non-suppurative myositis, which causes symmetrical weakness, and a unique rash. Immunological abnormalities are found in some cases and a vasculitis, which accounts for the pathological changes in skin and muscle, may also affect small nerves, the myocardium, the gastrointestinal tract and even the retina. The aetiology is unknown, but an unusual autoimmune response generated by a viral infection is often postulated.

Clinical features

Females are affected more frequently than males. Onset occurs mainly between 5 and 10 years of age but about 20% of the authors' cases had their onset before the age of 4 years. Although an acute onset with fever, muscle pain and swelling sometimes occurs, the onset is more frequently insidious, with increasing muscle weakness, fatigue, irritability and general debility. The cutaneous manifestations usually develop insidiously and may occasionally precede the muscle weakness by months or years. Occasionally they remain the sole clinical manifestation of the disease. The rash has a characteristic, indeed pathognomonic distribution, typically involving the upper eyelids, periorbital and malar regions and the extensor surfaces of the knuckles, elbows, knees and ankle malleoli. The facial rash is often described as violaceous or heliotrope. The nailfold capillaries are frequently dilated and tortuous in the active stages of the disorder. Sometimes the rash extends over the chest and trunk. Deposition of calcium in the dermis occurs later in the disease in up to two-thirds of patients. When extensive (calcinosis universalis) it may result in limitation of joint mobility and may cause ulcerations with extrusion of calcium through the skin.

Muscle weakness varies in severity but is usually progressive, mainly proximal and fairly symmetrical. It is often accompanied by pain or discomfort but tenderness and oedema are frequently absent. The child experiences difficulty in climbing stairs or onto chairs, rising from squatting or sitting and in using the arms to brush the hair or to dress. Swallowing difficulty is not uncommon. In severe cases there may be difficulty in breathing or in holding up the head. The tendon reflexes may be normal, depressed or occasionally quite brisk. Periarticular contractures tend to develop early and may produce joint deformities.

Gastrointestinal symptoms are present in about 20% of patients. Ulceration of the bowel may lead to haemorrhage and sometimes death.

Diagnosis

Muscle enzymes such as creatine kinase and aldolase are elevated in about two-thirds of patients. The erythrocyte sedimentation rate is often normal. Electromyographic findings often suggest the diagnosis because of the combination of changes indicative of denervation and primary muscle disease, namely fibrillations and positive waves at rest, and low-amplitude, brief, polyphasic action potentials on effort.

Muscle biopsy typically reveals a degree of atrophy in the periphery of the muscle fascicles (perifascicular atrophy). Intramuscular blood vessels are surrounded by mononuclear infiltrates and there is evidence of patchy degeneration and necrosis of muscle fibres. In a significant proportion of subjects, the biopsy is negative.

Prognosis

Prior to the advent of steroid therapy, the mortality of childhood dermatomyositis was approximately 30%. Half of the survivors were left chronically disabled.

With modern therapy, the mortality rate is less than 5% and the outcome of survivors is usually good, although a few are left with contractures, muscle atrophy and complications of therapy such as aseptic necrosis of the femoral head, cataracts, etc.

Treatment

General

Because of the tendency to joint and muscle contractures, an active physiotherapy programme is crucial from the early stages and should continue until the patient has entered a sustained remission. In cases presenting late with well-established contractures, prolonged hydrotherapy and gradual mobilization have been remarkably successful in reversing serious deformities.

Photosensitivity is frequent, so that patients must be instructed in the rigorous avoidance of ultraviolet light exposure.

Specific

Patients fall into three groups, as outlined by Spencer et al.[23] In the monocyclic group, constituting about one-third of patients, there is an early and sustained response to steroids, without relapse after cessation of treatment.

In the second, chronic polycyclic group, relapses occur after cessation or reduction of steroid therapy.

In the third, chronic continuous group, active disease continues despite high-dose steroid administration.

The mainstay of initial treatment is high-dose corticosteroid therapy, generally starting at approximately 2 mg/kg per day of prednisone. After 4–8 weeks of therapy, if there is strong evidence of improvement, the dose of steroids can be reduced, often to second daily administration, to minimize steroid complications. Steroids are then continued for 18–24 months.

If relapse occurs, prednisone can be recommenced or immunosuppression with azathioprine or methotrexate trialled.

In those patients exhibiting a poor response to steroids and azathioprine by 6 months, the response to cyclosporin has often been favourable. This chronic continuous group is the most challenging therapeutically. The drug therapy of calcinosis has been unrewarding but fortunately spontaneous resolution is common in childhood.

BOTULISM

Two main forms of botulism are seen in childhood. In classical botulism, the extremely potent toxin, produced by *Clostridium botulinum* in imperfectly sterilized contaminated preserves or canned foods, is ingested and produces neuromuscular blockade by binding presynaptically at cholinergic synapses, preventing acetylcholine release. Symptoms appear within hours of ingestion of the contaminated food. Vomiting, weakness, dizziness and dry mouth are followed by blurred vision, diplopia, dysphonia, dysphagia and eventually, in severe cases, by respiratory paralysis.

In infantile botulism, clostridial spores germinate and multiply in the gastro-intestinal tract of infants usually under the age of 6 months. Toxin produced by the organisms is then absorbed over a prolonged period. Constipation is frequently the earliest clinical sign and is followed in typical cases by lethargy, poor feeding, a weak cry and diminished motor activity. Ptosis and pooling of pharyngeal secretions supervene and, in severe cases, generalized weakness with or without respiratory paralysis. The condition often worsens over several months with eventual return to normal strength. The mortality is less than 3%.[25]

In both classical and infantile botulism, internal ophthalmoplegia with or without paralysis of the extraocular muscles may be seen.

Investigations

In both types of botulism, electromyography may reveal brief, small action potentials and evidence of a presynaptic defect at the motor end-plate.

Toxin can be demonstrated in ingested contaminated food samples and in the serum of patients with classical botulism. In infantile botulism, the diagnosis is established by the demonstration of clostridial organisms and toxin in the faeces of infected babies.

Management

The administration of honey to infants under 12 months is to be avoided because honey is often contaminated by *Clostridium* organisms. Admission to an intensive care unit is usually indicated in hospitalized cases. Meticulous respiratory care is paramount. Gavage feeding is appropriate for infants. Antitoxin administration is recommended in early cases of classical botulism, but it is not useful in infantile cases. Antibiotics do not appear to be of value and aminoglycosides may actually worsen the neuromuscular blockade.

With good respiratory and nutritional care, recovery within a few months is the rule. In cases of foodborne botulism, rapid notification and investigation are important in preventing further cases.

REFERENCES

1 Arnason B G W. Acute inflammatory demyelinating polyradiculoneuropathies. In: Dyck P J, Thomas P K, Lambert E H, Bunge R, eds. Peripheral neuropathy, Vol 2, 2nd edn. Philadelphia: Saunders, 1984: 2050–2100.
2 Hughes R A C, Winer J B. Guillain–Barré syndrome. Recent Adv Clin Neurol 1984; 4: 19–49.
3 Ouvrier R A, McLeod J G, Pollard J D (eds). Peripheral neuropathy in childhood. New York: Raven Press, 1990: pp 39–49.
4 McKhann G M, Cornblath D R, Griffin J W et al. Acute motor axonal neuropathy: a frequent cause of acute flaccid paralysis in China. Ann Neurol 1993; 33: 333–342.
5 Billard C, Ponsot G, Lyon G, Arthuis M. Polyradiculonevrites aigues de l'enfant. Arch Fr Pediatr 1979; 36: 149–161.
6 Becker W J, Watters G V, Humphreys P. Fisher syndrome in childhood. Neurology 1981; 31: 555–560.
7 Green S. Polyradiculitis (Landry–Guillain–Barré syndrome) with total external ophthalmoplegia: encephalo-myelo-radiculo-neuropathy. Dev Med Child Neurol 1976; 18: 369–380.
8 Prineas J W. Ann Neurol 1981; 9 (Suppl): 6–19.
9 Hughes R A C, Winer J B. Guillain–Barré syndrome. Recent Adv Clin Neurol 1984; 4: 19–49.
10 Ropper A M, Shahani B T. Arch Neurol 1984; 41: 511–514.
11 French Co-operative Group on Plasma Exchange in Guillain–Barré syndrome: role of replacement fluids. Ann Neurol 1987; 22: 753–761.
12 McKhann G M, Griffin J W, Cornblath O R, Mellits E D, Fisher R S, Quaskey S A and the Guillain–Barré Study Group. Plasmapheresis and Guillain–Barré syndrome: analysis of prognostic factors and the effect of plasmapheresis. Ann Neurol 1988; 23: 347–353.
13 Epstein M A, Sladky J T. The role of plasmapheresis in children with Guillain–Barré syndrome. Neurology 1991; 41: 1928–1931.
14 Yoshioka M, Shigekazu H, Hideshige M. Plasmapheresis in the treatment of Guillain–Barré syndrome in childhood. Paediatr Neurol 1985; 1: 329–334.
15 Lamont P J, Johnston H M, Berdoukas V A. Plasmapheresis in children with Guillain–Barré syndrome. Neurology 1991; 41: 1928–1931.
16 Van der Meche F B A, Schmitz P I M. The Dutch Guillain–Barré Study Group. A randomised trial comparing intravenous immunoglobulin and plasma exchange in Guillain–Barré syndrome. N Engl J Med 1992; 17: 1123–1129.
17 Shahar L, Murphy E G, Roifman C M. Benefit of intravenously administered immune serum globulin in patients with Guillain–Barré syndrome. J Pediatr 1990; 116: 141–144.

18 Al-Qudah A A. Immunoglobulins in the treatment of Guillain–Barré syndrome in early childhood. J Child Neurol 1994; 9: 178–180.

19 McDonald W I, Kocen R S. Diphtheritic neuropathy. In: Dyck P J, Thomas P K, Lambert E H, Bunge R, eds. Peripheral neuropathy, Vol II. Philadelphia: Saunders, 1984: pp 2010–2017.

20 Krugman S, Katz S L, Gershon A A, Wilfert C M. Diphtheria. In: Infectious diseases of children. St Louis: Mosby, 1992: pp 68–86.

21 Bradley W G. Myelopathies affecting anterior horn cells. In: Dyck P J, Thomas P K, Lambert E H, Bunge R (eds). Peripheral neuropathy, 2nd edn. Philadelphia: Saunders, 1984: pp 1351–1367.

22 Rubin G, Michowiz S D, Ashenasi A, Tadmor R, Rappaport Z H. Spinal epidural abscess in the pediatric age group: case report and review of the literature. Pediatr Infect Dis J 1993; 12: 35–75.

23 Spencer C H, Hanson V, Singsen B H, Bernstein B H, Jornreich H K, King K K. Course of treated juvenile dermatomyositis. J Pediatr 1984; 105: 399–408.

24 Pearn J H. The clinical features of tick bite. Med J Aust 1977; 2: 313–318.

25 Arnon S S. Infant botulism. Annu Rev Med 1980; 31: 541–560.

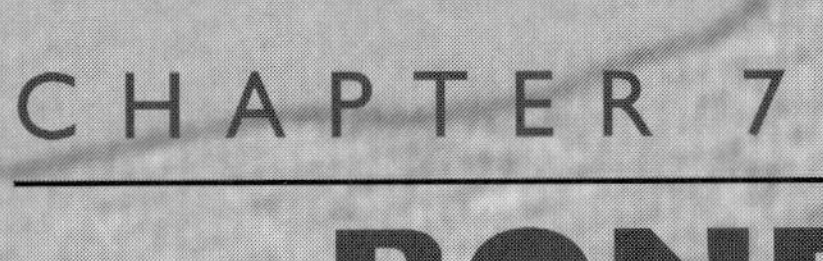

BONES

7.1. Bone and joint infections

7.1 — Bone and joint infections

INTRODUCTION

Early diagnosis is of paramount importance in the management of bone and joint infections in children. The immature skeleton is characterized by the presence of growth plates and epiphyses. The hyaline cartilage forming these structures is susceptible to irreversible damage by infection. Damage to these structures may result in growth disturbance or degenerative arthritis and permanent disability. Although antibiotic therapy is primarily responsible for the dramatic improvement in prognosis that has occurred over the last few decades, surgical drainage still plays an important role, particularly in the management of infection involving weight bearing joints.

ACUTE OSTEOMYELITIS

Epidemiology

Acute osteomyelitis is predominantly a disorder of childhood. Over the last two decades there has been a significant decrease in the overall incidence of osteomyelitis, possibly due to improvements in living standards and personal hygiene.[1,2] However, the establishment of neonatal intensive care units with consequent increased survival of preterm infants has resulted in a peak incidence in the first year of life. The mean age of presentation is 6 years, boys being more commonly affected than girls.[3]

Presentation

The classic presentation is that of an unwell child with a high fever and localized bone tenderness. There may be swelling, warmth and erythema at the site of the bone pain. Involvement of a lower limb manifests as a limp or reluctance to bear weight, whereas involvement of an upper limb will manifest as pseudoparalysis. The most common sites in order of frequency are:

- Femur
- Tibia
- Humerus
- Pelvis
- Calcaneus
- Phalanx
- Radius

Neonates with osteomyelitis often have multifocal bone involvement with less obvious signs and symptoms. They may present without fever or significant restriction of movement. The presentation of osteomyelitis involving the ilium is often late and sometimes misleading. Iliac fossa pain may precipitate an appendicectomy before the true diagnosis is made; or irritation of the upper trunk of the lumbosacral plexus causing low back pain and a limited straight leg raise may lead one to suspect a lumbar disc lesion.[4]

Pathogenesis

Acute osteomyelitis is most often a complication of a bacteraemia or septicaemia. In about a third of cases a primary focus of infection involving the respiratory tract or skin can be identified. Occasionally it may complicate an open fracture or penetrating injury. In acute haematogenous osteomyelitis the bacteria tend to lodge in the metaphyses of long bones, adjacent to the growth plates, because of sluggish blood flow in end capillaries (Fig. 7.1.1). Subsequent bacterial proliferation causes vascular occlusion and abscess formation. The abscess causes local bone destruction. A breach of the bone cortex allows pus to escape and form a subperiosteal abscess. This may discharge into surrounding soft tissues, or if the metaphysis is intracapsular, as is the case with the neck of the femur, septic arthritis may result. A less likely route of extension of the intraosseous abscess is through the growth plate to involve the epiphysis.

Osteomyelitis may result from a non-haematogenous route of infection, such as an open fracture or a penetrating injury. With early surgical exploration and debridement of traumatic wounds and appropriate antibiotic cover the incidence of bone infection is low.

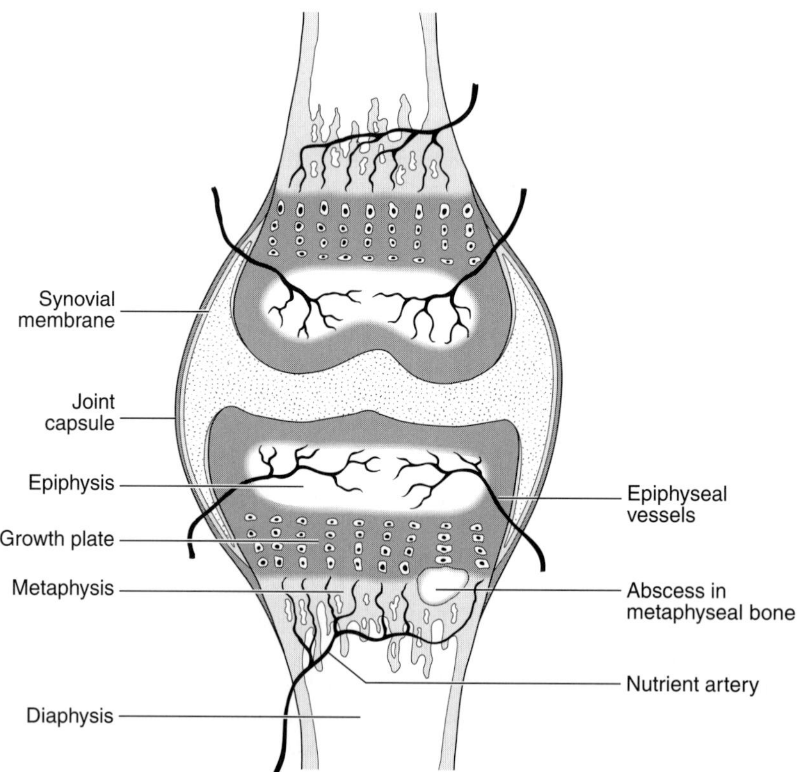

Fig. 7.1.1 Illustration of bone and joint anatomy in a child, demonstrating pathogenesis of acute haematogenous osteomyelitis.

Diagnosis

In a majority of cases the diagnosis can be made based on the clinical findings. The child will usually have a raised leucocyte count and an elevated erythrocyte sedimentation rate (ESR). The ESR, a sensitive but non-specific indicator of underlying infection, is usually greater than 50 mm/h. An X-ray taken soon after the onset of osteomyelitis will demonstrate soft tissue swelling and loss of normally defined tissue planes. Periosteal new bone formation becomes evident 7–10 days after onset. Localized bone rarefaction indicative of an intraosseous abscess may become evident after 10 days (Fig. 7.1.2a).

Ultrasonography is another readily available imaging technique which will demonstrate a periosteal reaction before it becomes evident radiologically. It is also useful in demonstrating the presence of a subperiosteal collection of pus or soft tissue abscess which may be difficult to detect clinically at some sites

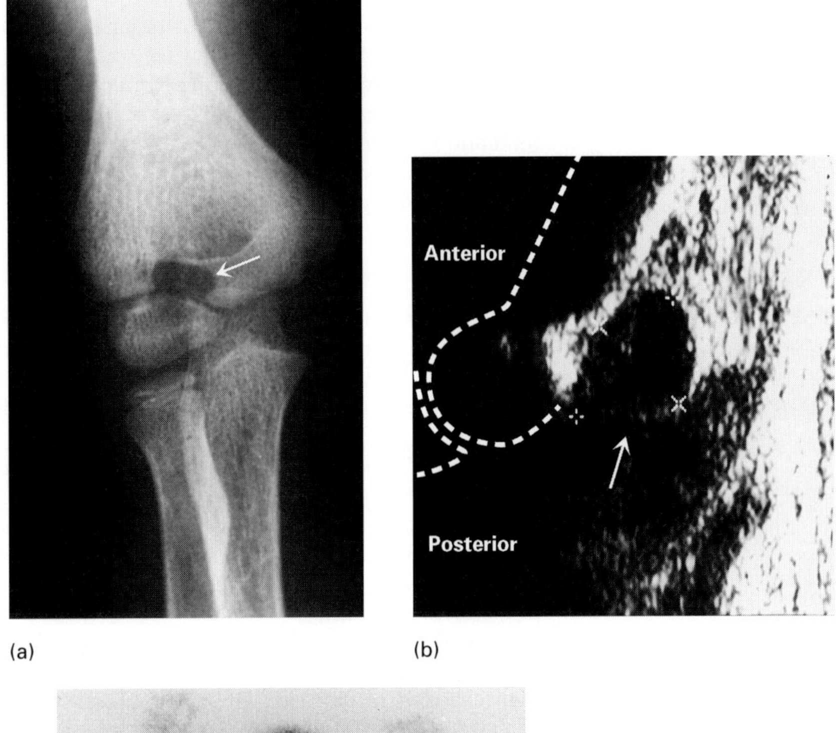

Fig. 7.1.2 Acute haematogenous osteomyelitis involving the distal humeral metaphysis of a 6-year-old boy. (a) X-ray demonstrating osteolytic lesion (anterior view). (b) Ultrasound scan demonstrating a subperiosteal abscess posteriorly (lateral view). (c) Bone scan demonstrating increased radionuclide uptake in the distal humerus.

(Fig. 7.1.2b). This imaging technique is non-invasive and does not involve exposure to radiation.

Bone scans are highly sensitive diagnostic aids but often serve only to confirm a clinically established diagnosis (Fig. 7.1.2c). Treatment should not be delayed unnecessarily awaiting bone scan results. Cellulitis and osteomyelitis can have a similar clinical picture and bone scans are valuable in making the correct diagnosis. In both cellulitis and osteomyelitis increased radionuclide uptake is seen at the affected site in the early phase scans (blood flow and blood pool images) indicative of increased vascularity, but focal increased radionuclide uptake in the late phase scans is seen only in osteomyelitis and is indicative of increased osteoblastic activity. Bone scans are also useful in localizing bone infection in less accessible sites such as the pelvis and spine.

An attempt should be made to isolate the causative organism before beginning treatment for acute osteomyelitis. Swabs should be taken from any infected lesions of the skin or upper respiratory tract. Blood cultures and aspiration of subperiosteal pus will yield an organism in 50–60% of cases. *Staphylococcus aureus* is the most common pathogen, accounting for 80% of cases.[5] Other pathogens include group A β-haemolytic streptococci, *Haemophilus influenzae* type b, *Streptococcus pneumoniae*, coagulase negative *Staphylococcus*, *Pseudomonas*, *Salmonella* and Gram-negative enteric rods. In osteomyelitis of the foot resulting from puncture wounds, *Pseudomonas* infection should be suspected. In cases with extensive bone destruction, especially involving the diaphysis, a bone biopsy should be performed to exclude a malignant bone tumour.

Treatment

Acute osteomyelitis with an early presentation can be expected to respond well to treatment with antibiotics. Success will be dependent upon selection of an appropriate antibiotic administered in an adequate dose for a sufficient duration. The treatment protocol used in our institution is derived from that reported by Cole et al.[6] The choice of antibiotics used within the first 24–48 h is based on the fact that *S. aureus* is the most commonly found organism and group A β-haemolytic *Streptococcus* the second most common. Cloxacillin in a dosage of 200 mg/kg per day and benzylpenicillin in a dosage of 200 mg/kg per day are given intravenously every 6 h. If the child is known to be allergic to penicillin, a cephalosporin is given instead. The antibiotic regime is modified according to the results of cultures and sensitivities, when available, and to the response to treatment. Intravenous antibiotics are continued until the child has been afebrile for 24 h, has decreased local signs and is systemically well. The medication is then changed to oral cloxacillin and phenoxymethylpenicillin (penicillin V) or cephalexin in a dosage of 100 mg/kg per day in four doses. The child should remain in hospital for at least 24 h on oral medication to ensure it is tolerated before discharge. A 3–6-week course of antibiotics is recommended.[1,6,7] The endpoint of therapy should be based mainly upon clinical assessment rather than haematological tests, X-rays or repeat bone scans. There should be no localized bony tenderness. The results achieved with a short course of intravenous antibiotics, followed by oral antibiotics, are as good as those achieved with prolonged intravenous therapy.[6] Also, the period of hospitalization is shortened and treatment costs considerably reduced. Oral therapy is not recommended for neonates because of erratic absorption.

Splinting of the affected limb, although an orthopaedic tradition, has not been shown to lead to a better outcome and is not practised routinely at our institution. It is occasionally indicated for patient comfort.

Surgical drainage is indicated whenever there is evidence of a soft tissue

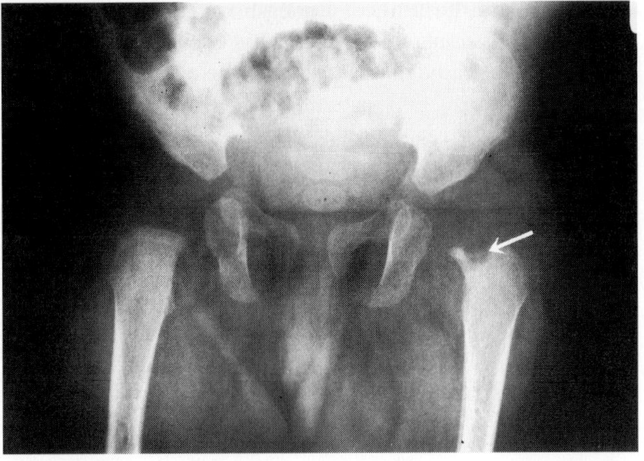

(a)

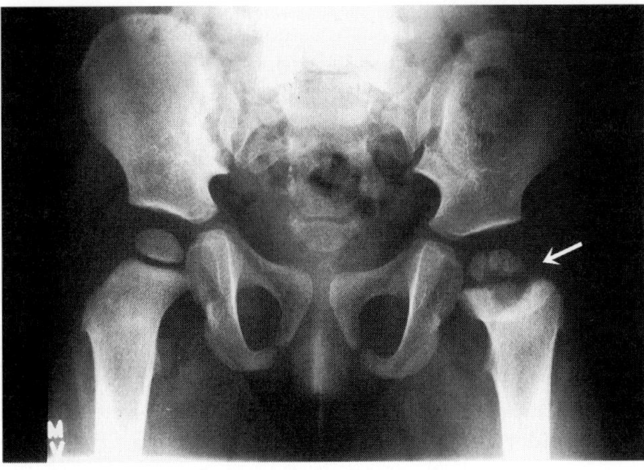

(b)

Fig. 7.1.3 Neonatal osteomyelitis of left neck of femur complicated by septic arthritis. (a) X-ray at 2 months of age demonstrating lytic lesion involving metaphysis of proximal femur. (b) X-ray at 2 years of age demonstrating abnormal ossification of epiphysis and a short femoral neck due to growth retardation. (c) X-ray at 5 years of age demonstrating progression of growth disturbance.

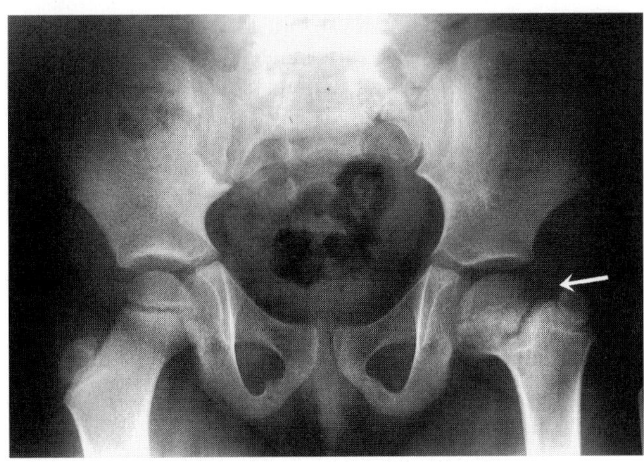

(c)

abscess. Drilling of bone should not be carried out routinely. Curettage of an intraosseous abscess cavity is occasionally required, but in so doing care should be taken to avoid damage to the adjacent growth plate.

Outcome

The success of treatment of acute osteomyelitis is related to the time of presentation. In patients with early presentation and treatment a cure can be expected in more than 90% of cases with the recommended treatment regime.[6] In patients with a late presentation and abscess formation a more prolonged course of antibiotics and surgical intervention are likely to be necessary to effect a cure. A late presentation is more likely in older children and when the pelvis and proximal humerus are involved. Acute osteomyelitis may cause growth plate damage leading to progressive limb shortening and sometimes angulatory deformity (Fig. 7.1.3). Chronic osteomyelitis is now a rare outcome.

CHRONIC OSTEOMYELITIS

Classification[8]

1. Non-specific
   a. Sequel to acute osteomyelitis
   b. Chronic unifocal osteomyelitis
   c. Chronic recurrent multifocal osteomyelitis
2. Specific
   a. Mycobacteria
   b. Mycoses
   c. Salmonella
   d. Other organisms

Non-specific

Sequel to acute osteomyelitis

Chronic osteomyelitis occurring as a sequel to acute osteomyelitis usually affects older children who present late. It may present as a flare, recurrent flares or a chronic discharging sinus. Boys are predominantly affected.

A bone cavity or sequestrum may be evident radiographically. Treatment should be directed to elimination of the dead bone and the dead space. Sequestrectomy, curettage of the cavity and long-term systemic antibiotic therapy may result in a cure. If these fail, local administration of high-dose antibiotics should be considered using either methyl methacrylate beads impregnated with gentamicin (Fig. 7.1.4) or an implantable pump loaded with amikacin.[9] The bony cavity can be eliminated by filling it with a vascularized muscle flap or a bone graft using the Papineau technique.

Chronic unifocal osteomyelitis

Chronic unifocal osteomyelitis, sometimes referred to as subacute osteomyelitis, is characterized by an insidious onset and a history of more than 2 weeks duration. The patient is not systemically unwell but complains of pain and may have a mild antalgic gait with lower limb involvement. There may be moderate local tenderness but not the exquisite tenderness seen in acute osteomyelitis. Chronic unifocal osteomyelitis does not have the same predilection for metaphyseal bone as acute osteomyelitis. It is classified according to site, as either epiphyseal, metaphyseal, diaphyseal or vertebral. Metaphyseal and diaphyseal lesions are not usually associated with marked soft tissue swelling. Epiphyseal lesions, however, are usually associated with a sympathetic joint effusion.

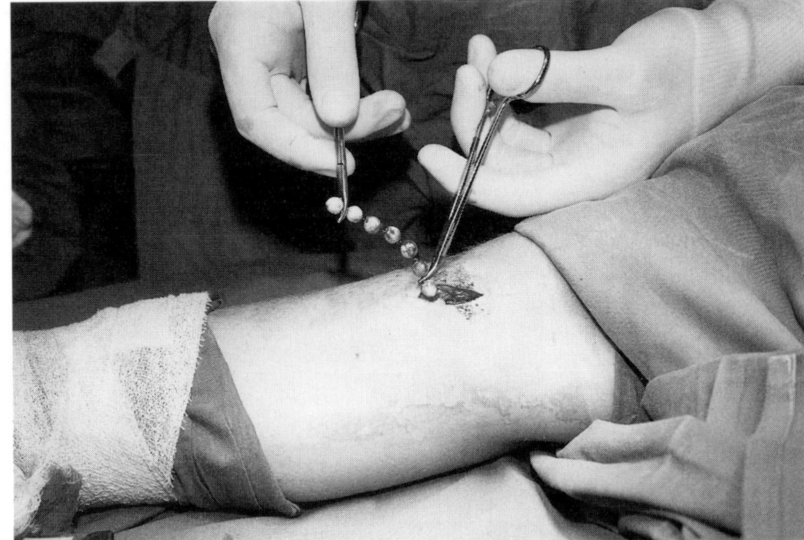

(a)

Fig. 7.1.4 Chronic unifocal osteomyelitis involving the proximal tibial metaphysis of an 8-year-old boy. (a) Methyl methacrylate (bone cement) beads impregnated with gentamicin inserted into bone cavity. (b) X-ray demonstrating multiloculated bone cavity involving proximal tibial metaphysis. (c) X-ray after curettage of bone cavity and insertion of gentamicin beads.

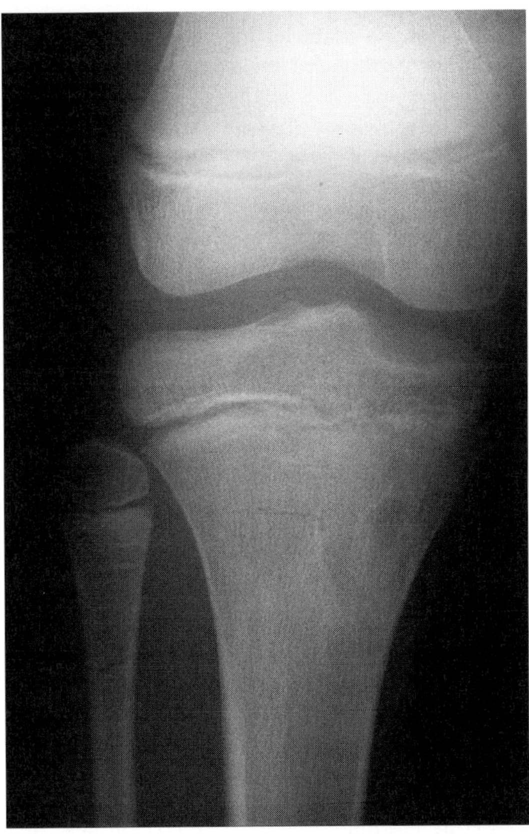

(b)

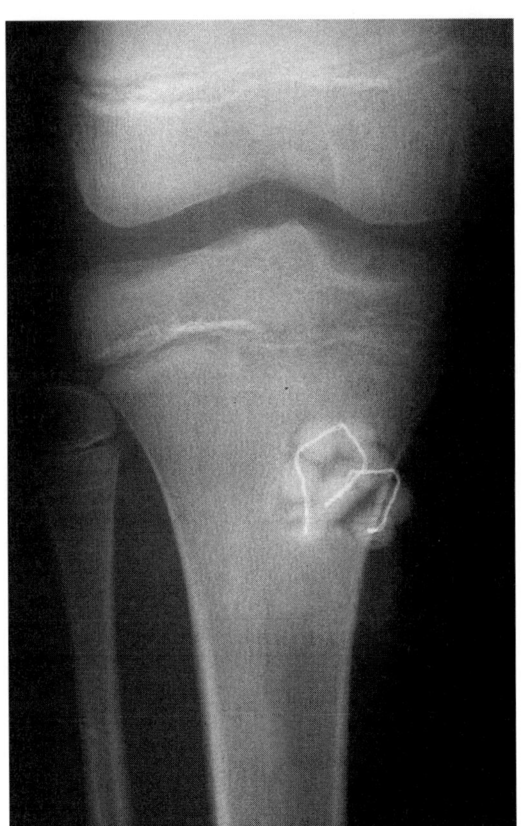

(c)

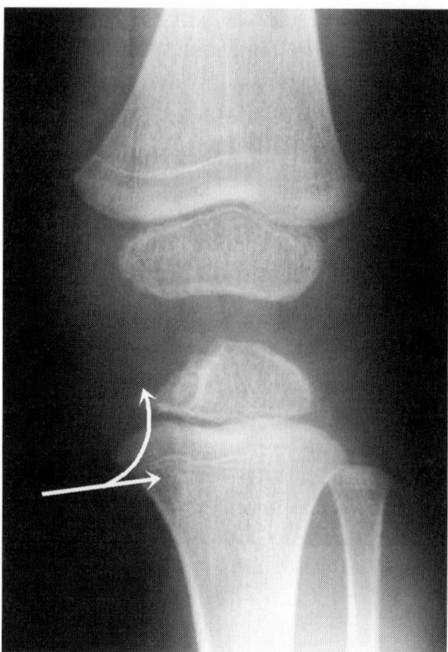

Fig. 7.1.5 X-ray of left knee. 18-month-old boy with acute haematogenous osteomyelitis involving proximal tibial metaphysis, extending across growth plate to involve the epiphysis and knee joint.

Epiphyseal and metaphyseal lesions have a characteristic radiographic appearance with an area of bone destruction surrounded by a fine sclerotic margin (Fig. 7.1.5). They can usually be distinguished from benign neoplasms and therefore in most cases biopsy is unnecessary.[10] Diaphyseal lesions show radiographic evidence of a periosteal reaction and create a diagnostic problem as malignancy must be excluded as a possible cause.[11,12] Routine investigations for osteomyelitis should be performed. Imaging techniques such as bone scans, computed tomographic scans and magnetic resonance imaging scans are useful in delineating the extent of bone changes. A biopsy should be performed on diaphyseal lesions to make a definitive histologic diagnosis.

Chronic recurrent multifocal osteomyelitis

Chronic recurrent multifocal osteomyelitis is a rare, poorly understood disorder. It occurs in late childhood and girls are affected more often than boys. It is characterized by an insidious onset of mild bone pain and soft tissue swelling, usually with fever. The clavicle and metaphyses of long bones are sites of predilection. As the name suggests, the affected child is likely to have multiple presentations over a few years with pain at different sites. Radiographs show a lytic lesion with a sclerotic margin. Bone scans demonstrate a focal increased uptake at affected sites, often before symptoms develop. In this disorder cultures are negative, but a biopsy is indicated, at least on initial presentation, to exclude bacterial osteomyelitis, histiocytosis X and neoplasia. Histology demonstrates acute and chronic inflammatory changes consistent with the diagnosis of osteomyelitis, but no organisms. The aetiology of this disorder remains unknown. Treatment modalities that have been tried include: prolonged antibiotic therapy, non-steroidal anti-inflammatory drugs, aspirin, systemic steroids and hyperbaric oxygen. None of these has consistently resulted in improvement.[13,14]

The natural history of chronic recurrent multifocal osteomyelitis is a slow spontaneous resolution of the osseous lesions without specific treatment, and decreased frequency of episodes with time.

Specific

Children with generalized debility which may be the result of prematurity, malnutrition, cytotoxic chemotherapy, immunodeficiency, drug addiction or any chronic illness, are susceptible to bone and joint infections. In these cases infection with an unusual organism needs to be considered. It is important to discuss this with a microbiologist and specifically to request that culture specimens be examined for the presence of acid-fast bacilli, fungi and anaerobic bacteria.

Mycobacteria

Bone and joint tuberculosis, although rare in developed countries, is being seen with increasing frequency because of migration from less well-developed countries. The causative organism is usually *Mycobacterium tuberculosis* and rarely *M. bovis.* In most cases it results from haematogenous spread after primary pulmonary infection. The spine, hip and knee are the most commonly affected sites, but any bone or joint may be involved.

The diagnosis should be considered in any patient with a slow insidious onset of bone pain and/or joint stiffness. A tuberculin test can be expected to be positive except in some seriously ill patients. A biopsy and positive culture are necessary to confirm the diagnosis. Treatment consists of prolonged combination chemotherapy.

Mycoses

Fungal infections of bones and joints are rare. Like tuberculous osteomyelitis, they are most likely to occur in patients with an immunodeficiency, e.g. chronic granulomatous disease or other neutrophil disorder, or a debilitating disease. Cytotoxic chemotherapy, steroid therapy and hyperalimentation also predispose. Causative organisms include *Candida albicans, Aspergillus* and *Cryptococcus.* The pathogenesis is usually haematogenous spread from a primary pulmonary focus with involvement of multiple viscera. Bone and joint infection is seen in only a minority of patients with multi-system disease.

The bone and joint involvement is characterized by local swelling and mild tenderness of insidious onset. Frequently the diagnosis is delayed because the clinical signs are less florid than with pyogenic infections and medical attention is directed towards treatment of the systemic illness.

The radiological changes seen in mycotic osteomyelitis are non-specific. The most common finding is a metaphyseal lytic lesion, sometimes with a periosteal reaction. Isolation of a mycotic organism from a joint aspirate or bone biopsy is essential to establish the diagnosis.

The diagnosis of mycotic osteomyelitis should be considered in cases of chronic osteomyelitis in which it has not been possible to culture a bacterial pathogen, in cases which fail to respond to routine antibiotics and osteomyelitis with fistulae.

Treatment consists of surgical debridement of bone followed by prolonged antimycotic therapy based on culture results. In the debilitated patient with a systemic mycotic infection the prognosis is poor.

Salmonella

Sickle cell disease is common in black Americans, black Africans and people of Mediterranean extraction. Sickled cells tend to lodge in the microvascular circulation of bones leading to thrombosis, infarction and sickle cell crises.

Bacteria commonly colonize infarcted bone following an episode of bacteraemia. Osteomyelitis is common in sickle cell anaemia and *Salmonella* is the causative agent in the majority of cases.[15]

Sickle cell osteomyelitis can be differentiated from a sickle cell crisis by the presence of positive cultures. Other distinguishing features include fever, multiple symmetrical bone involvement, an involucrum and longitudinal fissuring of the cortex.[16]

Salmonella osteomyelitis responds well to treatment with chloramphenicol.

An 8-week course is recommended.[15] Reticulocyte depression may complicate treatment. Ampicillin is used if the organism is sensitive.

Other organisms   Chronic osteomyelitis may also be seen in association with congenital infection with syphilis, cytomegalovirus and rubella.

ACUTE SEPTIC ARTHRITIS

Presentation

Acute septic arthritis in children occurs more commonly than acute osteomyelitis. Also, early diagnosis and treatment of septic arthritis are more imperative than with osteomyelitis. The epiphyses of infants and young children are largely cartilaginous. Therefore, they are easily damaged and sometimes totally destroyed by proteolytic enzymes found in pus.

The usual presentation is an unwell child with a fever and a painful, swollen joint. The hip and the knee are the most common sites of involvement and result in a refusal to bear weight. Joint swelling is usually not apparent clinically when the hip is involved but the affected child will tend to lie with the hip flexed and abducted because of increased tension within the joint. Swelling is a relatively late sign in septic arthritis of the shoulder because of overlying soft tissues. In older children joint movement is usually severely restricted in all directions by pain. Neonates most commonly present with decreased active movement of a limb, pseudopalsy, but have a moderate range of passive movement when examined. Neonates may also develop multiple joint involvement. Therefore, once the diagnosis of septic arthritis has been made, follow up examinations are important, looking for joint involvement at other sites.

Pathogenesis

Routes of infection:

1. Haematogenous spread
2. Contiguous spread from osteomyelitis
3. Penetrating injury

In most cases septic arthritis results from haematogenous spread of infection from a primary focus involving skin or the respiratory tract. Premature neonates and immunocompromised children are particularly at risk of developing septic arthritis. These children frequently require prolonged intensive care and umbilical catheters or intravenous cannulas may become a primary focus of infection.

Septic arthritis may occur as a complication of osteomyelitis. Acute haematogenous osteomyelitis usually involves metaphyseal bone. In children over 2 years of age the growth plate acts as a barrier preventing infection from extending into the epiphysis and joint (Fig. 7.1.1). However, in certain sites, such as the neck of femur and neck of humerus, the metaphysis is intracapsular, so that when the bone cortex is breached pus discharges into the joint (Fig. 7.1.3). In infants the growth plate is less well defined and blood vessels traverse the growth plate, allowing infection to spread from the metaphysis to the epiphysis and in some cases into the joint, resulting in septic arthritis (Fig. 7.1.5).

A penetrating injury to a joint may also introduce infection. This is sometimes iatrogenic but in most cases traumatic. The knee is the joint most susceptible to penetrating injuries. Synovitis following a penetration injury is not always due to sepsis. A foreign body reaction to organic material, such as a splinter of wood or pine needle, needs to be considered in the differential diagnosis, particularly in cases responding poorly to antibiotic therapy.

Diagnosis

The diagnosis of acute septic arthritis can usually be made on clinical assessment. The erythrocyte sedimentation rate (ESR) is a highly sensitive test, being elevated in 90% of cases.[17] Ultrasonography will demonstrate the presence of a joint effusion, and this is helpful at sites such as the hip and shoulder where joint swelling is difficult to detect clinically.

A technetium bone scan will demonstrate increased radionuclide uptake involving a joint, but cannot reliably distinguish septic arthritis from transient synovitis or other forms of inflammatory arthritis. However, a bone scan may be helpful in distinguishing septic arthritis from osteomyelitis. Gallium scans have been reported to be more accurate than technetium bone scans in detecting septic arthritis but they result in a greater delay in treatment and a higher radiation exposure.[18]

An arthrotomy or arthroscopic examination of the involved joint may be required to confirm the diagnosis of septic arthritis or exclude a foreign body synovitis. Particulate foreign bodies are characteristically sequestered in the synovial membrane and are rarely seen in synovial fluid.[19]

Treatment

The traditional treatment regime for septic arthritis has been drainage of pus and lavage of the joint, followed by immobilization and appropriate antibiotic therapy. Drainage of pus may be achieved by arthrotomy, arthroscopy or multiple joint aspirations. There are no controlled studies to show which is the most effective method of treatment. However, if the septic arthritis has been progressing for a few days then the production of fibrinous material may result in loculations of pus within the joint and in this situation aspiration is an ineffective method of drainage.

Resting infected joints is a time-honoured principle dating back to the treatment of tuberculous joints by Hugh Owen Thomas in the nineteenth century. Salter et al[20] have shown experimentally that continuous passive motion allows better healing of infected joints following drainage. In practice, children with septic arthritis are usually too young to cooperate with the use of a continuous passive motion machine. At our institution we have abandoned postoperative joint immobilization and encourage active joint movement when comfort allows.[21]

The causative organism in septic arthritis is age related. Initial antibiotic therapy in infants should provide cover against staphylococci, streptococci and Gram-negative bacteria. Between 6 months and 2 years of age, *H. influenzae* type b (Hib) was the most common causative organism, before routine immunization against Hib was introduced, followed by *S. aureus* and streptococci. A profound decrease in the incidence of *H. influenzae* type b disease has occurred since the introduction of vaccination[22] and hopefully this will be reflected in a decrease in the incidence of septic arthritis in children in this age group. In older children *S. aureus* and streptococci are the most common causative organisms.[17]

The choice of antibiotic may change when the results of Gram stain, cultures and sensitivities are available. Antibiotics should be administered intravenously initially and oral therapy commenced after a favourable clinical response. The duration of antibiotic therapy should be determined by response to treatment, type of organism and chronicity of infection prior to therapy, not by empiricism. A 3–6-week course is adequate for most cases.

Outcome

Although the majority of cases respond well to antibiotic therapy with a full recovery, in some cases damage to articular or growth plate cartilage may result in permanent joint deformity and disability (Fig. 7.1.3). In septic arthritis of the hip reported sequelae include premature closure of the triradiate cartilage, acetabular dysplasia, limb length discrepancy, premature closure of the proximal femoral growth plate, subluxation, dislocation, ischaemic necrosis of the femoral head, pseudarthrosis of the neck of femur and complete destruction of the femoral head.[23,24] Early diagnosis is imperative as delayed treatment will lead to a poor outcome.

DISCITIS

Discitis is a poorly understood disorder of childhood, characterized by restricted spinal mobility, elevated ESR and radiographic narrowing of the affected disc space. The aetiology is controversial, with proposed causes being an infectious process, a non-infectious inflammatory process or trauma. With no consensus on aetiology, treatment is equally controversial. There is general agreement, however, that the disorder has a benign self-limiting course.

Presentation

Most children with discitis present between 2 and 6 years of age. They are systemically well with no fever or only a slight fever. Back pain is the most common complaint but younger children will sometimes present with abdominal pain or an irritable hip. They walk with an abnormal gait and have a decreased lumbar lordosis. Movement in the lumbar spine is severely restricted. This can be nicely demonstrated by the dropped coin test, in which a child will flex the knees but hold the back straight to pick up a coin from the floor. The coin should be of a high enough denomination to attract the child's interest. Straight leg raising is limited by tight hamstrings.

Diagnosis

The ESR is nearly always raised but is not as high as is typically seen in osteomyelitis and septic arthritis. Attempts to isolate an organism are in most instances fruitless. Blood cultures are usually negative. Occasionally a positive blood culture may be found in the acute phase. Similarly percutaneous and open disc biopsies will usually demonstrate non-specific inflammatory changes but no organisms.[25-27] This certainly calls into question the proposed infectious aetiology.

Radiographs demonstrate disc space narrowing and this is usually evident at the time of presentation. The L4–5 disc space is the most common site. Later radiographic changes are resorption of vertebral end plates followed by sclerosis and irregularity of end plates in the healing phase. Tuberculous vertebral osteomyelitis needs to be considered in the differential diagnosis of a child with disc space narrowing. A clear chest X-ray and negative Mantoux test are helpful in making the correct diagnosis.

Bone scans show focal increased uptake at the affected disc level in 90% of cases. Tomograms, computed tomographic scans and magnetic resonance imaging scans further delineate the disc pathology.

Treatment

Treatment modalities for discitis in childhood include bed rest, traction, plaster cast immobilization and antibiotics. An uncertain aetiology creates a poor foundation for treatment. Furthermore, there is no consistent evidence that treatment has any bearing on the outcome.

The extent and duration of immobilization should be determined by the level of symptoms. In mild cases it is reasonable for children to limit their own activities according to their discomfort.

Several studies have shown no apparent value with antibiotic treatment.[25,27,28] Until further evidence becomes available it would seem appropriate to limit treatment with antibiotics to those patients who have a positive bacterial culture or who do not respond to adequate immobilization.

Outcome

Most patients remain pain free following healing of their discitis. Some will be troubled by recurrent mild or moderate back pain with strenuous activity. Significant scoliosis or kyphosis are usually not apparent.[27]

Follow-up X-rays show that the disc space usually remains narrowed. In some cases the disc space narrowing progresses to fusion of vertebral bodies. In others, a partial restoration of the disc space occurs.

CONCLUSION

Although laboratory investigations and organ imaging techniques have become more sophisticated during the last decade and new generation antibiotics are being made available, clinical vigilance remains the most important factor in the early diagnosis and management of bone and joint infections in children.

REFERENCES

1 Craigen M A C, Watters J, Hackett J S. The changing epidemiology of osteomyelitis in children. J Bone Joint Surg Br 1992; 74-B: 541–545.
2 Jones N S, Anderson D J, Stiles P J. Osteomyelitis in a general hospital: a five-year study showing an increase in subacute osteomyelitis. J Bone Joint Surg Br 1987; 69-B: 779–783.
3 Faden H, Grossi M. Acute osteomyelitis in children. Am J Dis Child 1991; 145: 65-69.
4 Beaupré A, Carroll N. The three syndromes of iliac osteomyelitis in children. J Bone Joint Surg Am 1979; 61-A: 1087–1092.
5 Nade S. Acute haematogenous osteomyelitis in infancy and childhood. J Bone Joint Surg Br 1983; 65-B: 109–119.
6 Cole W G, Dalziel R E, Leitl S. Treatment of acute osteomyelitis in childhood. J Bone Joint Surg Br 1982; 64-B: 218–223.
7 Gillespie W J, Mayo K M. The management of acute haematogenous osteomyelitis in the antibiotic era. J Bone Joint Surg Br 1981; 63-B: 126–131.
8 Cole W G. The management of chronic osteomyelitis. Clin Orthop 1991; 264: 84–89.
9 Perry C R, Pearson R L. Local antibiotic delivery in the treatment of bone and joint infections. Clin Orthop 1991; 263: 215–226.
10 Ross E R S, Cole W G. Treatment of subacute osteomyelitis in childhood. J Bone Joint Surg Br 1985; 67-B: 443–448.
11 Hoffman E B, de Beer J de V, Keys G, Anderson P. Diaphyseal primary subacute osteomyelitis in children. J Pediatr Orthop 1990; 10: 250–254.
12 Kozlowski K, Bellemore M, Marsden F W, Bale P, Kan A. Rare malignant mid-femoral tumours in the first decade of life. Pediatr Radiol 1992; 22: 493–497.
13 Manson D, Wilmot D M, King S, Laxer R M. Physeal involvement in chronic recurrent multifocal osteomyelitis. Pediatr Radiol 1989; 20: 76–79.
14 Yu L, Kasser J R, O'Rourke E, Kozakewich H. Chronic recurrent multifocal osteomyelitis. J Bone Joint Surg Am 1989; 71–A: 105–112.
15 Bennett O M, Namnyak S S. Bone and joint manifestations of sickle cell anaemia. J Bone Joint Surg Br 1990; 72-B: 494–499.
16 Engh C A, Hughes J L, Abrams R C, Bowerman J W. Osteomyelitis in the patient with sickle-cell disease: diagnosis and management. J Bone Joint Surg Am 1971; 53-A: 1–15.
17 Shaw B A, Kasser J R. Acute septic arthritis in infancy and childhood. Clin Orthop 1990; 257: 212–225.
18 Borman T R, Johnson R A, Sherman F C. Gallium scintigraphy for diagnosis of septic arthritis and osteomyelitis in children. J Pediatr Orthop 1986; 6: 317–325.

19 Reginato A J, Ferreiro J L, O'Connor C R et al. Clinical and pathologic studies of twenty-six patients with penetrating foreign body injury to the joints, bursae, and tendon sheaths. Arthritis Rheum 1990; 33: 1753–1762.

20 Salter R B, Bell R S, Keeley F W. The protective effect of continuous passive motion on living articular cartilage in acute septic arthritis: an experimental investigation in the rabbit. Clin Orthop 1981; 159: 223–247.

21 Bellemore M C. Bone and joint infections in children. Curr Opin Pediatr 1992; 4: 59–64.

22 Murphy T V, White K E, Pastor P et al. Declining incidence of *Haemophilus influenzae* type b disease since introduction of vaccination. JAMA 1993; 269: 246–248.

23 Choi I H, Pizzutillo P D, Bowen J R, Dragann R, Malhis T. Sequelae and reconstruction after septic arthritis of the hip in infants. J Bone Joint Surg Am 1990; 72–A: 1150–1165.

24 Little D G, Barrett I R. Septic arthritis of the hip in infancy. Aust NZ J Surg 1993; 63: 116–119.

25 Melenaus M B. Discitis. J Bone Joint Surg Br 1964; 46-B: 16–23.

26 Ryöppy S, Jääskeläinen J, Rapola J, Alberty A. Nonspecific diskitis in children. Clin Orthop 1993; 297: 95–99.

27 Crawford A H, Kucharzyk D W, Ruda R, Smitherman H C. Diskitis in children. Clin Orthop 1991; 266: 70–79.

28 Spiegel P G, Kengla K W, Isaacson A S, Wilson JC. Intervertebral disc-space inflammation in children. J Bone Joint Surg Am 1972; 54-A: 284–296.

JOINS

8.1. Infectious causes of arthritis

P. Malleson   S. Dobson

8.1 Infectious causes of arthritis

INTRODUCTION

In septic arthritis there are living bacteria (usually *Staphylococcus aureus*) actively invading the joint tissues. In several other arthritides there is good evidence that an infection is the cause of the inflammation, but the presence of viable organisms within the joint is uncertain. For instance in post-*Shigella* arthritis it seems clear that there are no bacteria in the joint; in Lyme disease, *Borrelia* are present in low numbers, and are probably viable; in post-*Yersinia* arthritis there is evidence that there are some, probably non-viable, fragments of the organism in the joint.

A list of the more common bacterial and viral infections associated with these forms of arthritis is given in Table 8.1.1.

Table 8.1.1   Infectious arthropathies

Bacterial
Infectious
  Lyme disease
  Gonococcus
  Brucellosis
Reactive
  1. HLA B27 independent
  Acute rheumatic fever/post-streptococcal reactive arthritis
  Meningococcus
  Tuberculous rheumatism (Poncet's disease)
  Mycoplasma
  2. HLA B27 associated
  Gastrointestinal: *Shigella, Salmonella, Yersinia, Campylobacter*
  Genitourinary: Chlamydia
Viral
  HIV
  Rubella
  Parvovirus
  Varicella
  Ross River

BACTERIAL ARTHRITIS

Lyme disease

Lyme disease is an important infectious cause of arthritis. However, its importance is almost as much due to the risk of over-diagnosis and inappropriate antibiotic treatment as to the risk of the disease itself.

The clinical manifestations of this multi-system illness are mainly related to direct tissue invasion with the spirochaete *Borrelia burgdorferi*. The vector for the spirochaete is usually a tick of the *Ixodes* species. Prevalence of the disease varies considerably across the world but it is endemic in parts of North America, Europe and Asia. Clinical features occur in stages though there is a degree of overlap and variation in latent periods (Fig. 8.1.2). The arthritis is a late manifestation in at least 50% of cases and occurs at between 2 and 15 months after initial infection, by which time many of the early signs of infection have settled.[1]

The classic clinical marker of Lyme disease is erythema migrans (EM), a skin lesion that begins days to weeks after the tick-bite as a red papule or macule that extends and expands over days and weeks to a large round lesion with partial central clearing (Fig. 8.1.1). It should have a diameter of at least 5 cm and may reach diameters of 20 cm or more.[2] It is not usually itchy. Unfortunately in children with Lyme disease EM is only present in 40–70%. Constitutional symptoms such as fever, lethargy, headache, stiff neck, fleeting myalgias and arthralgias and lymphadenopathy may occur as part of this early stage. The lesions of EM may be single or multiple and fade spontaneously over a period of weeks.

After a latent period of weeks to months, late manifestations may develop. Approximately 15% have central nervous system (CNS) involvement including meningitis and cranial nerve palsies, especially Bell's palsy. Peripheral radiculoneuropathy appears less common in children than in adults. Neurological symptoms are more common in the European experience than in North America. This and other disease variations may be related to differing tick species, infecting dose, host response and perhaps even spirochaete variation. Cardiac disease

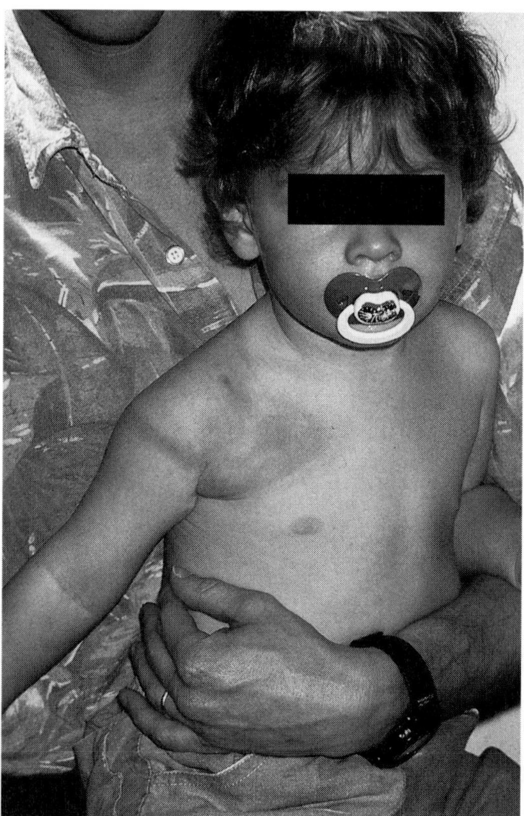

Fig. 8.1.1 Lyme disease. Erythema migrans with central clearing. See also colour plate.

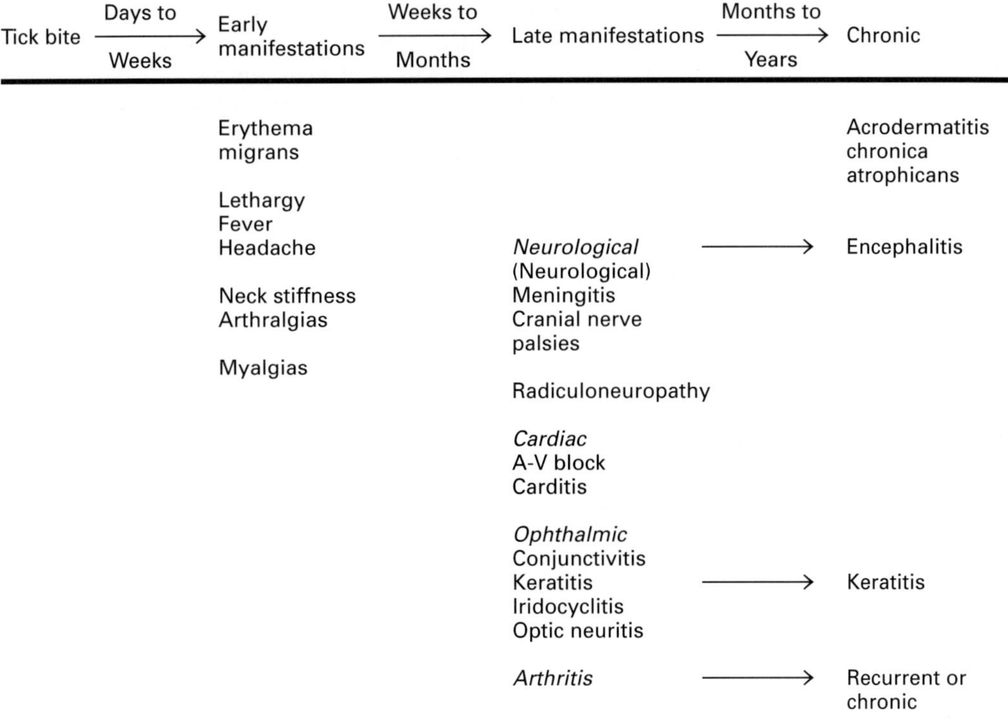

Fig. 8.1.2   Stages of Lyme disease.

also seems to be less common in children than adults. At most approximately 10% develop atrioventricular nodal block. A more diffuse carditis may occur.

The arthritis occurs several months after initial infection. It is acute, oligo-articular and episodic, with each episode usually lasting for less than 7 days. If untreated it can recur several times over the course of a year. The knee is the most usual joint involved and effusions may be massive. Other large joints such as shoulder, elbow, wrist, hip and ankle may be involved but small joints such as the hands rarely so. Aspiration reveals synovial fluid with an average of 30 000 cells/mm^2 predominantly neutrophils,[1] rather more than usually occurs in juvenile chronic arthritis. The natural history is for each acute episode to be short lasting and to resolve completely before a recurrence. Untreated acute episodes recur for several years but gradually decline in frequency and resolve completely.[3] Untreated, a small percentage of children may go, on to have chronic arthritis or episodes of subtle joint pain. Fortunately treatment with antibiotics is usually very effective in resolving arthritis. A small proportion of children have chronic arthritis in spite of treatment with antibiotics. This is associated with either HLA-DR4 or HLA-DR2 and with high antibody titres to the outer surface protein A of the spirochaete.[4,5] This, together with evidence of *B. burgdorferi* DNA being found in joint fluid during acute and recurrent episodes but not in chronic arthritis after multiple antibiotic courses, suggest that a host immunological response is more likely than persistent infection to be responsible for chronic arthritis.[6]

Consideration of the disease is easy if the child lives in or has travelled to an endemic area. The CDC case definition requires either erythema migrans to have been present or at least one late manifestation and laboratory evidence of infection.[2] Difficulty arises where EM has not been evident or clinical signs are vague and indistinct. The positive predictive value of serology depends so much on local disease prevalence. No widely available serological test is both highly specific and sensitive. In areas of high prevalence, where as much as 60% of the population has been exposed, clinical signs may be wrongly attributed to Lyme disease based on coincidentally positive serology. In areas of low prevalence false positives on a serology test become numerically important and a patient's symptoms again may be wrongly ascribed to Lyme disease. Serological results need to be interpreted in the context of the clinical and geographical setting and in consultation with the local reference laboratory. Both immunofluorescent assays (IFA) and enzyme-linked immunosorbent assays (ELISA) are widely used. IgM antibody to *B. burgdorferi* is detectable within 2 weeks of onset of erythema migrans and fades by 8 weeks. IgG is detectable by 3–4 weeks and gradually rises thereafter. The more accurate Western blot or immunoblot is available at reference laboratories and can be used to confirm or refute the first-line IFA or ELISA tests where the clinical setting requires it. Isolation of spirochaetes from joint fluid requires specialized laboratory help and is not routinely available.

Treatment of Lyme disease arthritis is with oral antibiotics for 30 days:[7]

- >9 years of age
  Doxycycline 100 mg twice daily.
- < 9 years of age
  Amoxycillin 30–50 mg/kg per day in three divided doses.
  Erythromycin 30 mg/kg per day in four divided doses.
  (if allergic to penicillin)

In children, response to antibiotics is usually excellent irrespective of time elapsing before the diagnosis is made. If oral antibiotics fail, then a 14–21-day intravenous course of antibiotics should be tried according to regimens used for CNS disease:

- Ceftriaxone 100 mg/kg per day i.v. once daily.
- Penicillin G 300 000 u/kg per day i.v. in four divided doses.
- Cefotaxime 200 mg/kg per day i.v. in four divided doses.

Failure to respond to antibiotics, as mentioned above, may be related more to host factors than to persistence of live organisms.

Gonococcus

Disseminated gonococcal infection is a cause of arthritis that is commonly diagnosed in the USA but is apparently less common in other developed countries. It should be considered in any sexually active adolescent particularly in patients with a migratory polyarthritis, and tenosynovitis of the hands and/or feet.[8,9] Systemic features may be marked or may be minimal. For reasons that are not clear, the arthritis often seems to occur during pregnancy or within a week of the onset of menses. A sterile vesiculopustular or haemorrhagic rash if present is almost pathognomonic, although a similar rash can be seen in chronic meningococcaemia. Because the gonococcus is a fastidious organism it is often difficult to culture the organism from the joints or other sites. The presence of Gram-negative intracellular diplococci on Gram stains from urethra, cervix, rectum, skin lesions or joints should raise the probability of disseminated gonococcus. However, non-pathogenic *Neisseria* species can be found, most frequently in the pharynx of young children, and therefore one must be somewhat cautious in making the diagnosis if the organism cannot actually be cultured.[10] Occasionally it is justified to give a therapeutic trial of antibiotics. The presence of gonococcal arthritis in younger children should raise the probability of sexual abuse.

Brucellosis

Brucellosis is a cause of arthritis of childhood that, although now uncommon in most developed countries, should be considered in children from countries or cultures where unprocessed dairy products are consumed; however, not all children with proven brucellosis have a history of eating such products. The arthritis develops in about one-third of infected children (considerably less frequently than in adults), is usually oligoarticular, affecting larger joints (hips, elbows, knees), and may be fairly low grade without significant systemic involvement suggestive of infection, so that the diagnosis is delayed for weeks or months.[11,12] Unlike adults the spine is never or only rarely affected, though sacroiliac disease does occur. Blood cultures may be positive for *Brucella* (usually *B. melitensis*) in a minority of children and rarely from synovial fluid cultures; the diagnosis is usually dependent on positive serological tests. Treatment with high dose co-trimoxazole appears to be efficacious and safe.[11]

Acute rheumatic fever and post-streptococcal reactive arthritis

Acute rheumatic fever (ARF) is the prototypic reactive arthritis. Although it is now an uncommon disease in the developed world, it is still a common cause of arthritis in much of the developing world. There have recently been some events that have resparked interest in ARF. Firstly, since 1984, there have been local epidemics of ARF in the USA.[13–15] Secondly, it has been recognized that there are individuals who develop arthritis following infection with group A streptococci, who have a more persistent form of polyarthritis than the flitting type of arthritis usually associated with ARF.[16,17] This form of arthritis has been termed post-streptococcal reactive arthritis (PSRA), and there has been controversy as to whether this is a forme fruste of ARF. Thirdly, there is strong evidence that the well-recognized genetic predisposition to ARF is linked to a B cell alloantigen recognized by a murine IgM monoclonal antibody known as D8/17.[18] This allo-antigen is not part of the major histocompatiblility complex, is only found on B cells, and although found in small amounts in normal subjects is found in much higher amounts in almost all patients with ARF and appears to be inherited in an autosomal recessive manner.

ARF develops following a pharyngeal infection with group A β-haemolytic streptococci. On the basis of the recent outbreaks in the USA it appears that:

- The majority of affected individuals are either asymptomatic, or only have a mild pharyngitis prior to the onset of ARF.
- Overt poverty may no longer be such an important risk factor as in the past, but overcrowding may still be important.
- Carditis, as defined by echocardiographic abnormalities, occurs in up to 90% of affected patients, although clinically detectable carditis is less frequent (30–50%).
- Arthritis is the most common manifestation of ARF, occurring in some 75% of patients.

Typically children with ARF develop arthritis of up to six joints, beginning about 3 weeks after the onset of pharyngitis. Each joint is inflamed for only a few days, and a new joint becomes involved as the inflammation subsides in the previously affected one. The arthritis usually responds rapidly to salicylates in anti-inflammatory doses (about 75 mg/kg per day in three to four divided doses), and it has been said that failure to obtain a rapid defervescence of the arthritis over a few days should put the diagnosis in doubt.

In PSRA the onset of arthritis is sooner (about 10 days) than with classical ARF and the arthritis is more prolonged, lasting several weeks, with a relatively poor response to aspirin, and affecting many joints in a symmetrical and cumula-

Table 8.1.2 Antibiotic treatment for ARF/post-streptococcal arthritis

Primary treatment	
Benzathine penicillin (i.m.)	(<27 kg) 600 000 units
	(>27 kg) 1 200 000 units
Penicillin V (oral)	250 mg 3 times daily × 10 day
Erythromycin (oral)	40 mg/kg/day in 4 divided doses × 10 days × 10 days
Prophylaxis	
Benzathine penicillin (i.m.)	1 200 000 units every 3 or 4 weeks
Penicillin V (oral)	250 mg twice daily
Erythromycin (oral)	250 mg twice daily

tive fashion. Although it was initially felt that PSRA might be separate from ARF, it is more likely that it is a variant of ARF, as several children with PSRA have developed carditis.[17]

Although the Jones criteria were introduced to try and reduce over-diagnosis, not all patients fulfilling them will have ARF; for example children with systemic onset juvenile chronic arthritis may have both polyarthritis and carditis and may have raised antistreptococcal antibodies (presumably as part of a polyclonal activation). Other diseases that can mimic ARF include systemic lupus erythematosus, viral arthropathies, and some other reactive arthropathies, particularly *Yersinia*-related arthritis. The diagnosis of a previous streptococcal infection can also be difficult. Streptococci in the throat may represent a carrier state, or conversely streptococci may have been eradicated from the throat, either spontaneously or due to antibiotic administration, prior to the onset of arthritis. The rapid tests for streptococcal antigens have a very low sensitivity. Not every child with ARF develops a raised titre to streptolysin O and unfortunately the streptozyme test, which is a rapid slide test measuring antibodies to five different bacterial products, is too unreliable to be useful.

Once a diagnosis of ARF or PSRA has been made, the aim of treatment is to eradicate streptococci which may still be present and then to prevent recurrences of streptococcal infections, as the risk of ARF is much greater in children who have already experienced one attack and the risk of cardiac involvement increases with the number of recurrences, although it is greatest with the first attack.

The treatment protocols recommended by the American Heart Association are shown in Table 8.1.2.[19] Whether to give intramuscular or oral prophylaxis is going to be influenced by both patient compliance and risk of recurrence, which is greater in the young child and in the first few years after the initial attack. The duration of prophylaxis is uncertain though should probably be for at least 5 years after the last attack, and life-long in anyone with significant rheumatic valvular abnormalities. Children with rheumatic heart disease should also receive endocarditis prophylaxis when having dental or other surgical procedures.

Meningococcus

Meningococcal disease occasionally can be associated with an acute arthritis in which bacteria can be isolated from the joint. More commonly (in up to 10% of infected children), a sterile oligoarthritis occurs about 1 week after onset of the acute infection as a complication of the convalescent period. It is probably a consequence of immune complex deposition. The arthritis resolves without sequelae after 2 or 3 weeks.

Tuberculosis (Poncet's disease)

Tuberculosis is usually a cause of a monoarthritis, with *Mycobacterium tuberculosis* being cultured from the joint. Occasionally a sterile polyarthritis known as

Poncet's disease can also occur. The aetiology of this form of arthritis is unknown but there is evidence for an exaggerated reaction of synovial fluid lymphocytes to purified protein derivative of *Mycobacterium* (PPD), similar to those seen against the infectious agent in other forms of reactive arthritis.[20]

HLA B27-related reactive arthritis

It has been recognized for many years that a sterile arthritis can occur following enteric infections with *Shigella flexneri*, *Salmonella* species, *Yersinia enterocolitica* or *Campylobacter jejuni,* or following genitourinary infection with *Chlamydia trachomatis*. In some cases there are other associated systemic features including inflammatory eye disease, and mucocutaneous lesions (balanitis, oral ulcerations and keratoderma blennorrhagica). Urethritis may also develop after an enteric precipitated episode and diarrhoea after a genitourinary precipitated one. The term Reiter's syndrome is often used to describe this more extensive symptom complex, but its use is more confusing than enlightening. The finding that links these conditions is that there is a greatly increased frequency of HLA B27 (40–80%) in patients who develop arthritis following infection with these organisms compared with the general population (about 8%). A number of patients with reactive arthritis develop a chronic arthritis with sacroiliac and spine involvement that is indistinguishable from ankylosing spondylitis. HLA B27 is found in about 90% of patients with ankylosing spondylitis. The possibility that ankylosing spondylitis is a form of reactive arthritis is intriguing, but as yet unproven.

In children, reactive arthritis usually follows an enteric infection[21] although *Chlamydia*-induced arthritis has been described even in young children.[22,23] Whether *Chlamydia*-induced arthritis always occurs as a result of sexual activity or abuse remains unclear, but the possibility of sexual abuse in a young child should certainly be investigated. Reactive arthritis generally occurs between 1 and 3 weeks after the preceding infection. It usually only involves a few lower limb joints, but affected joints can be extremely swollen and painful and mimic septic arthritis.

The frequency of arthritis following an infection with one of the above-mentioned organisms in children is not well known, but is probably between 1% and 5%, based mainly on adult studies. The frequency in patients who carry HLA B27 is about 20%. Although HLA B27 is a risk factor for the development of arthritis after a diarrhoeal illness or non-specific urethritis, the fact that only one in five patients with HLA B27 will develop arthritis means that it is not of great prognostic value in any individual. Reactive arthritis used to be considered a condition with an excellent prognosis; however, this is probably incorrect. It seems likely that a large proportion (perhaps even the majority) of adults with reactive arthritis has recurrent or persistent arthritis for many years that can significantly interfere with activities of daily living.[24] It is unknown whether the same is true for children, but this possibility should be borne in mind when the prognosis is discussed with the family.

Treatment

It is usually considered that reactive arthritis and the risk of arthritis persistence are unaffected by antibiotic therapy. Therefore antibiotics should only be given if the child is systemically unwell with the infection. There are, however, a couple of caveats. Firstly, both *Salmonella* and *Yersinia* infections can be associated with a true septic arthritis, which should be suspected if the arthritis develops in close temporal relationship to the onset of gastrointestinal symptoms, and if there is any doubt a joint aspiration must be performed for synovial fluid Gram stain and culture. Secondly, there is good evidence for the presence of chlamydial antigens in the joints of patients with Reiter's syndrome, and some evidence that there are actually viable organisms present.[25] There is also some evidence in adults that antibiotic treatment with tetracycline derivatives can shorten the duration of this form of reactive arthritis.[26] Therefore the rare child with *Chlamydia*-induced arthritis should probably receive antibiotic treatment.

VIRAL ARTHRITIS

Viral infections are a recognized cause of transient arthritis, and are also frequently postulated to be the cause of arthritis of unknown aetiology; for example, transient synovitis of the hip is often considered likely to be due to a viral infection.

Rubella

Rubella infection of both the wild-type and (less frequently) following immunization is a common cause of arthralgias or/and arthritis in adults or adolescents;[27] however, it is rare for rubella to be associated with musculoskeletal symptoms in children. Arthritis, if it occurs, does so about 7 days after the onset of rash, and between 2 and 4 weeks after immunization, most often affecting the joints and flexor tendon sheaths of the fingers and the knee joints.

Parvovirus B19

In an early synovitis clinic in the UK, parvovirus B19 was recently reported as the leading infectious cause of arthritis, usually in young women.[28] Like rubella, however, this virus rarely causes arthritis in children, even though it too is a common exanthem of childhood (Fifth disease).

Herpesviruses

Epstein–Barr virus (EBV), cytomegalovirus (CMV), varicella zoster and herpes simplex have all been reported to cause arthropathies. EBV and CMV sometimes cause systemic illness that may mimic systemic lupus erythematosus, with arthritis being one manifestation of a multi-system disease. Chickenpox occasionally causes a monoarthritis which develops a few days after the onset of rash; it has also been associated with the onset of psoriatic arthritis. When arthritis does occur in chickenpox it is much more likely to be a septic arthritis following secondary invasion of the skin lesions by *Staphylococcus aureus* or group A streptococcus.

Alpha viruses

Arthropod-transmitted alpha viruses are the cause of epidemics of polyarthritis in many parts of the world. In Australia, Ross River virus disease is such an infection, causing usually a mild arthritis of the wrists. A similar self-limited arthropathy known as O'nyong-nyong occurs in Africa.

Hepatitis B

Although in adults about 20% of hepatitis B infections are associated with arthritis and rash in a serum sickness-like illness, this seems to be rare in children. Significant arthropathy does not appear to be a complication of hepatitis B immunization in children.

Human immunodeficiency virus (HIV)

In adults there is increasing recognition of the occurrence of arthritis and other rheumatic symptoms in association with HIV infection. These include Reiter's syndrome, psoriatic arthritis and oligo- and polyarthritis. Cumulatively some

20% of patients appear to develop one or other of these forms of arthritis.[29] The evidence suggests that arthritis may be associated with more severe HIV disease. Arthritis in childhood HIV infection does not yet appear to have been described, but may be expected to occur as the prevalence of HIV infection in children increases. It should be remembered that several infections that are associated with HIV infection, namely gonococcus, *Chlamydia* and tuberculosis, can also cause arthritis, so arthritis should not be ascribed to HIV without first excluding other treatable causes.

SUMMARY

Both bacterial and viral infections can cause arthritis in children. The consequences of undiagnosed septic arthritis are such that this possibility should be considered in any child presenting with an acute-onset arthritis. Appropriate investigations would include blood cultures and cultures of synovial fluid, particularly if the child appeared at all systemically unwell or if the joint or contiguous bones were more than mildly tender. A physician should never be criticized for doing a joint aspiration, only for not doing one.

Tuberculosis should be considered in a child with monoarthritis if the child is from an at-risk group, and a chest radiograph and tuberculin skin test would be appropriate initial investigations, with a joint aspiration probably not being necessary to exclude this diagnosis if they are both negative.

Lyme arthritis is a diagnosis that should always be considered in a child who is from, or who has recently visited, an endemic area; however, *Borrelia* serology is difficult to interpret, side-effects from antibiotics are not insubstantial, so the risks should be carefully weighed when considering treating a child in whom the diagnosis is in doubt.

Cultures of the throat are part of the work-up for ARF, but a positive culture without raised ASO levels should not lead one to this diagnosis. As with Lyme arthritis, over-diagnosis may be more harmful than missing a case. Cultures of other sites such as rectum or faeces or the genitourinary tract are appropriate in children with arthritis occurring following an episode of diarrhoea, or if sexual abuse is suspected.

Culturing various sites for viruses or performing serological tests against a battery of viruses is usually a wasted effort. Viral cultures are very rarely positive, interpretation of a raised antibody level is often difficult, and most importantly from a clinical point of view, the results of such tests usually only become available long after the virus-associated arthritis has resolved.

Tests that are commonly used in the work-up of a child with arthritis such as antinuclear antibodies and rheumatoid factor may be transiently positive in children with some infections, and therefore are not tests that should be used to make a definite diagnosis of juvenile rheumatoid or juvenile chronic arthritis.[30]

REFERENCES

1 Zemel L S. Lyme disease: a pediatric perspective. J Rheumatol 1992; 19 (Suppl 34): 1–13.
2 Wharton M, Chorba T L, Vogt R L et al. Case definitions for public health surveillance. Morbidity Mortality Weekly Rep 1990; 39: 19–21.
3 Szer I S, Taylor E, Steeve A C. The long term course of Lyme arthritis in children. N Engl J Med 1991; 325: 159–163.
4 Steere A C, Dwyer E, Winchester R. Association of chronic Lyme arthritis with HLA-DR4 and HLA-DR2 alleles. N Engl J Med 1990; 323: 219–223.

5 Steere A C, Levin R E, Molloy P J et al. Treatment of Lyme arthritis. Arthritis Rheum 1994; 37: 878–888.

6 Nocton J J, Dressler F, Rutledge B J et al. Detection of *Borrelia burgdorferi* DNA by polymerase chain reaction in synovial fluid from patients with Lyme arthritis. N Engl J Med 1994; 330: 229–234.

7 Committee on Infectious Diseases. Treatment of Lyme borreliosis. Pediatrics 1991; 88: 176–178.

8 Fink C W. Gonococcal arthritis in children. JAMA 1965; 194: 237–238.

9 Brogadir S P, Schimmer B M, Myers A R. Spectrum of the gonococcal arthritis–dermatitis syndrome. Semin Arthritis Rheum 1979; 8: 177–183.

10 Committee on Infectious Diseases: American Academy of Pediatrics. Gonococcal infections. In: Peter G, Lepow M L, McCracken G H, Phillips C F, eds. Report of the committee on infectious diseases, 23rd edn. Elk Grove Village, IL: American Academy of Pediatrics, 1994.

11 Gomez-Reino F J, Mateo I, Fuertes A, Fomez-Reino J J. Brucellar arthritis in children and its successful treatment with trimethoprim–sulphamethoxazole (co-trimoxazole). Ann Rheum Dis 1986; 45: 256–258.

12 Gotuzzo E, Alarcon J S, Bocanegra T et al. Articular involvement in human brucellosis: A retrospective analysis of 304 cases. Semin Arthritis Rheum 1982; 11: 245–255.

13 Veasy L G, Wiedmeier S E, Orsmond G S et al. Resurgence of acute rheumatic fever in the intermountain area of the United States. N Engl J Med 1987; 316: 421–427.

14 Congeni B, Rizzo C, Congeni J, Sreenivasan V V. Outbreak of acute rheumatic fever in northeast Ohio. J Pediatr 1987; 111: 176–179.

15 Hosier D M, Craenen J M, Teske D W, Wheller J J. Resurgence of acute rheumatic fever. Am J Dis Child 1987; 141: 730–733.

16 Goldsmith D P, Long S S. Poststreptococcal disease of childhood: a changing syndrome. Arthritis Rheum 1982; 25 (Suppl 4): S18.

17 DeCunto C L, Giannini E H, Fink C W, Brewer E J, Person D A. Prognosis of children with post streptococcal reactive arthritis. Pediatr Infect Dis J 1988; 7: 683–686.

18 Khanna A K, Buskirk D R, Williams R C J, Gibofsky A, Crow M K, Menon A. Presence of a non-HLA B cell antigen in rheumatic fever patients and their families as defined by a monoclonal antibody. J Clin Invest 1989; 83: 1710–1716.

19 Dajani A S, Bisno A L, Chung K J et al. Prevention of rheumatic fever: a statement for health professionals by the committee on rheumatic fever, endocarditis and Kawasaki disease of the Council on Cardiovascular Disease in the Young, the American Heart Association. Pediatr Infect Dis J 1989; 8: 263–266.

20 Southwood T R, Hancock E J, Petty R E, Malleson P N, Thiessen P N. Tuberculous rheumatism (Poncet's disease) in a child. Arthritis Rheum 1988; 31: 1311–1313.

21 Singsen B H, Bernstein B H, Koster-King K G, Glovsky M M, Hanson V. Reiter's syndrome in childhood. Arthritis Rheum 1977; 20 (Suppl) 402–407.

22 Rosenberg A M, Petty R E. Reiter's disease in children. Am J Dis Child 1979; 133: 394–398.

23 Maximov A A, Shaikow A V, Lovell D J, Giannini E H, Soldatova S I. Chlamydia associated syndrome of arthritis and eye involvement in young children. J Rheumatol 1992; 19: 1794–1797.

24 Fox R, Calin A, Gerbo R C, Gibson D. The chronicity of symptoms and disability in Reiter's syndrome: an analysis of 131 consecutive patients. Ann Intern Med 1979; 91: 190–193.

25 Rahman M U, Cheema M A, Schumacher H R, Hudson A P. Molecular evidence for the presence of chlamydia in the synovium of patients with Reiter's syndrome. Arthritis Rheum 1992; 35: 521–529.

26 Silveira L H, Gutierrez F, Scopelitis E, Cuellar M L, Citera G, Espinoza L R. Chlamydia-induced reactive arthritis. Rheum Dis Clin North Am 1993; 19: 351–362.

27 Tingle A J, Allen M, Petty R E, Kettyls G D, Chantler J K. Rubella-associated arthritis: comparative study of joint manifestations associated with natural rubella infection and RA 27/3 rubella immunization. Ann Rheum Dis 1986; 45: 110–114.

28 Cohen B J, Buckley M M, Clewley J P, Jones V E, Puttick A H, Jacoby R K. Human parvovirus infection in early rheumatoid and inflammatory arthritis. Ann Rheum Dis 1986; 45: 832–838.

29 Calabrese L H, Kelley D M, Myers A, O'Connell M, Easley K. Rheumatic symptoms and human immunodeficiency virus infection: the influence of clinical and laboratory variables in a longitudinal cohort study. Arthritis Rheum 1991; 34: 257–263.

30 Allen R C, Dewez P, Stuart L et al. Anti-nuclear antibodies using HEp-2 cells in normal children and in children with common infections. Journal of Paediatrics and Child Health 1991; 27: 39–42.

EYES

9.1. Eyes: preseptal and orbital cellulitis, conjunctivitis, uveitis and panophthalmitis

C. Donaldson   F. Martin   J. Smith

9.1 Eyes: preseptal and orbital cellulitis, conjunctivitis, uveitis and panophthalmitis

PRESEPTAL AND ORBITAL CELLULITIS

Infection of the preseptal space of the eyelids is referred to as preseptal or peri-orbital cellulitis. The orbital septum is a thin fibrous membrane that extends from the tarsal plate to the orbital margin and, together with the tarsal plates, separates the soft tissues of the eyelid from the orbit. Although thin it is a relatively effective barrier to the spread of infection. Infection posterior to the septum is termed orbital cellulitis. This distinction is important because if left untreated this latter condition can result in cavernous sinus thrombosis, blindness and even death.

Preseptal cellulitis

The majority of patients are younger than 10 years. The mode of infection may be internal spread from the respiratory tract, sinuses or middle ear. The most common agents include *Haemophilus influenzae* and *Streptococcus pneumoniae*, which are thought to be spread by venous lymphatic channels. It is important to note that *H. influenza*e type b is most commonly seen in children between 6 months and 2 years of age[1] due to lack of effective antibodies to the capsular antigen. Typically a sharply demarcated area of reddish purple discoloration is found. It can produce serious invasive disease including meningitis, facial cellulitis and epiglottitis.

External infection may, for example, occur secondary to conjunctivitis, dacryocystitis or trauma. In this situation the more commonly encountered organisms are *Staphylococcus aureus, Streptococcus, Peptococcus, Bacteroides* (following bites) and herpes simplex and varicella zoster viruses.

The onset is usually relatively rapid such as overnight. There is lid oedema, tenderness, pain and erythema. Little discharge is found and the globe appears uninflamed and white unless there is a conjunctivitis (Fig. 9.1.1). The child can be feverish, irritable and lethargic. Upper respiratory tract infection, lid wound or dacryocystitis may be present and there is often regional lymphadenopathy. It is of the utmost importance to assess the entire child.

Critically, there is no proptosis, motility disturbance or marked conjunctival chemosis. The vision is normal, as are pupillary responses and fundoscopy.

Special subgroups

Impetigo: This is caused by *Staphylococcus aureus* or less commonly *Streptococcus pyogenes* (group A), is usually in children under 6, there is an association with poor hygiene and it may complicate pre-existing skin lesions such as varicella. Red macules develop into serous vesicles surrounded by a thin erythematous margin. The material dries to form a characteristic thick yellow crust.

Herpes simplex: This may be primary or recurrent and is more common in

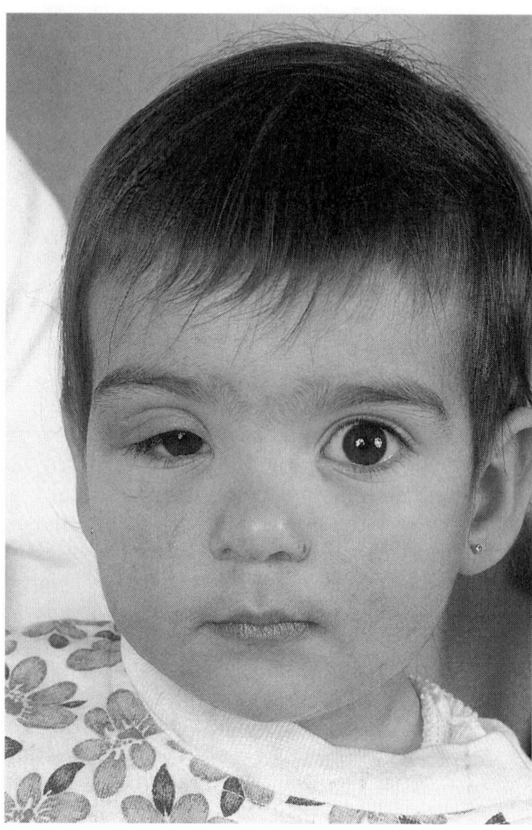

Fig. 9.1.1 Preseptal cellulitis. See also colour plate.

immunocompromised patients. It may be associated with conjunctival and/or corneal disease. Single or multiple small, thin-walled vesicles are present which proceed through pustular and crusted stages. There may be secondary bacterial infection.

Varicella zoster: Usually confluent areas of vesicular eruption and associated findings make this diagnosis straightforward. There can be conjunctival and/or corneal ulceration. Secondary bacterial infection may develop.

Erysipelas: This is due to *Streptococcus pyogenes* group A and is not common. It commences as a raised red plaque which is sharply demarcated from the surrounding skin. The child is unwell, with high fever. Toxins from the infection diffuse to the orbit causing orbital signs: mild proptosis, conjunctival chemosis and perhaps limitation of ocular movement.

Investigation

Enquire as to Hib immunization status. Conjunctival and nasopharyngeal swabs are taken for bacteriology. If a vesicle is present this may be swabbed for virology. In all but the mildest cases a full blood count, electrolytes, creatinine and blood culture are obtained. Computed axial tomographic (CAT) scan of the sinuses and orbits is performed if it is not possible to examine the globe or if within 24 h the infection does not respond to intravenous antibiotic therapy or if signs of orbital extension develop. In young children the sinuses can be hard to interpret and experienced review of the films should be sought when the diagnosis is in question.

Management

Ophthalmic review is essential. Very mild cases in systemically well, afebrile children can be treated on an outpatient basis with oral antibiotics and daily review. Otherwise admit the child to hospital and explain to the often anxious parents the reasoning behind the need for the therapy. Check tetanus prophylaxis if there is associated injury. Intravenous antibiotics providing appropriate spectrum coverage are commenced, e.g. cefotaxime and flucloxacillin. If the patient is allergic to these medications then possible alternatives are clindamycin, vancomycin or chloramphenicol.

Monitor patient response at least twice daily and continue or modify therapy according to patient response and results of investigations. If there is complicating conjunctivitis then treat this as well with broad-spectrum topical antibiotic eye drops: chloramphenicol, framycetin sulphate or neomycin/polymyxin.

In neonates keep gonorrhoea and chlamydia in mind if there is marked conjunctival inflammation — see below.

If sinusitis is present, or if the condition is not settling as anticipated, then an ear, nose and throat (ENT) review should be immediately sought. Surgical drainage of an abscess may be necessary.

Following 48–72 h of intravenous therapy with resolution of infection, change to oral antibiotics such as amoxycillin/clavulanic acid, flucloxacillin or erythromycin for a further 5–7 days.

Following discharge the patient is reviewed in a few days or immediately if any deterioration.

Special subgroups

- Impetigo: depends on severity. Flucloxacillin i.v.i.; oral flucloxacillin, erythromycin or amoxycillin/clavulanic acid; topical mupirocin 2% ointment and attend to hygiene.[2]
- Herpes simplex: ophthalmic review and acyclovir ocular ointment five times daily.
- Varicella zoster: as for herpes simplex.
- Erysipelas: penicillin G or erythromycin i.v.i.

Orbital cellulitis

In this situation the orbit proper (i.e., posterior to the thin orbital septum in the eyelid) is infected (Fig. 9.1.2), with a resultant decrease in normal function of the contained structures. It is extremely important to recognize this condition as, if left untreated, there is a high risk of death from intracranial sepsis and an even greater risk of permanent visual loss in the affected eye. In about 10% of cases subperiosteal or orbital abscess may occur.

Epidemiology

Orbital cellulitis is uncommon and more frequent in children older than 5 years. It is rarely bilateral.

Mode of infection

The vast majority are secondary to bacterial sinusitis, especially the ethmoid. The bones of the paraorbital sinuses are thin and infection can pass readily through these or via the foramina into the orbit. Here the veins do not possess valves, and haematogenous retrograde spread of infection is possible. Less common causes are penetrating injuries, systemic sepsis, dental infections and necrotic malignant tumours.[3]

Causative organisms

These include *Staphylococcus aureus*, *Streptococcus pyogenes*, *Streptococcus pneumoniae*, *Haemophilus influenzae* (especially in infants), fungi (e.g. mucormycoses) in immunocompromised and diabetic subjects, and parasitic infections, e.g. echinococcosis.

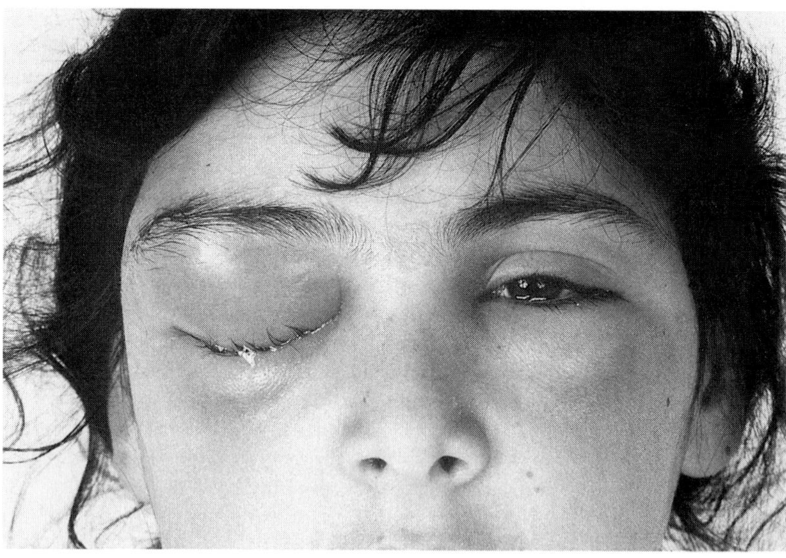

Fig. 9.1.2 Orbital cellulitis with oedema, redness and proptosis. See also colour plate. (Fig. 1A.6.8)

Clinical presentation

The child is febrile and unwell, with a painful red eye, with marked eyelid oedema and erythema. The signs of paramount importance are those suggesting orbital involvement. These include limitation of ocular motility, conjunctival chemosis, decreased visual acuity, pupillary dysfunction and proptosis (this is usually axial but may be non-axial, especially with abscess formation). There may be a recent history of respiratory tract infection or sinusitis.

Note: Orbital fungal infection is rare but devastating. It is usually seen in ketoacidotic diabetic or immunocompromised patients. The fungi tend to invade and thrombose arteries, causing a typical blackened, necrotic skin. Therapy involves amphotericin B and surgical debridement. The prognosis is poor.

Complications

Decreased vision may be due to corneal surface changes, but permanent loss is usually due to optic nerve damage and corneal exposure from proptosis. Orbital or subperiosteal abscess is difficult to detect clinically, but more likely if there is non-axial proptosis or a poor response of cellulitis to adequate antibiotic therapy. Meningitis or intracranial abscess, cavernous sinus thrombosis or septicaemia may develop.

Cavernous sinus thrombosis is an emergency and without appropriate treatment the mortality rate approaches 100%. It is rare, but should be suspected if the following signs develop: more severe orbital pain with rapidly increasing proptosis; development of bilaterality; deeply erythematous upper lid discoloration; decreasing vision; cranial nerve palsies; pupillary dysfunction; or decreasing consciousness. Immediately seek neurological assistance.

Investigation

This is as for preseptal cellulitis, but in this scenario a CAT scan of the brain and orbits with fine cuts should be ordered on an urgent basis and ENT consultation is mandatory. Dental consultation may also be indicated. Magnetic resonance imaging (MRI) provides further information in some cases.[4]

Management

This is as for preseptal cellulitis although antibiotic therapy will have to be maintained for a longer period of time, depending on clinical response. Subperiosteal or orbital abscess requires surgical drainage of the abscess and involved sinus.

Cavernous sinus thrombosis is treated with high-dose intravenous antibiotics, and in some cases anticoagulants and/or systemic steroids.

CONJUNCTIVITIS

Conjunctivitis is inflammation of the conjunctiva — the thin mucous membrane that lines the anterior aspect of the globe to the corneal limbus and the posterior surface of the eyelids. It has many possible aetiologies; however, the majority of these can be readily diagnosed clinically. In some situations microbiological examination is more crucial than others.

As with all ocular disease it is important to assess the entire child as sometimes conjunctivitis can be a manifestation of a systemic process.

Neonatal (ophthalmia neonatorum)

This refers to conjunctivitis that occurs during the first month of life. It may be aseptic (usually chemical) or septic. The infective types result from exposure in the birth canal. Neonatal conjunctivitis is put into a separate category due to its relative frequency in the past and, more importantly, because of its potentially devastating complications in certain cases. It is often helpful to take into account the period of time since birth until the development of the conjunctivitis. Although not a hard and fast rule, different organisms tend to appear at different times after birth.

Chemical conjunctivitis (e.g. silver nitrate) most commonly occurs during the first few days of life. There is a mild watery discharge and spontaneous resolution over a short period of time.

Gonococcal infection tends to develop in the first week. This is now fortunately uncommon, but due to this organism's ability to penetrate intact epithelial surfaces it can lead to severe ocular damage. There tends to be a copious purulent discharge with this infection (see Fig. 12.1.14) as opposed to the milder, watery discharge associated with the chemical type. A conjunctival swab and Gram stain should be performed, looking for Gram-negative intracellular diplococci and treatment consisting of systemic third-generation cephalosporin and saline eye irrigation instituted.[5] The possibility of coexistent syphilitic or chlamydial infection must be borne in mind. The parents are screened and treated for venereal disease.

Other bacteria that may be causative agents include *Haemophilus* species, *Staphylococcus aureus* and *Streptococcus pneumoniae*. Topical antibiotic therapy with chloramphenicol, framycetin sulphate or neomycin/polymyxin is usually all that is needed. More severe infections will need systemic therapy.

Chlamydia

Chlamydial conjunctivitis more usually develops after the first week. Clinically there is a watery discharge that becomes more purulent over time. Marked lid oedema may occur, as may pseudomembrane formation. In many cases laboratory tests are needed to distinguish this from other types of conjunctivitis. If left untreated the condition generally resolves in about 8 months. However, there is a risk of conjunctival and/or corneal scarring, with resultant decreased vision. It is also associated with a neonatal pneumonitis or otitis which may typically occur in the first 2 months. A conjunctival swab is taken for ELISA antigen detection or PCR, or a scraping for microscopy and culture. Therapy consists of a 2-week course of erythromycin syrup (50 mg/kg per day in divided doses) as well as topical erythromycin.[6] The parents are treated with either erythromycin or tetracycline orally.

Herpes simplex

Herpes simplex infection is less common but may develop in the neonatal period, with vesicles developing on the eyelids and maybe on other parts of the body. There is a risk of potentially lethal disseminated disease and in likely cases vesicle fluid culture should be performed and systemic acyclovir administered.

Non-neonatal

Bacterial

Acute bacterial conjunctivitis is very common and will be seen frequently in the casualty department. The most commonly encountered organisms are *Staphylococcus aureus* and *Staph. epidermidis*, *Haemophilus aegyptius* and streptococci. The majority of these infections if left untreated will resolve spontaneously within about 14 days. However, the condition can be most uncomfortable as well as potentially serious, and prompt appropriate therapy is in the patient's best interests.

These patients present with a short history of moderate discomfort, mucopurulent ocular discharge and sticking of the lids together after sleeping. One eye is affected first and the other shortly after. There is often a history of contact with a similarly affected person. It is not painful per se and any visual loss is mild and alleviated by gentle eye wash. The cornea remains clear but the conjunctiva is injected. The injection generally becomes more intense away from the cornea, which is the opposite of what one usually finds in cases of acute iridocyclitis. The upper lids should be everted in order to assess further the degree of inflammation and exclude other causes such as subtarsal foreign body.

A conjunctival swab is taken and the patient started on topical antibiotic drops whilst waiting for the result. Appropriate therapies are chloramphenicol, framycetin sulphate or neomycin/polymyxin eye drops.

Resistant cases may occur due to resistant organisms, anatomical abnormality (e.g. lacrimal duct obstruction with dacryocystitis), medicamentosal, ocular rosacea, etc. and warrant ophthalmological review.

Note: Gonococcal conjunctivitis is even rarer in children outside the neonatal period. There is a copious amount of purulent discharge and a risk of corneal invasion and visual loss. Child abuse should be suspected. A positive Gram stain should lead to the patient being admitted and commenced on systemic therapy.

Viral

Viral conjunctivitis is most commonly caused by the adenovirus family, and less commonly by herpes simplex, varicella zoster, enterovirus, molluscum contagiosum, Epstein–Barr and measles viruses.

Adenoviral conjunctivitis ranges from an unnoticed mild infection to a debilitating, uncomfortable condition with marked conjunctival inflammation, lid oedema and corneal infiltration that may scar. This latter, less frequent situation may last for many weeks. The usual presentation is that of gritty discomfort, conjunctival injection and watery ocular discharge with maybe a coexistent flu-like illness or sore throat. The conjunctiva shows a follicular response. Regional lymphadenopathy is often present. There is no specific treatment and the majority of cases resolve within 10 days. Great care must be taken by the health worker as well as other patient contacts, because it is highly contagious for about 2 weeks. It is spread by finger-to-eye contact. Swabs are generally not indicated, except perhaps in those cases that are more severe, persistent, or for whom the diagnosis is in doubt. A topical lubricant drop may promote comfort and/or a topical antibiotic (e.g. chloramphenicol) may be used to help prevent confusing superinfection.

Herpes simplex virus conjunctivitis is associated with eyelid vesicles and a follicular conjunctivitis as well as possible corneal ulceration. Treatment is with topical acyclovir but urgent ophthalmic review must be sought.

Varicella zoster virus has associated cutaneous manifestations that aid in making the diagnosis. With zoster, the ophthalmic division of the trigeminal nerve is the second most commonly affected region. The virus can affect virtually any part of the eye and ophthalmic review should be arranged urgently as a matter of routine.

Enterovirus may cause a haemorrhagic conjunctivitis that is self-limiting over about 10 days. Its appearance is most alarming as large, bright red areas of subconjunctival haemorrhage quickly develop with a marked watery discharge. Although it is highly contagious it tends to run a benign course and over-treatment with antibiotics or steroids is generally not indicated. A simple artificial tear preparation may help symptomatically.

UVEITIS

The highly vascular uveal tract consists, from anterior to posterior, of the iris, ciliary body and choroid. Inflammation of this tract may be referred to as anterior, intermediate or posterior uveitis. If the iris is primarily affected then the term iritis may be used, as may iridocyclitis with involvement of the ciliary body and similarly choroiditis. Inflammation of all the components is termed panuveitis.

Uveitis is a distinctly important clinical entity because, apart from being potentially sight threatening, it can have systemic associations that may be life threatening. The majority of cases of uveitis are not of an infective nature; however, when they are, the risk of systemic disease is relatively high.

Anterior uveitis

In the acute type, the patient develops symptoms of pain, redness and photophobia which may have been present for weeks. The older child may complain of decreased or blurred vision.

Typically there is ciliary injection which is seen as a reddish hue surrounding the cornea. This decreases with increasing distance from the cornea, in contradistinction to conjunctivitis. On slit lamp examination there are white blood cells circulating in the anterior chamber. These may attach to the cornea, forming aggregations referred to as keratic precipitates. If enough white cells are recruited by the inflammatory stimulus then a layer may develop inferiorly called a hypopyon. Adhesions (posterior synechiae), can build between the iris and the anterior lens surface leading to pupil irregularity and sometimes, if complete, severe intraocular pressure rises. Fundoscopy in purely anterior disease is usually normal.

In the chronic form the symptoms may be quite mild and may have been present for years. Cataract, glaucoma, corneal degeneration and cystoid macular oedema are often encountered.

One of the most common causes of anterior uveitis in children is trauma and the possibility of intraocular foreign body must be kept in mind. Other common causes include idiopathic, juvenile rheumatoid arthritis, Fuchs' heterochromic iridocyclitis, herpes simplex and zoster, ankylosing spondylitis and sarcoidosis.[7,8] Other infectious agents include measles, mumps and Epstein–Barr viruses, syphilis, tuberculosis, leprosy and Lyme disease.

The possibility of a masquerade syndrome with overflow inflammation from the posterior segment must be excluded. The possibilities include retinoblastoma,[3] leukaemia, intraocular foreign body and retinal detachment.

Management necessitates ophthalmic evaluation followed by investigation depending on the clinical picture. Mumps, measles, chickenpox and infectious mononucleosis have characteristic systemic findings. Herpes simplex and zoster-induced anterior uveitis usually accompanies a keratitis. Syphilis and Lyme disease will often display posterior segment signs.

Treatment depends on the cause. Frequent ophthalmic evaluation is mandatory to follow the process and prevent permanent visual loss. Misdiagnosis and poor management increase the possibility of complications such as cataract, corneal scarring, glaucoma and blindness. Therapy consisting of topical steroid and mydriatic eye drops may be adequate in some cases (e.g. zoster) but contraindicated in others (e.g. simplex) and consequently this condition should not be managed by non-specialist practitioners.

Posterior uveitis

In this condition there is inflammation of the choroid. The preverbal child may not present until permanent visual loss has occurred secondary to retinal scarring. This decreased vision may result in strabismus. The older child may complain of fuzzy vision. The teenager may describe floaters due to vitreous inflammatory debris. Systemic features often direct the medical officer's attention to the eyes.

There are usually anterior chamber cells and flare in addition to vitreous cells; however, the eye frequently appears externally quiet and not inflamed. The retina displays areas of inflammatory exudate as well as variable amounts of retinal oedema, haemorrhage and scarring.

Causes of infective posterior uveitus include the TORCH infections (i.e., toxoplasmosis, congenital rubella, cytomegalovirus and herpes simplex), toxocariasis, congenital syphilis, AIDS, tuberculosis and fungi. The systemic manifestations of these infections are described elsewhere in this book and will not be reviewed again.

Ocular *Toxoplasma gondii* (an intracellular parasite) is usually acquired in utero with maternal infection. A chorioretinal scar with a hyperpigmented border results and it is often in the macular region with considerable visual loss (Fig. 12.1.7). Any part of the retina may be involved with re-excitation of a congenital lesion, at which stage a focus of inflammatory exudate is seen adjacent to the pigmented border. The optic disc may become involved, with the appearance of optic neuritis. Diagnosis is usually made by fundal examination and associated toxoplasmosis serology.[9] Treatment is indicated for posterior, larger lesions with accompanying visual loss. Smaller peripheral lesions can be carefully monitored.

Therapy consists of clindamycin and/or pyrimethamine and/or sulphonamide and/or systemic corticosteroid.[10,11] Corticosteroids should not be given without antimicrobial cover. The exact regime depends on the severity of the infection and the patient's immune capabilities. If pyrimethamine is used then the patient is also given folinic acid to avoid leucopenia and thrombocytopenia, and a white cell and platelet count is performed weekly.

Congenital rubella may result in a mottled pigmentary retinopathy (Fig. 12.1.4). Other ocular manifestations include bilateral or unilateral cataract, microphthalmos, keratitis and glaucoma.[12]

Congenital cytomegalovirus usually does not result in ocular disorders but possible manifestations include chorioretinitis, keratitis, cataract and microphthalmus.

Ocular manifestations of herpes simplex infection include blepharoconjunctivitis, keratitis, uveitis and secondary cataract and retinal necrosis. This latter condition is usually associated with zoster.[12]

Congenital syphilis may result in chorioretinitis, keratitis, iridocyclitis and secondary cataract, optic atrophy and glaucoma. The chorioretinitis results in a salt and pepper type retinopathy.

HIV infection can result in retinal cotton wool spots as well as a number of secondary infections. Among these are cytomegalovirus, *Pneumocystis carinii*, *Cryptococcus neoformans*, *Toxoplasma gondii*, herpes simplex and syphilis.[13]

PANOPHTHALMITIS

This term refers to inflammation of all the ocular structures, including Tenon's capsule. The infection may be exogenous (e.g. penetrating injury) or endogenous, and causative agents include bacteria, fungi and parasites.

Bacterial panophthalmitis is not common in children. The most commonly encountered organisms include *Staphylococcus aureus*, *Staph. epidermidis*, *Streptococcus*, *Pseudomonas* and *Proteus*. Endogenous cases may be bilateral and meningococcus and pneumococcus are most commonly encountered.[14] Clinically there is ocular pain with marked swelling and injection of the lids and conjunctiva and a hypopyon. Occasionally malignant tumours such as retinoblastoma may present with a similar clinical picture. Systemic infections such as meningitis may dominate.

Treatment consists of immediate admission and ophthalmic review. Conjunctival swab, full blood count, electrolytes, creatinine and blood culture are taken and intravenous access is attained. The patient is fasted and provisions made by the ophthalmic team for aqueous and vitreous biopsies. These specimens are plated on glass slides for urgent Gram stain as well as on blood, chocolate and Sabouraud's agar and in meat broth. Initial therapy is broad spectrum consisting of intravitreal, subconjunctival and systemic gentamicin and cephalothin. Topical atropine is given. The role of initial vitrectomy is controversial. Treatment is directed by the results of the cultures.

Fungal infections are rare and usually found in association with *Candida* septicaemia. The initial ocular complication is generally a discrete, fluffy white retinal lesion with overlying vitreous activity.

Lyme disease may present as a panophthalmitis and is caused by the spirochaete *Borrelia burgdorferi*. Other ocular manifestations include conjunctivitis, uveitis, vitritis, optic neuropathy, papilloedema and cranial nerve palsies.

REFERENCES

1 Molarte A B, Sherwin J I. Periorbital cellulitis in infancy. J Paediatr Ophthalmol Strabismus 1989; 26(5): 232–234.
2 Hogan P A. Impetigo: topical or systemic therapy? Curr Ther 1994; 55: 65–67.
3 Sheilds J A, Sheilds C L, Suvarnamani C, Schroeder R P, DePotter P. Retinoblastoma manifesting as orbital cellulitis. Am J Ophthalmol 1991; 112: 442–449.
4 Hopper K D, Sherman J L, Boal D K, Eggli K D. CT and MR imaging of the paediatric orbit. Radiographics 1992; 12: 485–503.
5 Jakobeic F A, Azar D. Neonatal conjunctivitis. Int Ophthalmol Clin 1992; 32(1).
6 Taylor H R, Fitch C P, Murillo-Lopez F, Rapoza P. The diagnosis and treatment of chlamydial conjunctivitis. Int Ophthalmol 1988; 12: 95–99.
7 Wakefeild D, McCluskey P J, Dunlop I, Penny R. Uveitis: aetiology and disease associations in an Australian population. Aust NZ J Ophthalmol 1986; 14: 181–187.
8 Rothova A, Buitenhuis H J, Meenken C et al. Uveitis and systemic disease. Br J Ophthalmol 1992; 76: 137–141.
9 Phaik C S, Seah S, Ong S G, Chandra M T, Hui S E. Anti-toxoplasma serotitres in ocular toxoplasmosis. Eye 1991; 5: 636–639.

10 Lam S, Tessler H H. Quadruple therapy for ocular toxoplasmosis. Can J Ophthalmol 1993; 28: 58–61.
11 Engstrom R E Jr, Holland G N, Nussenblatt R B, Jabs Da. Current practices in the management of ocular toxoplasmosis. Am J Ophthalmol 1991; 111: 601–610.
12 Yoser S L, Forster D J, Rao N A. Systemic viral infections and their retinal and choroidal manifestations Survey Ophthalmol 1993; 37(5).
13 Morinelli E N, Dugel P U, Lee M, Klatt E C, Narsing A R. Opportunistic intraocular infections in AIDS. Trans Am Ophthalmol Soc 1992; 90: 97–108.
14 Okada A A, Johnson R P, Liles W C, D'Amico D J, Baker A S. Endogenous bacterial endophthalmitis; report of a ten year retrospective study. Ophthalmology 1994; 101: 832–839.

SKIN

F. Bell   A. Finn

10.1   Exanthemata

INTRODUCTION

A great many childhood infectious diseases are accompanied by a rash or other cutaneous manifestation. The term exanthem is usually used to describe an acute infectious disease accompanied by a rash. It may alternatively describe the skin appearance itself, as enanthem is used to describe the appearance of the mucous membranes, for example Koplik's spots in measles.

Six 'classical' childhood exanthemata were described in the last century. The first two were scarlet fever and measles. Rubella was later recognized as a distinct entity. A fourth disease, scarlatina, was probably a milder form of scarlet fever. To these infections were later added erythema infectiosum or 'fifth disease' and roseola infantum, 'sixth disease'. This chapter describes these illnesses together with chickenpox and a number of enteroviral infections which may be accompanied by a rash.

In clinical practice, rashes are associated with many other infectious agents, including bacteria (e.g. staphylococcal or meningococcal disease, typhoid, Lyme disease), mycoplasma, rickettsiae, a wide variety of viruses (e.g. Epstein–Barr virus (EBV), adenovirus, cytomegalovirus (CMV)), fungi (e.g. candida), protozoa (e.g. toxoplasma) or parasitic infestation (e.g. scabies). In some children the relationship between rash and infection is less clear (e.g. erythema multiforme) or an infectious agent is suspected but not identified (e.g. Kawasaki disease, pityriasis rosea). Finally, infection may precipitate the presentation of underlying disease (e.g. guttate psoriasis following streptococcal upper respiratory tract infection or perianal disease).

Rash and fever may be presenting features of a wide variety of non-infectious processes. Rash may accompany food or drug sensitivity, autoimmune or collagen vascular disease (e.g. systemic lupus erythematosus (SLE), dermatomyositis, juvenile chronic arthritis), result from environmental factors (e.g. sunburn, contact sensitivity) or dermatological disease (e.g. atopic dermatitis, psoriasis). Even in the child at particular risk of infection, other factors may be responsible for the rash (e.g. infiltration by donor lymphocytes in graft-versus-host disease).

Cutaneous appearances, in particular the timing and distribution of rash, may provide important clues but are not always diagnostic in themselves: while the rash of measles begins behind the ears and progresses downwards in a characteristic fashion, in many children with erythematous rashes a specific diagnosis is not made and is unimportant as affected individuals make rapid and uneventful recoveries.

STREPTOCOCCAL INFECTION AND THE SKIN

In its most dramatic presentation streptococcal infection is responsible for the

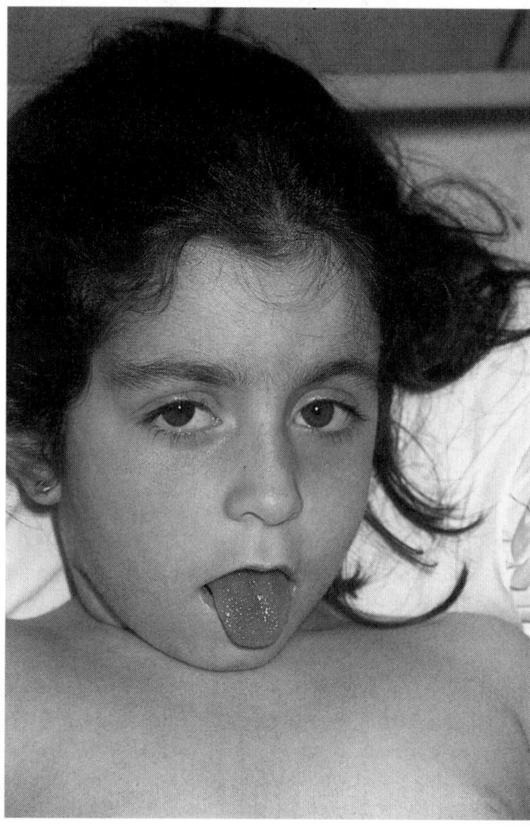

Fig. 10.1.1 This child presented with fever, sore throat and rash. A throat swab grew group A streptococcus. The rash of 'scarlatina' does not show all the features of classical scarlet fever. Note the 'strawberry tongue'. See also colour plate.

striking appearance of scarlet fever. Once a much feared childhood disease occurring in epidemics, scarlet fever is now relatively unusual but may be associated still with septic shock and fatal outcome. The illness results from infection with occasional strains of group A β-haemolytic streptococcus (*Streptococcus pyogenes*) which produce an erythrogenic exotoxin responsible for the rash. Lesser forms of the disease are common and the term scarlatina is sometimes used for infection in which the rash does not develop the classical appearance (Fig. 10.1.1). The site of infection is usually the pharynx or tonsils but the exanthem may result from infected burns, wound or skin infections. Scarlet fever and scarlatina may follow chickenpox. Occasionally infection with toxigenic staphylococci can produce a very similar clinical picture.

Group A streptococci are also an important cause of local skin sepsis. The term erysipelas is used to describe a superficial streptococcal cellulitis often involving the face or a limb, typified by a tender oedematous plaque of erythema with a sharply demarcated leading edge.

Scarlet fever

Epidemiology and spread

Infection is most common among school-age children and is unusual under 2 years of age. Transmission usually occurs by direct contact or respiratory droplets but is occasionally food-borne. The incubation period is short, between 2 and 5 days. Untreated cases remain infectious for a prolonged period but further spread is unlikely after 24 h of appropriate antibiotic therapy.

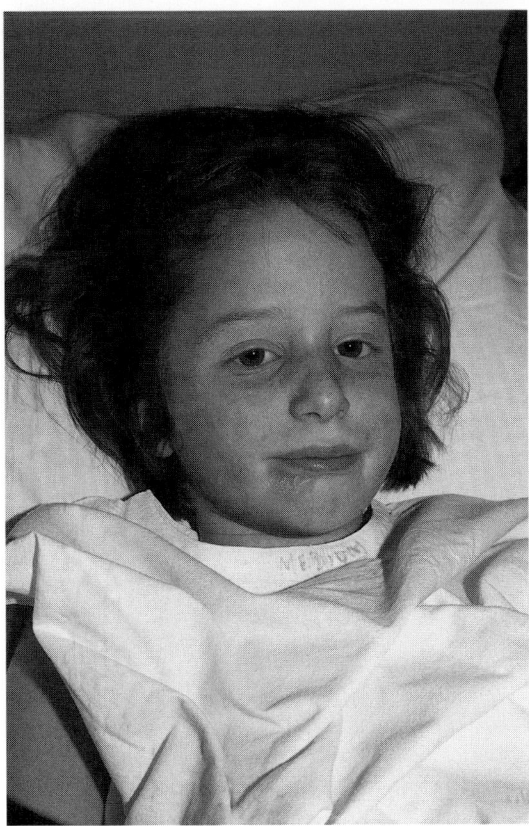

Fig. 10.1.2   Scarlet fever. Diffuse erythroderma with circumoral pallor. See also colour plate.

Clinical features and management

The illness is of abrupt onset with fever, vomiting, sore throat and abdominal pain. The severity of the pharyngitis is variable, often accompanied by tender lymphadenopathy and occasionally petechial palatal haemorrhages. The rash develops quickly, often within 12 h and always within 2 days of the onset of symptoms. The cheeks and forehead become flushed, and there is circumoral pallor (Fig. 10.1.2). A generalized confluent rash follows on the neck and trunk, sparser on the limbs but usually involving the palms and soles of the feet. The punctate rash feels like coarse red sandpaper — a background of erythema with superimposed tiny, raised, intensely red spots blanching on pressure. Pinpoint petechiae may occur in the flexures and produce a pathognomonic linear purpuric pattern (Pastia's lines) in the folds of the axillae and cubital fossae. The tongue is characteristically involved, initially coated with a thick, white layer through which swollen red papillae protrude ('white strawberry tongue'), followed several days later by peeling of the white layer to reveal the raw ('red strawberry') tongue. After a week the rash typically starts to desquamate, particularly on the hands and feet.

Occasional complications include otitis media or other focal sepsis, particularly if antibiotic treatment has been delayed. Non-suppurative complications, appearing some 2 weeks after infection, are unusual but include acute glomerulonephritis, rheumatic fever and erythema nodosum. Immunologically mediated, these complications are no more likely to follow scarlet fever than other group A streptococcal infection.

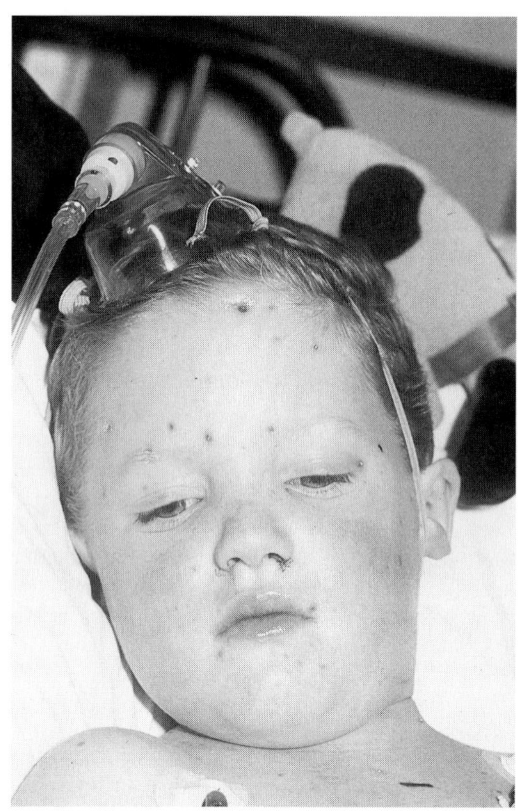

Fig. 10.1.3 Scarlet fever complicating chickenpox. Chickenpox lesions on forehead and rash with circumoral pallor. See also colour plate.

Treatment

Treatment with penicillin is indicated on clinical diagnosis or following bacterial culture. A 10-day course is needed to eradicate the organism and to prevent rheumatic fever. This requires careful discussion with the child and parents as clinical recovery will be complete before this time.

Diagnostic testing

Investigations should include a throat swab for bacterial and viral culture as clinical features may be difficult to distinguish from viral exanthemata (particularly adenovirus or EBV infection). In some centres rapid tests for group A streptococci are used. However, the organism may colonize the throat without symptoms and be isolated in the course of intercurrent illness. The blood count usually shows a neutrophilia. Antibody is produced to a number of bacterial products following streptococcal infection. The demonstration of raised anti-streptolysin 'O' or anti-DNase B titres some weeks later may be useful in confirming previous streptococcal infection, but these tests are not specific for group A disease.

MEASLES

Most adults have both heard of and had measles. This will not be so for very much longer. The spread of this ancient disease may have been increased by urbanization in the nineteenth century but now has been drastically reduced in the industrialized world by immunization. Measles is theoretically eradicable in that the virus is antigenically uniform and stable, there is no non-human reservoir, no carrier state and there is a highly effective vaccine. However, globally, problems with measles are far from over and it remains a leading cause of childhood mortality in many parts of the world.

Clinical features and management

In classical measles, a young child develops coryzal symptoms, exudative conjunctivitis, fever and malaise 10–14 days after exposure and may be markedly unwell with irritability and cough. A day or two later, Koplik's spots — white spots 1–2 mm across, sitting on an area of inflamed red buccal or labial mucosa — appear and may be the only clue to the diagnosis in a sick child. The rash — brick red, maculopapular and erythematous — appears 1–2 days later behind the ears and on the face and spreads down onto the trunk and limbs over 3–4 days, initially as discrete spots which coalesce to form large confluent red areas of skin (Fig. 10.1.4a). In black skin the erythema is not obvious; the rash is merely papular and followed by desquamation (Fig. 10.1.4b). The infectious period is approximately 3 days before to 4 days after the onset of the rash.

Measles in developed countries is often complicated by otitis media (2.5%), pneumonia (4%) and rarely by postinfectious encephalitis (2–10 per 10 000 cases). In the developed world, deaths occur at a rate of about 1 in 10 000 cases. Subacute sclerosing panencephalitis, a severe late progressive neurological form of the infection, has an incidence of 1 in 1 000 000 cases of measles, but is preventable by immunization. Measles is more serious in infants and young children in developing countries where malnutrition is common. The rash may be haemorrhagic and the infection complicated by stomatitis, candidiasis, diarrhoea, pneumonia and other problems. A complex association between the infection, associated anorexia, malnutrition and immunodeficiency (decreased T cell immunity) results in a mortality rate of around 10%, and increased mortality for up to a year following measles, in children in developing countries.

At present, measles is rare in countries where immunization rates are high but may be contracted when travelling abroad. Unvaccinated individuals previously protected by herd immunity may develop the classical syndrome, which tends to increase in severity with advancing age. Cases may occur in previously immunized individuals, some of whom have partial immunity and develop a mild modified form of the disease which is hard to distinguish from other exanthemata.

There is no specific therapy for measles. Cases in normal individuals are usually best managed out of hospital with antipyretic and analgesic therapy. When it occurs in severely immunocompromised patients there may be no rash, since T cells appear to be responsible for the rash, and disease may progress to involve multiple organs, in particular a giant cell pneumonitis which is almost uniformly fatal. The importance of an effective immunization programme in protecting this small but growing population should not be forgotten. All staff working with immunocompromised patients should be shown to be immune to measles. Such patients exposed to measles can be protected by administration of intramuscular immunoglobulin if it is given within 6 days. In such cases it may be valuable to seek expert advice.

Diagnostic testing

No one would have considered a diagnostic test necessary in the days of classical measles in toddlers. With mild modified measles and the importance of investigating outbreaks thoroughly this has changed. The standard approach has been to demonstrate seroconversion of anti-measles IgG or the presence of anti-measles IgM in blood. A test for specific IgM in saliva is reliable and less invasive. Immunofluorescence for measles antigen can be performed on nasopharyngeal secretions.

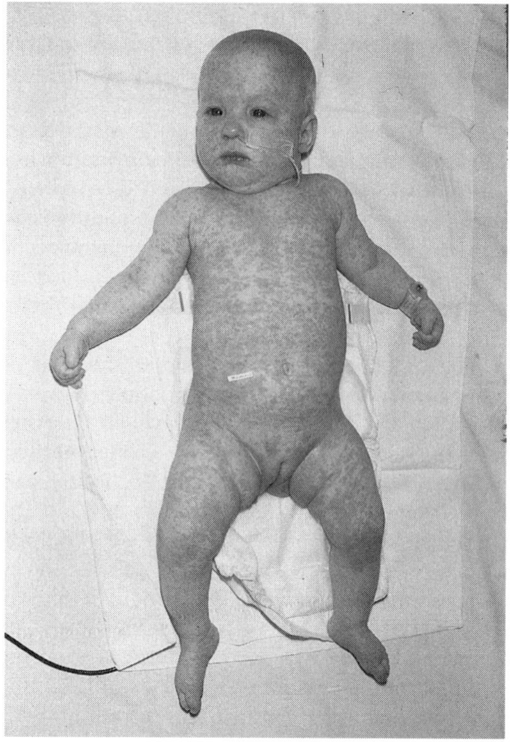

(a)

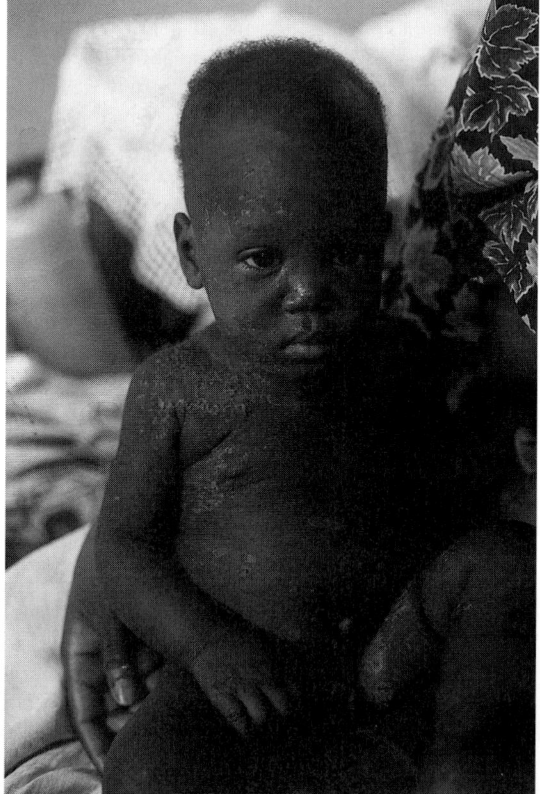

(b)

Fig. 10.1.4 (a) Maculopapular rash, confluent in places, of measles. (b) Measles in a black child: desquamating rash. See also colour plate.

Epidemiology and immunization

The effectiveness of measles vaccine has been established in the USA. In 1963, before the vaccine was licensed, there were 400 000 cases reported each year, but a national vaccination programme has resulted in a 99% reduction in cases.

In 1968 immunization with live attenuated measles vaccine was begun in the UK. For 15 years uptake rates remained low at around 50% and although the incidence of measles fell somewhat, it continued to occur widely in preschool children, so that one way or another more than 90% of children had measles antibody by the age of 10. During the 1980s, vaccine uptake rates increased steadily to over 90%, initially as measles vaccine and from 1988 as measles, mumps, rubella vaccine given as one dose during the second year of life.

Notifications of measles have fallen dramatically but the proportion of cases in older children has risen due to outbreaks among a large cohort of susceptible school-age children who had not been immunized or who were primary vaccine failures (vaccine efficacy is around 95%). Large outbreaks of measles among such populations have been reported in other countries. Many countries give children two doses of measles vaccine routinely, the first at 12–15 months and the second at school entry or at 10–16 years. A previous clinical diagnosis of measles does not contraindicate immunization.

RUBELLA (GERMAN MEASLES)

Rubella is another childhood illness which has become rare in many countries due to immunization. In childhood it is a mild disease and its main clinical significance is the spontaneous abortion or severe multisystem disease induced in babies infected transplacentally when a susceptible woman acquires the infection in early pregnancy. Thus a current shift in epidemiology towards infection during childbearing years is clearly of extreme importance. Congenital rubella is discussed in Chapter 12.1.

Clinical features and management

The clinical syndrome of rubella is often non-specific although there are sometimes characteristic features. Clinical diagnosis is unreliable, as other viruses including parvovirus B19 and enteroviruses can cause a rubelliform rash. Many infections are asymptomatic. A 2- or 3-day prodrome of malaise, fever, conjunctivitis and pharyngitis is common in adults and adolescents but rare in children, who generally develop a central, maculopapular, erythematous rash about 17 days after exposure, classically of discrete spots, which spread onto the limbs. Fever is mild and there is often characteristic postauricular or suboccipital lymphadenopathy, particularly in older patients in whom the rash is sometimes pruritic and accompanied by joint pains or arthritis. Encephalitis and thrombocytopenia are rare complications.

There is no specific therapy for rubella. Patients may be given antipyretics and analgesics as necessary. Intramuscular immunoglobulin has been used in rubella-exposed susceptible pregnant women but is far from reliable in preventing congenital rubella. Rubella may be infectious up to 7 days after the onset of the rash. Congenital cases may be infectious for up to a year or more.

Diagnostic testing

A specific diagnosis of rubella can be made by culture from upper respiratory secretions on special cell lines, but such cultures are not routinely available. In practice, however, the only situations where a specific diagnosis is imperative is in a pregnant woman or newborn suspected of having been congenitally infected and this is usually done serologically. In the former case a rising IgG titre may be documented and, in both, rubella-specific IgM may be detected. The diagnosis of congenital rubella is very difficult to confirm after infancy.

Epidemiology and immunization

The significance of congenital rubella syndrome became fully appreciated and led to the development of live attenuated rubella vaccine in the 1960s. Initially this vaccine was given to prepubescent schoolgirls in both the UK and Australia — a policy which had a significant impact on the incidence of congenital disease but not childhood rubella, despite relatively low initial uptake rates. In 1988, rubella vaccine was included in the universal childhood programme in the UK, and is given at 12–15 months to all children mixed with measles and mumps vaccine, as has been done elsewhere, e.g. the USA, for some years. This, combined with rising immunization rates, has resulted in effective herd immunity and rubella is now rarely seen in children.

ERYTHEMA INFECTIOSUM (FIFTH DISEASE, 'SLAPPED CHEEK' DISEASE)

Erythema infectiosum is the most frequent clinical manifestation of infection with human parvovirus B19. Striking erythema of the face, the 'slapped cheek' appearance, is followed by a rash which spreads to trunk and limbs.

Epidemiology and spread

Erythema infectiosum usually affects school-age children. It is often recognized in outbreaks but sporadic illness may occur. The incubation period is commonly 6–14 days but may extend to 3 weeks. Infection is spread by respiratory droplets. The illness is highly infectious in the early stage but viral shedding has usually ceased by the time of the appearance of the rash, rendering infectious precautions unnecessary. Attack rates within households may approach 40%. Infection is often asymptomatic; some 50% of the adult population show serological evidence of past infection with parvovirus B19.

Clinical features

A febrile non-specific prodrome may precede the appearance of the rash by a week. The characteristic exanthem develops in three stages. A confluent fiery red erythema first appears on the cheeks, accompanied by circumoral pallor. The outer margins of this area may be slightly raised. Over the next 1–3 days the rash spreads as a discrete maculopapular eruption, initially involving the proximal extensor surface of the limbs and later moving onto the flexor aspects and the trunk (Fig. 10.1.5). The rash fades over the next few days with central clearing giving rise to a lace-like or reticular pattern (Fig. 10.1.5), and has usually resolved within a week. In the third stage, lasting a further 1–3 weeks or more, the rash may continue to reappear and fade, often induced by environmental factors such as warmth and sunlight. Most children are not unwell and have little more than mild fever. In older children and adults the illness may be accompanied by more significant debility and an arthritis affecting hands, wrists and knees. Uncomplicated erythema infectiosum requires no treatment.

Diagnostic testing

Diagnosis is usually clinical and is straightforward when the disease occurs within an outbreak. Confirmation is obtained by demonstrating antibody to the infecting agent (IgM antibody is usually detectable with the onset of rash). It may be possible (e.g. in the immunosuppressed) to demonstrate the presence of the virus by electron microscopy or using the polymerase chain reaction.

Complications of parvovirus B19 infection

The virus has a predilection for infecting and destroying erythroid precursor cells, resulting in mild transient anaemia. This is of significance only in indivi-

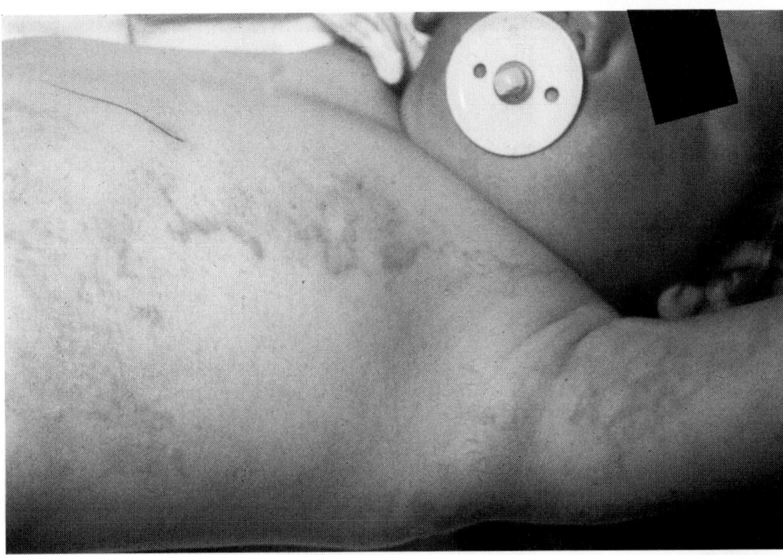

Fig. 10.1.5 Fifth disease. Slapped cheek appearance and lacy rash on trunk. See also colour plate.

duals with shortened red cell survival such as hereditary spherocytosis, sickle cell disease or thalassaemia, where infection may lead to severe aplastic crisis necessitating blood transfusion. Infection in the immunocompromised child may give rise to chronic anaemia. Maternal infection in pregnancy may lead to stillbirth or fetal hydrops due to fetal anaemia. This can be treated with intrauterine blood transfusion.

ROSEOLA INFANTUM (EXANTHEM SUBITUM, SIXTH DISEASE)

Roseola infantum is a common exanthem in childhood. As many as 30% of children may be affected and almost all cases present before the age of 2 years.

Clinical features

The illness is characterized by the sudden onset of fever (often 39–40°C) without prodrome. Typically the fever resolves after 3–5 days, followed by the appearance of a widespread macular or maculopapular rash. The timing of the resolution of fever, followed often within hours by the striking appearance of the rash, typifies the disease. Infection is seldom accompanied by significant constitutional disturbance, although children are often irritable until the fever settles.

The rash affects principally the neck and trunk, often extending to the face and proximal extremities. The lesions are erythematous, 2–5 mm across, sometimes surrounded by a pale area. The rose-coloured macules remain discrete and rarely become truly confluent (Fig. 10.1.6). The rash may be present for a few hours or remain for up to 2 days. It is not pruritic and does not desquamate. There are few other consistent physical findings, although red throat and lymphadenopathy are sometimes seen. The rash closely resembles measles, but when it appears the child is well and afebrile, in contrast to the child with measles rash who is febrile and irritable. Investigations may show leucopenia with relative lymphocytosis after the initial stage of the illness.

Commonly these infants come to medical attention following a seizure associated with high fever. Other complications are unusual but meningoencephalitis and thrombocytopenia have been reported. Management simply involves the use of antipyretic agents and supportive measures.

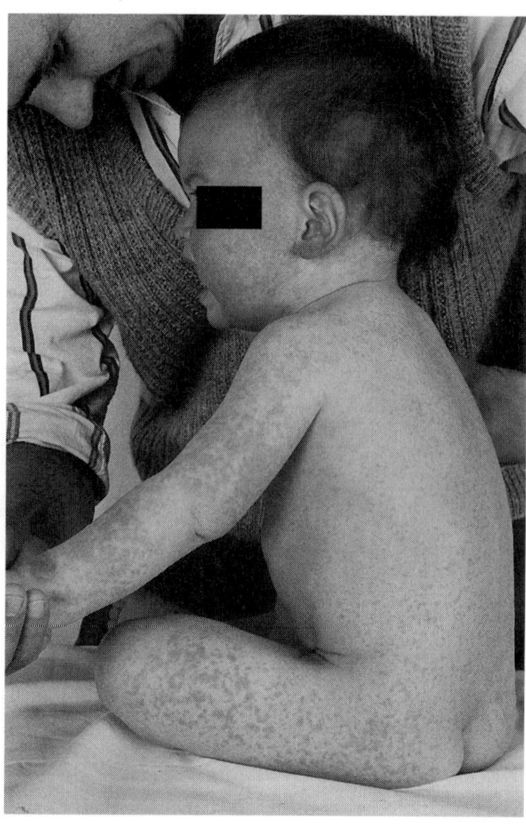

Fig. 10.1.6 Roseola infantum exanthem subitum or sixth disease. Morbilliform rash. See also colour plate.

Epidemiology and aetiology

Roseola is usually a sporadic illness, and although outbreaks have been described, direct spread is unusual. It is most common between the ages of 7 and 13 months. Human herpesvirus type 6 is thought to be responsible for the majority of cases of roseola infantum, although human herpesvirus type 7 has been implicated in a small number.

Young children with unexplained fever are sometimes given treatment with antibiotics. Recognizing roseola infantum as the cause of a rash appearing on the fourth or fifth day of a febrile illness may be important in avoiding labelling these children as antibiotic allergic.

ENTEROVIRAL INFECTION AND THE SKIN

Non-polio enteroviruses are a frequent cause of exanthemata in children, particularly through the summer and autumn. The agents responsible belong to the picornavirus (small RNA virus) family which includes the Coxsackie and echoviruses. The incubation period is usually short, between 3 and 5 days. Infection may occur in outbreaks.

Clinical features

Enteroviral infection may present in a variety of ways. Signs and symptoms are commonly non-specific, e.g. malaise and fever, but may include those of meningoencephalitis, myocarditis, conjunctivitis, hepatitis and stomatitis. Rash frequently accompanies infection and is particularly common in the younger child and in infection with certain subtypes, e.g. Coxsackie B5 and echo 9. There are, however, a wide spectrum of cutaneous manifestations even with infections caused by a single agent. Enteroviral rashes may be morbilliform (confluent measles-like), vesicular, urticarial, papular (Ch. 10.2), or even petechial. The latter can lead to concerns about possible meningococcal infection and such children should be closely observed and sometimes treated with intravenous antibiotics as a precaution. The rash accompanying echovirus infection is usually non-specific — a widespread but fleeting, fine, maculopapular eruption.

Diagnostic testing

Diagnosis usually depends on viral isolation from appropriate samples, e.g. throat swab or cerebrospinal fluid (CSF). Enteroviruses may be found in the stools of asymptomatic children and excretion frequently persists for some months after infection. Isolation of virus from faeces during a febrile illness does not therefore confirm causation. Paired serology may then be useful in demonstrating a rise in titre, but a group-specific complement fixation test, of relatively low sensitivity, is the serological test usually used, because of the large number of possible strains. Specific IgM against, say, Coxsackie B virus strains can be detected when a strain is grown or suspected.

Hand, foot and mouth disease

Hand, foot and mouth disease is a common enteroviral infection associated with characteristic cutaneous features. Coxsackie A16 is the agent most frequently responsible, although a number of other Coxsackieviruses and echoviruses may produce an identical clinical picture.

Epidemiology and spread

Transmission is via respiratory droplets, infected stools, or direct contact with the rash. It occurs as minor epidemics among preschool and younger school-age children.

Clinical features

Vesicles appear in the anterior mouth, most commonly on the tongue and buccal mucosa. These are often painful and accompanied by fever. The mouth lesions ulcerate and may be as large as 1 cm across. Shortly afterwards macules or vesicles surrounded by erythema involve the hands and feet (Fig. 1A.6.5), particularly on fingers and toes, lateral aspects of the palms, sides and soles of the feet. A maculopapular rash on the buttocks extending onto the thighs is often present but does not become vesicular. Children are seldom unwell and do not report other symptoms. There is no specific treatment. Skin lesions typically resolve within 1 week but may recur.

CHICKENPOX (VARICELLA) AND HERPES ZOSTER (SHINGLES)

Primary infection with the varicella zoster virus is responsible for chickenpox, usually a mild self-limiting systemic illness. Reactivation of latent varicella zoster virus gives rise to the cutaneous eruption of shingles. Thus, chickenpox and shingles, once thought to be caused by different viruses, are different manifestations (primary and secondary) of infection with the same virus.

Chickenpox

Epidemiology and spread

Chickenpox is a highly infectious disease usually affecting children between 2 and 8 years old. Most individuals have contracted infection and acquired immunity by adult life. Infection is spread by respiratory droplets or direct contact with a case. The disease is infectious from 1 day preceding the first appearance of the rash until the last vesicles are dry. The incubation period may be between 10 and 21 days but is usually approximately 16 days.

Clinical features and management

In young children there is no prodrome, the illness presenting first with fever and a macular rash on the scalp, face and trunk. In the early stages of the disease when it is not certain whether or not a child has chickenpox, the presence of lesions in the scalp, under the hair, can be very helpful. These are often itchy. The rash develops rapidly over the next 3–5 days with cropping of new lesions over the whole body in central distribution, more predominant on the trunk than limbs (Fig. 10.1.7). The skin lesions progress rapidly, becoming papular and then vesicular. Vesicles are typically round or elliptical, containing clear fluid with a margin of erythema. The rash is intensely pruritic and, if scratched as they form, vesicles may not be recognized. The contents become pustular, then lesions crust, dry and separate without residual scarring. The progression from macule to crust may be very rapid and typically lesions within crops coexist at various stages. Mucous membranes of the mouth, oropharynx and conjunctivae are usually involved. Fever of 38–39°C persists for 2–3 days, followed by gradual resolution.

The commonest complication is secondary staphylococcal infection of skin lesions. This may produce lesions of bullous impetigo spreading out from a centrally placed chickenpox vesicle. Bullous varicella can look quite alarming (see Fig. 10.1.8) but responds readily to antistaphylococcal antibiotics. Encephalitis, usually with predominantly cerebellar involvement is a well-recognized complication. Pneumonia is rare in children; resolution may lead to nodular calcification

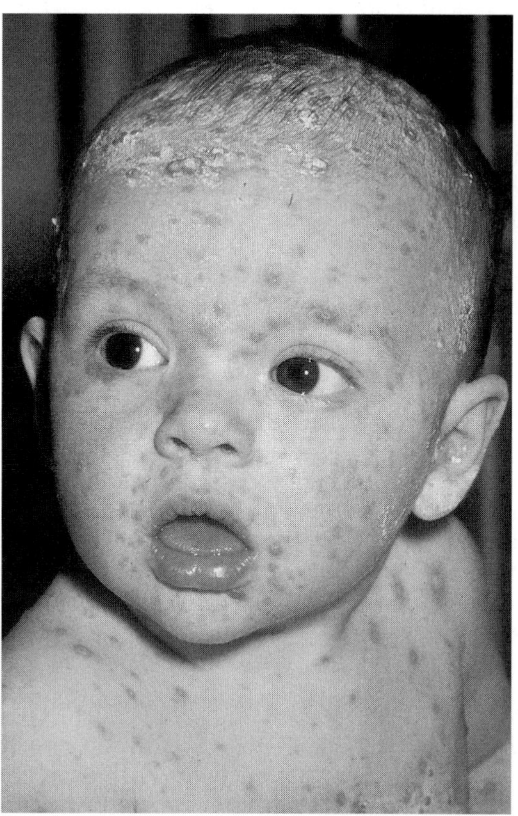

Fig. 10.1.7 Chickenpox. Vesicular lesions at different stages of development. White scalp due to calamine lotion to reduce itching. See also colour plate.

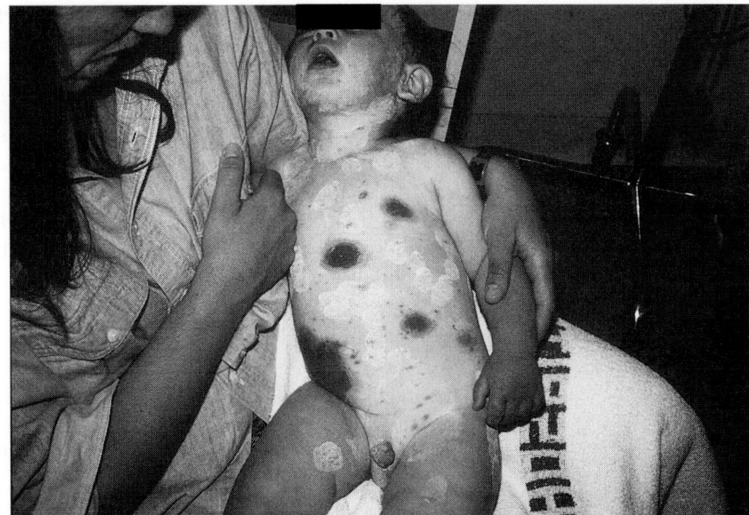

Fig. 10.1.8 Bullous varicella. Alarming appearance caused by staphylococcal superinfection of chickenpox. See also colour plate.

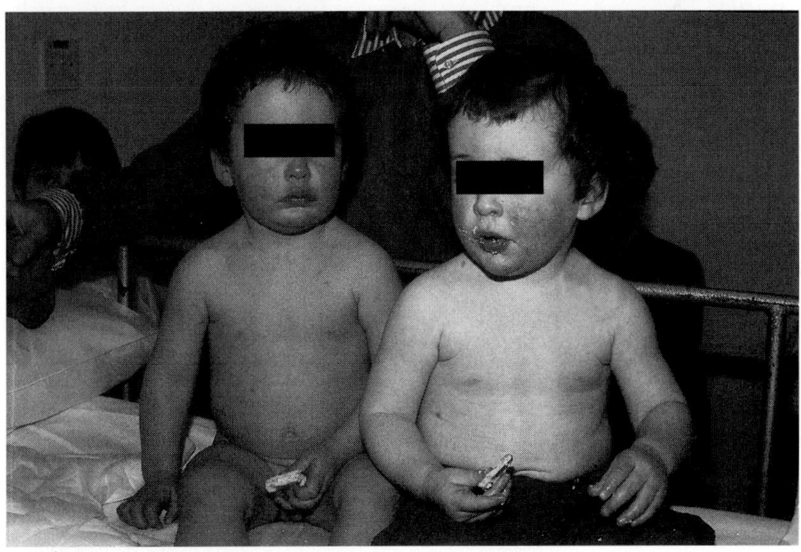

Fig. 10.1.9 Varicella and ampicillin. Ampicillin can cause a diffuse rash, here seen in one of twins with chickenpox, in VZV as well as EBV infections. See also colour plate.

on chest X-ray. Thrombocytopenia, hepatitis, arthritis, nephritis and pancreatitis may also complicate the disease. There is an association with Reye's syndrome, particularly in children who have received aspirin. Ampicillin may cause an erythrodermic rash with VZV infection (Fig. 10.1.9) albeit less frequently than with EBV.

Chickenpox may be a serious disease in the immunocompromised child. The illness is often prolonged, with crops of new vesicles appearing for several weeks. Varicella may disseminate with multiple organ involvement or may be complicated by severe bleeding and disseminated intravascular coagulation (haemorrhagic chickenpox). Some protection may be afforded by previous infection but children without detectable varicella antibody, with severe immunosuppression or significant immunodeficiency should be considered at risk. If in contact with chickenpox or zoster these individuals should be considered for prophylaxis with specific immunoglobulin (zoster immunoglobulin, ZIG) as soon as possible.

If lesions subsequently appear, treatment with acyclovir will modify disease and intravenous therapy is indicated in those with severe disease or complications. All staff working with immunocompromised patients should be shown to be immune to varicella. A live attenuated vaccine is available in some countries.

Because of high infectivity and danger to the immunocompromised, children with chickenpox should be managed away from hospital if possible. Should admission be necessary they require barrier nursing with appropriate control measures to avoid transmission of infection. Children with chickenpox are not infectious in the incubation period, an important point when deciding what constitutes a chickenpox contact.

Diagnostic testing

Diagnosis is usually clinical but may be difficult in the immunocompromised or in those in whom disease has been modified by treatment with ZIG or acyclovir. Confirmation by identification of varicella virus in vesicle fluid by electron microscopy or immunofluorescence may be helpful in these circumstances. The virus is labile and may not always be cultured successfully.

Varicella in pregnancy

Non-immune mothers exposed to chickenpox in pregnancy present a number of problems. Pregnant women are themselves at risk of fulminant disease and their infants may be also be affected. Infection between 8 and 20 weeks gestation may on rare occasions give rise to an embryopathy with limb hypoplasia, cicatricial skin scarring and CNS or eye malformations (Fig. 12.1.10). Infants exposed in utero and unaffected at birth may subsequently develop herpes zoster as maternal antibody declines. Maternal chickenpox around the time of birth may lead to

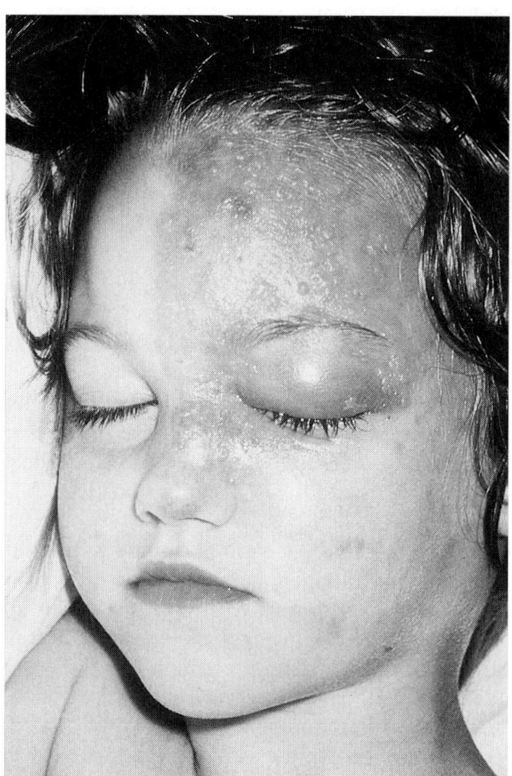

Fig. 10.1.10 Ophthalmic zoster: Herpes zoster of the ophthalmic division of the trigeminal nerve. See also colour plate.

severe neonatal varicella with a high incidence of pneumonitis and mortality of up to 20%. Infants particularly at risk are those born within 5 days of the appearance of maternal rash or whose mothers develop clinical disease within 48 h of delivery. These infants are at risk of transplacental infection before acquisition of protective maternal antibody. They should be given zoster immune globulin (ZIG) at birth and some authorities recommend additional prophylactic treatment with acyclovir. Infants should remain with their mother but both require isolation from other mothers and babies. Infection later in the neonatal period carries higher risks than childhood disease but is rarely life threatening.

Herpes zoster

Reactivation of virus latent in the dorsal root ganglion leads to a vesicular rash in the distribution of the affected sensory dermatome (shingles or zoster). This may reflect a suppression of cell-mediated immunity but may be seen in normal children.

Characteristically children who develop zoster have had primary chickenpox in early infancy, or were exposed to varicella in utero. The rash typically involves one to three unilateral dermatomes. The thoracic nerves are most commonly affected but any nerve root may be involved, including the cranial nerves. Involvement of the ophthalmic division of the trigeminal nerve may result in ocular damage (Fig. 10.1.10). This is likely if the rash extends to the tip of the nose, indicating involvement of the nasociliary branch of the fifth nerve. Advice from an ophthalmologist should be sought in this situation. Involvement of the geniculate ganglion can lead to vesicles on the pinna of the ear, the Ramsay-Hunt syndrome (Fig. 10.1.11).

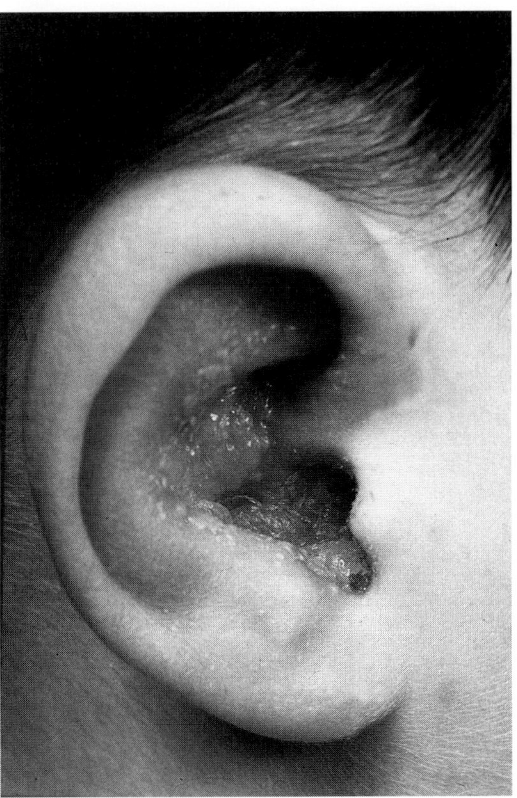

Fig. 10.1.11 Ramsay-Hunt syndrome: herpes zoster of the geniculate ganglion causing eruption on the pinna.

The vesicles are often larger than those of chickenpox and may coalesce. They progress through the same stages of crusting and healing as in primary infection. Isolated vesicles may appear away from the main eruption. The rash may be preceded by pain or paraesthesiae, diagnosis becoming clear when vesicles subsequently appear in the same distribution. Pain persisting after healing of the rash (post-herpetic neuralgia) is unusual in childhood.

Zoster is infectious; susceptible individuals in contact with shingles may subsequently develop chickenpox.

Acyclovir given as vesicles first appear is effective in shortening the course of the eruption which may otherwise persist for 2–3 weeks. Acyclovir should be used intravenously for ophthalmic herpes, but use of acyclovir is otherwise controversial.

FURTHER READING

Report of the committee on infectious diseases (1994 Red book), 23rd edn. American Academy of Pediatrics, 1994.
Plotkin S A, Mortimer E A, eds. Vaccines. Philadelphia: Saunders, 1988.
Feigin R D, Cherry J D, eds. Textbook of pediatric infectious diseases, 3rd edn. Philadelphia: Saunders, 1992.
Cherry J D. Contemporary infectious exanthems. Clin Infect Dis 1993; 16: 199–207.

10.2 Non-specific patterns of viral exanthem

There are many situations in which similar rashes can be produced by a variety of different viruses and where the same virus can produce a variety of different exanthemata.

The viruses particularly involved are enteroviruses, adenoviruses, hepatitis A and B, Epstein–Barr virus and cytomegalovirus. The most prominent of these are the enteroviruses.

The patterns seen can be divided into macular, papular, urticarial, purpuric, vesicular and/or pustular and erythrodermic. Various combinations of these may occur.

MACULAR EXANTHEMATA

These are usually very widespread and are characteristically difficult to differentiate from allergic reactions to drugs. In general, the occurrence of lesions in a linear distribution along scratch marks, exaggeration in areas of sunburn, under arm-bands, or on prior skin disease, and the presence of lymphadenopathy favour a viral over a drug aetiology.

PAPULAR EXANTHEMATA

The papules may be few or multiple and vary in size from tiny pinpoint lesions to 0.5–1.0 cm in diameter. The lesions in an individual case tend to be uniform in size. Pruritus is prominent. A linear distribution of groups of lesions is commonly seen and the limbs are usually affected more than the trunk. There is a special variant in which the lesions are restricted to the acral parts of the limbs and occasionally the face and in which occasional lesions may be vesicular (Fig. 10.2.1). This is called the papulovesicular acrolocated syndrome (PALS), and is the reaction pattern originally described as Gianotti–Crosti syndrome, an exanthem of hepatitis B. It is now clear that an identical pattern can occur with a variety of viruses and that the predominant cause varies from area to area. In Sydney, Australia, enteroviruses are by far the commonest cause and it is characteristically a reaction pattern of the 2–4-year age group. The condition may take up to 10 weeks to resolve and it is important that parents are made aware of this prolonged course at the outset.

URTICARIAL EXANTHEMATA

It is important to appreciate that in over 90% of cases of urticaria in children in

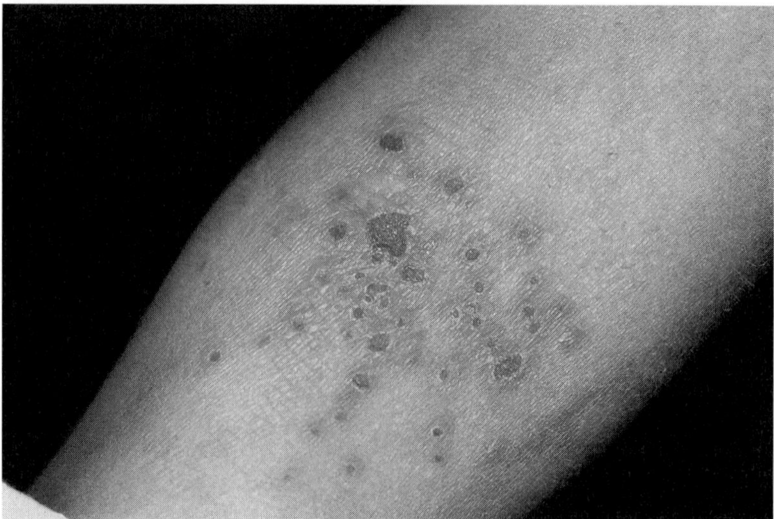

Fig. 10.2.1 Papular acro-located syndrome (PALS). See also colour plate.

the first 5 years of life the cause is a viral illness. Urticaria of viral origin is usually less pruritic than urticaria due to food or drug allergy. There is often some purpura in the centre of severe urticarial lesions in young children leading to a 'target-like' appearance that is frequently confused with erythema multiforme (Figs 10.2.2–10.2.5). The alteration in shape, and often disappearance of the erythematous component of individual lesions over a 12–24 h period, confirms the diagnosis of urticaria. The bruising colour change from the purpura takes a few more days to settle.

PURPURIC EXANTHEMATA

Enteroviruses are the commonest causes of purpuric exanthemata (Fig. 10.2.6).

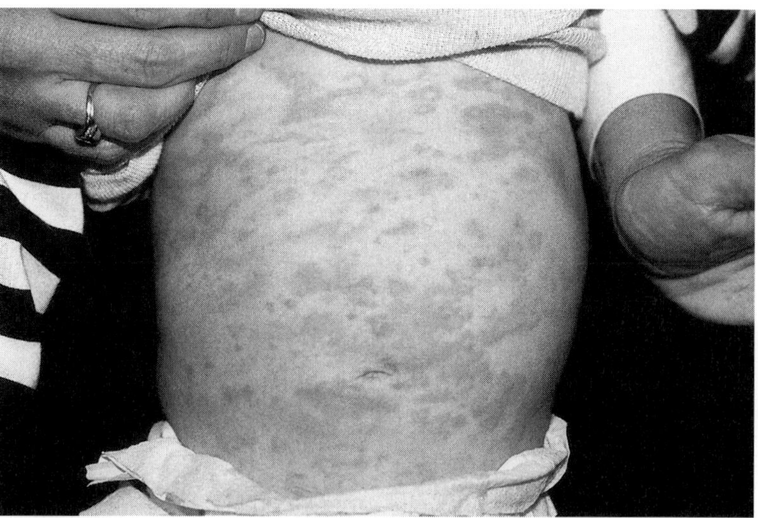

Fig. 10.2.2 Purple urticaria. Urticarial rash with purpura in some lesions; common and benign. See also colour plate.

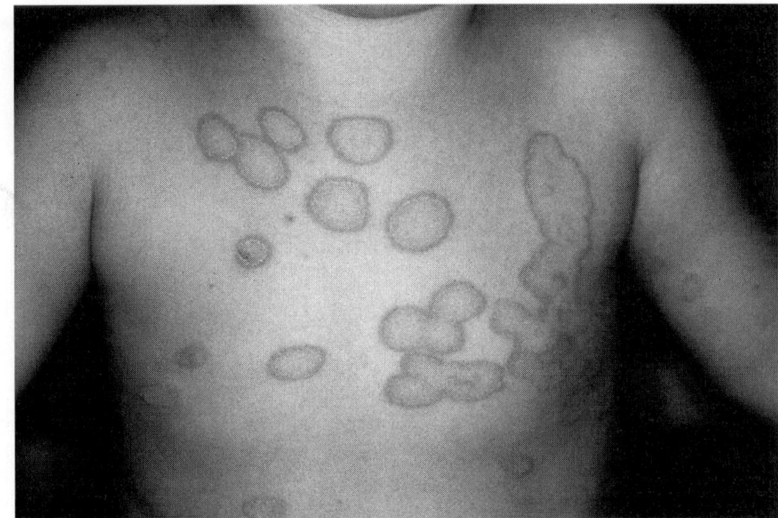

Fig. 10.2.3   Urticaria. Diffuse lesions, with central sparing, which migrate.

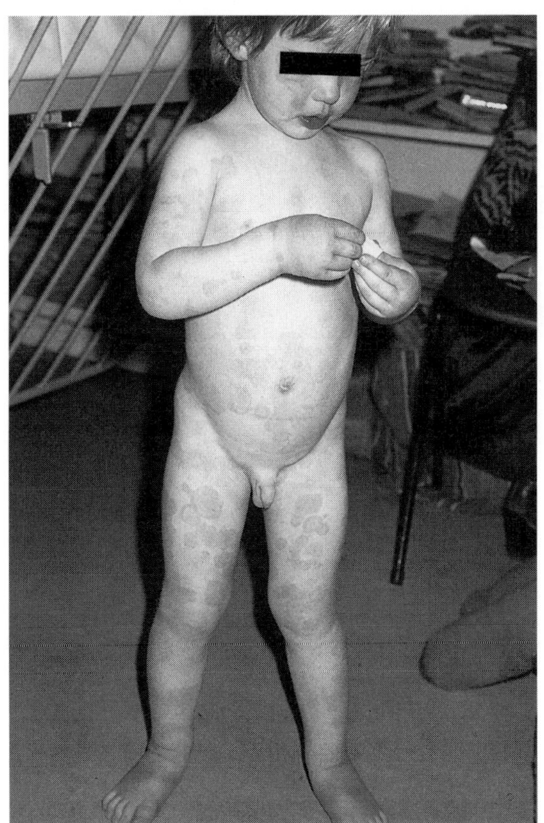

Fig. 10.2.4   Urticarial rash with joint swelling.

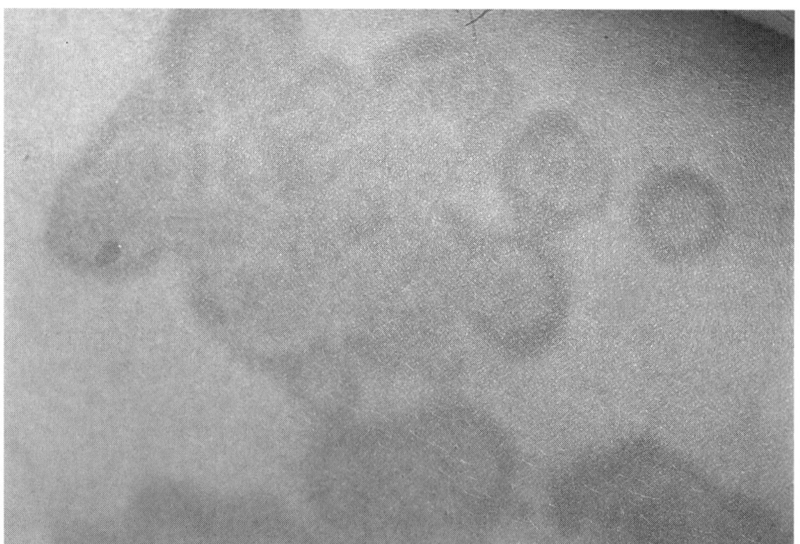

Fig. 10.2.5 Urticarial rash. Close-up.

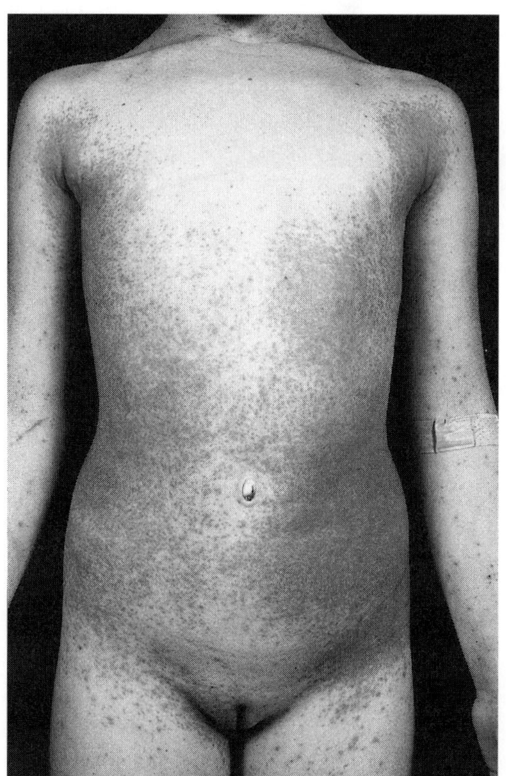

Fig. 10.2.6 Enterovirus exanthem. Dramatic rash, purpuric in places. See also colour plate.

Clearly the most important condition to be differentiated is meningococcal septi-caemia. The purpuric lesions caused by enteroviruses tend to be monomorphic, small petechial macules but larger, angulated lesions sometimes occur.

VESICULAR AND/OR PUSTULAR EXANTHEMATA

These lesions start as vesicles but often, as in varicella, become pustular and an admixture of lesions is seen. They often have an oval shape, which is unusual in varicella, and may become purpuric, leading to a characteristic grey colour of the pustule. The lesions are often concentrated mainly on the limbs. Hand, foot and mouth disease is a characteristic example. The buttocks are another common site of involvement.

ERYTHRODERMIC EXANTHEMATA

A rare exanthem presents with a generalized erythema, occasionally with super-imposed papules or pustules. The usual cause is staphylococcal or streptococcal toxin. It also mimics a variety of primary skin diseases, in particular erythrodermic psoriasis or generalized pustular psoriasis.

10.3 Cutaneous infections

IMPETIGO

Impetigo is caused by group A β-haemolytic streptococcus (GABHS) and *Staphylococcus aureus*, either alone or in combination. It occurs particularly in children under 6 years and is commonest in summer and autumn.

Impetigo is traditionally divided into two clinical types: bullous, and non-bullous or crusted.

Bullous impetigo

This presents, often on previously normal skin, as small vesicles which may develop into large bullae, with little or no surrounding erythema. They are filled initially with clear fluid which then becomes pustular (Fig. 10.3.1. The thin roof

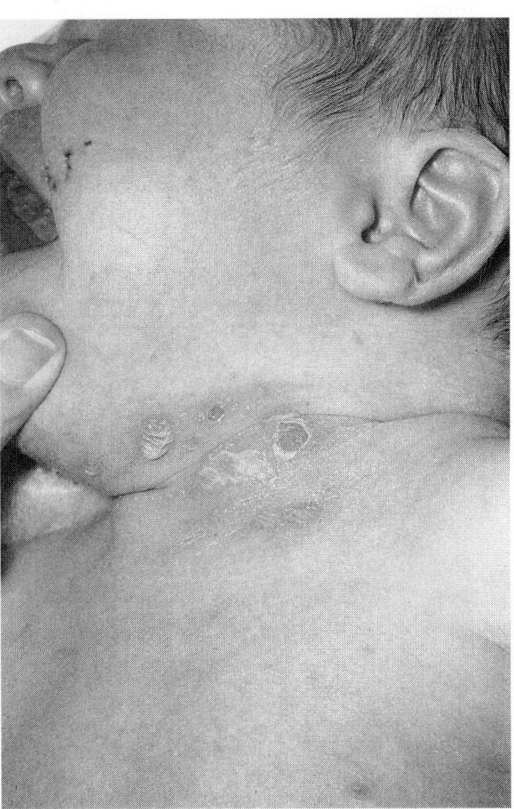

Fig. 10.3.1 Bullous impetigo in a neonate. Note pus-filled blisters.

of the bulla soon breaks and the base dries, leaving a lacquered appearance. The remains of the roof form a peripheral collarette of scale. The denuded lesions may expand to cover large areas in just a few days. The condition is usually painless, with no lymphadenopathy or systemic toxicity. Bullous impetigo is always caused by *S. aureus*, with the usual strain involved being group II, phage type 71.

The diagnosis of bullous impetigo is usually clinically obvious but bacterial culture is recommended for confirmation and to identify the sensitivity profile of the causative organism. The treatment of choice is a penicillinase-resistant penicillin, given orally. The incidence of erythromycin resistance of *S. aureus* is increasing but varies from area to area and one must be aware of the status of the local *S. aureus* strains before considering this agent as initial treatment.[1,2]

Of particular importance is bullous impetigo in the neonate. Rarely, in the setting of premature rupture of the membranes, lesions may be present at birth. Most cases, however, develop in the second week of life and the usual source is a cord infection in situations where the antistaphylococcal cord care practices in the neonatal nursery are suboptimal. Early treatment of neonatal bullous impetigo with systemic antibiotics is very important as, unlike in older children, it may be complicated by septicaemia, septic arthritis, osteomyelitis and other serious systemic infections.

Non-bullous or crusted impetigo

This may occur on normal skin or be superimposed on other skin diseases such as atopic dermatitis, insect bites and scabies. The earliest lesion is a small vesicle or pustule which soon ruptures to be replaced by an expanding yellow-brown crust (Fig. 10.3.2).

Studies prior to the late 1970s suggested that GABHS was the primary aetiological agent in most cases of non-bullous impetigo and that when *S. aureus* was cultured it represented a secondary invader or contaminant. However, recent studies, based on both increased frequency of isolation of *S. aureus* and treatment failures with penicillin, indicate that in many parts of the world *S. aureus* must now be regarded as the primary pathogen of non-bullous as well as bullous impetigo. However, in some areas, including the Pacific Islands and the Northern Territory of Australia, GABHS does persist as an important pathogen in impetigo.

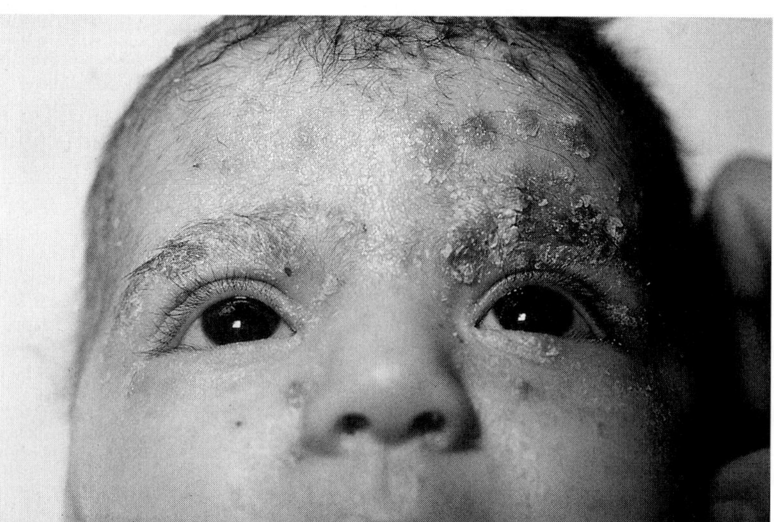

Fig. 10.3.2 Impetigo. Weeping and crusted lesions.

Non-bullous impetigo is usually superficial and heals without scarring. Occasionally streptococcal disease becomes invasive, producing deep punched-out ulcers (ecthyma), with local cellulitis and lymphadenopathy and scarring sequelae. Group A streptococcal infection of the skin may cause a spreading cellulitis, with a sharply demarcated edge, called erysipelas (Fig. 10.3.3), once a dreaded disease with a high mortality. Rheumatic fever has not occurred following streptococcal impetigo but acute glomerulonephritis is a well-recognized complication.[3] Repeated urinalyses should be performed whenever a streptococcal skin infection is diagnosed.

It is important to be aware of the situation in one's own local area to make appropriate decisions regarding investigation, treatment and follow-up. Ideally, bacterial culture and sensitivity testing should be obtained. If an antibiotic is commenced prior to the results being available, an agent which covers both GABHS and *S. aureus* should be chosen, using a penicillinase-resistant penicillin, a cephalosporin or erythromycin in those areas where resistance of *S. aureus* to this agent is rare. If GABHS is cultured penicillin V is the treatment of choice. There is recent enthusiasm for the use of topical mupuricin in impetigo as an alternative to oral antibiotics. Mupirocin in a 2% concentration has anti-bacterial activity against *S. aureus* and GABHS. Development of resistance is uncommon. It may have a place as sole therapy in some cases of localized impetigo but its effectiveness is doubtful when the disease occurs in inaccessible areas such as the nares, in the napkin area and periorally in a child who constantly licks the area. It is inappropriate in widespread disease.

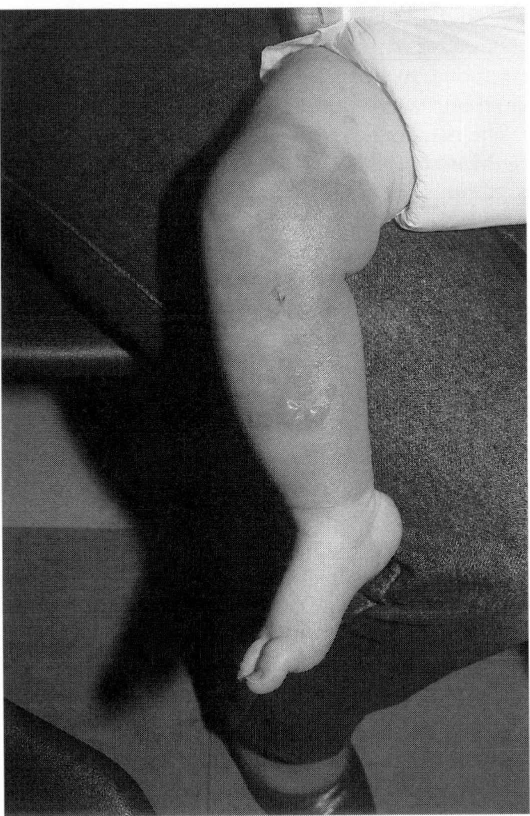

Fig. 10.3.3 Erysipelas. Group A streptococcal cellulitis with sharp leading edge. See also colour plate.

SECONDARY INFECTION OF ATOPIC DERMATITIS

Staphylococcus aureus is a frequent invader of damaged skin. Colonization by *S. aureus* is an almost constant phenomenon in atopic dermatitis. In a recent study *S. aureus* was isolated from the affected areas in 90% of a group of children with atopic dermatitis as compared with an isolation rate of 5% from the skin of controls.[4] Secondary staphylococcal infection of atopic dermatitis may present as clinical impetigo but more commonly simply as a worsening of the dermatitis with increased redness, exudation and itching. This reaction may be explained not only by the actual infection but also by both immediate and delayed hypersensitivity reactions to the staphylococccal antigens. Secondary infection of atopic dermatitis usually responds well to appropriate antibiotics used in conjunction with standard therapy for the underlying disease. It is important to note that an early herpes simplex infection superimposed on eczema may be mistaken for a bacterial infection and this condition should be considered if the response to antibiotics is not as expected.

FURUNCULOSIS

Furuncles or boils are cutaneous abscesses centred around hair follicles, caused by certain species of coagulase-positive *S. aureus*. While boils may occur in previously normal skin, local predisposing factors are cutaneous injury, friction and sweating. Patients with anaemia, diabetes mellitus, neutrophil chemotactic defects and hypogammaglobulinaema are at particular risk, but most patients are otherwise clinically well.

Episodes of furunculosis are often recurrent and many patients with recurrences are found to carry furuncle-producing strains of *S. aureus* in nostrils, axilla or groin or to have close contact with someone who does.

The management of furuncles depends on their maturity. Early lesions should be treated with warm compresses and oral penicillinase-resistant penicillins. Erythromycin may be used in patients allergic to the preferred antibiotics but is no longer a treatment of choice due to the development of bacterial resistance, which is particularly prevalent in the strains of *S. aureus* causing furunculosis. Incision into early lesions should be avoided but once the lesions have matured and pointed, incision and drainage may occasionally be indicated in conjunction with the use of antibiotics. Incision should, however, be avoided in lesions located in the areas of upper lip, nose, central brow and external auditory canal, where uncontrolled infection may cause cavernous sinus thrombosis.

Chronic and recurrent furunculosis should be treated with a course of antibiotics of several weeks duration. While the patient is on antibiotics all clothing, towels and bed linen which have contacted the affected areas should be washed in hot water. Attempts should be made to deal with the carrier state in the patient and/or close contacts, who should always be investigated also. Washing of the groin, axilla and hands with an antiseptic soap can help, as can topical nasal antibiotics such as mupirocin. Oral rifampicin has also been successful in reducing carriage but should not be used alone because of the rapid development of resistance.

PERIANAL STREPTOCOCCAL DISEASE

This is a distinctive perianal eruption due to group A β-haemolytic streptococcus

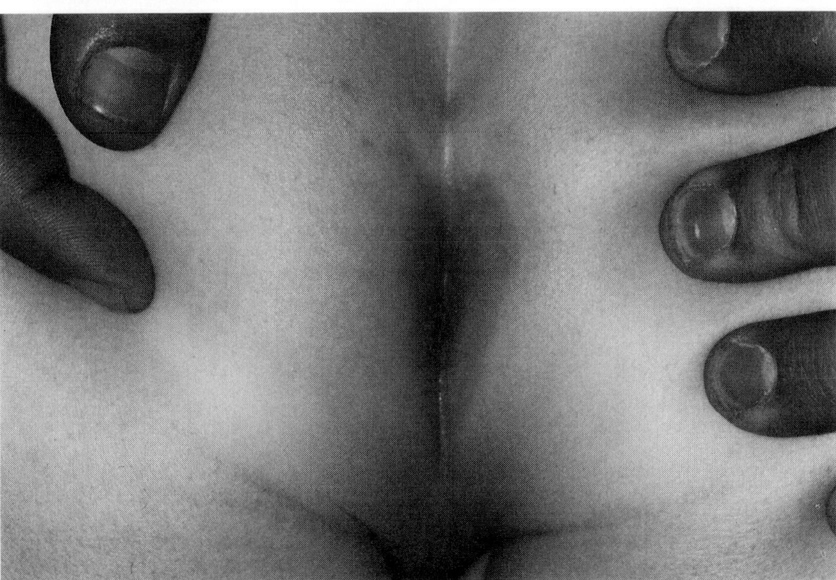

Fig. 10.3.4 Perianal streptococcal disease.

(GABHS). It was originally designated perianal streptococcal cellulitis. More recently, as its superficial nature has been recognized, the terms perianal streptococcal disease and perianal streptococcal dermatitis have been used.[5]

The peak incidence is in children 3–4 years of age but it may occur in infants. A likely mode of transmission is digital contamination from an infected oropharynx, and many patients have positive pharyngeal cultures of the same streptococcal strain isolated from the perianal area, although symptoms of pharyngitis are rarely present. The child complains of pain on defaecation and often refuses to open the bowels; bright blood is frequently seen on the stool. On examination a bright pink erythema extends from the anal rim, which is often fissured and macerated, out 2–3 cm from the anus (Fig. 10.3.4); the skin is tender but not indurated, and lymphangitis and lymphadenopathy are absent.

The diagnosis is established by culture, on blood agar, of GABHS from a swab of the perianal skin. The laboratory should be specifically requested to culture for GABHS as many routinely process perianal swabs on selective media designed to identify the common enteric pathogens. Patients may demonstrate an associated GABHS balanitis or vulvovaginitis.

The treatment of choice is oral penicillin V 50 mg/kg per day in four divided doses combined with the use of topical mupirocin twice a day. Recurrences are very frequent without this combined therapy, which should be continued for 10 days. Erythromycin is appropriate in penicillin-allergic patients.

STAPHYLOCOCCAL SCALDED SKIN SYNDROME

Staphylococcal scalded skin syndrome (SSSS) is a generalized blistering and peeling condition caused by an exfoliative toxin produced by certain strains of *Staphylococcus aureus* (Fig. 10.3.5).[6] The site of the infection may be a purulent pharyngitis, rhinitis, conjunctivitis, wound or neonatal umbilical infection. The condition is most often seen in children under 5 years. It begins with irritability

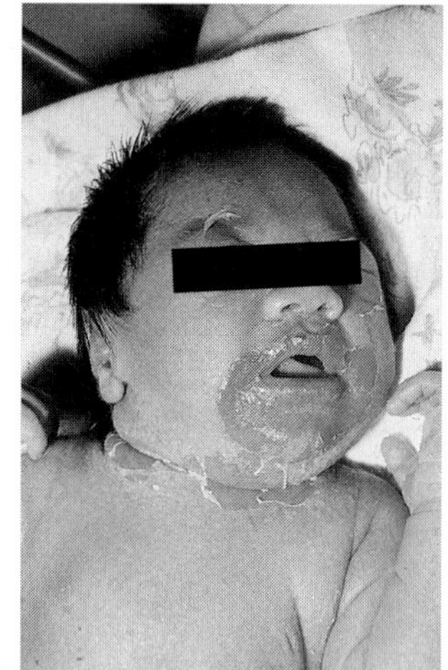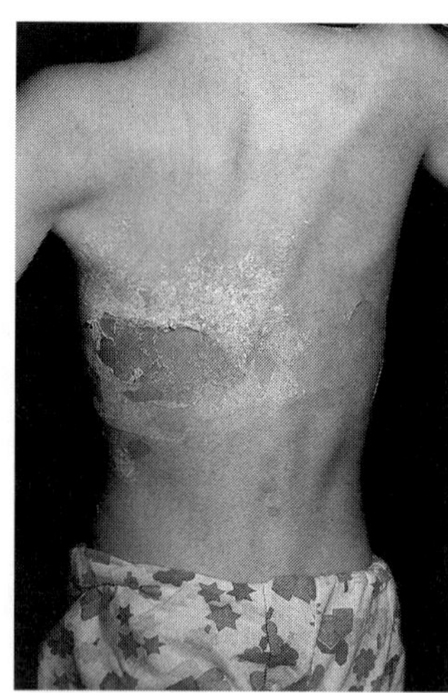

Fig. 10.3.5 Staphylococcal scalded skin syndrome. **A** In a neonate. **B** In an 8-year-old boy.

and fever. There is a marked skin tenderness and macular erythema beginning around the lips and nose and then becoming generalized, being most prominent in the flexures. The mucosae remain unaffected. After 1–2 days, the tender skin begins to wrinkle and occasionally flaccid bullae develop. The skin then peels off in large superficial wet sheets. The denuded areas become dry, crusted and fissured and heal without scarring.

Cultures of skin and blister fluid are negative and a site of primary staphylococcal infection should be sought. This will reveal the responsible *S. aureus* usually phage group II and particularly types 3A, 3C, 55 and 71.

During the early erythrodermic phase the differential diagnosis includes staphylococcal scarlet fever, Kawasaki disease and toxic shock syndrome. In the blistering stage Stevens Johnson syndrome (SJS) and toxic epidermal necrolysis (TEN) must be differentiated. In these conditions the split is subepidermal, whereas in SSSS it occurs high in the epidermis. The clinical apppearance in SJS and TEN usually attests to the deeper level of the split in the skin but rapid histological studies can be used if necessary for confirmation.

Management of SSSS includes supportive measures such as non-stick sterile sheets, analgesia and intravenous fluids if oral fluids are not adequately ingested. Handling, even by parents, should be kept to an absolute minimum as an extreme tenderness is a universal finding. Treatment with penicillinase-resistant antibiotics is important but may not significantly alter the clinical course if started too late. It will, however, reduce the chance of septic complications. Systemic steroids are absolutely contraindicated. Emollients may be helpful later in the course of the illness but should be avoided in the early stages.

ERYTHEMA MARGINATUM

This is a distinctive urticarial eruption which is seen in about 25% of patients with rheumatic fever. The lesions are initially erythematous papules which spread to form annular and polycyclic configurations. They are transient, lasting only for several hours, and are seen most often in the evening in febrile patients. Unlike common urticaria the lesions are not itchy. The aetiology remains obscure.

ERYTHEMA ANNULARE CENTRIFUGUM

This is the distinctive eruption seen at the onset of infection with the Lyme disease spirochaete, *Borrelia burgdorferi*, which is introduced by the bite of a tick. An itchy red papule appears at the site of the bite and after some days an erythematous ring develops around the papule. The ring slowly expands and may reach over 30 cm in diameter, with the central papule usually persisting (Fig. 8.1.2). Whether secondary lesions occur or whether all lesions originate at the site of a bite remains controversial. The expansion of the cutaneous lesion is accompanied by the onset of the systemic symptoms and signs of the disease, which are described elsewhere in this text (Ch. 8.1).

PEDICULOSIS

Human lice, being ectoparasites, are dependent on man for survival. They are six-legged insects without wings, grey in colour or brown-red when engorged with blood. The body louse and the head louse have a thin body 2–4 mm long and three similar pairs of legs; the pubic louse is wider and shorter and the second and third pair of legs are larger than the first, producing a crab-like appearance. The ova (nits) appear as oval grey-white 0.5 mm specks, attached by a firm chitin ring to hairs or clothes (Figs 10.3.6, 10.3.7).

Pediculosis capitis (head lice) is a common infestation, often occurring in epidemics in schools. The occipital area of the scalp is preferentially involved and may be the only site affected. The condition is itchy, leading to scratching with excoriations and also eczematization and secondary infection which may mask the underlying infestation. Permethrin shampoos are effective pediculicides but may not destroy ova, and a repeat application after a few days is recommended to kill further hatched lice. Removal of nit cases with a fine comb is easier if the chitin is softened by a prior application of vinegar.

Pediculosis corporis (body lice) is rare in children except in severely overcrowded conditions with poor hygiene. The organism infests bedding and clothing and the nits are not found on the human host. The lice hatch with body warmth

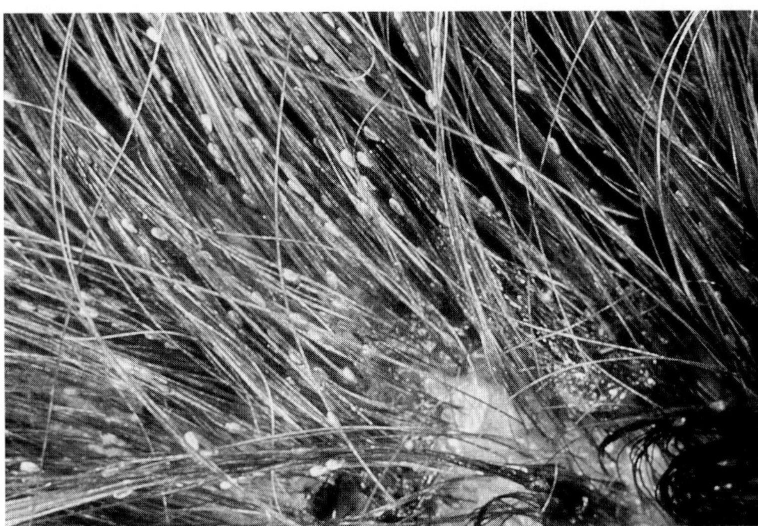

Fig. 10.3.6 Head lice. Note eggs cases (nits).

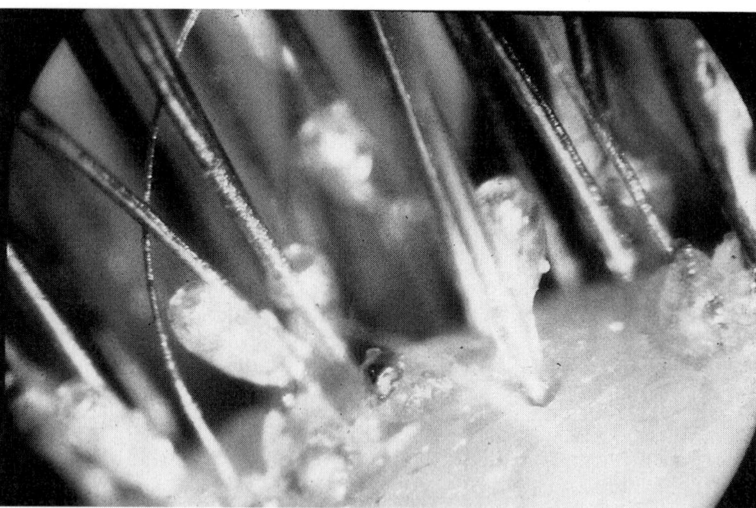

Fig. 10.3.7 Eyelash lice. Close-up of egg cases.

and puncture the skin, producing very itchy, small, red papules with haemorrhagic puncta. Spots of dried blood may be found on the clothing and bed linen. Treatment is directed towards removal of the organisms from materials with hot water laundering and hot ironing or the use of a hot electric drier.

Pediculosis pubis (pubic lice, crab lice) is mainly an adult disease. The pubic louse has as its normal habitat the anogenital area, but in children it is particularly seen on the eyelashes and occasionally at the anterior scalp margins. Eyelash infestation in children may occur from innocent close contact with an affected adult but the possibility of sexual abuse must always be considered. Pediculosis of the eyelashes is best treated with petroleum jelly applied thickly twice a day for a week.

SCABIES

This is an infection caused by the mite *Sarcoptes scabei* and transmitted under circumstances of close physical contact. A small number of mites burrow into the skin in several characteristic sites; these are palms and soles in infants and at any age between the fingers, wrists, axillae, nipples, penis and scrotum (Fig. 10.3.8). The pathognomonic curved 2–3 mm long burrow (Fig. 10.3.9) is often masked by scratch marks, secondary eczema and secondary bacterial infection (Fig. 10.3.10). Other markers of the sites of mite invasion are small papules and blisters. The secondary eruption of scabies is often the presenting feature, with multiple, excoriated papules most prominent on abdomen, buttocks and inner thighs. Severe nocturnal irritation is characteristic and a marked dermographism at the sites of scratching is a particular feature in infants.

Large inflammatory nodules may occur at the sites of burrows or as part of the secondary eruption and sometimes they are the predominant feature, leading to diagnostic difficulties.

Available scabicides vary from country to country but the ideal treatment is with a single 8–14 h application of 5% permethrin cream. This has proved effective, safe and of low irritability.[7] No disinfection of clothing is required. It is important to treat everyone in close physical contact with the patient also.

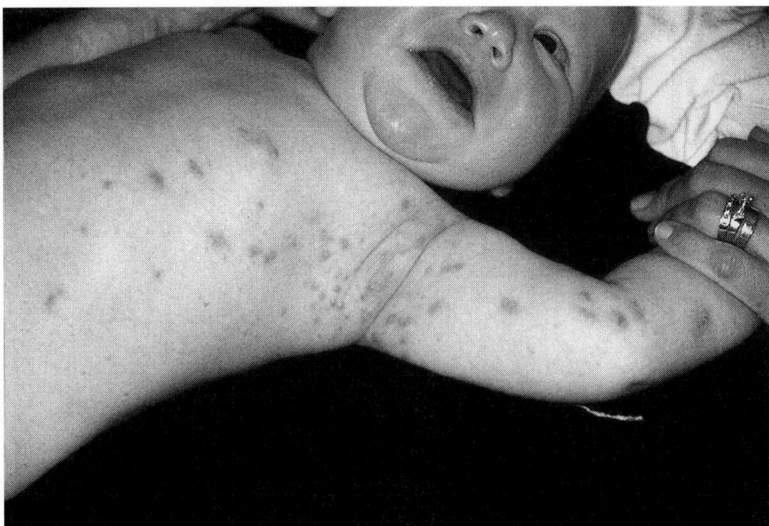

Fig. 10.3.8 Scabies. Note nodules around axilla

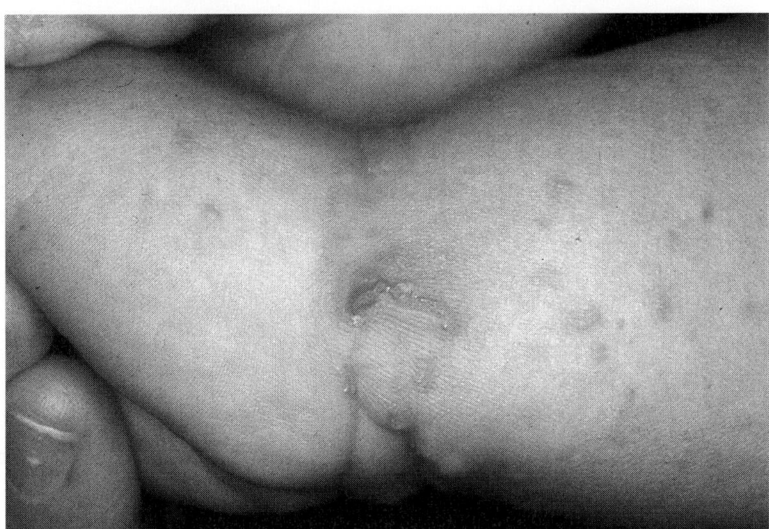

Fig. 10.3.9 Scabies. Characteristic burrow.

Nodules, which may persist despite successful treatment, usually respond to a 20% coal tar solution applied daily.

TINEA

Tinea is an infection due to dermatophyte fungi from human, animal or soil sources. It occurs on any part of the skin surface and may involve nails and hair.

On the skin the characteristic lesions are erythematous and scaly, often studded with papules or pustules, with a tendency to clear centrally and spread peripherally, producing annular or geographical configurations (Fig. 10.3.11). The lesions are asymmetrically distributed, which is a useful differentiating point

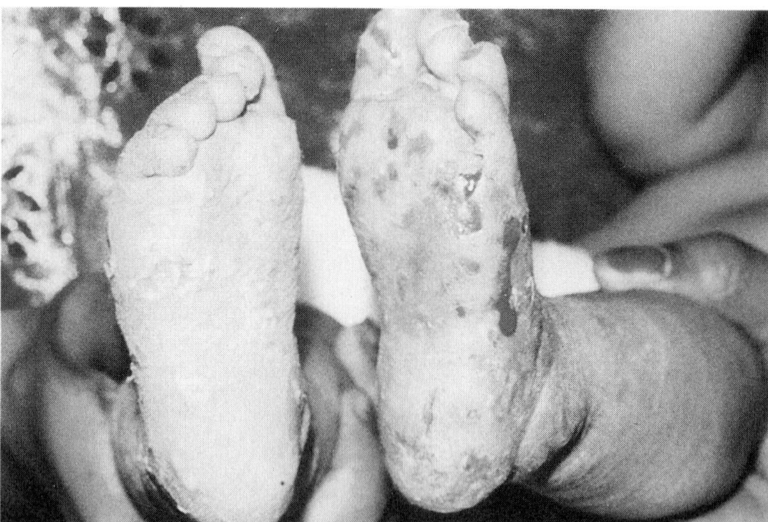

Fig. 10.3.10 Infected scabies. Impetiginous infection of the foot complicating scabies. See also colour plate.

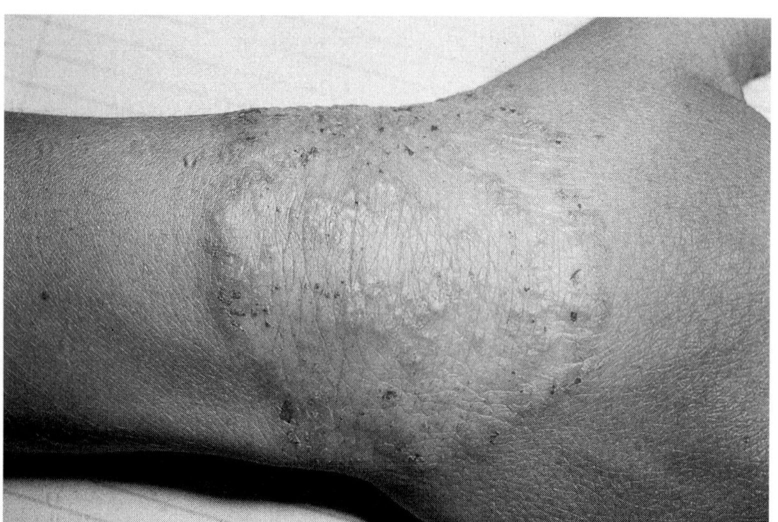

Fig. 10.3.11 Tinea corporis on back of hand, where cat may have rubbed, showing papules and pustules.

from discoid eczema and psoriasis which may also present as annular scaly lesions. Nail tinea, which is rare in children, produces a white crumbling nail plate and subungual scale.

On the scalp there is a characteristic combination of inflammation and alopecia with short broken hairs. Depending on the type of hair invasion by the fungus the hairs are broken off almost flush with the scalp or at 2–5 mm (Fig. 10.3.12). The signs of inflammation vary from a mild erythema and scale to a pustular carbuncle-like lesion (kerion) (shown in Fig. 10.3.13).

The Wood's light is useful in the diagnosis of some types of scalp tinea, with the infected hairs fluorescing a bright-green colour. Other varieties of scalp tinea do not fluoresce and the Wood's light has no place in the diagnosis of tinea of the skin surface. The diagnosis of tinea is confirmed by scraping scales or hair

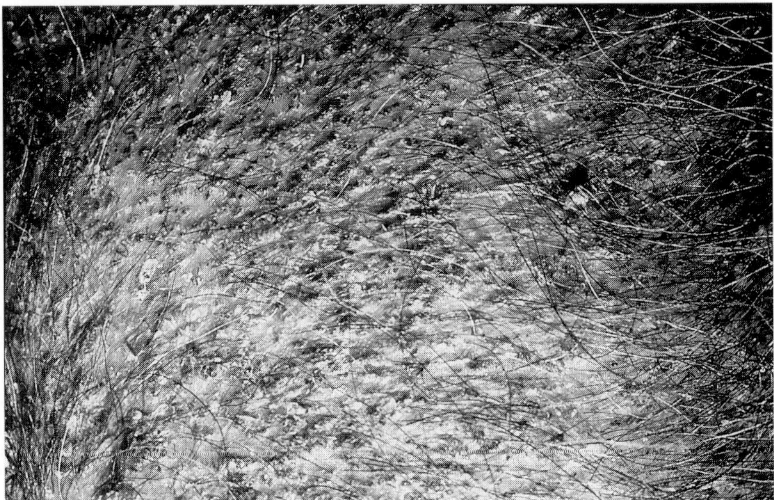

Fig. 10.3.12 Black dot tinea capitis. Hairs broken flush with scalp form black dots.

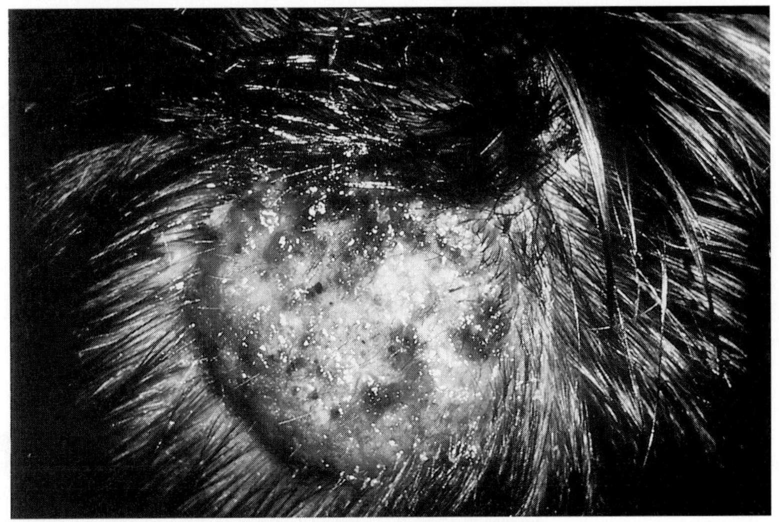

Fig. 10.3.13 Boggy swelling of the scalp due to tinea capitis with superinfection.

onto a slide, adding 20% potassium hydroxide and examining microscopically. Septate branching hyphae are seen in the scales and massed spores in or around the hairs. The fungus can be cultured on appropriate media.

Topical antifungals may be effective for small localized patches of tinea on the skin but oral griseofulvin is the treatment of choice for hair and nail tinea and extensive cutaneous disease. In general a 3-month course of griseofulvin is used but nail disease requires longer treatment.

MOLLUSCUM CONTAGIOSUM

This is a poxvirus infection, occurring particularly in the 2–5-year age group. Outbreaks occur in children who bath together or swim in heated pools.

The lesions are spherical and pearly white, usually 1–3 mm in diameter but sometimes larger, with a central umbilication. Common sites are the axillae and sides of the trunk and the anogenital area. When they occur on the eyelids they may cause conjunctivitis and punctate keratitis. A secondary eczema often occurs around lesions, especially in atopics, and scratching spreads the mollusca. The lesions may become inflamed, tender and finally crusted and this heralds spontaneous resolution, which occurs in most lesions within several months.

Mollusca are resistant to chemical therapy. The most satisfactory approach is de-roofing of the lesion with a cutting-edged needle and wiping out the contents. The lesion itself is anaesthetic, so this is painless if the lesion is large enough for the needle to be introduced into the molluscum without penetrating the surrounding skin. With multiple tiny lesions spontaneous disappearance should be awaited ideally. However, if the lesions are troublesome due to site or perpetuation of eczema, removal under a general anaesthetic may rarely be considered.

HERPES SIMPLEX VIRUS INFECTION

Recurrent herpes simplex

Recurrent herpes simplex of the face is common in children, often precipitated by sunburn, fever or local trauma. Less commmonly recurrent herpes occurs at other sites, e.g. herpetic whitlow of the finger (Fig. 10.3.14). Recurrent genital herpes is a very rare occurrence in children; when it occurs the possibility of sexual abuse as the source of the herpes in this area must be considered. It is important to appreciate that where the causative organism is type 1 herpes simplex virus the possibility of abuse as the aetiology is not excluded. Local recurrences of herpes are best treated with simple saline bathing. Topical antiviral agents are of very limited value.

Erythema multiforme (EM) following herpes simplex

The commonest cause of EM minor is recent herpes simplex infection.[8] It has its onset 7–10 days after the onset of the herpes. It comprises fixed red papules or plaques which often show some central duskiness followed by blistering and/or

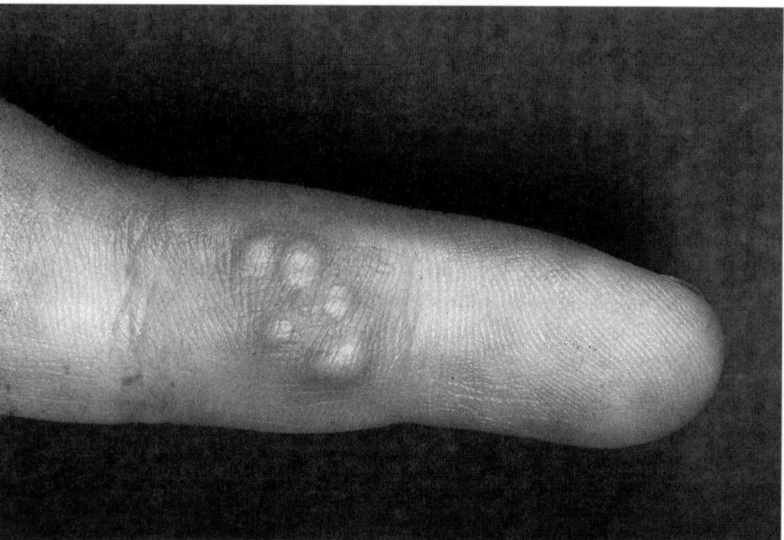

Fig. 10.3.14 Herpes simplex on volar aspect of finger.

necrosis. The lesions do not alter their shape within hours and disappear within 24 h as do the lesions of urticaria. The lesions of EM minor tend to be symmetrically distributed and are often most prominent on the limbs. Oral erosions are few in number or absent. The condition usually resolves spontaneously in 1–2 weeks but may recur with subsequent attacks of herpes simplex. If the frequency of recurrences of EM is disabling, the use of prophylactic oral acyclovir to prevent development of herpes may be considered. Using the polymerase chain reaction, herpes simplex DNA has recently been demonstrated in lesions of EM from patients without a history of prior herpes, suggesting that many apparently idiopathic cases of EM minor are in fact herpes-associated.[8]

Disseminated herpes simplex infection in the atopic

Patients with atopic dermatitis are more susceptible to certain infections, including herpes simplex. There is a tendency for this condition to spread rapidly in these patients, both by surface and haematogenous dissemination. The condition has been called eczema herpeticum and Kaposi's varicelliform eruption. It may originate from a primary or recurrent infection or from an exogenous reinfection. The lesions are vesicles or pustules 2–4 mm across which evolve into deep punctate erosions (Fig. 10.3.15). The lesions have a tendency to coalesce to produce geographical configurations. The condition may spread with alarming rapidity, producing large, bleeding, eroded areas. Fever and systemic toxicity are usual. If significant spread has occurred, the child should be hospitalized and treated with intravenous acyclovir; oral acyclovir is rarely able to contain fast-spreading disease. Topical preparations should be avoided as their use may

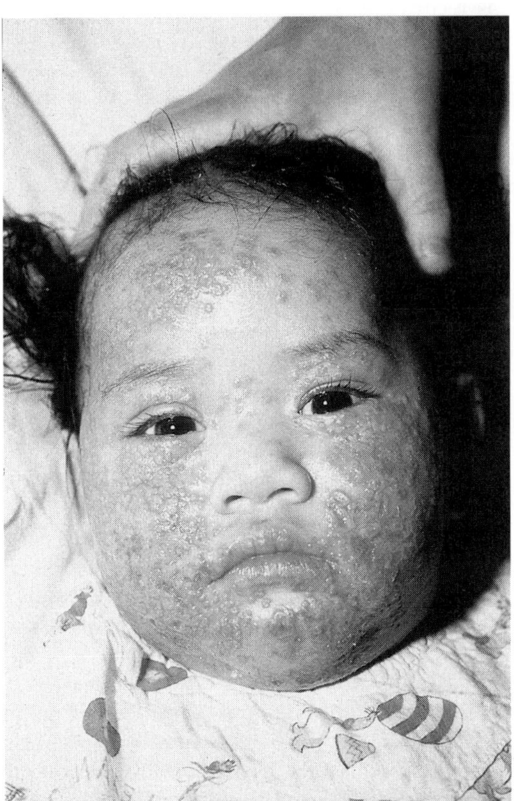

Fig. 10.3.15 Eczema herpeticum (Kaposi's varicelliform eruption). Vesicular and umbilicated lesions. Note sparing of nose. See also colour plate.

spread the virus. Tap water or saline packs relieve discomfort and systemic antibiotics may be required to deal with secondary infection. The condition usually resolves with remarkably little scarring.

VIRAL WARTS

Viral warts or verrucae are caused by a variety of human papilloma viruses (HPV). Different types of HPV have a predilection for certain anatomical sites and a tendency to produce certain clinical types of warts, although there is much overlap.

The major types seen in childhood are:

- Common warts
- Plantar warts
- Plane warts
- Filiform warts
- Anogenital warts

Common warts, the well-known, raised, rough-surfaced papules or tumours, occur particularly on the hands, especially on the fingers. They are often clustered around and under the nails and over the finger joints. Other commmon sites are the knees and elbows and the dorsa of the feet. Various topical keratolytic preparations, often combined with adhesive plaster occlusion and paring, are effective in a small percentage of cases. Liquid nitrogen cryotherapy is useful but too painful for younger children. Cautery and diathermy should be avoided, as recurrences are common, and scarring is a significant risk over finger joints and on the palms. Recently the use of oral cimetidine in a dose of 25–40 mg/kg per day has been found to be a safe and remarkably successful therapy for multiple, long-standing, refractory warts in children and may well become the treatment of choice.[9]

Plantar warts appear initially as small, pale papules on the sole, often over the metatarsal heads. They enlarge to produce well-defined keratotic lesions, lacking the skin markings of the surrounding normal skin. They are usually flush with the surface of the sole but palpation reveals that they may extend deeply. They are more tender on lateral compression than on direct pressure, which enables differentiation from a corn or callus. Multiple contiguous or separate lesions may occur. Cautery, diathermy and excision of plantar warts are contraindicated because of the considerable risk of producing painful scars, particularly if the lesions are over pressure points. Keratolytic agents may be used under plaster occlusion or the wart can be hardened by application of formalin and repeatedly pared.

Plane warts are flat, skin-coloured or brownish papules, occurring particularly on the face and the dorsa of the hands. They demonstrate the Koebner isomorphic phenomenon, occurring in areas of trauma, such as along scratch marks or in the area of a graze or other dermatosis. Very large numbers of lesions may be present. This type of wart usually responds well after 1–2 weeks to the topical application of retinoic acid overnight. This preparation must be avoided in the daytime as it causes a sun sensitivity.

Filiform warts are long frond-like lesions occurring particularly around the nose and mouth. They may reach over 1 cm in length. These lesions tend to be refractory to topical agents and, if multiple or causing considerable cosmetic distress, are usually best treated by diathermy or cautery, which will require general anaesthesia in a young child.

Anogenital warts are usually pink, soft and elongated and are often pedunculated. They occur separately or in large masses. When they occur in children the possibility of sexual abuse must always be addressed. Because of the different sites of predilection for individual HPV types, the presence of multiple hand warts in a child with anogenital warts does not enable the possibility of sexual abuse to be ignored. One well-recognized source is intrapartum transmission from cervical or vaginal warts in the mother. Topical podophyllin or podophyllotoxin, very carefully applied according to strict instructions, may be effective in some cases, but if lesions are multiple, diathermy under general anaesthesia is the usual treatment of choice.

REFERENCES

1 Rogers M, Dorman D, Gapes M et al. A three year study of impetigo in Sydney. Med J Aust 1987; 147: 59–62.
2 Gonzalez A, Schachner L A, Cleary T et al. Pyoderma in childhood. Adv Dermatol 1989; 4: 127–141.
3 Barnett B O, Frieden I F. Streptococcal skin diseases in children. Semin Dermatol 1992; 11: 3–10.
4 Hoeger P H, Lenz W, Boutonnier A et al. Staphylococcal skin colonization in children with atopic dermatitis: prevalence, persistence and transmission of toxigenic and non-toxigenic strains. J Infect Dis 1992; 165: 1064–1068.
5 Krol A L. Perianal streptococcal dermatitis. Pediatr Dermatol 1990; 7: 97–100.
6 Resnick S D. Staphylococcal toxin-mediated syndromes in childhood. Semin Dermatol 1992; 11: 11–18.
7 Schultz M W, Gomez M, Hansen R C et al. Comparative study of 5% permethrin cream and 1% lindane lotion for the treatment of scabies. Arch Dermatol 1990; 126: 167–170.
8 Weston W, Brice S, Jester J, Lane A et al. Herpes simplex virus in childhood erythema multiforme. Pediatrics 1992; 89: 32–34.
9 Orlow S, Paller A. Cimetidine treatment for multiple viral warts in children. J Am Acad Dermatol 1993; 28: 794–796.

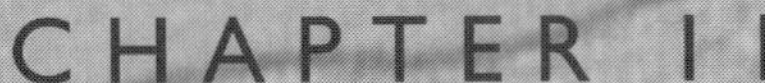

FEVER

M. Levin   N. Klein

11.1   An approach to the child with fever

INTRODUCTION

Fever is the commonest childhood symptom seen by primary health care professionals in the developed world. In most cases, the fever signifies a self-limiting viral illness which requires no more than symptomatic management. In a minority of cases there is a more serious cause which must be correctly diagnosed and treated. The problem facing paediatricians is how to identify the relatively few children with potentially serious disease from the vast majority with benign infections. This chapter will present a practical approach to managing febrile children.

WHAT CAUSES FEVER?

Body temperature is regulated by the anterior hypothalamus, which balances heat loss and heat production to maintain a constant internal temperature of about 36.8°C. Fever results from an upward shift in the hypothalamic thermostat so that the balance between heat loss and heat production will be altered to raise the body's internal temperature. Many substances can induce fevers. These may be exogenous, including lipopolysaccharide (LPS), enterotoxins and other exotoxins, or endogenous pyrogens such as interleukins 1 and 6 (IL-1, IL-6), tumour necrosis factor (TNF) and interferons.[1] Endogenous pyrogen production may be stimulated by a wide range of stimuli including bacteria, fungi, viruses, neoplasms, connective tissue disorders, drugs and trauma.[2,3] Fever per se does not identify the underlying stimulus but merely signifies its presence.

THE PITFALLS OF DEFINITIONS

A number of definitions have in the past been used as aids in the diagnosis of febrile episodes. These have been simplified in recent years to: (a) fevers with localizing signs; (b) fevers without localizing signs; and (c) fevers of unknown origin. The former two definitions are usually applied to fevers of recent onset while fever of unknown origin usually refers to children with fevers lasting longer than a week which has defied initial investigations. These definitions can be helpful practically and are essential for epidemiological studies.[4,5] However, they may also lead to misdiagnosis and delay in the recognition of some diseases. This is particularly true of the causes of prolonged fevers in which attempts to establish the diagnosis at an early stage may be critical to providing appropriate and adequate treatment (e.g. Kawasaki disease).

RULES FOR MANAGEMENT OF FEBRILE CHILDREN

1. History and examination are the most valuable guides to the aetiology and severity of disease. Diagnosis cannot be made over the telephone.
2. The diagnosis of a 'viral illness' which is so frequently made by health care workers is usually a statement of statistical probability and not based on factual information. While this diagnosis may be suspected, a management plan must be instituted which will guard against missing other, more serious conditions.
3. No single general physical finding or laboratory investigation can reliably distinguish between a viral or bacterial infection. The degree of temperature elevation, white blood cell count, response to antipyretics, acute-phase reactants and age of the patient may provide important clues to the underlying diagnosis but are not in themselves diagnostic. A combination of history, examination, and where appropriate laboratory investigations, is required to adequately assess and manage febrile children.

MANAGEMENT OF FEBRILE CHILDREN

There are numerous approaches to the management of children with fever. To a large extent the locally available facilities will play an important role in dictating policy. In this section the principles of management are outlined in preference to rigid guidelines which may be inappropriate in some settings.

History and examination

It cannot be stressed enough that the first step in investigating a child is to take a thorough history and perform a careful examination. In addition to a general history and examination, establishing the nature, onset and duration of the fever, it is particularly important to answer the following questions:

1. Where has the infection come from?
   - Travel history
   - Contact with infectious diseases
   - Trauma with penetrating injuries
   - Dietary history
   - Contact with animals
   - Insect bites
2. Is the child predisposed to infections?
   - Recurrent infections/severe infections in the past
   - Underlying disorder, e.g. nephrotic syndrome, sickle cell disease, malignancy
   - Primary immunodeficiencies—consanguineous parents
   - Aquired immunodeficiencies—blood transfusions, risk of HIV
   - Shunts/cannulae/Hickman lines
   - Immunization history
3. What are the likely pathogens?
   - Season, e.g. influenza in winter, enteroviruses in summer
   - Prevalent organisms in the community
   - Age-related pathogens, e.g. respiratory syncytial virus (RSV) in infants
4. Are there subtle clues on examination as to the aetiology of the fever?
   - Rash
   - Bone tenderness/joint swelling

- Presence of tonsillar tissue (suggesting severe combined immunodeficiency)
- Trauma

Initial management and the development of a management plan

Fever with localizing signs

Even if after the history and examination it is clear that there are localizing symptoms and signs of an infection, a management plan should be formulated. If the child appears severely ill it is advisable to admit the child to hospital until there is evidence of improvement. If the child is thought to be well enough to stay at home, clear instructions about what to do if the child deteriorates are essential. The appropriate treatment for each condition, including antibiotics, is described in the relevant chapters of this book.

Fever with vague or absent localizing symptoms and signs

Children presenting with an acute onset of high fever but without localizing signs present a difficult management problem. The vast majority of such children will be suffering from trivial viral illnesses or be in the prodromal phase of childhood exanthems. However, in a small percentage (less than 10%) they will be suffering from bacteraemia due to organisms such as *Haemophilus influenzae*, *Streptococcus pneumoniae* or *Neisseria meningitidis*.[6,7] If the fever is caused by a bacteraemic illness, a significant proportion of the affected children will develop a severe localized infection such as meningitis, septic arthritis or osteomyelitis, or features of septic shock. The clinical findings, in those children who are suffering from a bacteraemic illness, are overlapping, and often indistinguishable, from the majority of children whose fever is caused by trivial viral illnesses. A number of clinical features may increase the likelihood that bacterial infection is present. These include the height of the fever, the presence of signs of systemic toxicity and the presence of features of peripheral underperfusion, including pallor, cool periphery, mottled skin, tachycardia and prolonged capillary refill time. Laboratory markers which predict an increased risk of bacterial infection include an elevation of the white cell count above $15 \times 10^9/l$, an increased proportion of neutrophils, or the presence of an abnormally low white cell count ($< 2.5 \times 10^9/l$). Elevation of the erythrocyte sedimentation rate or C-reactive protein may also be helpful in predicting the presence of a bacterial infection. However, while these clinical features and laboratory markers may help in the detection of children who are suffering from a bacteraemic or septicaemic illness they do not reliably distinguish bacterial from viral illnesses.[7,8]

Because of the difficulty in detecting, on clinical grounds, the small proportion of children who are bacteraemic, from the vast majority who have trivial viral illnesses, and because of the serious complications which may occur if bacterial infection is not detected and treated, a number of authorities have suggested that all children and infants who are febrile and appear clinically ill should have blood cultures and urine cultures taken together with a full blood count, and should then be commenced on parenteral antibiotics active against the common childhood pathogens.[7-9] Antibiotics are continued for those who are found to have positive blood cultures and discontinued for those whose blood cultures are negative. While this approach has the advantage of detecting and treating the majority of febrile children who are suffering from bacterial infection, it also has a number of disadvantages.[10] A very large number of children who have viral illnesses will be treated with antibiotics in order to detect the small number who have bacterial infections. The discomfort, cost and potential adverse effects of treating large numbers of children with antibiotics are considerable, and there are concerns that widespread use of short courses of broad-spectrum antibiotics may induce bacterial resistance. In addition, a single blood culture may fail to detect a bacteraemic illness (particularly in the case of *N. meningitidis*) and may result in an inadequate course of antibiotics being given to some patients.

An alternative approach which is favoured by many authorities is to investigate only those children who have high temperatures and features of systemic toxicity but to withhold antibiotics until cultures become positive, or there are clear clinical or laboratory features to suggest a septicaemic illness. While this approach may decrease the number of children receiving unnecessary antibiotics, there are undoubtedly some patients who will deteriorate and become critically ill while awaiting the results of cultures.

Which of these two approaches is preferable depends on a number of different factors, which must be assessed for each patient. These include the experience of the clinician, the reliability of family members or nursing staff in observing the child and bringing to medical attention any changes in the child's condition. In addition the frequency of particular pathogens in each country needs to be considered. In countries where *N. meningitidis* is a major cause of community-acquired septicaemic illnesses, a lower threshold for antibiotic administration should be adopted, as children with meningococcaemia may deteriorate with frightening rapidity.

In those children who are felt to be well enough to be observed at home, a detailed plan of management should be discussed with the family. The parents or guardians must have a clear understanding of the clinical features to observe, and of what actions should be taken if there is deterioration or a failure to improve. Ready access to further medical consultation must always be arranged if febrile children are to be managed at home.

Table 11.1.1   Causes of prolonged fever in children

INFECTIOUS DISEASES	**Viral**
Systemic bacterial infections	Cytomegalovirus
Salmonella (typhoid/non-typhoid)	Hepatitis viruses
Mycobacteria	Human immunodeficiency virus
Brucellosis	Epstein–Barr virus
Leptospirosis	Human herpesvirus type 6
Spirochaete infections	
Yersinia	**Chlamydia**
Borrelia	**Rickettsia**
Rochalimaea	
	Fungi
Focal bacterial infections	**Parasitic infection**
Absesses	Malaria
Sinusitis	Toxoplasmosis
Osteomyelitis	Leishmania
Endocarditis	
Urinary sepsis	

NON-INFECTIOUS	
Collagen vascular disease	Familial Mediterranean Fever
Malignancies	*Kawasaki disease
Drugs	Still's disease
Inflammatory bowel disease	CNS/autonomic abnormalities
Erythrophagocytic lymphocytic histiocytosis	Sarcoidosis

*Maybe infectious

PROLONGED FEVERS

While the likely causes of prolonged fevers may be distinct from the majority of causes of acute fevers, all causes of fever should be considered at the time of presentation. If a child is still pyrexial after 48 h from presentation and no cause has been found, active investigation to exclude the less common causes of fever should be judiciously initiated. This must include continuous re-evaluation of the patient. Table 11.1.1 shows the main categories to consider in children with persistent fevers. While intial investigations may be serological and non-invasive, including cardiac echo, abdominal ultrasonography, failure to find the cause of a fever may require isotope bone and/or gallium scans, bone marrow aspirate, lymph node biopsy, colonoscopy, liver biopsy and magnetic resonance imaging scans. Investigation should be proportional to the severity of the child's illness.

REFERENCES

1 Dinarello C A, Wolff S M. The role of interleukin-1 in disease. N Engl J Med 1993; 328: 106–113.
2 Dinarello C A, Wolff S M. Pathogenesis of fever and the acute phase response. In: Mandell G L, Bennett J E, Dolin R, eds. Principles and practice of infectious diseases. 4th Edition. New York: Churchill Livingstone, 1995; pp 531–536.
3 Lorin M. Fever: pathogenesis and treatment. In: Feigin R D, Cherry J D, eds. Textbook of pediatric infectious diseases. 3rd Edition. Philadelphia: Saunders, 1992; pp 130–136.
4 Lorin M, Feigin R D. Fever of unknown origin. In: Feigin R D, Cherry J D, eds. Textbook of pediatric infectious diseases. 3rd Edition. Philadelphia: Saunders, 1992; pp 1012–1022.
5 Gelfand J A, Wolff S M. Fever of unknown origin. In: Mandell G L, Bennett J E, Dolin R, eds. Principles and practice of infectious diseases. New York: Churchill Livingstone, 1995; pp 536–549.
6 Jaffee D M, Tanz R R, Davis T et al. Antibiotic administration to treat possible occult bacteremia in febrile children. N Engl J Med 1987; 317: 1175–1180.
7 Baraff L J, Bass J W, Fleisher G R et al. Practice guidelines for the management of infants and children 0–36 months of age with fever without source. Pediatrics 1993; 92: 1–12.
8 Bass J W, Steele R W, Wittler R R. Antimicrobial treatment of occult bacteremia: a multicentre co-operative study. Pediatr Infect Dis J 1993; 12: 466–473.
9 Fleisher G R, Rosenberg N, Vinci R, et al. Intramuscular versus oral antibiotic therapy for the prevention of meningitis and other bacterial sequelae in young, febrile children at risk from occult bacteremia. J Pediatr 1994; 124: 504–512.
10 Long S S. Antibiotic therapy in febrile children. J Pediatr 1994; 124: 585–588.

M. Levin   N. Klein

11.2 Kawasaki disease

INTRODUCTION

It is over 25 years since Dr Tomisaku Kawasaki's original description of the disease that now bears his name.[1] Kawasaki disease (KD), which was first thought to be a benign, self-limited febrile illness, is now known to be associated with sudden death in up to 1% of affected children, and is one of the most common causes of acquired heart disease in children in the USA and Japan. This is now known to be due to an acute coronary vasculitis which occurs in up to 30% of children with the disorder.[2,3]

EPIDEMIOLOGY

The epidemiology of KD has been well documented. It is a disease of young children. Eighty-five per cent of affected children are less than 4 years of age, with a peak incidence in children at the end of the first year of life. Many of the epidemiological features suggest that KD has an infectious aetiology. In Japan the disease occurs in epidemics at approximately 3-yearly intervals. These spread in wave-like fashion over a period of several months.[4,5] Similar epidemicity is described in the USA, Canada and Europe.

Oriental races, particularly Japanese and Koreans, appear to be at greatest risk of KD, followed by blacks at intermediate risk and Caucasians with the lowest risk. Males are more commonly affected than females.[6]

Despite the obvious epidemic nature of KD, there is little evidence of person-to-person spread of the illness. However, siblings of affected children are at greater risk than the general population and may develop the illness within days of the index case, suggesting a common exposure to the aetiological agent rather than secondary transmission.[6,7]

CLINICAL FEATURES

The clinical features (Fig. 11.2.1, Table 11.2.1) are high fever, rash, conjunctivitis, mucositis and lymphadenopathy. This is associated with changes in the peripheral extremities such as erythema and induration of the skin of the hands and feet, with later desquamation of the fingers and toes. These changes are accompanied in many cases by arthritis, aseptic meningitis, a sterile pyuria and derangements in liver function with a mild hepatitis. Laboratory features during the acute phase of the illness are those of a marked acute-phase response, with neutrophilia, elevation of the erythrocyte sedimentation rate, C-reactive protein and other acute-phase proteins. There is often a mild normochromic, normocytic

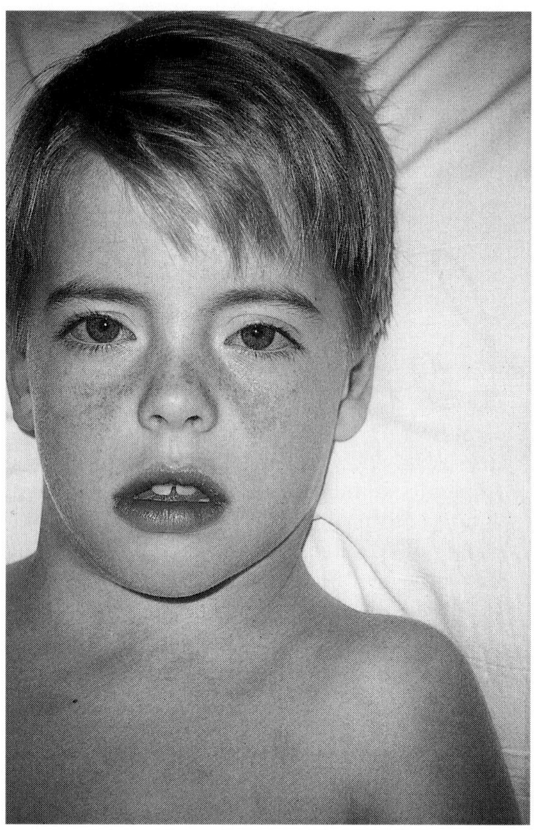

Fig. 11.2.1 Child with Kawasaki disease. Note red, cracked lips ("lipstick sign") and bilateral conjunctivitis (see also colour section)

Table 11.2.1 Diagnostic criteria for Kawasaki disease

(A) Fever of 5 or more days' duration
(B) Presence of four of the following five conditions:
    (1) Bilateral conjunctival injection
    (2) Changes in the mucous membranes and upper respiratory tract, such as injected pharynx, dry cracked lips, strawberry tongue[a]
    (3) Changes of the peripheral extremities including oedema, erythema, desquamation (may occur later)[a]
    (4) Polymorphous rash
    (5) Cervical lymphadenopathy
(C) Exclusion of: staphylococcal and streptococcal infection, measles, leptospirosis and rickettsial disease

[a]One of these is sufficient.
Note: in the presence of coronary artery aneurysms detected echocardiographically, (A) plus three of the four criteria in (B) is diagnostic.

anaemia and hypoalbuminaemia. These findings resolve, but are often followed by a marked thrombocytosis which occurs in the subacute phase of the illness.[8]

The major pathological feature of KD is an acute multi-system vasculitis affecting small- and medium-sized musculoelastic arteries. As part of this multi-system disease, of greatest concern is the presence of coronary artery involvement including coronary artery dilatation or frank aneurysm formation, which has been documented in up to 30% of children with KD. Accompanying the changes in the coronary arteries, there is evidence of myocarditis. Severe myocardial involvement may account for a small proportion of the early deaths in KD. The majority of these, however, are due to acute myocardial infarction secondary to thrombus formation in the affected vessels. Myocardial infarction, or ischaemia, with papillary muscle dysfunction may be the cause of acute mitral insufficiency.[3]

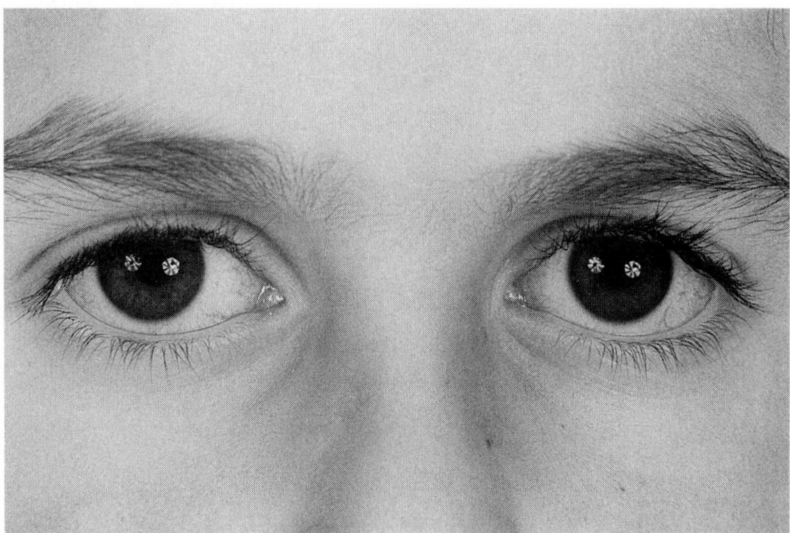

Fig. 11.2.2 Conjunctivitis: non-exudative with limbal sparing.

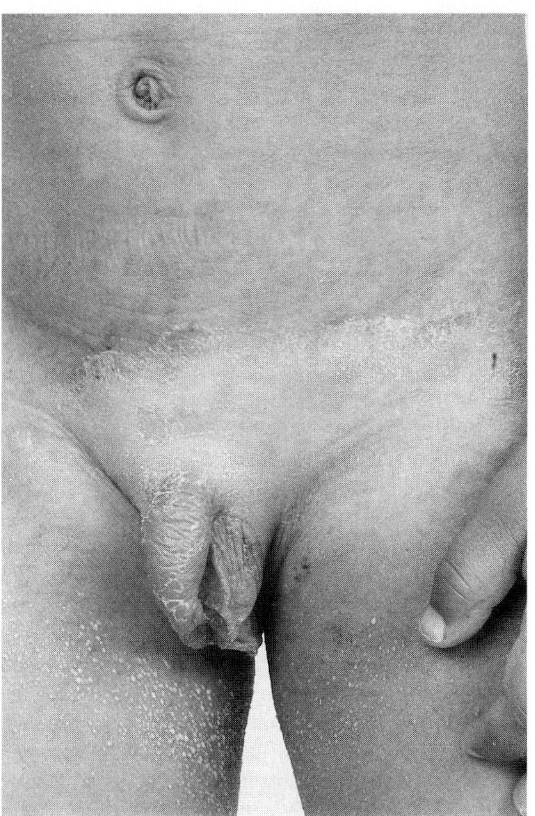

Fig. 11.2.3 Peeling groin rash, highly suggestive of Kawasaki disease.

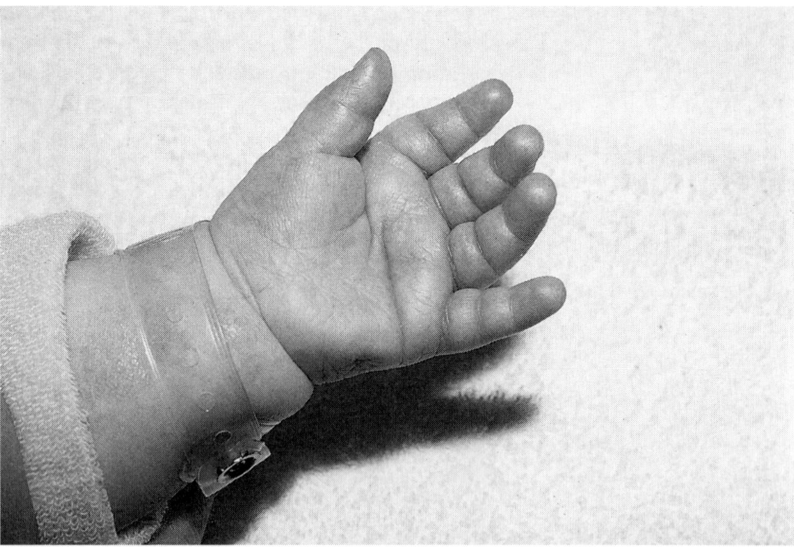

Fig. 11.2.4 Non-pitting peripheral oedema, particularly seen in infants with KD.

The diagnosis of KD requires four of the five recognized clinical criteria (Table 11.2.1);[8] however, there are increasingly frequent reports of atypical KD in which not all of the clinical criteria are met.[9] These cases are usually diagnosed retrospectively in children who have had unusual febrile illnesses associated with coronary artery abnormalities typical of KD. Coronary artery disease may present in adolescence or early adult life,[10] when a long period has passed since the acute illness, and the memory of the disease by the patient or the patient's family may have faded. Because of the occurrence of coronary disease in children who have not fulfilled the classical criteria, the possibility of KD should be considered in the differential diagnosis of any unusual febrile illness in early childhood, where other causes have been ruled out.[6]

PATHOPHYSIOLOGY

Immunological studies indicate that KD is associated with a marked activation of the immune system. There are increased circulating levels of cytokines including interleukin 1 (IL-1), interleukin 6 (IL-6), tumour necrosis factor α (TNF-α) and interferon γ (IFN-γ). Circulating soluble CD4, CD8 and interleukin 2 (IL-2) receptors, together with polyclonal hypergammaglobulinaemia and high levels of IgG and IgM circulating immune complexes, have also been demonstrated in the acute phase of KD. These changes are accompanied by evidence of neutrophil activation.[6,11]

The histological lesion is an intense perivasculitis with endothelial cell swelling, endothelial cell proliferation, adhesion of polymorphonuclear leucocytes (PMLs) to the endothelial wall and endothelial necrosis. This is associated with infiltration by PMLs and mononuclear cells. These histological features suggest a role for cytokine-mediated vascular endothelial cell injury.[11]

The clinical and laboratory findings in KD are characteristic of diseases that are caused by bacterial toxins that act as 'superantigens'. These diseases, such as streptococcal scarlet fever, staphylococcal scalded skin syndrome and the streptococcal and staphylococcal toxic shock syndromes, have many striking clinical and laboratory similarities to KD.[12] Streptococcal exotoxins and staphylo-

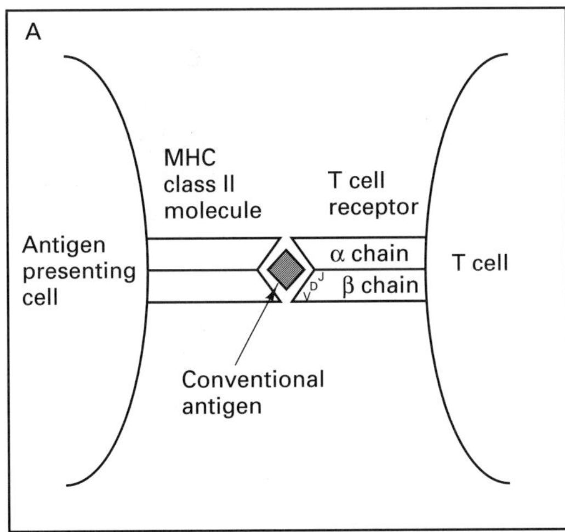

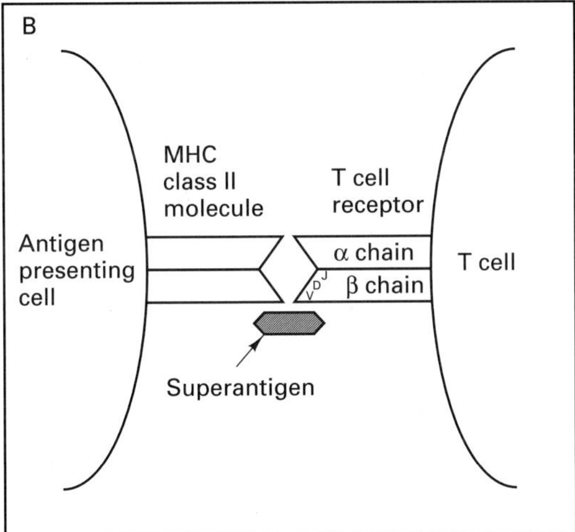

Fig. 11.2.5   (A) T cell stimulation by a conventional antigen. (B) T cell stimulation by a superantigen.

coccal enterotoxins are prototypic superantigens which stimulate populations of T cells that express particular T cell receptor, β chain-variable (Vβ) gene segments. Superantigens bind to the Vβ region of the T cell receptor, in conjunction with MHC class 2 antigens, and induce T cell proliferation and subsequent cytokine release (Fig. 11.2.5). For example, staphylococcal toxic shock toxin 1 (TSST-1) induces massive expansion of Vβ 2+ T cells.[13]

The clinical, laboratory and immunological changes which occur in KD suggest that a toxin acting as a superantigen may be the cause of KD. Based on these observations, a study by Abe et al[14] of Vβ gene expression on T cells in the acute and convalescent phases of KD has demonstrated elevated levels of circulating Vβ 2+ and Vβ 8.1+ T cells in the acute phase of KD, with a reduction in the abnormal levels of these cells in the convalescent phase. The findings of Vβ 2 expansion in the acute phase of KD has been confirmed in a study by Curtis et al,[15] but has not been confirmed in some other studies. The detection of Vβ expression is dependent on the timing of the investigation, and this may explain the failure of some studies to confirm the findings of Abe et al.

AETIOLOGY

Although the epidemiological evidence strongly suggests an infectious aetiology, attempts to identify the causative agent of KD have so far been unsuccessful. Published evidence implicating *Rickettsia*, retroviruses, environmental toxins and skin commensals have all failed to be confirmed on subsequent studies.[6] However, in view of the possibility of a toxin acting as a superantigen as the cause of KD several groups have investigated the possibility that the disorder is caused by superantigens, similar to those produced by streptococci and staphylococci. Leung et al reported that toxic shock toxin producing staphylococci could be isolated from a significantly greater proportion of children with KD than controls.[16] Curtis et al have also reported the presence of superantigen-producing bacteria in the nose and throat cultures of children with KD.[17] However, toxic shock toxin was only responsible for the superantigen activity in some of the cases. In others a range of other known enterotoxins were detected, and in some no known toxin could be isolated. This suggests that a range of different superantigen toxins, including perhaps a novel toxin, may be responsible for the disorder. Further research will undoubtedly define the aetiology in the coming years.

TREATMENT

There is now good evidence that intravenous immunoglobulin administered within the first 10 days of the illness reduces the risk of coronary artery aneurysms. A single high dose (2 g/kg) of intravenous immunoglobulin has been shown to be more effective in the prevention of coronary artery aneurysms than the intermittent dosage regimen.[18] Aspirin, in anti-inflammatory doses (30–80 mg/kg per day) is recommended during the acute phase of the disease, and low-dose aspirin (2 mg/kg per day) is given as an anti-platelet agent once the fever and acute inflammatory response have subsided. In patients who have developed coronary artery aneurysms, aspirin is continued on a long-term basis to reduce the risk of coronary artery thrombosis.

The mechanism by which intravenous immunoglobulin acts to reduce the risk of coronary artery aneurysms is not well understood. Intravenous immuno-globulin has immunomodulatory effects in decreasing activation of a number of inflammatory cells. Intravenous immunoglobulin may also potentiate the removal of circulating immune complexes, and may also interrupt platelet adhesion to the sub-endothelium. A direct effect in inhibiting a causative toxin may also be involved. It is of interest that pooled adult serum contains antibodies against superantigen toxins such as toxic shock toxin.

In patients with severe coronary artery involvement, other anti-platelet agents such as dipyridamole and prostacyclin may be beneficial. Thrombolytic treatment is indicated in patients who have impending coronary artery occlusion.

OUTCOME

The occurrence of coronary vasculitis has important implications for long-term prognosis in KD. The prognosis for coronary artery lesions is closely related to the maximal luminal diameter in the affected vessel. Although over 50% of aneurysms have been demonstrated to regress over a period of 1–2 years, it is doubtful whether affected arteries ever return to normality. Abnormalities in histological features, reactivity and coronary flow reserve have been demonstrated in arteries that appear normal on coronary angiography. There have now been several reports of juvenile atherosclerosis, premature-onset ischaemic heart disease and sudden death occurring several years after apparent recovery from KD. Fortunately, follow-up of the very large number of children with KD has, so far, suggested that the majority of affected children have an excellent prognosis and that deaths are very rare after the first 2 months of the illness.[19] However, the long-term prognosis of KD remains uncertain especially for those children who have demonstrable coronary artery abnormalities. These children require long-term follow-up with serial echocardiography and in some cases coronary angiography.

CONCLUSION

Although it may be difficult to distinguish KD from other acute febrile exanthems in childhood, the existence of effective therapy in the form of high-dose intravenous gamma globulin makes early diagnosis imperative. The absence of any diagnostic test for KD, and the recent recognition of atypical cases, makes a high index of suspicion essential in any child with an atypical febrile illness. Continuing research into the pathophysiology will lead to improvements in diagnostic techniques, thus allowing earlier therapy, and therefore prevention of the significant long-term consequences of KD.

REFERENCES

1 Kawasaki T. Acute febrile mucocutaneous syndrome with lymphoid involvement with specific desquamation of the fingers and toes in children (Japanese). Jpn J Allergy 1967; 16: 178–222.
2 Kato H, Koike S, Yamamoto M, Ito Y, Yano E. Coronary aneurysms in infants and young children with acute febrile mucocutaneous lymph node syndrome. J Pediatr 1975; 86: 892–898.
3 Nakamura Y, Fujita Y, Nagai M et al. Cardiac sequelae of Kawasaki disease in Japan: statistical analysis. Pediatrics 1991; 88: 1144–1147.
4 Yanagawa H, Nakamura Y, Kawasaki T, Shigematsu I. Nationwide epidemic of Kawasaki disease in Japan during winter of 1985–86. Lancet 1986; ii: 1138–1139.
5 Nakamura Y, Yanagawa I, Kawasaki T. Temporal and geographical clustering of Kawasaki disease in Japan. Prog Clin Biol Res 1987; 250: 19–32.
6 Levin M, Tizard E J, Dillon M J. Kawasaki disease: recent advances. Arch Dis Child 1991; 66: 1369–1372.
7 Fujita Y, Nakamura Y, Sakata K et al. Kawasaki disease in families. Pediatrics 1989; 84: 666–669.
8 Diagnostic guidelines for Kawasaki disease. American Heart Association Committee on Rheumatic Fever, Endocarditis, and Kawasaki Disease. Am J Dis Child 1990; 144: 1218–1219.
9 Rowley A H, Gonzalez C F, Gidding S S, Duffy C E, Shulman S T. Incomplete Kawasaki disease with coronary artery involvement. J Pediatr 1987; 110: 409–413.
10 Pounder D J. Coronary artery aneurysms presenting as sudden death 14 years after Kawasaki disease in infancy. Arch Pathol Lab Med 1985; 109: 874–876.
11 Nonoyama S. Immunological abnormalities and endothelial cell injury in Kawasaki disease. Acta Paediatr Jpn 1991; 33: 752–755.
12 Cone L A, Woodward D R, Schlievert P M, Tomory G S. Clinical and bacteriological observations of a toxic shock-like syndrome due to Streptococcus pyogenes. N Engl J Med 1987; 317: 146–149.
13 Marrack P, Kappler J. The staphylococcal enterotoxins and their relatives. Science 1990; 248: 705–711.
14 Abe J, Kotzin B L, Jujo K et al. Selective expansion of T cells expressing T-cell receptor variable regions V beta 2 and V beta 8 in Kawasaki disease. Proc Natl Acad Sci USA 1992; 89: 4066–4070.

15 Curtis N, Zheng R, Lamb J R, Levin M. Evidence for a superantigen mediated process in Kawasaki disease. Arch Dis Child 1995; 72: 308–311.
16 Leung D Y M, Meissner H C, Fulton D R, Murray D L, Kotzin B L, Schlievert P M. Toxic shock syndrome toxin-secreting Staphylococcus aureus in Kawasaki syndrome. Lancet 1993; 342: 1385–1388.
17 Curtis N, Chan B, Levin M. Toxic shock syndrome toxin-secreting Staphylococcus aureus in Kawasaki syndrome (letter). Lancet 1994; 343: 299.
18 Newburger J W, Takahashi M, Beiser A S et al. A single intravenous infusion of gamma globulin as compared with four infusions in the treatment of acute Kawasaki syndrome. N Engl J Med 1991; 324: 1633–1639.
19 Nakamura Y, Yanagawa H, Kawasaki T. Mortality among children with Kawasaki disease in Japan. N Engl J Med 1992; 326: 1246–1249.

M. Levin   N. Klein

11.3   Shock in the febrile child

INTRODUCTION

Shock is a pathophysiological state of impaired cardiovascular function, resulting in inadequate tissue and organ perfusion.[1] Diminished supply of oxygen and nutrients to the tissues leads to local hypoxia, anaerobic metabolism and impaired cellular function. Shock is one of the commonest paediatric emergencies, and occurs in a wide variety of infections, as well as in non-infectious conditions. Effective treatment of shock requires identification and treatment of the initiating disorder, and measures to correct the disordered physiology.

AETIOLOGY AND PATHOPHYSIOLOGY

Shock can be initiated by four main groups of disorders: (1) fluid, blood or electrolyte loss (which may be either external or internal); (2) cardiac failure; (3) loss of vascular tone; (4) combinations of all the above. Although there are numerous non-infectious processes which may initiate shock through each of these mechanisms, infections are amongst the most common precipitants. For example, gastroenteritis, due to either bacterial or viral infection, may produce shock through severe diarrhoea and vomiting; infections primarily affecting the myocardium such as viral myocarditis, or cardiac tamponade due to pericardial infection or tuberculosis, can severely reduce cardiac output; and abnormalities of vascular tone, either pathological vasodilatation or profound vasoconstriction, may be seen in bacterial sepsis. Septicaemic disorders such as meningococcaemia produce shock due to a combination of fluid and electrolyte loss, depressed cardiac function and abnormalities of vascular tone.

Impaired cardiac output and/or abnormal blood flow distribution are common to all forms of shock. Cardiac output is dependent on heart rate, preload, myocardial contractility and afterload. Bacterial infections may adversely affect cardiac output through diminished preload as a consequence of diminished venous return to the heart, reduced myocardial contractility (due to the myocardial depressant effects of sepsis and acidosis) or alterations in afterload due to pathological vasodilatation or vasoconstriction. Regardless of the initiating event, the body will respond to reduction in cardiac output by a series of homeostatic vasoconstrictor responses, which attempt to maintain cerebral and coronary perfusion at the expense of less vital tissues (Fig. 11.3.1). If the initiating insult is maintained, the compensatory vasoconstriction leads to a progressive reduction in organ perfusion. Hypoxia in the underperfused tissues results in impaired cellular metabolism and ultimately in cell death. Proteolytic enzymes and other toxins are released from damaged cells, which increase vascular permeability, activate the clotting and kinin pathways, and diminish vascular tone.

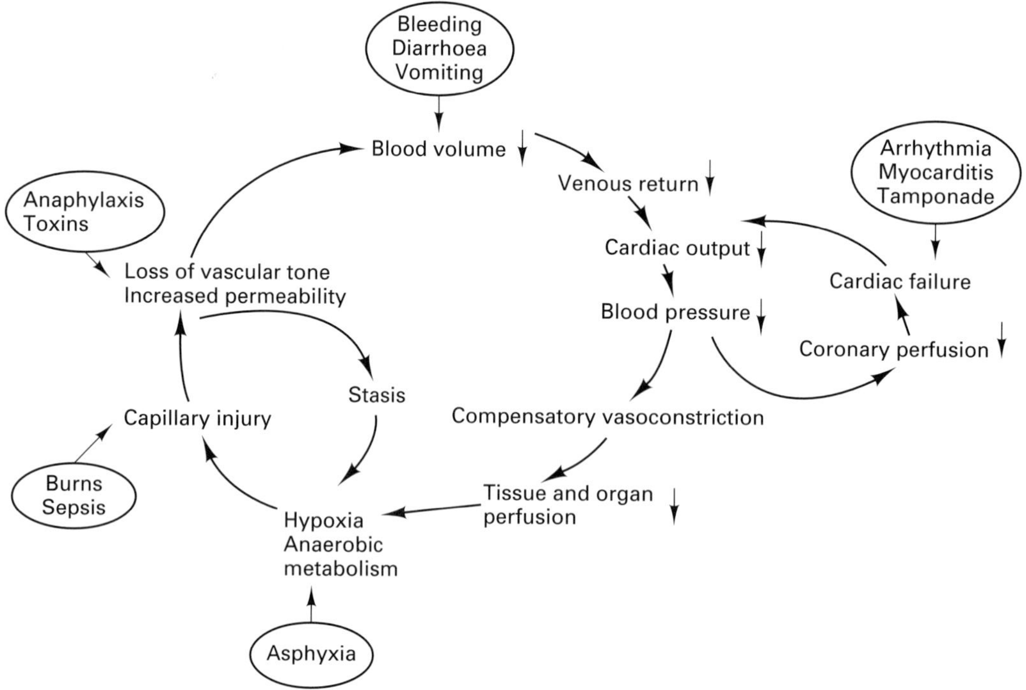

Fig. 11.3.1 Cyclic mechanisms in septic shock. (Modified from Hackel et al 1974 and Ledingham 1976)

Increased capillary permeability leads to further losses of colloid from the vascular space. Platelets and coagulation pathways are activated by damaged endothelium resulting in the formation of microthrombi in the capillaries of the lung, kidneys and other organs. Late shock is characterized by generalized hypoperfusion, increasing acidosis and disseminated intravascular coagulation. Respiratory, renal and hepatic failure cause further metabolic derangements. Cardiac function is impaired by hypoxia and acidosis as well as the reduced cardiac filling and elevated peripheral resistance. Ultimately the compensatory mechanisms are overwhelmed, coronary and cerebral perfusion fall, and irreversible cardiac and cerebral damage occur.

MICROBIOLOGY

The microbial causes of shock differ depending on the age of the patients, their immunological status and their country of residence. All the causes of severe gastroenteritis may precipitate shock and are discussed in detail in Chapter 3.1. Non-diarrhoeal causes of shock in the neonatal period are septicaemia due to group B streptococcus or coliforms. Less commonly, staphylococcal sepsis, salmonella or enteroviral infection may be the precipitant. In infants and older children *Neisseria meningitidis* is the commonest cause of community-acquired septicaemia and shock in many countries. *Streptococcus pneumoniae* and *Haemophilus influenzae*, group A streptococcus and *Staphylococcus aureus* septicaemia are less common causes. In the immunocompromised, or those severely ill with underlying renal, hepatic or pulmonary disorders, *Pseudomonas aeruginosa* or other Gram-negative organisms, as well as staphylococci, group A streptococci and *Streptococcus pneumoniae*, must be considered. In asplenic patients *S. pneumoniae* is the commonest cause of septic shock. In tropical countries, shock may be seen in association with severe malaria, salmonella sepsis, meliodosis, and viral infections such as dengue and the viral haemorrhagic fevers. Rickettsial infections, such as Rocky Mountain spotted fever, should be considered in certain geographic locations.

IMMUNOPATHOGENESIS

Each of the infections listed above as triggering shock has distinct immuno-pathogenic features. However, host immune responses are probably involved in all forms of infection-associated shock. Having gained access to the bloodstream, infectious agents trigger an intense inflammatory response which is responsible for much of the tissue and organ damage.[2] In the case of Gram-negative bacteria, endotoxin is probably the most important bacterial component triggering the inflammatory response,[3] and infusions of endotoxin produce all of the features commonly seen in septic shock. In the case of Gram-positive infections other cell wall fragments, including teichoic acid, are important precipitants. Specific enzymes or toxins may play a role in initiating shock in some infections. Levels of endotoxin correlate with the severity of disease in infections such as meningo-coccaemia.[3] Endotoxin appears to act by triggering the release of a range of inflammatory mediators from macrophages, including the cytokines, tumour necrosis factor and interleukin 1 and platelet-activating factor.[4] Activation of macrophages, neutrophils and platelets occurs concurrently with activation of complement and the clotting cascade. Endotoxin increases the expression of adhesion molecules on neutrophils and endothelium. Neutrophils adhere to the endothelium and initiate endothelial injury through the release of proteolytic enzymes and reactive oxygen metabolites. A combination of cytokine, complement and proteolytic enzyme-mediated damage to the endothelium results in disruption of endothelial function as well as depressed myocardial function.[5]

CLINICAL PATHOPHYSIOLOGY

There are few medical conditions which present as complex an array of clinical problems as is found in children with septic shock. Although cardiorespiratory failure is the predominant clinical problem, this coexists with multi-organ failure, severe coagulopathy and a complex metabolic derangement, with acidosis and electrolyte disturbance. Although the precise sequence of events leading to this derangement is not well understood, most of the abnormalities are explained by four primary processes:[6] (1) severe capillary leak resulting in loss of circulating volume; (2) vasodilatation of some vascular beds coexisting with vasoconstriction of others; (3) intravascular thrombosis; (4) severe depression of myocardial function.

Increased vascular permeability (capillary leak) is one of the earliest events in septic shock. Leakage of albumin and other plasma proteins from the intra-vascular compartment into the interstitium results in hypovolaemia and diminished venous return to the heart. Reduced filling of the left and right ventricles results in diminished cardiac output, as predicted by Starling's law (Fig. 11.3.2). The importance of hypovolaemia has been well documented in meningococcal sepsis: patients who do not survive the disease have persistently low central venous and pulmonary and capillary wedge pressures, and are resistant to volume replacement.[7] It is not uncommon for patients with severe septic shock to require

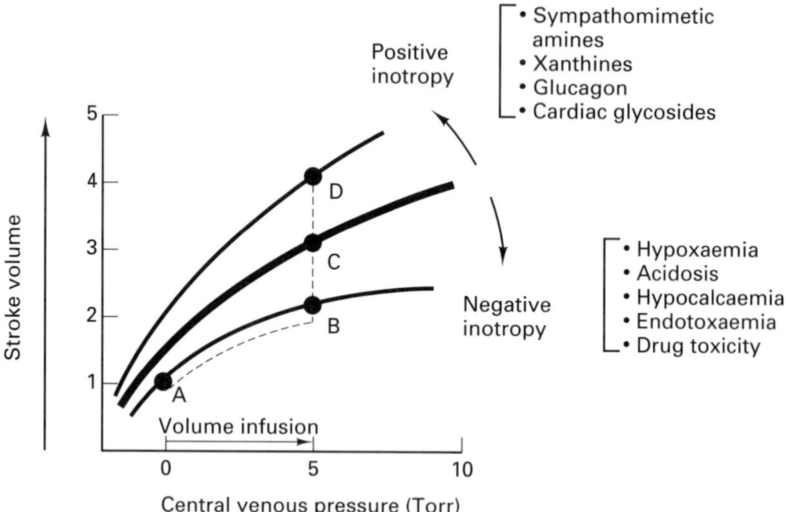

Fig. 11.3.2   Starling's law. The Starling curve relates cardiac output (or stroke volume) to the filling pressure of the left and right ventricles. Patients presenting with meningococcal septicaemia are usually at point A, with a low central venous pressure and low cardiac output. Volume replacement increases cardiac output (point B), but myocardial contractility remains impaired due to the negative inotropic effects of acidosis, electrolyte imbalance and endotoxaemia. Correction of the myocardial depressant factors and the use of exogenous inotropic agents improves the cardiac output achieved at the same filling pressure (points C and D).

very large volumes of colloid to restore their circulating volume. Marked peripheral oedema is the inevitable consequence of the profound capillary leak.

Intense vasoconstriction is usually present in children with septic shock. The warm shock commonly seen in adults with Gram-negative sepsis is uncommon in children with disorders such as meningococcal sepsis, but may be seen later in the disease after adequate volume resuscitation, and in immunocompromised children with other forms of Gram-negative sepsis. Most children with septic shock have high peripheral vascular resistance and a diminished cardiac output.[7] Following adequate volume replacement and the use of inotropes, a different picture may emerge which may more closely resemble the warm shock usually seen in adults. Peripheral vasodilatation, wide pulse pressure, hypotension and progressive acidosis may develop despite evidence of elevated cardiac output. The mechanisms responsible for the vasoconstriction and inappropriate vasodilatation of some vascular beds are not well understood. Vasoconstrictor substances such as catecholamines and renin, aldosterone, thromboxane A2 and endothelin are elevated in septic shock.[8] Excessive production of vasodilator substances such as nitric oxide and prostacyclin may explain vasodilatation seen in patients with warm shock.[9]

Disturbances in haemostasis are invariably present in patients with septic shock. Thrombocytopenia, prolongation of prothrombin time, KPTT and thrombin time, and reduction of plasma fibrinogen with elevation of fibrin degradation products are usually present.[10] There is often a picture of disseminated intravascular coagulation which is supported by the finding of elevated levels of fibrinopeptide A and depletion of coagulation pathway factors.[10] Reduction of coagulation inhibitors, antithrombin III, protein C and protein S is common, as are abnormalities in fibrinolysis.[11,12] Patients with septic shock may paradoxically simultaneously have problems of excessive bleeding and thrombosis. Those with severe disseminated intravascular coagulation (DIC) have evidence of bleeding from venepuncture sites or mucous membranes. This may coexist with microvascular thrombosis, producing the picture of purpura fulminans; in severe cases gangrene of limbs or digits and thrombosis of internal organs may occur.

The mechanisms responsible for myocardial dysfunction in septic shock are complex. Although hypovolaemia may be the major initiating event, myocardial function may remain depressed following adequate volume resuscitation. A variety of factors may contribute to poor myocardial contractility, including hypoxia, acidosis and electrolyte imbalance.[6,13]

Dysfunction of other organs invariably occurs in patients with severe sepsis. Respiratory failure is extremely common in patients with shock and is due to a combination of capillary leak affecting the pulmonary vasculature and alveoli, and occlusion of pulmonary capillaries with thrombi composed of platelets, fibrin and inflammatory cells. Early manifestations of pulmonary involvement include elevated respiratory rate, intercostal recession and hypoxia.[14] In severe cases progressive hypoxia occurs and pulmonary oedema may develop suddenly with cyanosis and frothy pulmonary oedema fluid filling the airway. Respiratory failure is likely in shocked patients who are not electively ventilated.

Oliguria is one of the earliest events in septic shock. Initially this is prerenal in origin but if shock persists intense renal vasoconstriction and reduced renal perfusion result in established renal failure. Abnormalities of gastrointestinal and hepatic function are common and in severe cases diminished brain perfusion results in coma.

CLINICAL FEATURES

The early clinical features of septic shock reflect the compensatory vasoconstrictor responses which maintain vital organ perfusion at the expense of peripheral perfusion. A low blood pressure is not a feature of early shock, and arterial blood pressure may be maintained by vasoconstriction even in severely shocked patients. Some children become hypertensive in response to volume loss. Reduction of blood pressure may only occur when the compensatory vasoconstriction is overwhelmed and is often a preterminal event. In early shock, the child is restless and anxious. Tachycardia is one of the earliest findings and may coexist with tachypnoea. Peripheral perfusion is poor, with a gradient above 4°C between the central temperature and the peripheral temperature. Capillary filling is sluggish. It is best assessed by pressure over the skin or nail beds and observation of the time for the capillaries to fill. Oliguria is usually present, and parents frequently note that their child has not passed urine for several hours.

LABORATORY FINDINGS

In early shock haemoconcentration with elevation of haemoglobin and packed cell volume is common. However, anaemia may also be present if bleeding or haemolysis has occurred. Elevation of urea and creatinine may indicate renal under-perfusion.

Advanced shock

Clinical features in advanced shock reflect severely diminished perfusion of all tissues and organs.[1] Peripheral perfusion is extremely poor, with an increasing difference between central and peripheral temperature (often above 10°C). Capillary filling is often slow and areas of blue discoloration, due to stagnation of blood in dilated capillaries, are superimposed upon areas of extreme pallor. There is increasing tachycardia, hypotension and signs of cardiac failure. The respiratory rate rises as shock and acidosis worsen. Cyanosis develops. Later, as the child becomes exhausted, breathing becomes laboured and respiratory arrest occurs unless assisted ventilation is initiated. Restlessness and confusion are followed by drowsiness, coma and occasionally by convulsions. Once coma is present cerebral damage and death are imminent unless cerebral perfusion is rapidly restored. Severe shock is invariably accompanied by oliguria or anuria. Abdominal distension and ileus are common and watery or bloody diarrhoea is often a preterminal event.

Laboratory findings in advanced shock

Haemoglobin and platelet counts fall. Coagulopathy is present with thrombocytopenia, and prolongation of partial thromboblastin time, prothrombin time and thrombin time. Fibrinogen is reduced and fibrin degradation products elevated, indicating disseminated intravascular coagulation. Electrolyte imbalance with hypokalaemia or hyperkalaemia, abnormalities of plasma sodium, and elevation of urea and creatinine are common. Derangement of blood glucose, calcium, phosphate and magnesium is common. Ischaemia of the liver and pancreas results in elevation of plasma transaminases and pancreatic enzymes. Blood gases show a progressively falling oxygen tension (pO_2), rising carbon dioxide tension (pCO_2) and metabolic acidosis. The chest X-ray may show the appearance of pulmonary oedema and acute respiratory distress syndrome.

DIAGNOSIS

If prognosis is to improve, shock should be diagnosed and treated by recognition of early signs of peripheral under-perfusion as described above. If treatment is withheld until advanced shock has developed, the process may be extremely difficult to reverse and the mortality is high. Clinical features alone are sufficient to enable the diagnosis of early shock to be made. Identification of the causative infectious agent is seldom possible on clinical grounds alone and depends on the results of cultures of blood or other sites. Treatment of both the underlying infection and of shock itself should be initiated as soon as the child has been recognized to be in shock, and should not await the identification of the causative agent.

MANAGEMENT

General principles

The shocked child presents a complex array of clinical and metabolic derangements. It may be difficult to decide which to treat first. Those conditions which immediately threaten life must be identified at the onset. The ABC of resuscitation is always part of the initial assessment of shock. Maintenance of the airway, effective ventilation and exclusion of a profound disturbance of cardiac rate and rhythm are always primary objectives. The aims of treatment are:

1. to improve oxygenation, oxygen-carrying capacity, cardiac output and blood flow distribution;
2. to treat the cause of shock by administering antibiotics to cover the likely pathogen and searching for and removing any focus of infection;
3. to support vital organ function while awaiting recovery.

Vascular access

Vascular access for fluid and drug administration as well as for monitoring is an essential early step in the management of shock. In severely shocked children it may be difficult to secure even a peripheral venous line. Percutaneous cannulation of internal or external jugular, femoral or subclavian veins can be rapidly performed by those familiar with the techniques. However, there is a high risk of complication (pneumothorax, carotid artery puncture and haematoma) when these routes are attempted by the inexperienced. Surgical cut-down onto the saphenous vein may be a safer alternative. Intraosseous infusion should be commenced in patients in whom vascular access cannot be obtained. Rapid volume expansion with plasma or 0.9% sodium chloride will often improve perfusion sufficiently to enable more secure access to be obtained.

Initial resuscitation

Supplemental oxygen should be administered by face mask. The initial dose of antibiotics should be administered as soon as vascular access has been obtained or may be initiated by the intramuscular route if any delay in obtaining vascular access is expected. The initial antibiotic choice will depend on the age of the patient, and whether they have an underlying immunosuppressive disorder. In the neonatal period cefotaxime and ampicillin will provide cover for most of the expected pathogens, with flucloxacillin or vancomycin added if staphylococcal infection is strongly suspected. Beyond the neonatal period a third-generation cephalosporin plus β-lactamase-resistant penicillin (such as flucloxacillin) will provide cover for most of the likely pathogens. In the immunocompromised a wide variety of organisms are possible, including *Pseudomonas*, and initial treatment should therefore include an aminoglycoside plus piperacillin and either vancomycin or flucloxacillin to cover Gram-positive organisms. An alternative regimen would be ceftazidime, plus aminoglycoside, and flucloxacillin.

Volume replacement

The correction of hypovolaemia is the single most important therapeutic measure in the treatment of shock. Even in cardiac failure, the failing myocardium may require a higher than normal filling pressure to achieve optimal cardiac output, and a trial of volume expansion with careful monitoring is justified unless pulmonary oedema is present at the time of initial presentation. The aim of volume replacement is to adjust the preload on the left and right ventricles in order to achieve maximum cardiac output (Fig. 11.3.2).[15] Patients with severe septic shock generally have an ongoing capillary leak, and very large volumes of colloid may be required to restore circulating volume. Several times the estimated total blood volume may be required in the first 24 h and such volumes can only be administered safely with careful monitoring of central venous pressure (CVP) or pulmonary capillary wedge pressure along with continuous clinical assessment.

Volume replacement should commence as soon as the diagnosis of shock has been made, and vascular access established. A number of different resuscitation fluids are available for initial resuscitation. Although resuscitation may be initiated with crystalloid solutions such as 0.9% saline, colloid-containing solutions are generally preferred as they remain longer in the intravascular space, and their use is associated with less interstitial and oedema; 4.5% albumin is our preferred resuscitation solution, although synthetic colloids such as hydroxyethyl starch or gelatine may be used if albumin is not immediately available. An initial volume of 20 ml/kg should be infused rapidly over 10–30 min. If this improves perfusion, a further 20–40 ml/kg can be given over the next hour. If initial volume replacement results in correction of the signs of shock and improved peripheral perfusion, no invasive monitoring or additional inotropic support is necessary. However, if signs of shock persist following initial volume replacement, this may indicate either severe volume depletion or continuing losses which require additional volume replacement. However, failure to respond to volume resuscitation may also be due to severe cardiac failure or the development of pulmonary oedema. The clinical distinction between these two possibilities may be extremely difficult, and invasive monitoring of CVP or pulmonary wedge pressure is then essential to guide further volume replacement and the use of inotropes. With careful monitoring of CVP, peripheral perfusion, and central and peripheral temperature, volume expansion should be continued until the CVP reaches levels at which ventricular preload is adequate (Fig. 11.3.3). Cardiac output is generally optimal at a CVP between 8 and 15 mmHg or a pulmonary wedge pressure of between 15 and 20 mmHg. More information is obtained from serial measurements of CVP following fluid challenge than from a single reading. Once the optimal preload has been achieved as indicated by an adequate CVP, fluids should be given to cover maintenance requirements, ongoing losses from stool, urine or secretions, and to replace any ongoing volume deficit occurring through the capillary leak.

Measures to improve myocardial contractility

Once volume deficits have been corrected, further improvement in cardiac output and tissue perfusion may be obtained by improving myocardial contractility.[1,15] This can be achieved by correction of acidosis, hypoxia, anaemia and electrolyte imbalance, all of which may depress myocardial function. Inotropic agents are useful in improving cardiac output, as well as improving the distribution of blood to the tissues, and further improvement in cardiac output may be achieved by the use of vasodilators which reduce afterload. During the initial resuscitation, before central vascular access has been obtained, dopamine (5–10 µg/kg per minute) or dobutamine (5–10 µg/kg per minute) should be commenced through a peripheral vein. Higher doses of dopamine or dobutamine are best delivered through a central line once access has been obtained. While inotropes will improve myocardial contractility, they should only be used concurrently with volume resuscitation and vigorous treatment of metabolic factors which depress contractility, such as hypoxia, anaemia, acidosis and electrolyte imbalance. The available inotropes have differing degrees of activity on alpha and beta adrenergic and dopaminergic receptors in the cardiovascular system. Stimulation of alpha adrenergic receptors is associated with cutaneous, splanchnic and renal vasoconstriction, and elevation of peripheral vascular resistance. Beta I receptor activation increases heart rate and contractility, but also increases cardiac work and oxygen consumption. Beta II receptors mediate peripheral and skeletal muscle vasodilatation and bronchodilatation and therefore reduce peripheral vascular resistance. Dopaminergic receptors mediate splanchnic and renal vasodilatation. Although sympathomimetic agents with a mixture of alpha and beta receptor activities (such as adrenaline) will improve cardiac output through their beta agonist effect, their effect on alpha receptors may result in a rise in peripheral vascular resistance, vasoconstriction, increase in afterload and myocardial work, and diminished perfusion of the tissues.

Most children with septic shock already have intense vasoconstriction, and the addition of an alpha stimulating agent may further reduce peripheral and organ perfusion. Initial treatment with dopamine (5–10 µg/kg per minute) in combination with dobutamine (10–20 µg/kg per minute) may be adequate to correct signs of shock in most patients. In patients with profound septic shock who remain hypotensive despite the administration of dopamine or dobutamine,

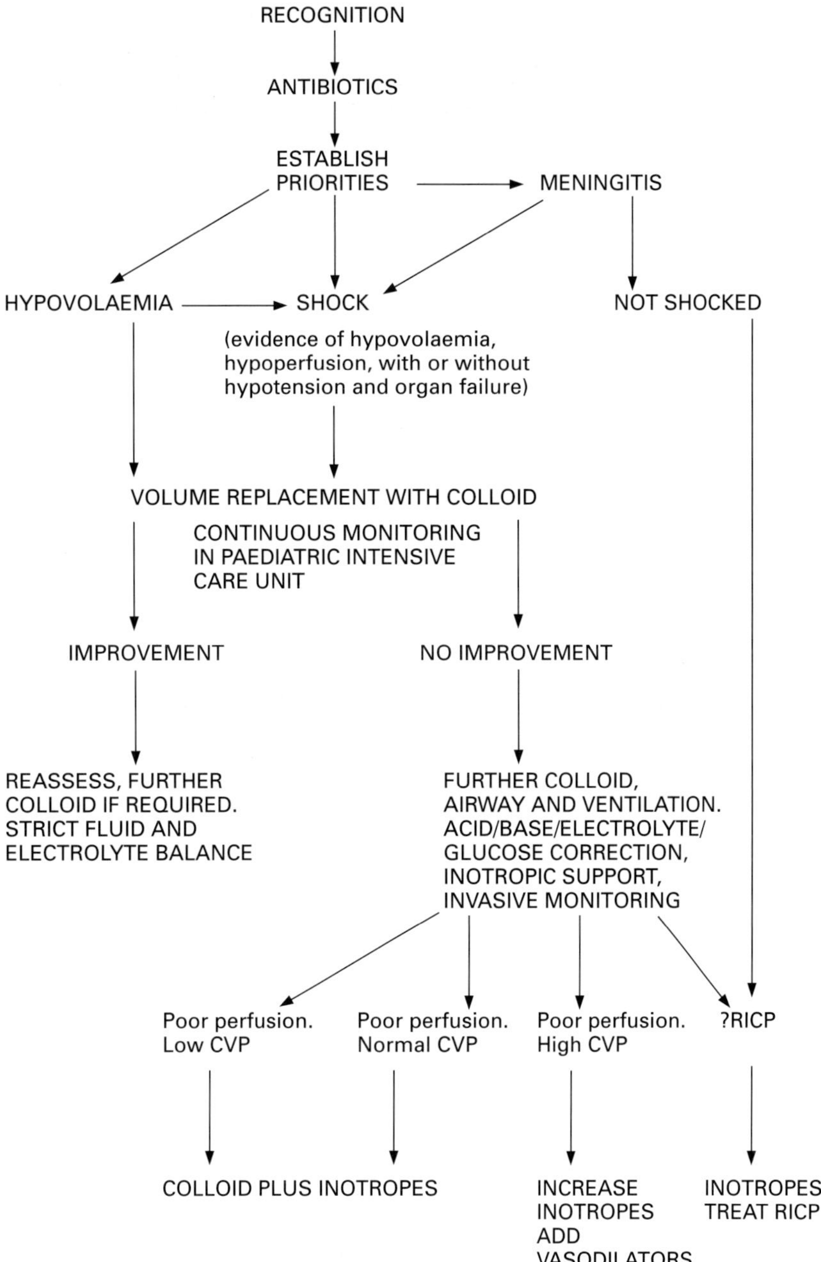

Fig. 11.3.3 Treatment of shock flow diagram. CVP, central venous pressure; RICP, raised intracranial pressure.

or in those who have signs of severe cardiac failure, adrenaline in doses of 0.02–3 µg/kg per minute may be required.

In patients with continued peripheral vasoconstriction, despite adequate cardiac filling pressure and arterial blood pressure, vasodilators are a logical and effective treatment in improving perfusion and reducing the afterload on the heart. Prostacyclin (5–20 ng/kg per minute) or nitroprusside are the most commonly used vasodilators, and are particularly indicated in patients with severe vasoconstriction and impending peripheral gangrene. Vasodilators, however, should be administered with extreme caution. Unless venous filling has already been optimized and careful haemodynamic monitoring is in place, severe hypotension may result. The phosphodiesterase inhibitor inoximone has also been advocated for its positive inotropic and vasodilatory activity in patients with refractory shock, but there is so far not much experience with its use.

Respiratory failure

Pulmonary oedema may occur suddenly in patients with severe septic shock. Elective ventilation should be initiated in any child with severe shock requiring large volumes (> 60 ml/kg) of colloid and those who have signs of persistent shock despite initial volume replacement. Control of the airway and administration of positive pressure ventilation allows volume resuscitation to proceed safely, with a reduced risk of sudden development of pulmonary oedema. Some patients present in profound respiratory failure, even if they have not received volume resuscitation. Such patients should be ventilated immediately to prevent acute respiratory collapse developing.

Correction of acidosis and electrolyte imbalance

Low glucose is common in severely shocked children and should be detected and treated early. Metabolic acidosis is almost always present in patients with severe septic shock. Mild degrees of metabolic acidosis are adequately compensated by hyperventilation, but in severe shock the pH falls. Reduction of the pH below 7.2 is associated with impaired myocardial function, arrhythmia and a poor cardiovascular response to inotropic drugs. Mild reductions in pH will respond to improvement of perfusion following volume replacement and the use of inotropes. However, severe acidosis should be corrected by the infusion of sodium bicarbonate. Respiratory acidosis must always be treated by ventilation before administration of bicarbonate. Bicarbonate should be given as an infusion of 1–2 mmol/kg over 10 min and subsequent correction of acidosis should be guided by the frequent determination of blood gases.

Hypokalaemia is common in patients with septic shock, while hyperkalaemia may occur in those in established renal failure. Rapid correction of hypokalaemia should be undertaken in patients with potassium levels below 3 mmol/l with 0.5 mmol/kg of KCl infused over 30 min with careful monitoring. Hypocalcaemia is common in shock and should be corrected by slow infusion of 10% calcium chloride 0.1–0.2 ml/kg. Hypomagnesaemia and hypophosphataemia should also be corrected.

Treatment of organ failure

Ventilation

Respiratory failure is invariably present in severe shock and is a common cause of death. In early shock patients usually hyperventilate and have a normal pO_2, low pCO_2 and normal chest X-ray. However, as shock worsens increased interstitial oedema results in a fall of lung compliance. Obstruction of lung capillaries by platelet and fibrin microthrombi causes increasing ventilation perfusion imbalance. There is a progressive fall in pO_2, increase in oxygen requirement and ultimately a rise in pCO_2. Pulmonary oedema and a picture of acute respiratory distress syndrome follow and respiratory arrest may occur suddenly. Control of the airway and positive pressure ventilation allows resuscitation to continue without fear of sudden arrest and also allows sedation and paralysing agents to be administered which decrease oxygen requirements. Elective ventilation should be undertaken in all severely shocked patients if the level of consciousness declines, and there is no response to simple volume expansion. Any reduction in oxygen saturation or rise in pCO_2 should immediately be treated with oxygen and ventilation.

Renal support

Impaired renal perfusion and oliguria occur early in shock. Initially the kidneys respond by maximal sodium and water retention. If renal hypoperfusion persists, acute renal failure occurs. In early shock, volume expansion and inotropic support will improve urine flow. Dopamine in doses of 1–6 µg/kg per minute is useful in improving renal blood flow. However, once renal failure is established, peritoneal dialysis or haemofiltration should be started. Dialysis is urgently indicated if urine flow is less than 0.5 ml/kg per hour or if there is a rise in potassium or if acidosis or fluid overload supervenes.

Central nervous system

Deterioration of cerebral function manifested by restlessness, confusion and coma is common in shock. It may be the result of the initiating insult, or of cerebral hypoperfusion. Elective intubation and ventilation must be performed early in comatose patients. Electrolyte imbalance, hypoglycaemia and hypocalcaemia should be corrected and convulsions controlled. Cerebral oedema should be treated by controlled ventilation to maintain the pCO_2 between 2.5 and 3.5 kPa. Limitation of extravascular fluid accumulation and the use of diuretics may be helpful in reducing cerebral oedema. Mannitol infusions (0.5–1 g/kg) effectively reduce intracranial pressure acutely, but should be used with considerable caution in patients with renal failure and severe capillary leak.

Monitoring

All patients with sepsis-associated shock require careful clinical assessment of central and peripheral temperature, capillary refill time, pulse rate and volume, blood pressure, urine output and level of consciousness. In severely shocked patients, and those who do not respond to initial volume replacement or those who have multi-organ failure, invasive monitoring of CVP or pulmonary wedge pressure is necessary to guide volume replacement. In severely shocked patients continual arterial pressure should be monitored through an intra-arterial catheter and measurement of core and peripheral temperature via rectal and big toe temperature probes should be undertaken. Urine output should be monitored hourly through an indwelling venous catheter. Pulse oximetry is extremely useful in detecting changes in respiratory status and oxygenation. Table 11.3.1 and Figure 11.3.3 indicate how data derived from clinical assessment and haemodynamic parameters can be used to guide volume replacement and inotropic support.

Table 11.3.1 Use of haemodynamic parameters to guide management

BP	CVP	Central/peripheral temperature gradient > 5°C (> 41°F)	Diagnosis	Management
↓	↓	↑	Volume depleted	Plasma/saline infusion
↓	↑	↑	Cardiogenic shock	Inotropic support, consider vasodilators
N or ↑	N or ↑	↑	Vasoconstricted	Vasodilators
N or ↑	↑	N	Overloaded	Diuretics, dialysis, fluid restriction

BP, blood pressure; CVP, central venous pressure; N, normal.

Prognosis

Patients with all forms of septic shock have a significant risk of death. Mortality rates for patients with meningococcal sepsis and septic shock are 20–50% in most series. However, with aggressive intensive care and support of multi-organ failure, survival may occur even in patients with profound shock. Management of all patients with severe septic shock should be undertaken on a paediatric intensive care unit familiar with the shock and its complications, to provide the best possible chance of survival.

FEBRILE SHOCK SYNDROMES

Introduction

The general principles described above for the management of septic shock are applicable to most bacterial as well as viral disorders causing shock. However, there are a number of distinct syndromes in which shock occurs as part of an infective process, which require separate discussion, either because they have distinct clinical features and pathophysiology, or because they occur in particular geographic regions and have epidemiological features differing from those of the usual forms of bacterial septic shock. A partial list of these syndromes and some of their distinguishing features is shown in Table 11.3.2.

Staphylococcal toxic shock syndrome

Staphylococcal toxic shock syndrome is a systemic illness characterized by fever, shock, erythematous rash, diarrhoea, confusion and renal failure.[16] The disorder was first described by Todd et al in 1978.[17] During the 1980s hundreds of cases were reported in the USA, mostly in menstruating women and associated with tampon use. Although the majority of cases worldwide are seen in women and are associated with menstruation, children of both sexes and all ages are affected.

The illness usually begins suddenly with high fever, diarrhoea and hypotension, together with a diffuse erythroderma. Mucous membrane involvement with hyperaemia and ulceration of the lips and oral mucosa or vaginal mucosa, strawberry tongue, and conjunctival injection are usually seen. Desquamation occurs in the convalescent phase of the illness. Confusion is often present in early stages and may progress to coma in severe cases. Multi-organ failure with evidence of impaired renal function, elevated hepatic transaminases, thrombocytopenia and disseminated intravascular coagulation are frequently seen. The diagnosis is made on the basis of the clinical features, and the exclusion of other disorders causing a similar picture, such as Rocky Mountain spotted fever, leptospirosis, measles and streptococcal infection.

The staphylococcal toxic shock syndrome is now known to be due to infection or colonization with strains of *Staphylococcus aureus* which produce one or more protein exotoxins. Most cases in adults are associated with toxic shock toxin 1, but in children many isolates associated with this syndrome produce other enterotoxins (A–F). The staphylococcal enterotoxins appear to induce disease by acting as superantigens, which activate T cells bearing specific V beta regions of the T cell receptor, and causing proliferation and cytokine release.[18] The systemic illness and toxicity are believed to be largely the result of an intense inflammatory response induced by the toxin. The site of toxin production is often a trivial focus of infection or simple colonization, and bacteraemia is infrequently observed.

The management of staphylococcal toxic shock syndrome depends on early diagnosis, aggressive cardiovascular support with volume replacement, inotropic support and in severe cases elective ventilation. If oliguria persists, despite optimization of intravascular volume and administration of inotropes, dialysis should be commenced early.

Table 11.3.2 Shock syndromes in childhood

Disease	Age	Fever	Rash	Shock	Encephalo-pathy	DIC	Thrombo-cytopenia	Renal pathology	Geographic localization	Predisposing factors
Gram-negative sepsis	All	√	–	√	± Occasional meningitis	√	√	Vasomotor nephropathy	No	Neonates Immuno-compromised Renal tract abnormalities
Gram-positive sepsis Pneumococcus *Staphylococcus aureus*	All	√	Occasional erythema	√	–	√	√	Vasomotor nephropathy	No	Asplenia focal infection
Staphylococcal toxic shock syndrome	All	√	Erythematous Late desquamation Conjunctivitis	√	√	√	√	Vasomotor nephropathy	No	Menstruation Tampons
Streptococcal toxic shock syndrome	All	√	Mucous membrane involvement	√	√	√	√	Vasomotor nephropathy	No	Local infection
Meningococcal sepsis	Young children Young adults	√	Petechiae, purpura	√	Meningitis may coexist	√	√	Vasomotor nephropathy Cortical necrosis	Worldwide	Complement deficiency Generally none
Leptospirosis	Older children Adults	√	Erythematous Mucous membrane involvement Conjunctivitis	√	Meningitis Encephalitis	√	√	Tubular interstitial nephritis + vasomotor nephropathy	Yes	Contact with infected water
Rocky Mountain spotted fever + other rickettsia	Older children Adults	√	Erythematous Petechiae Conjunctivitis Mucosal involvement	√	±	√	√	Vasomotor nephropathy	Yes	Tick–bite
Brazilian purpuric fever	Children	√	Petechiae Purpura	√	–	√	√	? Vasomotor nephropathy	South America	Conjunctivitis
Haemorrhagic shock and encephalopathy	Infants	√	Occasionally petechiae, usually none	√	Severe	√	√	Vasomotor nephropathy	No	No
Heat stroke Malignant hyperthermia	All Mostly infants	Hyperpyrexia	–	√	√	√	√	Vasomotor nephropathy	No	Overheating

Table 11.3.2 (*contd*)

Disease	Age	Fever	Rash	Shock	Encephalopathy	DIC	Thrombocytopenia	Renal pathology	Geographic localization	Predisposing factors
Reye syndrome	Infants and children	Biphasic preceding illness	No May follow varicella	Only very late	Severe	Coagulopathy of liver failure	Later	Seldom involved Late vasomotor nephropathy	No	Chickenpox Aspirin usage
Dengue shock syndrome	Children	√	Erythematous maculopapular petechiae rash Occasional desquamation	√	Yes ? Secondary to shock	√	√	Vasomotor nephropathy + viral immune complex injury	Tropical Africa South America Asia	Mosquito bite
Hantaan virus, haemorrhagic fever and renal syndrome	Children or adults	√	Conjunctival injection Petechiae Purpura	√	√	√	√	Vasomotor nephropathy + interstitial nephritis	Worldwide Mild Scandinavian form. Severe disease in Eastern Europe Asia, China	Aerosol infection from rodent execreta
Congo Crimean haemorrhagic fever	Older children Adults	√	Purpura	√	√	√	√	Vasomotor nephropathy + interstitial nephritis	Africa Asia Eastern Europe	Tick–bite
Lassa fever	Older children Adults	√	Purpura Erythema	√	√	√	√	? Vasomotor nephropathy	West Africa	Aerosolized rodent excreta
Yellow fever	Older children Adults	√	Conjunctival infection Flushed face	Late	Later with liver failure	√	√	Vasomotor nephropathy	Africa South America	Mosquito bite
Vasculitis SLE	Older children	√	Petechiae Purpura Erythema	Occasionally	Occasionally	Sometimes	Sometimes	Glomerulonephritis Vasculitis	No	No

DIC, Disseminated intravascular coagulation; SLE, systemic lupus erythematosus.

Antistaphylococcal antibiotics should be started as soon as the diagnosis is suspected, and the site of infection identified. If there is a focus of infection such as a vaginal tampon, surgical wound or infected sinus, drainage of the site should be undertaken early to prevent continued toxin release into the circulation. There is some evidence from both human and animal studies that steroids shorten the duration of the illness. Intravenous immunoglobulin, which contains neutralizing antibodies against toxic shock toxin and other enterotoxins, may be beneficial, but has not been subjected to controlled trials. With aggressive intensive care most affected patients survive; recovery may be seen even in patients who have had severe shock and multi-organ failure.

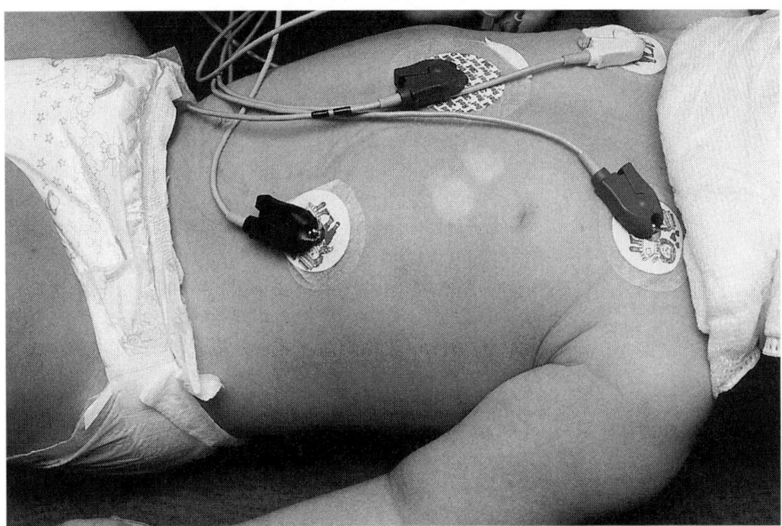

Fig. 11.3.4 Toxic shock syndrome. Intense erythema with prolonged blanching on fingertip pressure. See also colour plate.

Streptococcal toxic shock syndrome and invasive group A streptococcal infection

Since 1988 there have been several reports of an illness which has many similarities to the staphylococcal toxic shock syndrome, occurring in both children and adults, associated with invasive group A streptococcal disease.[19] Patients with this syndrome present with high fever, erythematous rash and mucous membrane involvement, hypotension and multi-organ failure. Unlike staphylococcal toxic shock syndrome, in which the focus of infection is usually trivial and bacteraemia is seldom seen, the streptococcal toxic shock syndrome is usually associated with bacteraemia or a serious focus of infection such as septic arthritis, myositis, fasciitis or osteomyelitis. Laboratory findings of anaemia, neutrophil leucocytosis, thrombocytopenia and disseminated intravascular coagulation are often present, together with impaired renal function, hepatic derangement and acidosis.[20]

The reasons for the emergence of streptococcal toxic shock syndrome, and the increasing number of cases with invasive disease due to group A streptococcus, are not clear. Strains causing toxic shock syndrome and invasive disease appear to differ from common isolates of group A streptococcus, in producing large amounts of pyrogenic toxins, which may have superantigen-like activity. The pathophysiology of staphylococcal toxic shock syndrome and that caused by the streptococcal toxins are similar in that both organisms produce superantigen toxins which induce release of cytokines and other inflammatory mediators.

Treatment of streptococcal toxic shock syndrome depends on administration of appropriate antibiotics, aggressive circulatory support, and treatment of multi-organ failure if present. As a focus of infection is often present, surgical intervention to drain the infective focus in muscle, bone or joints or body cavities is often required. Renal failure is usually self-limited and recovery of renal function occurs in patients who respond to treatment of shock and support of multi-organ failure.

Haemorrhagic shock and encephalopathy

The syndrome of haemorrhagic shock and encephalopathy was first described in 1983 and the disorder has now been reported from many countries.[21] Haemorrhagic shock and encephalopathy usually affect infants in the first year of life, with a peak onset of 3 to 4 months of age.[22] A prodromal illness with fever, irritability, diarrhoea or upper respiratory tract infection occurs 2–5 days before the onset in two-thirds of cases. Affected infants develop profound shock, coma, convulsions, bleeding and evidence of disseminated intravascular coagulation, diarrhoea and oliguria. Laboratory findings include acidosis, falling haemoglobin and platelets, elevated urea and creatinine and elevated hepatic transaminases. Despite vigorous intensive care the prognosis is poor, and most affected infants have died or have been left severely neurologically damaged. However, a small number of patients have been reported to survive without residual sequelae.

The aetiology of the disorder is at present unknown. Exhaustive studies have failed to identify specific infectious agents, toxic or metabolic disorders. There is evidence that defective protease inhibitor production may be involved in the pathogenesis of the disorder, and it has been suggested that a failure to produce the normal acute-phase rise in protease inhibitors such as α_1-antitrypsin may predispose to the development of severe shock during otherwise trivial infections.

The clinical and laboratory findings in patients with haemorrhagic shock and encephalopathy overlap those seen in infants with many other fulminant infections, as well as toxic or metabolic disorders. The diagnosis can therefore only be made following the exclusion by appropriate cultures and metabolic studies, of fulminant bacterial infections, and viral infections such as disseminated enteroviral infection or disseminated herpes simplex.[23] The staphylococcal and streptococcal toxic shock syndromes are usually distinguished by the absence of rash and mucous membrane involvement. A number of metabolic diseases including the organic acidaemias and fatty acid oxidase deficiencies may produce similar pictures and must always be excluded. Malignant hyperthermia or heat-stroke due to over-wrapping, as well as unrecognized hypoxic insults, must also be excluded. Reye syndrome may present a similar picture of a severe encephalopathy and deranged liver function tests, but profound shock and severe capillary leak of the sort seen in haemorrhagic shock and encephalopathy syndrome are seldom seen in Reye syndrome except as a preterminal event, once cerebral coning has occurred.

Viral haemorrhagic fevers

The possibility of infection with haemorrhagic fever viruses should be considered in patients who present with fever, shock and bleeding if they reside in regions of the world where haemorrhagic fevers are known to exist, or if they have recently travelled to these regions. The term haemorrhagic fever is used to describe at least 12 distinct RNA viruses, which have in common the propensity to cause severe disease with prominent haemorrhagic manifestations.[24] The viral haemorrhagic fevers are widely distributed through both temperate and tropical regions of the world, and in many countries are important causes of mortality and morbidity. Most viral haemorrhagic fevers are zoonoses (with the possible exception of dengue virus) in which the virus is endemic in animals and human infection is acquired through the bite of an insect vector. Transmission by aerosol and nosocomial transmission from infected patients are important for Lassa, Junin, Machipo, Congo Crimean haemorrhagic fever, Marburg and Ebola viruses.

The different viral haemorrhagic fevers have many clinical similarities, but also important differences in their severity, major organs affected and prognosis in response to treatment. In all viral haemorrhagic fevers, severe cases occur in only a minority of those affected, and subclinical infection or non-specific febrile illnesses occur in the majority of those infected.[25] Fever, myalgia, headache, conjunctival suffusion and erythematous rashes occur in all the viral haemorrhagic fevers. Haemorrhagic manifestations range from petechiae and bleeding from venepuncture sites, to severe haemorrhage into the gastrointestinal tract, kidney and other organs. The capillary leak syndrome, with evidence of haemoconcentration, pulmonary oedema, oliguria and ultimately shock occurs in the most severely affected cases. Renal involvement occurs in all the haemorrhagic fevers, proteinuria is common, and prerenal failure occurs in all severe cases complicated by shock. However, in Congo Crimean haemorrhagic fever and haemorrhagic fever with renal syndrome, an interstitial nephritis, which may be haemorrhagic, is characteristic, and renal impairment is a major component of the illness.[26]

Dengue haemorrhagic fever and dengue shock syndrome

Dengue is endemic and epidemic in tropical America, Africa and Asia where the mosquito vector *Aedes aegypti* is present. There are four distinct dengue viruses (types 1–4) which exhibit only short-term cross-immunity, and thus repeated infection may occur. Classical dengue fever is a self-limited non-fatal disease; dengue haemorrhagic fever and dengue shock syndrome, which occur in a minority of dengue-infected patients, have a high mortality.[27] After an incubation of 5–8 days, the illness begins with fever, headache, arthralgia, weakness, vomiting and hyperaesthesia. The face is usually flushed, and a generalized transient macular rash which blanches on pressure may be noticed. In uncomplicated dengue the fever usually last 5–7 days, and shortly after onset a maculopapular rash appears, sparing the palms and the soles and occasionally followed by desquamation. Fever may reappear at the onset of the rash.

In dengue haemorrhagic fever/dengue shock syndrome, the typical febrile illness is complicated by haemorrhagic manifestations, ranging from a positive tourniquet test or petechiae, to purpura, epistaxis and gastrointestinal bleeding. Laboratory investigations reveal thrombocytopenia and evidence of a consumptive coagulopathy. Increased capillary permeability is suggested by haemoconcentration, oedema and pleural effusions. In severe cases hypotension and shock supervene largely as a result of hypovolaemia. Renal manifestations include oliguria, proteinuria, haematuria and rising urea and creatinine. Acute renal failure occurs in patients with severe shock, largely as a result of renal underperfusion.[28]

The pathophysiology of dengue haemorrhagic fever and dengue shock syndrome remains poorly understood. There is evidence that the disorder may be the result of immune activation due to sequential infection by different strains of dengue.[29] The increased capillary permeability and haemorrhagic manifestations suggest widespread endothelial injury. The diagnosis of dengue is made by exclusion of bacterial infections, leptospirosis and rickettsial disease, and by virus isolation from blood or serology. There is no specific antiviral treatment and management of patients with dengue shock syndrome or dengue haemorrhagic fever depends on aggressive circulatory support and volume replacement with colloid and crystalloid. With correction of hypovolaemia, renal impairment is usually reversible, but dialysis may be required in patients with established acute renal failure.

Other haemorrhagic fevers

A number of other haemorrhagic fevers are important causes of serious illness in particular geographic locations. These include: Congo Crimean haemorrhagic fever, which is distributed throughout Eastern Europe, Asia and Africa; haemorrhagic fever and renal syndromes caused by Hantaan virus, which is distributed worldwide and has caused major problems in parts of Europe and Asia; yellow fever (seen in Africa and in South America); Rift Valley fever (Sub-Saharan Africa); Lassa fever (West Africa); and Argentinean, Bolivian and Venezuelan haemorrhagic fevers found in South America. Rare causes of fulminant disease are Marburg and Ebola viruses occurring in parts of Africa. These infections frequently have a common presentation with fever, headache, muscle ache and rigors together with nausea, vomiting and diarrhoea. There is often conjunctival injection and bleeding manifestations ranging from petechiae to cutaneous ecchymoses, and bleeding from mucous membranes or gastrointestinal tract in severe cases. The possibility of these infections should be considered in patients who have resided in or travelled to areas of the world where they are endemic. Treatment is in general supportive, as outlined above for patients with septic shock. There is evidence that ribavirin is effective in some of the viral haemorrhagic fevers, including Lassa fever.

REFERENCES

1 Levin M. Shock. In: Black D, ed. Paediatric emergencies, 2nd edn. London: Butterworth, 1987; pp 87–116.
2 Bone R C. The pathogenesis of sepsis. Ann Intern Med 1991; 115: 457–469.
3 Brandtzaeg P, Kierulf P, Gaustad P et al. Plasma endotoxin as a predictor of multiple organ failure and death in systemic meningococcal disease. J Infect Dis 1989; 159: 195–204.
4 Waage A, Brandtzaeg P, Halstensen A, Kierulf P, Espevik T. The complex pattern of cytokines in serum from patients with meningococcal septic shock. J Exp Med 1989; 169: 333–338.
5 Parrillo J E. Pathogenetic mechanisms of septic shock. N Engl J Med 1993; 328: 1471–1477.
6 Nadel S, Levin M, Habibi P. Current management of meningococcal septicaemia and meningitis. In: Cartwright K, ed. Meningococcal disease, Vol. 9. Chichester: Wiley, 1995; pp 207–243.
7 Mercier J-C, Beaufils F, Hartman J-F, Azéma D. Hemodynamic patterns of meningococcal shock in children. Crit Care Med 1988; 16: 27–33.
8 Voerman H J, Stehouwer C D A, van Kamp G J, van Schijndel R J M S, Groeneveld A B J, Thijs L G. Plasma endothelin levels are increased during septic shock. Crit Care Med 1992; 20: 1097–1101.
9 Cobb J P, Cunnion R E, Danner R L. Nitric oxide as a target for therapy in septic shock. Crit Care Med 1993; 21: 1261–1263.
10 Thijs L G, de Boer J P, de Groot M C M, Hack C E. Coagulation disorders in septic shock. Intensive Care Med 1993; 19: s8–s15.
11 Powars D R, Rogers Z R, Patch M J, McGehee W G, Francis R B. Purpura fulminans in meningococcemia: associated with acquired deficiencies of proteins C and S. N Engl J Med 1987; 317: 571–572.
12a Brandtzaeg P, Joø G, Brusletto B, Kierulf P. Plasminogen activator inhibitor 1 and 2, alpha-2-antiplasmin, plasminogen, and endotoxin levels in systemic meningococcal disease. Thromb Res 1990; 57: 271–278.
12b Brandtzaeg P, Sandset P M, Joø G B, Ovstebo R, Abildgaard U, Kierulf P. The quantitative association of plasma endotoxin, antithrombin, protein C, extrinsic pathway inhibitor and fibrinopeptide A in systemic meningococcal disease. Thromb Res 1989; 55: 459–470.

13 Parrillo J E, Buret C, Shelhamer J H et al. Circulation myocardial depressant substance in humans with septic shock: septic shock patients with a reduced ejection fraction have a circulating factor that depresses in vitro myocardial cell performance. J Clin Invest 1985; 76: 1539.
14 Repine J E. Scientific perspectives on adult respiratory distress syndrome. Lancet 1992; 399: 466–469.
15 Perkin R M, Levin D L. Shock in the pediatric patient. J Pediatr 1982; 101: 319–332.
16 Chesney P J, Bergololl M S, Davis J P, Vergerant J M. The disease spectrum, epidemiology and aetiology of toxic shock syndrome. Annu Rev Microbiol 1984; 38: 315.
17 Todd J, Fishaut M I, Kapral F, Welch T. Toxic shock syndrome: associated with phage group 1 staphylococci. Lancet 1978; ii: 1116–1118.
18 Marrack P, Kappler J. The staphylococcal enterotoxins and their relatives. Science 1990; 248: 705–711.
19 Cone L A, Woodward D R, Schlievert P M, Tomory G S. Clinical and bacteriologic observations of a toxic shock-like syndrome due to Streptococcus pyogenes. N Engl J Med 1987; 317: 146–149.
20 Torres-Martinez, Mehta D, Butt A, Levin M. Streptococcus associated toxic shock. Arch Dis Child 1992; 67: 126–130.
21 Levin M, Kay J D S, Gould J G, Mathews D J, Dinwiddie R. Haemorrhagic shock and encephalopathy: a new syndrome with high mortality in young children. Lancet 1983; ii: 64–67.
22 Levin M, Pincott J R, Hjelm M. Haemorrhagic shock and encephalopathy: clinical, pathologic, and biochemical features. J Pediatr 1989; 114: 194–203.
23 Chesney P J, Chesney R W. Haemorrhagic shock and encephalopathy: reflections about a new devastating disorder that affects normal children. J Pediatr 1989; 114: 254–256.
24 LeDuc J W. Epidemiology of haemorrhagic fever viruses. Rev Infect Dis 1989; 11: 5730–5735.
25 Gear J H S. Clinical aspects of African viral haemorrhagic fever. Rev Infect Dis 1989; 11 (Suppl 4): 777–782.
26 Gear J H S. Clinical aspects of African viral haemorrhagic fever. Rev Infect Dis 1989; 11 (Suppl 4): 777–782.
27 Hayes E B, Gubler D J. Dengue and dengue haemorrhagic fever. Paediatr Infect Dis J 1992; 11: 311–317.
28 Halstead S B. Dengue and dengue haemorrhagic fever. In: Feigin R D, Cherry J D, eds. Textbook of pediatric infectious diseases. Philadelphia: Saunders, 1987; pp 1510–1521.
29 Halstead S B. Antibody, macrophages, dengue virus infection, shock, haemorrhage: a pathogenetic cascade. Rev Infect Dis 1989; 11 (Suppl 4): 830–839.

M. Levin   N. Klein

11.4   The child with a petechial rash and fever

INTRODUCTION

The descriptive term petechial rash is used to describe the appearance of small discrete areas of haemorrhage seen within the subcutaneous tissues. In their early stages new areas of petechiae may be visible as areas of reddening ranging from pinpoint in size to a few centimetres. Fresh petechiae are difficult to distinguish from erythematous macules commonly seen in a variety of viral illnesses. The essential feature which distinguishes a petechial rash from other erythematous rashes is their response to pressure. Whereas erythematous rashes blanch on pressure (as dilated blood vessels are emptied), petechial rashes persist as blood has extravasated from the capillaries. It is often helpful to view the rash through a glass slide or drinking glass, and this enables persistence of the bruising to be seen during the application of pressure. Within a few hours of their appearance, petechiae often become blue/black in colour and may easily be confused with traumatic bruises. Larger areas of subcutaneous haemorrhage are termed purpura which if extensive and confluent are given the name 'purpura fulminans'.

Petechiae and purpura are a common cutaneous manifestation of a wide range of different disorders, including bacterial and viral infections, inflammatory disorders and neoplasms (Table 11.4.1). Although some of the causes of petechial rashes are self-limited conditions (such as enteroviral infections) others may be fulmi-nant and life-threatening (such as meningococcal sepsis or leukaemia) and the appearance of petechiae must therefore always be treated as an emergency, which requires immediate investigation to define the cause, and treatment.

PATHOGENESIS AND PATHOLOGY

Petechiae and purpura may occur as a result of three distinct pathological processes. Bleeding from the capillaries, venules and arterioles may occur simply as a result of severe thrombocytopenia. The histopathological appearances of thrombocytopenia-associated purpura are simply those of extravasation of blood cells from the microvasculature and are indistinguishable from traumatic bruises. The commonest causes of thrombocytopenia-associated petechiae are immunologically mediated platelet destruction occurring in idiopathic thrombocytopenic purpura, marrow infiltrative conditions such as acute lymphoplastic leukaemia, thrombocytopenia occurring following acute viral illnesses and drug-induced thrombocytopenia due to marrow suppression.

The second pathological process resulting in petechial or purpuric rash is a primarily thrombotic process resulting in thrombosis within the capillaries or venules and haemorrhagic infarction of the surrounding tissues. Histopathological appearances are those of dilatation of capillaries and venules, occlusion

Table 11.4.1   Causes of petechial or purpuric rash

Infections	*Congenital* CMV, rubella, toxoplasmosis
	Bacterial *Neisseria meningitidis* or septicaemia due to other organisms
	Viral Enterovirus, CMV, EBV, HHV6, HIV, viral haemorrhagic fever
	Fungal Disseminated candidiasis or other fungal sepsis
	Focal infection Bacterial endocarditis
Immune-mediated	Idiopathic thrombocytopenic purpura 'Postinfectious' purpura fulminans Schönlein–Henoch purpura SLE Vasculitis, e.g. polyarteritis nodosa
Decreased platelet production	Marrow infiltration (leukaemia) Drug-induced
Coagulation abnormalities	*Prothrombotic* Protein C and S deficiency
	Defective coagulation DIC Haemophilia
Vessel wall fragility	Collagen disease

CMV, cytomegalovirus; DIC, disseminated intravascular coagulation; EBV, Epstein–Barr virus; HHV6, human herpesvirus type 6; HIV, human immunodeficiency virus; SLE, systemic lupus erythematosus.

of non-inflamed capillaries by venous thrombi and haemorrhage into the surrounding tissues. This form of purpura occurs in association with septicaemic shock, particularly that due to meningococcal infection.[1] It is often associated with gangrene of limbs or digits. It is also seen in postinfectious purpura fulminans, a condition in which purpura occurs 1–3 weeks after an otherwise trivial bacterial or viral infection, the most common of which are varicella and streptococcal infections.[2] This form of purpura is often associated with deficiencies of protein C and S, evidence of DIC, and is probably mediated by autoantibodies directed against protein S.[3,4]

The third pathological process leading to purpura is that of an inflammatory vasculitis with infiltration and destruction of the walls of capillaries, venules and arterioles by neutrophils and macrophages. This form of purpura is seen in meningococcal disease and other forms of bacterial sepsis, in Schönlein–Henoch purpura and in the purpura occurring in autoimmune diseases such as systemic lupus erythematosus and polyarteritis nodosa.[5]

In septic shock, a variety of different immunological mechanisms may contribute to the onset of purpura. Vasoconstriction and poor blood flow through the cutaneous tissues facilitate venous thrombosis. Depletion of the coagulation inhibitors, antithrombin III, protein C and protein S occurring in sepsis together with upregulation of procoagulant factors favours venous thrombosis, and inflammatory cell activation with neutrophil and macrophage adherence to endothelium may result in disruption of the vessel wall.[6] All of these mechanisms probably play a role in the purpura of meningococcal sepsis.

CLINICAL APPROACH TO THE CHILD WITH PETECHIAL RASH AND FEVER

The presence of a petechial or purpuric rash in a child is always an emergency. Although there are many possible causes, bacterial sepsis, particularly due to *Neisseria meningitidis*, should always be considered first, as a delay in the diagnosis of meningococcal sepsis may increase the chance of death. Although in general children with meningococcal sepsis or other forms of bacterial sepsis who develop petechiae will have a high fever and signs of systemic toxicity, this is not always the case, and in the early stages of meningococcal sepsis petechiae may be present in a child who does not appear particularly ill. It is therefore preferable to consider all children with petechial or purpuric rashes to have bacterial sepsis, and to entertain the possibility of non-infectious inflammatory or thrombocytopenic disorders only once the possibility of bacterial infection has been excluded. If a child with petechial rash and fever is seen outside a hospital, penicillin should be administered prior to transfer of the child to hospital. If a child is first seen in hospital, blood cultures should be obtained and intravenous antibiotics administered by the first doctor to see the patient, without awaiting any additional investigation results. Other investigations including full blood count, coagulation studies, urea, electrolytes and creatinine, and morphological examination of the blood film should be obtained. In patients with known congenital heart disease, the possibility of bacterial endocarditis should be considered, and at least two sets of blood cultures should be obtained before commencing antibiotics. Serum should also be stored for antibody studies which would be necessary should the diagnosis of bacterial sepsis not be confirmed, Nasopharyngeal secretions, stool and urine should be obtained for viral culture. Secure venous access should be obtained, and in patients who appear severely ill and toxic at least two venous lines should be secured in case shock develops later in the illness.

CHOICE OF ANTIBIOTICS

Although meningococcal septicaemia is the most likely cause of a petechial rash, other bacterial infections including *Haemophilus influenzae*, *Streptococcus pneumoniae* and other Gram-negative bacilli may occasionally cause purpura. In immunosuppressed patients *Pseudomonas* should also be considered. The initial choice of antibiotics should therefore cover other possibilities in addition to *Neisseria meningitidis*. A third-generation cephalosporin (cefotaxime or ceftriaxone) is appropriate for community-acquired infections. In the immunocompromised and those with underlying disorders, ceftazidime plus an aminoglycoside or ceftazidime and flucloxacillin would be appropriate alternatives. If history of tick-bites or travel is obtained then the possibility of rickettsial infection should be considered and chloramphenicol or tetracycline should be administered as well.

INITIAL MANAGEMENT OF PURPURA ASSOCIATED WITH SEPTIC SHOCK

All children with suspected meningococcal sepsis or purpura fulminans associated with bacterial sepsis should be closely monitored on a high-dependency or intensive care unit. Even if the child appears only moderately unwell initially, patients with meningococcal sepsis may progress to fulminant shock within the space of a few hours and meticulous monitoring is therefore essential.[7] All febrile children with petechial rash should have the following parameters monitored:

blood pressure, pulse rate and respiration, capillary refill time and urine output. Any patients who have signs of early shock (see above) should be aggressively managed with the correction of volume deficits, intensive care monitoring and, if necessary, inotropic support.

Patients with petechiae who show signs of systemic toxicity or shock will usually turn out to have meningococcal sepsis or other forms of bacterial septicaemia. Their management has been described in detail above. Laboratory findings will usually be those of anaemia, moderate thrombocytopenia, and evidence of disseminated intravascular coagulation with prolongation of prothrombin time (PT), KPTT and thrombin time, and elevated fibrin degradation products. Despite the presence of thrombocytopenia, platelet transfusions are rarely required, and may be detrimental in patients who have a predominantly consumptive disorder. Management of the purpura and disseminated intravascular coagulation (DIC) is predominantly treatment of the infection, treatment of the shock, and if necessary replacement of fibrinogen and clotting factors with fresh frozen plasma infusions.[7] Prostacyclin may be beneficial in patients with impending peripheral gangrene in improving peripheral perfusion and preventing platelet aggregation. Heparin has been suggested as being beneficial in the treatment of severe purpura with DIC and peripheral thrombosis[8] but is often associated with an increased risk of haemorrhage. In severely affected patients low-dose heparin (10 units/kg/per hour) helps to reduce the risk of peripheral gangrene with little increase in the risk of haemorrhage. Other experimental treatments include infusions of antithrombin III and protein C concentrate, but these require further evaluation in control trials.[9,10]

MANAGEMENT OF PATIENTS WITH PURPURA WHO DO NOT HAVE SHOCK OR SYSTEMIC TOXICITY

Patients with purpura who have no signs of shock or systemic toxicity are likely to have an alternative diagnosis to acute bacterial sepsis. Patients with idiopathic thrombocytopenic purpura or marrow infiltrative conditions are usually afebrile, and appear generally well apart from the bruising. Profound thrombocytopenia is usually the sole abnormality on initial investigations. Bone marrow examination may be required to exclude the possibility of marrow aplasia or an infiltrative disorder. Further discussion on the management of idiopathic thrombocytopenic purpura or marrow infiltrative thrombocytopenias can be found in haematology texts.

A variety of viral infections, particularly those caused by enteroviruses, but occasionally due to cytomegalovirus or Epstein–Barr virus, may present with petechiae. Patients are generally less ill than those with meningococcal sepsis. The correct diagnosis is often only made after an initial period of treatment for presumed meningococcal sepsis. If no evidence of acute bacterial infection is found on blood culture or cultures of throat, CSF or urine, and if the full blood count and acute-phase proteins do not suggest acute bacterial sepsis, these alternative diagnoses should be vigorously searched for. Enteroviral infection is usually self-limited and the diagnosis is often only confirmed when the results of stool or nasopharyngeal cultures become available once the patient has already recovered. Epstein–Barr virus infection should be diagnosed by serological studies, the detection of atypical lymphocytes, and a positive monospot. All of the congenital infections can produce petechiae and their diagnosis and management are discussed in detail elsewhere. Henoch Schönlein purpura can easily be confused with meningococcal sepsis as both disorders can present with purpura, arthralgia, and abdominal pain. Most patients with Henoch Schönlein are however afebrile, but this diagnosis should only be made only after exclusion of chronic meningococcaemia or early stages of meningococcal sepsis.

POSTINFECTIOUS PURPURA FULMINANS

If extensive purpura is present without signs of shock or systemic toxicity, the possibility of postinfectious purpura fulminans should be considered (Fig. 11.4.1). This devastating disorder occurs 1–3 weeks after an otherwise uncomplicated childhood infection. Chickenpox and streptococcal infection are the most common antecedent infections. Large areas of blue-black discoloration may appear on the skin with terrifying rapidity, and may progress to gangrene of limbs and digits rapidly. Haematological studies usually show evidence of DIC, with prolonged coagulation indices, low fibrinogen and elevated fibrin degradation products. The disorder is associated with severe protein S deficiency, probably due to production of autoantibodies against protein S.[4] Treatment is with heparinization, fresh frozen plasma and, in cases complicated by major vessel thrombosis, thrombolytic treatment with tissue plasminogen activator. Skin grafting and amputations of gangrenous digits may be required in some patients.

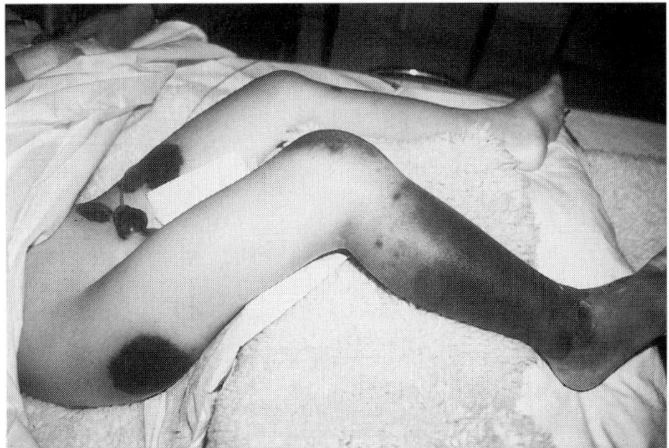

Fig. 11.4.1   A child with purpura fulminans following varicella. Sharply demarcated areas of blue-black discoloration are present on legs. There is impending gangrene of the lower leg.

REFERENCES

1 Dahle J S. Pathogenesis of hemorrhagic skin lesions in meningococcal disease. NIPH Ann 1983; 6: 49–55.
2 Adcock D M, Hicks M J. Dermatopathology of skin necrosis associated with purpura fulminans. Semin Thromb Hemostas 1990; 16: 283–292.
3 Francis R B. Acquired purpura fulminans. Semin Thromb Hemostas 1990; 16: 310–325.
4 Levin M, Eley B S, Louis J, Cohen H, Young L, Heyderman R. Postinfectious purpura fulminans caused by an autoantibody directed against protein S. J Pediatr 1995; 123: 355–363.
5 Seiden M V. Case records of Massachusetts General Hospital. N Engl J Med 1995; 333: 862–867.
6 Levi M, Cate H T, Poll T, Deventer S J H. Pathogenesis of disseminated intravascular coagulation in sepsis. JAMA 1993; 270: 975–979.
7 Nadel S, Levin M, Habibi P. Treatment of meningococcal disease in childhood. In: Cartwright K, ed. Meningococcal disease, vol. 9. Chichester: Wiley, 1995; pp 207–243.

8 Bick R L. Disseminated intravascular coagulation. Med Clin North Am 1994; 78: 511–543.
9 Fourrier F, Chopin C, Huart J J, Runge I, Caron C, Goudemand J. Double-blind, placebo-controlled trial of antithrombin III concentrates in septic shock with disseminated intravascular coagulation. Chest 1993; 104: 882–888.
10 Rivard E G, David M, Farrell C, Schwarz H P. Treatment of purpura fulminans in meningococcemia with protein C concentrate. J Pediatr 1995; 126: 646–652.

CHAPTER 12

CONGENITAL

12.1. Congenital infections and their postnatal effects

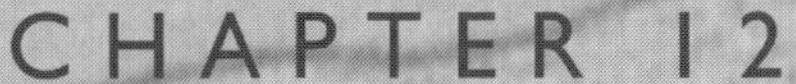

J. M. Forrest   M. A. Burgess

12.1   Congenital infections and their postnatal effects

INTRODUCTION

Congenital infection results from maternal infection during pregnancy. If this occurs early in the pregnancy, by the haematogenous transplacental route, placentitis and fetal infection may occur. If it occurs in the first trimester, at the time of organogenesis, structural congenital malformations may accompany the congenital infection (rubella, cytomegalovirus (CMV), toxoplasma and herpes simplex virus (HSV)). However, the distinction between defects caused by arrested development and those resulting from chronic fetal infection is often difficult to make.

Viral infections are common during pregnancy. The vast majority involve the upper respiratory and gastrointestinal tracts and have no effect on the fetus. However, a number of viruses can cause fetal and chronic perinatal infection. Only four viruses are accepted as causing both chronic infection and true congenital malformations: rubella, CMV, varicella zoster and HSV. Others, including vaccinia, variola, Coxsackie B group, hepatitis viruses, western equine encephalitis and Japanese B encephalitis, may cause chronic intrauterine infection and resultant defects or illness. Some enteroviruses, arboviruses and the attenuated rubella vaccine virus also cross the placenta at times, as may the human immunodeficiency virus (HIV) and human parvovirus.

Congenital infection may also occur as a result of peripartum maternal infection (HSV, enteroviruses, *Listeria*), reaching the infant either across the placenta (*Listeria*) or by direct spread from the mother's genital tract (HSV, *Chlamydia*, gonorrhoea, group B streptococcus). Congenital tuberculosis, malaria and syphilis still occur, although uncommonly in the Western world.

Maternal infection may be clinical or subclinical. It is important to realize that subclinical maternal infection may be just as damaging to the fetus as clinical infection. Congenital infection should be suspected during pregnancy when there has been a suspicious maternal illness or contact, when there is unexplained intrauterine growth retardation or stillbirth, or when a neonate has congenital defects, hydrops, growth retardation, jaundice, splenomegaly, thrombocytopenia or unexplained fever or rash.

Symptoms of congenital infection may not be apparent at birth, but may develop later, months or even years after birth. Infants with congenital infection may have continuing infection, with postnatal development or exacerbation of defects (pulmonary artery stenosis in rubella, deafness in CMV infection, chorioretinitis in toxoplasmosis).

Some congenitally infected infants may be infectious after birth, and may pass their infection on to attendants and others (rubella, CMV).

The microorganisms which can cause congenital infection are listed in Table 12.1.1.

Table 12.1.1 Microorganisms which cause congenital infection

Viruses	Bacteria	Protozoa	Others
Rubella[a]	*Treponema pallidum*	Toxoplasma	*Chlamydia*
Cytomegalovirus	Group B streptococcus	Malaria	*Mycoplasma*
Herpes simplex virus[a]	*Listeria monocytogenes*		*Coxiella burnetii*
Herpes virus 6	Gonococcus		
Varicella zoster[a]	*Mycobacterium tuberculosis*		
Parvovirus (B19)			
Human immunodeficiency virus			
Hepatitis A, B, C			
Influenza			
Epstein–Barr virus			
Enteroviruses			
Measles			
Mumps			
Rubella vaccine virus			

[a] Also causes congenital malformations.

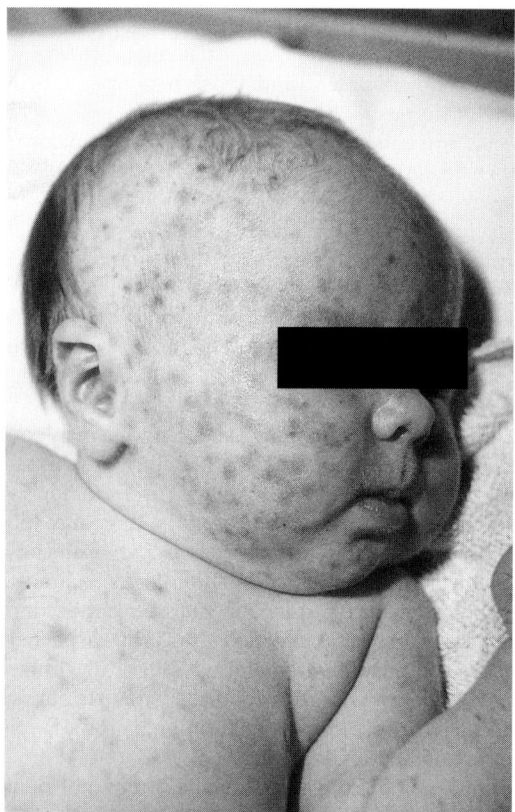

Fig. 12.1.1 Rash of congenital infection. Appearance is due to areas of extramedullary erythropoiesis in skin, sometimes referred to as blueberry muffin. Suggestive of rubella or toxoplasmosis. See also colour plate.

CONGENITAL RUBELLA

The first indication that the placenta was not an impervious barrier to viral infection came in 1941 when Sir Norman Gregg, an Australian ophthalmologist, described congenital cataracts in children whose mothers had had rubella early

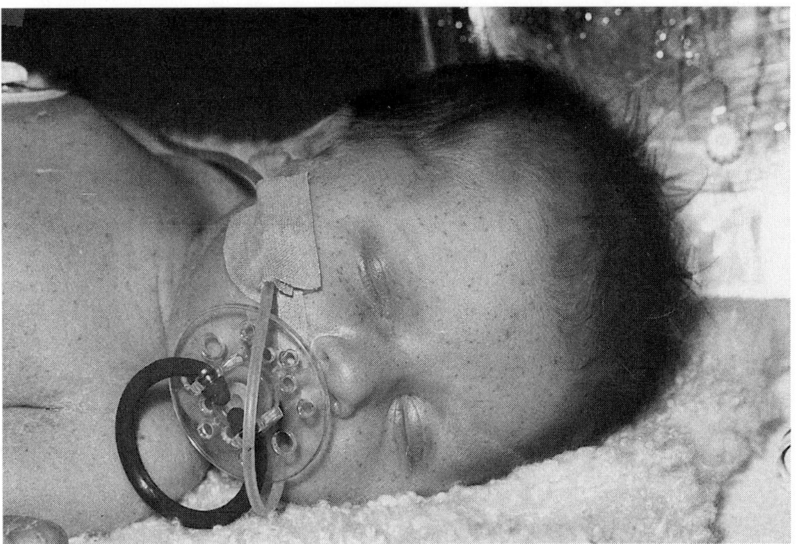

Fig. 12.1.2 Congenital CMV infection, age 2 days. Jaundice and fine petechial rash. See also colour plate.

in their pregnancies. This trivial, often subclinical, maternal infection can cause devastating malformations as well as continuing infection in the developing fetus.[1]

Primary infection during the first trimester almost always results in fetal infection, with a high incidence of congenital defects (heart, eyes, hearing and central nervous system (CNS)). Infection between 12 and 17 weeks (from the last menstrual period) may cause deafness — after 17 weeks damage is rare (Table 12.1.2).[2] Growth retardation often follows infection in early pregnancy, and the fetus is usually chronically infected. Virus can be isolated from many fetal organs and from liveborn infants, often for months, despite the presence of specific antibody. Very rarely, congenital rubella may follow subclinical reinfection in women with natural or vaccine-induced immunity.[3]

The clinical manifestations of congenital rubella can be divided into those due to developmental malformation; transient effects of persisting infection presenting early in postnatal life; and late onset manifestations.

Developmental defects include low birth weight due to intrauterine growth

Table 12.1.2 Risk of congenital rubella defects

Weeks since last menstrual period	Defects	Percentage affected
0–12	Heart[a] Eye[b] Deafness[c] Central nervous system	80%
13–16	Deafness Mental retardation	35%
17+	Deafness ? Mental retardation	1%

Adapted from Gilbert G L. Infectious disease in pregnancy and the newborn infant. Melbourne: Harwood, 1991: pp 34–50.
[a] Patent ductus arteriosus: 25–62 days.
[b] Retinopathy: 16–131 days.
[c] Deafness: 16–131 days.

retardation; cardiovascular defects (pulmonary and renal artery stenosis, patent ductus arteriosus, septal defects, coarctation of the aorta); ocular defects (cataracts, cloudy cornea, pigmentary retinopathy, microphthalmia, glaucoma); sensorineural deafness; neurological defects (microcephaly, psychomotor retardation, and rarely foci of cerebral calcification); genitourinary abnormalities (polycystic kidney, hydronephrosis), undescended testes, cleft palate and bony defects.

Effects of persisting infection include encephalitis with persistent abnormalities of the CSF (virus has been isolated from the CSF for up to 18 months), lymphadenopathy, hepatosplenomegaly, interstitial pneumonitis, thrombocytopenia and osteitis (alternating linear densities in the metaphases of long bones, without periosteal reaction). Almost any organ can be affected.

Many congenitally infected infants are apparently normal at birth, but growth retardation, deafness, epilepsy, cataracts (Fig. 12.1.3) (rubella virus can be isolated

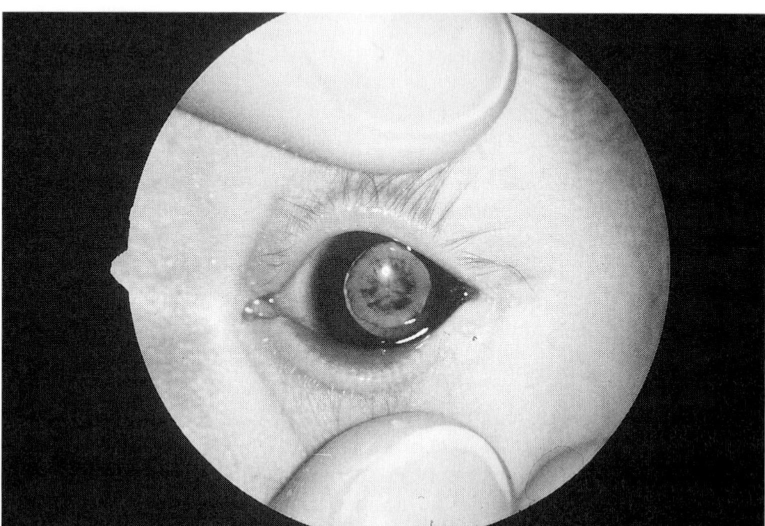

Fig. 12.1.3 Congenital rubella infection. Cataract.

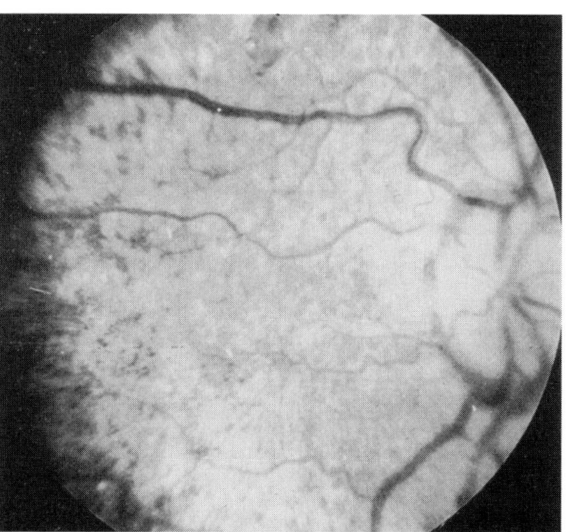

Fig. 12.1.4 Congenital rubella infection. 'Salt and pepper' retinopathy.

from lenses removed up to three years after birth), retinopathy (Fig. 12.1.4), pulmonary artery stenosis, and neurological (motor and intellectual) deficiencies can appear or progress in the postnatal period. Sensorineural deafness, often progressive, may occur without other abnormalities, so hearing should be tested regularly. Deafness is the commonest manifestation of congenital rubella.

Immunological abnormalities have been described in some children with congenital rubella: hypogammaglobulinaemia, very high and rising IgM levels, circulating immune complexes, reduced complement levels and abnormalities of cell-mediated immunity. Occasionally, affected infants develop a rash and progressive pneumonitis ('late-onset disease') late in the first year of life. A rare progressive panencephalitis in the second decade, with high CSF IgM levels and rubella virus isolated from the brain, has been described. Long-term immune-mediated sequelae of congenital infection include hypothyroidism, thyroiditis and growth hormone deficiency. Diabetes mellitus occurs in 10% of long-term survivors.

Diagnosis

Primary maternal rubella can be diagnosed serologically by seroconversion, a rising titre of IgG antibodies, or demonstration of rubella-specific IgM. Pregnant women who are exposed to rubella or have a suspicious illness should have serum collected as soon as possible. Ideally both acute and convalescent sera should be obtained. In some instances a third specimen may be indicated about a month after the contact. Occasionally, expert advice is needed to interpret results.

The diagnosis of congenital rubella can be made by detecting rubella-specific IgM in fetal serum or cord blood, or by cultivating the rubella virus from throat, conjunctiva, urine or lens. If laboratory data are incomplete, presence of two of (cataracts/congenital glaucoma; congenital heart disease; hearing loss; pigmentary retinopathy), plus one of (purpura; splenomegaly; jaundice; microcephaly; mental retardation; meningoencephalitis; radiolucent bone disease) are compatible with the diagnosis.[4]

Persistence of rubella IgG beyond 6 months of age in a child with compatible defects is also diagnostic.

Babies with congenital rubella may be infectious for 12 months or more. Non-immune pregnant women should not feed or change them.

Prevention

Congenital rubella can be prevented by vaccination of susceptible women before they become pregnant (see Ch. 18.1). In some countries all children are vaccinated at 12–15 months; in others adolescent schoolgirls and non-immune women after delivery are vaccinated. Some countries now combine these two approaches. In Europe, North America and Australia, vaccination programmes commenced in the late 1960s, and the incidence of congenital rubella has fallen from about one in 2000 live births to close to zero.[5,6] However, vaccination is not carried out in most developing countries, so immigrants from these countries are likely to be non-immune.[7]

All susceptible women of childbearing age should be vaccinated, but not during pregnancy, because the vaccine contains live attenuated virus, which can cross the placenta and infect the fetus. Although rubella vaccine virus has been isolated from eye and CNS of aborted fetuses from susceptible women who were vaccinated during pregnancy, no cases of congenital rubella syndrome have been found among a large number of infants carried to term after maternal vaccination during pregnancy,[8] so termination is not indicated.[9]

CONGENITAL CYTOMEGALOVIRUS INFECTION

Now that vaccination has reduced the incidence of congenital rubella, CMV is the commonest cause of congenital infection in developed countries. It contributes significantly to the incidence of brain damage, deafness and occasionally visual impairment. The estimated incidence of prenatal CMV infection ranges from 0.2–2.2% of live births in industrialized countries. Like other herpesviruses, CMV can cause persistent infection and can become reactivated, especially in immunosuppressed individuals.

Primary maternal CMV infection during pregnancy (which is often either asymptomatic or non-specific) results in viraemia, with transmission to the fetus in 20–50%[10] and of sequelae in 10–25% after maternal infection during the first 6 months of pregnancy.[11] Fetal infection can occur at any stage of pregnancy, although the first trimester is the major risk period. Fetal infection can also follow reactivation of maternal CMV infection, but the risk of sequelae is much less than after primary maternal infection (8% compared with 25%).[11]

Infants may acquire the infection perinatally from maternal secretions (throat, urine or cervix), infected blood transfusions, or from breast milk during the first months of life.

Symptomatic congenital CMV infection usually occurs only in infants infected during primary maternal infection and, even in this group, 80–90% are normal at birth. Clinical manifestations include intrauterine growth retardation, hepatosplenomegaly with jaundice and abnormalities of liver function, and thrombocytopenia with petechial rash (Fig. 12.1.2). The CNS is often involved (microcephaly, increased cerebrospinal fluid (CSF) protein levels, intracranial calcification, hydrocephalus). Sensorineural deafness is common, though often unrecognized in the neonatal period. Chorioretinitis is the commonest ocular manifestation — it resembles the chorioretinitis of congenital toxoplasmosis (Fig. 12.1.7) but rarely progresses in later life (Table 12.1.3). Defects in tooth enamel are common. Mortality is as high as 30% among the severely affected infants. Most infants with symptomatic congenital CMV at birth, especially neurological involvement, have long-term sequelae such as mental retardation, cerebral palsy, deafness (which may be progressive) and eye defects.[12]

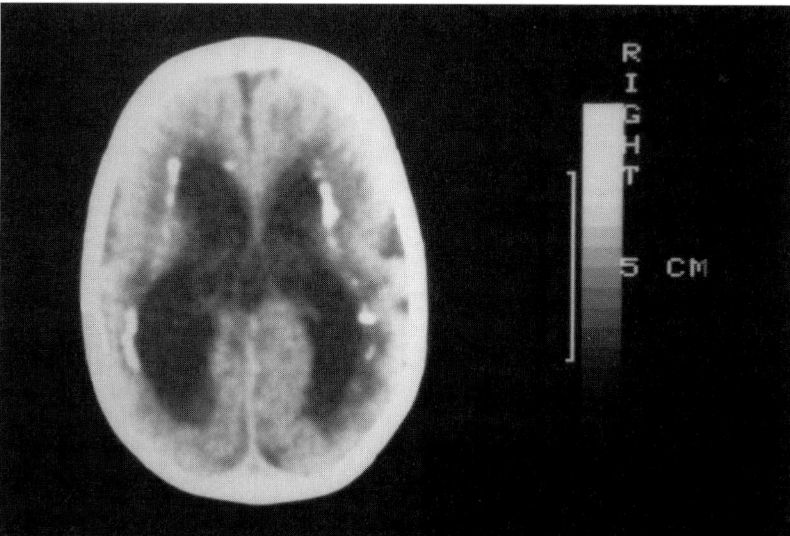

Fig. 12.1.5 Congenital CMV infection. CT scan showing dilated ventricles and periventricular calcification.

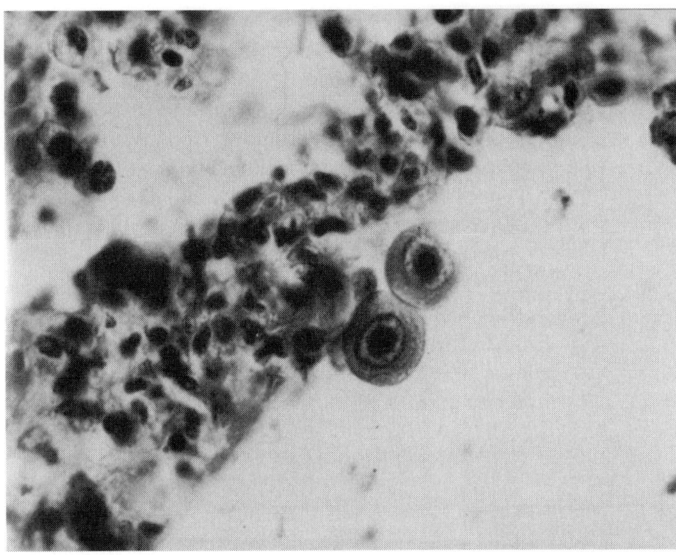

Fig. 12.1.6   CMV pneumonitis. CMV inclusion bodies in cells in alveolar space.

Table 12.1.3   Intrauterine infections which can cause congenital eye defects

Cataracts	Chorioretinopathy
Rubella	Rubella (usually does not affect vision)
	Cytomegalovirus
Toxoplasmosis	Toxoplasmosis
Varicella zoster	Varicella zoster
	Herpes simplex virus

Far fewer (5–15%) infants with asymptomatic disease have sequelae. These usually become apparent in the first 2 years of life. The most common defect which follows asymptomatic congenital infection is deafness, which occurs in about 5%.[13] It may progress, usually in the first 3 years of life, but occasionally as late as 8–14. Uncommonly, microcephaly, psychomotor retardation, chorioretinitis and dental defects may develop in infants who were asymptomatic at birth.

All babies with congenital CMV infection should be carefully followed up with regular hearing tests. They are infectious: virus may be present in saliva, tears, urine and other secretions. Pregnant women should either avoid contact with these infants or protect themselves by careful handwashing.

Diagnosis

Culture of virus from the baby's urine, throat or nasopharyngeal aspirate in the first week of life indicates congenital infection, as does detection of CMV-specific IgM in cord blood. After the first week of life it may be difficult to tell whether positive viral cultures indicate prenatal or postnatal infection.

Prenatal diagnosis may be established by identifying virus in amniotic fluid,[14] and abnormalities consistent with but not diagnostic of CMV infection may be detected by fetal ultrasound. The possibility that ganciclovir therapy may lessen the incidence and/or severity of sequelae is being investigated by controlled trials in symptomatic neonates.[15]

Prevention

Although 'protection of women of childbearing age by vaccination is the logical approach',[16] the situation is not as straightforward as with rubella. A live attenuated vaccine (Towne 125) was developed in 1975, but concerns about reactivation of the vaccine virus and its possible oncogenic potential have limited its use, although preliminary trials in normal volunteers and renal transplant volunteers were encouraging. Subunit inactivated vaccines are also under trial. If successful, these will avoid some of the potential problems with live vaccines.

Pregnant women should be counselled about possible sources of infection (young children in day care centres, family transmission, blood products, etc.). Screening of all pregnancies is not indicated.[17] In developing countries most adult women will be immune. In developed countries 40–60% of young adults are immune. Pregnant women who have a contact or a suspicious glandular fever-like illness should be tested for seroconversion, presence of IgM antibody or viraemia.

TOXOPLASMOSIS

Congenital infection with the protozoa *Toxoplasma gondii* may clinically resemble congenital rubella and congenital CMV, but the incidence in most countries is much less (2–6/1000 pregnancies).

The definitive host is the cat family. Oocytes in cat faeces may remain infective for up to 1 year in warm moist soil. If ingested by humans or domestic animals they release trophozoites which can invade any nucleated cell to form tissue cysts. Human toxoplasmosis is acquired by ingestion of raw or under-cooked meat, especially pork and lamb (hence the high incidence of toxoplasmosis in France) or soil contaminated by faecal oocysts (unwashed vegetables, or soil on hands after gardening). Oocysts in meat are destroyed by freezing. They may be present in cat fur or cat litter. Infection can also be acquired by blood transfusion or transplantation. It is not transmitted by simple direct contact with acute or congenitally infected persons.

When acquired in pregnancy, toxoplasmosis can cause fetal infection with potentially serious consequences. Infants of mothers with a primary infection in pregnancy, which is usually asymptomatic or a non-specific flu-like illness, are at risk. Infection is transplacental. The later in pregnancy the infection occurs, the more likely is spread to the fetus, but the most severe fetal effects follow maternal infection early in pregnancy. Reactivation and subsequent fetal infection may occur in women who are immunosuppressed (transplant recipients or patients with HIV).[18]

Congenital toxoplasmosis is usually asymptomatic — only about 10% of cases are symptomatic at birth.[19] The classical triad of chorioretinitis, intracranial calcification and hydrocephalus is not common, but 90% of those infants who are symptomatic will have intellectual impairment.[20] Hydrocephalus is usually associated with other severe brain lesions.

Infants with generalized infection may have anaemia, blueberry muffin appearance (Fig. 12.1.1), thrombocytopenic purpura (Fig. 12.1.2), jaundice, hepato-splenomegaly, lymphadenopathy, pneumonitis and myocarditis — clinically resembling congenital CMV infection. Chorioretinopathy may be apparent at birth, as active lesions or retinal scars. Microphthalmia, squint, nystagmus and cataracts occur less commonly.

Children with proven congenital toxoplasmosis should be carefully followed up, because neurological defects and deafness may develop in later years. Chorioretinitis in particular may not become apparent until childhood or early

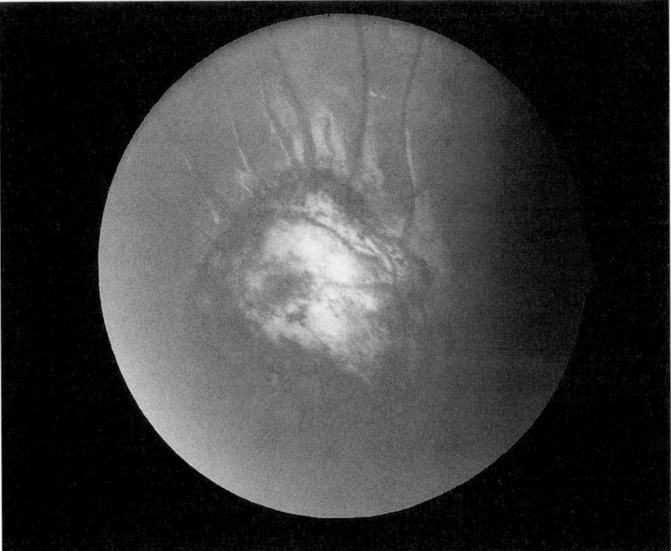

Fig. 12.1.7 Congenital toxoplasmosis. Classical appearance of retinopathy with peripheral pigmentation.

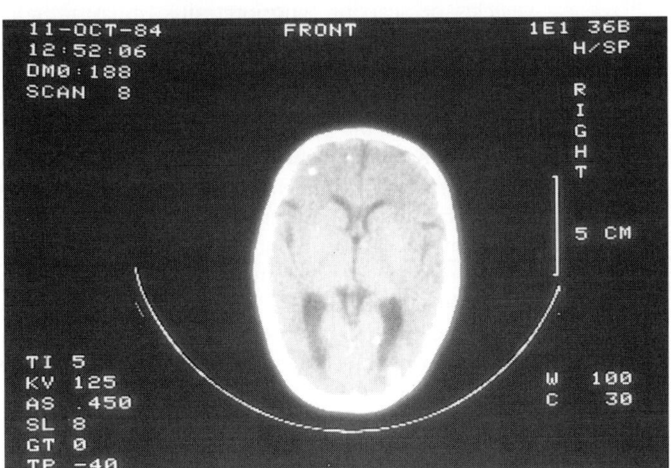

Fig. 12.1.8 Congenital toxoplasmosis. CT scan showing punctate areas of calcification.

adult life. Treatment of subclinical congenital toxoplasmosis (see below) has been shown to reduce the incidence of sequelae.[21] Many authorities recommend treatment of all cases to limit progression of damage.

Diagnosis

Detection of toxoplasma-specific IgM or IgA in cord blood or fetal sera, or culture of placental tissue, will provide a diagnosis if congenital toxoplasmosis is suspected. The levels of IgG and IgM often rise after birth in infected infants. Cerebral computed tomographic (CT) scanning may show hydrocephalus and intracranial calcification (Fig. 12.1.8).

Antenatal screening for toxoplasmosis has been carried out in France and Austria for many years.[19] Seronegative women are tested repeatedly during pregnancy. Studies in these countries have shown that treatment of the mother with antiprotozoal agents (spiramycin; pyrimethamine plus a sulphonamide) during pregnancy can reduce the risk of transmission to the fetus.

All pregnant women who have a suspicious illness should have acute and convalescent sera tested.

Prevention

In those countries where congenital toxoplasmosis is rare, and screening is not carried out because it is not cost-effective,[22] pregnant women should be advised to avoid ingestion of resistant forms of the parasite which may be found in cat faeces and soil, or in raw and undercooked meat or poultry.

There is no vaccine against toxoplasmosis.

CONGENITAL HERPES SIMPLEX VIRUS INFECTION

Like other herpesviruses, herpes simplex virus (HSV) can remain latent for months or years. HSV-1 causes mainly oral and pharyngeal lesions; HSV-2 mainly affects the genital area. Both types can affect the genital area and infect the fetus.

Intrauterine HSV infection causing congenital fetal abnormalities is uncommon but well documented. It is said to account for only about 5% of all neonatal HSV infections.[23] Infants infected in utero may have some combination of skin vesicles or scarring, chorioretinitis, microphthalmia, microcephaly or hydranencephaly. Subsequent mental retardation with defects of vision and hearing is common.

Intrauterine infection may occur late in pregnancy, but most infections are transmitted to the fetus from infected maternal secretions during delivery, or from ascending infection after premature rupture of the membranes. Infants born to mothers with active primary genital herpes are at greatest risk. Maternal reactivation of genital herpes is less likely to result in neonatal herpes, though cases have been documented. Since most maternal and recurrent HSV infections are asymptomatic, preventing infection of the infant is difficult.

Skin involvement is the commonest manifestation in the infant. Early recognition and treatment (with acyclovir or adenosine arabinoside) may prevent dissemination of infection, pneumonitis or meningoencephalitis. Some authorities

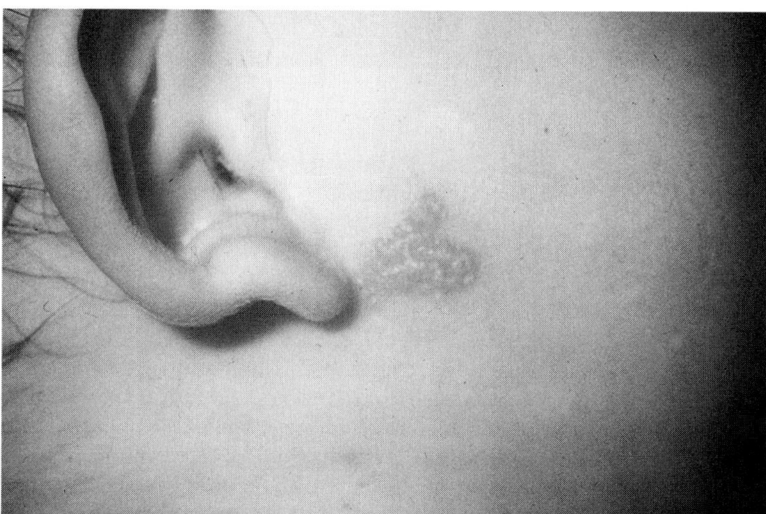

Fig. 12.1.9 Congenital HSV infection. Without urgent treatment, this baby has a 70% risk of disseminated HSV infection, encephalitis and death.

recommend continued administration of acyclovir in maintenance doses to prevent recurrence of infection at least throughout the first year of life.

Diagnosis

Virus may be cultured from mucocutaneous lesions, CSF, urine, nasopharyngeal aspirates or pharyngeal swabs. Immunofluorescent techniques can provide a rapid diagnosis.

Primary genital herpes in the third trimester poses a significant risk to mother and baby, and should be treated with acyclovir.

Opinions vary, but delivery by caesarean section, especially if lesions are present in the perineal region, should be considered to decrease the risk of exposure to the neonate.[24] Such infants should be carefully observed for any sign of illness until 6 weeks of age.[23]

CONGENITAL HERPESVIRUS 6 INFECTION

This typical herpesvirus, one of the seven recognized human herpesviruses, causes exanthem subitum or roseola infantum, a common febrile illness with rash in the first 2 years of life.

The presence of herpesvirus 6-specific IgM in cord blood,[25] and its isolation from the thymus of a fetus obtained through induced abortion from an HIV-positive woman,[26] suggest that congenital infection can occur. Herpesvirus 6 has also been detected in villous tissue of two women with herpesvirus 6 IgM antibodies who spontaneously aborted at 6–12 weeks of pregnancy.

However, since most adults are immune, the risk of congenital infection is probably minute.

CONGENITAL VARICELLA ZOSTER INFECTION

Varicella zoster virus infection during pregnancy, causing either chickenpox or, less commonly, shingles in the mother can lead to congenital varicella.

About 95% of women of childbearing age are immune to varicella. A primary infection in the first half of pregnancy can lead to spontaneous abortion, in the third trimester to premature labour. Severe varicella pneumonia at any stage of pregnancy can cause fetal death.

The relationship between maternal varicella in early pregnancy and congenital defects in the offspring was first described by La Foret and Lynch in 1947. Typical features are hypoplasia of one limb with cicatricial skin lesions in a dermatomal distribution affecting that limb (Fig. 12.1.10). Intrauterine growth retardation, neurological abnormalities (microcephaly, hydrocephalus and cerebellar hypoplasia), eye lesions (microphthalmia, cataracts, Horner's syndrome, chorioretinitis and scars), and gastrointestinal and genitourinary abnormalities may also be present.[27]

Recent prospective studies suggest that the absolute risk of congenital embryopathy after maternal varicella infection in the first 20 weeks of pregnancy is about 2%.[28,29] There are only occasional reports of fetal damage after maternal zoster.

Varicella virus has not been isolated from affected infants. This may mean that fetal infection does not persist, as with CMV and rubella. However, it is possible that the virus may have become latent in dorsal sensory nerve ganglia and other neural tissues and become reactivated, so that fetal damage depends on the stage of gestation at which reactivation, not maternal varicella, occurs.[30]

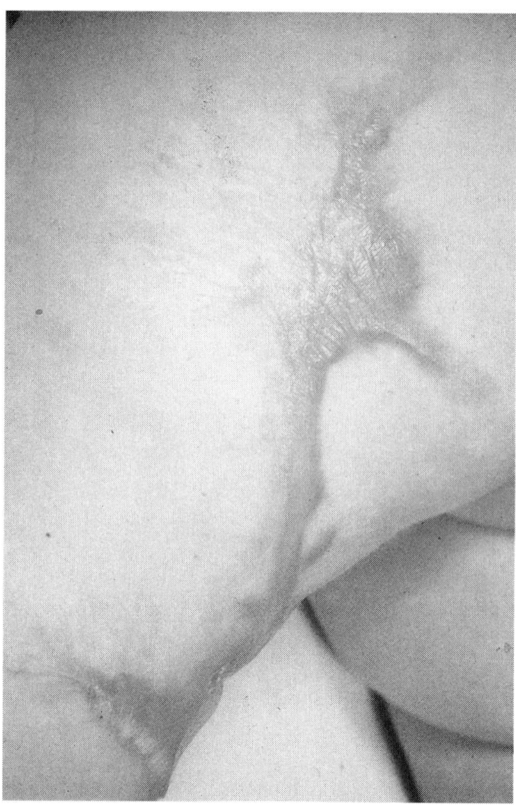

Fig. 12.1.10 Congenital varicella infection. Circumferential scarring of limb.

Maternal chickenpox in the last 3 weeks of pregnancy may cause perinatal infection. If the mother's rash appears 5 days before to 2 days after delivery, the infant is at risk of severe neonatal chickenpox, which carries a high mortality rate. Such infants have been exposed to a large transplacental viral inoculum without the protection of maternal antibody. They may be well at birth but become severely ill at 5–10 days. Babies whose mothers develop chickenpox rash up to and including 5 days before delivery or up to 2 days after delivery should be given intramuscular zoster immune globulin as soon as possible.[31]

Treatment of severe neonatal or maternal infection is with intravenous acyclovir.

Diagnosis

This may be established by (1) evidence of maternal infection — clinical, virological, serological; (2) presence of typical skin lesions, in a dermatomal distribution, in the infant; (3) presence of varicella-specific IgM in the infant, or the occurrence of typical herpes zoster in the first few months of life, or persistence of varicella IgG antibodies.

CONGENITAL HUMAN PARVOVIRUS (B19) INFECTION

This small virus causes erythema infectiosum (fifth disease), a febrile illness associated with a distinctive rash (a slapped cheek appearance and a lacy rash on the trunk and extremities) and occasional arthralgia (Ch. 10.1). Asymptomatic infection may occur. The virus infects erythroid cells and replicates in the bone marrow, so in people with shortened red cell survival it can cause aplastic crises.

Fifty per cent of women of childbearing age are susceptible. Intrauterine infection, which may be clinical or subclinical, may cause spontaneous abortion, non-immunological hydrops fetalis or fetal death, because of anaemia secondary to infection of red cell progenitors.

Most reports of sequelae have followed maternal infection in the first half of pregnancy. Third-trimester maternal infections followed by the birth of anaemic newborns have been described.[32]

Intrauterine transfusion in B19-infected hydropic fetuses has resulted in the birth of healthy babies,[33] and there has been one report of spontaneous resolution of B19-induced hydrops.[34]

A prospective British study suggested a transplacental transmission rate of 33%, and a risk of fetal death in an infected pregnancy of 9%.[35]

Diagnosis

Detection of specific IgM antibody or viral antigen is the most sensitive way to diagnose recent infection in the mother, and their presence in cord blood establishes the diagnosis of congenital B19 infection.

If maternal infection has occurred, an increased maternal serum α-fetoprotein is a useful, sensitive but non-specific predictor of a possible unfavourable fetal outcome.

CONGENITAL HIV INFECTION

It is known that women with HIV infection may transmit this to their infants, but the frequency with which this occurs is uncertain, and the relative risks of transplacental versus perinatal transmission are likewise unclear. 'Evidence is accumulating that intrauterine transplacental transmission of HIV is the commonest route'.[36] HIV has been detected in placentas, in tissues of aborted fetuses and in cord blood. Postnatal infection from breast milk has been demonstrated (see Ch. 15.1).

The existence of a characteristic syndrome of growth failure, microcephaly, hypertelorism, dysmorphic craniofacial features, lymphadenopathy and hepatomegaly due to intrauterine infection has been suggested,[37] but remains controversial.

Congenitally infected children usually develop symptoms earlier than those who have acquired the infection after birth. They are more likely than adults to have severe recurrent bacterial infections and lymphoid interstitial pneumonitis, but Kaposi's sarcoma and reactivation of latent infections are rare in children. Progressive encephalopathy occurs in most infected children, and haematological abnormalities are common.

A large multicentre trial (59 sites in the USA and France) involving 364 infants and their mothers showed that treatment of HIV-infected mothers and their babies with zidovudine significantly reduced HIV transmission from mother to baby by two-thirds, the regimen being well tolerated by both mothers and infants.[38]

In developed countries where bottle-feeding is safe, HIV-infected mothers should not breast-feed, but in places where there is a high infant mortality from infectious disease or malnutrition, WHO/UNICEF recommend that all women, including those known to have HIV, should breast-feed their infants.[39]

OTHER VIRUSES WHICH MAY CAUSE CONGENITAL INFECTION

Hepatitis B

Acute maternal hepatitis B in the first trimester does not cause congenital malformations or spontaneous abortion. If it occurs in the third trimester there is a 50–70% chance of transmission of infection to the infant, and premature labour is more likely.

Routine antenatal screening should be carried out to detect chronic carriers, whose infants should receive hepatitis B immune globulin and hepatitis B vaccine at birth. This is 90–95% effective in preventing neonatal infection. Most transmission of infection from carrier mothers to their infants occurs around the time of delivery.

Caesarean section may offer additional protection for infants of highly infectious carrier mothers.

The virus is present in the breast milk of carriers and, in those infants in whom vaccination fails, breast milk may be a source of infection.

Hepatitis A

This virus is rarely transmitted to the fetus. Infection in the third trimester may increase the risk of preterm delivery and fetal death.

Hepatitis C

Recent reports from Japan indicate that hepatitis C virus can be vertically transmitted from mother to infant, and the risk of transmission is correlated with the titre of HCV RNA in the mother,[40] but transplacental transmission has not been proved.

Enteroviruses

This family of small RNA viruses includes the polio viruses, the echoviruses, Coxsackie A and B viruses and enteroviruses 68–71.

Neither polioviruses nor live attenuated polio vaccines have been implicated in congenital anomalies.

Occasional intrauterine infection can be associated with severe maternal infection, but the placenta is usually a significant barrier. The onset of various enterovirus infections, including paralytic polio, in the first 3 days of life, and isolation of virus from amniotic fluid or cord blood, show that intrauterine infection can occur.

Influenza

Intrauterine influenza can occur, but is exceptional, probably because maternal viraemia is rare. A reported association between maternal influenza in the first trimester and congenital anencephaly may have been related to the effects of hyperthermia on the fetus.[41]

Influenza vaccine containing inactivated virus may be safely given to pregnant women if indicated.[42]

Epstein–Barr virus

Infection with the Epstein–Barr virus during pregnancy is not usually associated with an adverse effect on the fetus — intrauterine infection is very uncommon, because only 5% of women of childbearing age are susceptible.

Measles and mumps

Measles is rare during pregnancy. Severe maternal infection can result in abortion, fetal death and premature labour. If the mother develops measles near term, the infant may be born with congenital measles, which may have a high fatality rate, especially in premature infants.

Measles is not associated with congenital abnormalities.

There are no data about the effect of immunization against measles during pregnancy, but since the vaccine virus is a live attenuated one it should not be used during pregnancy.

Mumps is also uncommon during pregnancy. It may cause congenital malformations in animals, and there have been anecdotal reports of central nervous system abnormalities in humans. Its suggested association with endocardial fibroelastosis in infants is unproved.

Congenital mumps with parotitis, pneumonia and virus isolated from nasopharyngeal aspirates, has been reported.

Mumps vaccine virus can cross the placenta, so should not be given during pregnancy.

CONGENITAL SYPHILIS

This infection should be preventable by screening during pregnancy. The risk of fetal infection depends on the stage of pregnancy, and the stage of the syphilitic infection in the mother. Organisms reach the fetus when the mother is bacteraemic.

Most congenital syphilitic infections are asymptomatic at birth and are diag-

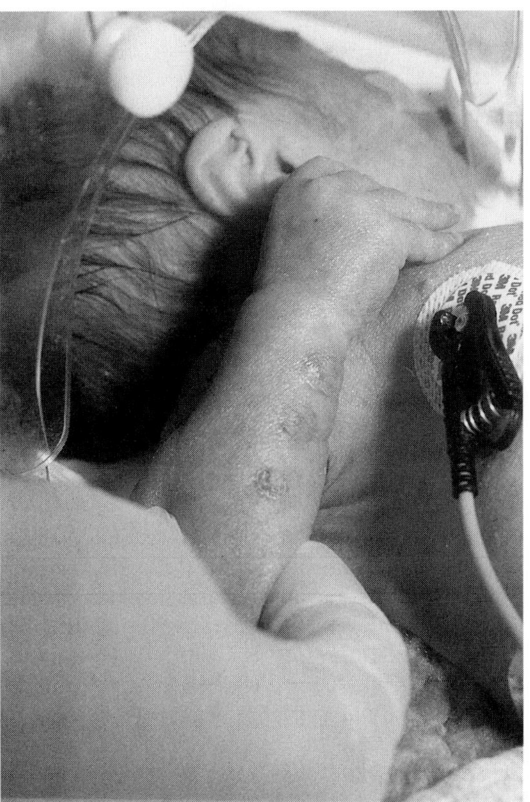

Fig. 12.1.11 Congenital syphilis. Baby born with blistering lesions, which turn brown as they heal. See also colour plate.

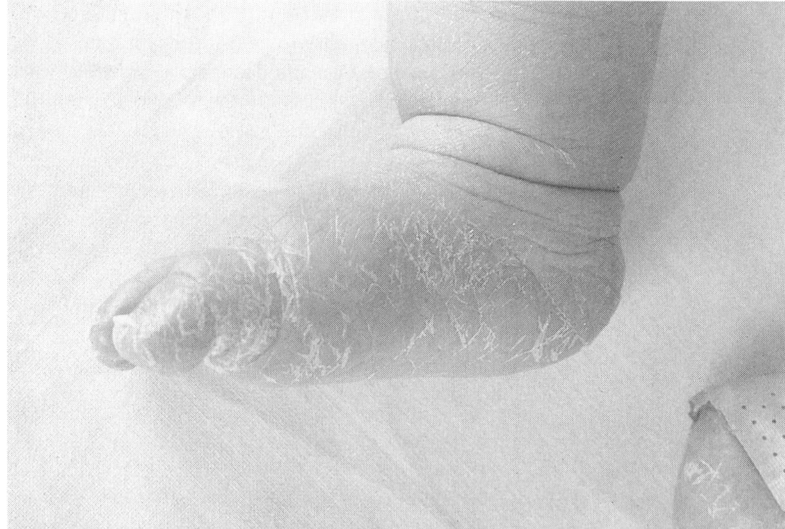

Fig. 12.1.12 Congenital syphilis. Late presentation (age 4 months) with anaemia, oedema, hepatosplenomegaly and this appearance of red, dry feet. See also colour plate.

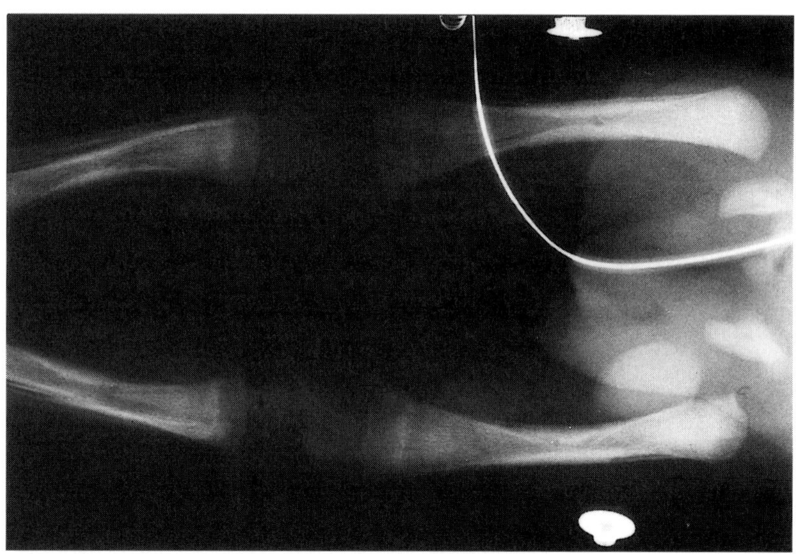

Fig. 12.1.13 Congenital syphilis. Marked bilateral osteitis.

nosed by serological means or by X-ray changes in the long bones. In untreated children who have symptoms at birth the mortality is as high as 54%.

Symptoms of early congenital syphilis (diagnosed in the first 2 years of life) usually appear during the first 3 months. Any organ may be involved. Typical changes include nasal discharge, rashes on palms and soles, bony lesions, hepatosplenomegaly, anaemia, hydrops, growth retardation and microcephaly. Congenital neurosyphilis is hard to diagnose, but is important because involvement of the CNS determines the long-term prognosis.

Late congenital syphilis (diagnosed after 2 years of age) includes classic stigmata due to scars of earlier tissue damage plus lesions from continuing infection. Dental defects (Hutchinson's teeth and 'mulberry molars'), eye changes (interstitial keratitis and anterior uveitis), mid-face defects including a 'saddle nose', fissures around the mouth and nostrils, Clutton's joints and other bony changes may be found. Mental retardation and other manifestations of congenital neurosyphilis are fortunately rare.

Once the diagnosis is made, treatment with penicillin and long-term follow-up can commence.

CONGENITAL GONORRHOEA, CHLAMYDIA AND GENITAL MYCOPLASMAS

Both gonorrhoea and chlamydia can cause neonatal conjunctivitis. They may be transmitted together. If the conjunctivitis is severe it is more likely to be gonococcal. Intrauterine infection is very rare.

Intrauterine ureaplasma infection is also rare, but chorioamnionitis with intrauterine growth retardation and premature delivery has been reported, and congenital pneumonia is well documented.

CONGENITAL LISTERIOSIS

This Gram-positive bacillus (*Listeria monocytogenes*) is a relatively uncommon human pathogen. It usually affects only those who are very young, very old, pregnant or immunocompromised.

Sources of infection include contaminated food (milk, cheese, uncooked vegetables, shellfish, pâté, poultry). A faecal–oral route is usual, and asymptomatic faecal carriage is not uncommon.

Maternal infection is usually a mild self-limited flu-like illness. Intrauterine infection usually occurs during the second or third trimesters causing premature delivery or stillbirth in 20%. Most liveborn infants develop symptoms soon after delivery. Respiratory distress due to congenital pneumonia is the most common manifestation. Fits, hepatosplenomegaly, a rash and conjunctivitis indicate disseminated infection.

Symptoms developing within the first 2–3 days of life are usually associated

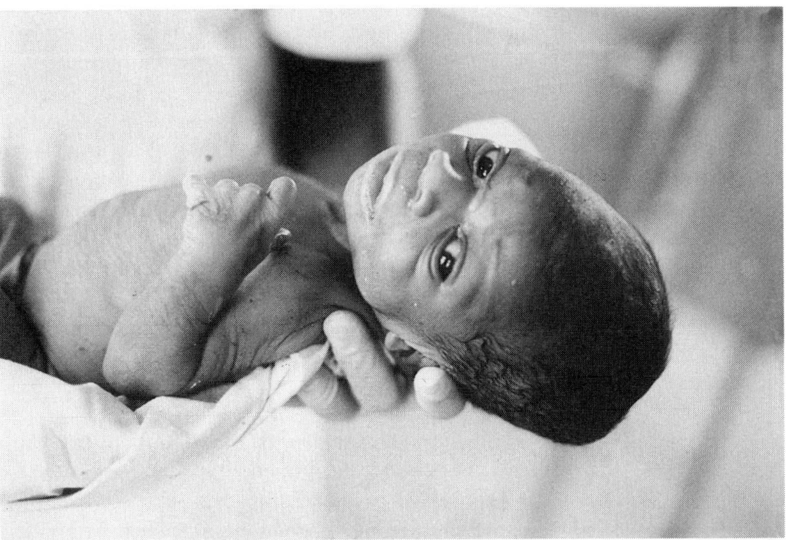

Fig. 12.1.14 Neonatal gonorrhoea. Baby born with pus trickling from eye.

with meningitis. Neonatal mortality of congenital listeriosis may approach 30%; the overall perinatal mortality may be as high as 50–60%.

Diagnosis may be made by isolation of the organism from cultures of blood or CSF. Treatment with ampicillin and gentamicin should continue for 2 weeks.

GROUP B STREPTOCOCCUS

This organism is an opportunistic pathogen in compromised hosts, especially neonates. It colonizes the pharynx, gut and genitourinary tracts of 5–40% of healthy individuals.

Intrauterine fetal infection occurs by the ascending route, and causes chorio-amnionitis. Mothers who are vaginal carriers have an increased risk of mid-trimester abortion and premature delivery. Intrauterine pneumonia has been found at autopsy in infected infants. About 50% of infected infants develop symptoms within a few hours of birth.

TUBERCULOSIS

It is difficult to distinguish intrauterine tuberculosis from early postnatal infection. The placenta is usually an effective barrier against intrauterine infection. Infection may reach the fetus by the haematogenous route or by direct extension from endometrial tuberculosis.

The criteria for congenital tuberculosis include a proven diagnosis of tuberculosis in an infant with one of the following four: development of lesions in the first week of life; a primary complex in the fetal liver or a caseating hepatic granuloma; tuberculosis of the placenta or maternal genital tract; and exclusion of the possibility of postnatal transmission from a contact.[43]

Infection in the first trimester may lead to spontaneous abortion or to stillbirth or neonatal death from extensive caseating tuberculosis.

Affected infants may appear well at birth, but develop symptoms days or weeks after birth. Some may develop fulminant disease and die within hours; others may survive without treatment for up to 2 years.

Symptoms may be non-specific (failure to thrive, fever, respiratory distress) or include cough, pneumonia, jaundice, hepatosplenomegaly, lymphadenopathy or skin tubercles. Meningitis is uncommon.

Diagnosis and prevention

Once diagnosed congenital tuberculosis can be successfully treated. Thinking of the diagnosis, especially extrapulmonary tuberculosis, is the hardest part.

Infants should not be cared for by persons with active tuberculosis.

Routine antenatal chest X-rays may be wise in countries with a high background incidence of tuberculosis. The use of routine or selective maternal Mantoux testing has been debated.

MALARIA

In areas where malaria is endemic there is a high frequency of placental infection, but congenital infection is uncommon in the infants of mothers who have a high level of 'immunity'. In such an immune population, the incidence of clinically significant congenital malaria is about 0.3%, compared with 1–4% in infants of non-immune mothers. However, infants in such areas have larger spleens than infants in non-endemic areas, and placental infection is associated with impaired fetal growth.[44]

Congenital malaria is more likely in infants of non-immune mothers, and in mothers whose immunity has begun to wane, often because they have left an endemic area.

Clinical features resemble those of neonatal sepsis: fever, irritability, anorexia, diarrhoea, jaundice, hepatosplenomegaly, fits, anaemia and thrombocytopenia.

Once diagnosed and treated, congenital malaria does not relapse because there is no exoerythrocytic stage, since the congenital infection is bloodborne.

Q FEVER

Coxiella burnetii may infect the placenta and cause abortion and stillbirth, but it is very uncommon.[45]

CONCLUSIONS

A surprisingly wide range of microorganisms is capable of infecting the fetus. Although some cause chronic infection, some result in severe fetal disease. Only rubella, CMV, varicella zoster, HSV-1 and 2 appear to cause structural congenital malformations.

In fewer than 5% of children born with congenital malformations is congenital infection a cause of their defects. In countries with rubella vaccination programmes this proportion is even lower.

The last few years have seen the emergence of HIV and the identification of parvovirus as important fetal pathogens. It is likely that others will be identified in the future. We must remain alert to this possibility.

We must also encourage the development and use of appropriate screening and vaccination programmes to prevent fetal infection.

REFERENCES

1 Burgess M A. Gregg's rubella legacy 1941–1991. Med J Aust 1991; 155: 355–357.
2 Miller E, Cradock-Watson J E, Pollock T M. Consequences of confirmed rubella at successive stages of pregnancy. Lancet 1982; ii: 781–784.
3 Burgess M A. Rubella reinfection: what risk to the fetus? Med J Aust 1992; 156: 824–825.
4 Gilbert G L. Infectious disease in pregnancy and the newborn infant. Melbourne: Harwood, 1991: p 41.
5 Cochi S L, Edmonds L E, Dyer K et al. Congenital rubella syndrome in the United States, 1970–1985: on the verge of elimination. Am J Epidemiol 1989; 129: 349–361.
6 Condon R J, Bower C. Rubella vaccination and congenital rubella syndrome in Western Australia. Med J Aust 1993; 158: 379–382.
7 Miller E, Waight P A, Vurdien J E, Jones G, Tookey P A, Peckham C S. Rubella surveillance to December 1992: second joint report from the PHLS and National Congenital Rubella Surveillance Programme. CDR Rev 1993; 3: R35–R40.
8 Pass R F. Commentary: is there a role for prenatal diagnosis of congenital cytomegalovirus infection? Pediatr Infect Dis J 1992; 11: 608–609.
9 Burgess M A. Rubella vaccination just before or during pregnancy. Med J Aust 1990; 152: 507–508.
10 Gilbert G L. Infectious disease in pregnancy and the newborn infant. Melbourne: Harwood 1991: p 72.
11 Fowler K B, Stagno S, Pass R F, Britt W J, Boll J J, Alford C A. The outcome of congenital cytomegalovirus infection in relation to maternal antibody status. N Engl J Med 1992; 326: 663–667.

12 Gilbert G L. Infectious disease in pregnancy and the newborn infant. Melbourne: Harwood, 1991: p 79.

13 Stagno S. Cytomegalovirus. In: Remington J S, Klein J O, eds. Infectious diseases of the fetus and newborn infant, 3rd edn. Philadelphia: Saunders, 1990: pp 241–181.

14 Grose C, Meehan T, Weiner C P. Prenatal diagnosis of congenital cytomegalovirus infection by virus isolation after amniocentesis. Pediatr Infect Dis J 1992; 11: 605–607.

15 Hayes K. Prenatal cytomegalovirus infection: differing data and attitudes. Personal communication, 1993.

16 Yow M D, Demmler G J. Congenital cytomegalovirus disease: 20 years is long enough. N Engl J Med 1992; 326: 702–703.

17 Schoub B D, Johnson S, McAnerney J M et al. Is antenatal screening for rubella and cytomegalovirus justified? S Afr Med J 1993; 83: 108–110.

18 Hall S M. Congenital toxoplasmosis. Br Med J 1992; 305: 291–297.

19 Antenatal screening for toxoplasmosis in the UK (editorial). Lancet 1990; 336: 346–348.

20 Gilbert G L. Infectious disease in pregnancy and the newborn infant. Melbourne: Harwood, 1991: p 205.

21 Daffos F, Forestier F, Capella-Pavlovsky M et al. Prenatal management of 746 pregnancies at risk for congenital cytomegalovirus. N Engl J Med 1988; 318: 271–275.

22 Walpole I R, Hodgen N, Bower C. Congenital toxoplasmosis: a large survey in Western Australia. Med J Aust 1991; 154: 720–724.

23 Carmack M A, Prober C G. Neonatal herpes: vexing dilemmas and reasons for hope. Curr Opin Pediatr 1993; 5: 21–28.

24 McIntosh D, Isaacs D. Herpes simplex virus infection in pregnancy. Arch Dis Child 1992; 67: 1137–1138.

25 Dunne W M, Demmler G J. Serological evidence for congenital transmission of human herpesvirus 6. Lancet 1992 ; 340: 121–122.

26 Aubin J-T, Poirel L, Agut H et al. Intrauterine transmission of human herpesvirus 6 . Lancet 1992; 340: 482–483.

27 Alkalay A L, Pomerance J J, Rimoin D L. Fetal varicella syndrome. J Pediatr 1987; 111: 320–323.

28 Pastuszak A L, Levy M, Schick B et al. Outcome after maternal varicella infection in the first 20 weeks of pregnancy. N Engl J Med 1994; 330: 901–905.

29 Enders G, Miller E, Cradock-Watson J, Bolley I, Ridehalgh M. Consequences of varicella and herpes zoster in pregacy: prospective study of 1739 cases. Lancet 1994; 343: 1547–1550.

30 Gilbert G L. Chickenpox during pregnancy. Br Med J 1993; 306: 1079–1080.

31 McIntosh D, Isaacs D. Varicella zoster virus infection in pregnancy. Arch Dis Child 1993; 68: 1S–2S.

32 Committee on Infectious Diseases (American Academy of Pediatrics). Parvovirus, erythema infectiosum, and pregnancy. Pediatrics 1990; 85: 131–133.

33 Soothill P. Intrauterine blood transfusion for non-immune hydrops fetalis due to parvovirus B19 infection. Lancet 1990; 336: 121–122.

34 Morey A L, Nicolini U, Welch C R, Economides D, Chamberlain P F, Cohen B J. Parvovirus B19 infection and transient fetal hydrops. Lancet 1991; 337: 496.

35 Public Health Laboratory Service Working Party on Fifth Disease. Prospective study of human parvovirus (B19) infection in pregnancy. Br Med J 1990; 300: 1166–1170.

36 Gilbert G L. Infectious disease in pregnancy and the newborn infant. Melbourne: Harwood, 1991: p 139.

37 Marion R W, Wiznia A A, Hutcheon R G, Rubinstein A. Human T-cell lymphotropic virus type III (HTLV-III) embryopathy. Am J Dis Child 1986; 140: 638–640.

38 Banatvala J E, Chrystie I L. HIV screening in pregnancy: UK lags. Lancet 1994; 343: 1113–1114.

39 Ziegler J B. Breast feeding and HIV. Lancet 1993; 342: 1437–1438.

40 Ohto H, Terazawa S, Sasaki N et al. Transmission of hepatitis C virus from mothers to infants. N Engl J Med 1994; 330: 744–750.

41 Edwards M J. Influenza, hyperthermia, and congenital malformation. Lancet 1972; i: 320–321.

42 CDC. Prevention and control of influenza: recommendations of the Immunization Practices Advisory Committee (ACIP). MMWR 1992; 41 (No. RR-9): 1–17.

43 Cantwell M F, Shebab Z M, Costello A M et al. Brief report: congenital tuberculosis. N Engl J Med 1994; 330: 1051–1054.

44 Macgregor J D, Avery J G. Malaria transmission and fetal growth. Br Med J 1974; 2: 433–436.

45 Raoult D, Stein A. Q fever during pregnancy: a risk for women, fetuses, and obstetricians. N Engl J Med 1994; 330: 371.

CHAPTER 13

THE NEONATE AND YOUNG INFANT

13.1. Assessment and management of the young, febrile infant (30–90 days)

P. Hewson

13.1 Assessment and management of the young, febrile infant (3–90 days)

INTRODUCTION

All experienced clinicians dealing with children have seen rapid deterioration in young infants from being apparently well to near death when infected with agents such as group B streptococcus, Gram-negative organisms and respiratory syncytial virus. One traumatic, tragic experience may influence many years of clinical practice.

Equally, experience and attention to clinical detail has successfully allowed careful review rather than investigation and hospitalization in many situations.

A large amount of data is now accumulating to help determine the risks of serious disease in early infancy. By using the data now available, and understanding the clinical, psychosocial and geographical context of the febrile young infant, it is increasingly possible to suggest practical and reasoned guidelines for the most appropriate management in each situation.

Our task is to identify:

1. those babies and situations where there is an increased risk of serious infection with possible rapid demise;
2. where serious infection may not be recognized; and
3. where the serious infection may not be managed appropriately.

This chapter outlines the data which help us achieve these tasks and attempts to delineate the issues which determine where an aggressive or conservative approach is indicated in this vulnerable age group.

EPIDEMIOLOGY

Many illnesses are presumed to be infective, though only 10–20% of infants under 90 days of age presenting to a paediatric outpatient setting had fever.[1,2] However, 46% of presenting infants were perceived as hot by parents, and the final clinical diagnosis was infective in 50% of all infants.[1]

Of those infants in Boston and Melbourne with a documented fever, between 10% and 15% had serious infective illness, i.e. were culture positive, or required intravenous or nasogastric fluids, oxygen therapy or parenteral antibiotics on perceived clinical grounds. In Melbourne 76% of infections were viral and 24% had documented bacterial disease. Of the presumed total infective group, only 4.4% had bacterial illness. In an earlier study, 12% of infections were bacterial in the neonatal period, while 6% of infections in 1–2-month infants were bacterial.[3] The risk of sepsis in term neonates is generally quoted as one per 1000 births.[4]

Of all infants presenting, 2–6% have a significant infective illness, with a majority of these being viral. Another 2–6% have serious non-infective illness.[1]

Of those infants who look well clinically but have a rectal temperature above 38°C, 5–8% have a bacterial illness.[5] Half of these have a urinary tract infection or a positive bacterial stool culture and approximately 1–3% of all well-looking infants under 3 months are bacteraemic. These figures vary from community to community depending on the race involved, the nutritional status and standard of hygiene, and from season to season depending on the presence of an epidemic of an infectious disease such as bronchiolitis, gastroenteritis or bacterial enteritis.

FEVER

In the community, the presence of a fever strongly suggests the presence of infective illness. Other causes of a raised temperature in young babies include being over-clothed or over-wrapped, maternal fever in the breast-fed baby, dehydration, or more rarely, central nervous system (CNS) disease such as intracranial haemorrhage.[6–9] Although the presence of a fever generally indicates infective illness, not all infective illness causes a fever.[10] Specifically, 25–30% of infants with bacterial infection do not have a fever at the time of presentation.

Measurement

Normal body temperature ranges from 36.0 to 37.2°C per axilla (taken for 5 min) and from 36.7 to 37.9°C when taken rectally (3 cm past the anal verge and for 2 min).[11] The rectal temperature has been found to be more reliable than axillary temperature,[11] though the axillary temperature is often recommended because of its convenience, while in some smaller studies the difference in reliability was minimal.[12,13] Tympanic membrane temperature measurements are unreliable in early infancy and young children.[14]

Significance

Young infants tend not to develop very high fevers despite serious infection. In fact, not infrequently they become hypothermic. The reason for this is uncertain, though it may be associated with their poorer immune response. Fever itself is thought to be an adaptive response to infective stress, and antipyretics are inappropriate unless fever is excessively high for age, i.e. above 39.5°C rectally.

Severity

In infants under 3 months of age, as in older infants, the higher the fever, the more likely the presence of bacterial illness.[2,15] However, infants under 3 months are less likely to have high fevers even if they have bacterial infections.

Duration

It is difficult to predict the cause of the illness on the basis of the duration of fever. Both viral and bacterial illness have variable fever duration. Parainfluenza and rhinoviral infection have the shortest fever duration though respiratory viral infection can be prolonged. The mean fever duration for parainfluenza 1, 2 and 3 viral infections was 4.0, 2.5 and 3.1 days respectively, in one study.[16]

Fever, or lack of fever in itself, can be misleading and it is the associated clinical findings which should influence management decisions.[10]

Treatment

Medication for the fever is unnecessary unless associated with significant irritability or if the temperature is above 39.5°C. Minimal clothing and light wrapping is the first option. Treatment of the fever with antipyretics such as paracetamol (acetaminophen) is usually unnecessary, however, and concentration on assessment of the cause and management of the illness takes priority.

CONCEPTS OF SICKNESS AND BEING WELL: CLINICAL, HAEMATOLOGICAL–IMMUNOLOGICAL AND MICROBIOLOGICAL

Clinical

Because so many babies with infective illness (including bacterial infection) do not have a fever, any triaging system needs to identify infective illness by using more than a thermometer. Clinical markers of decreasing function and indicators of physiological stress or decompensation in a clinical setting consistent with known infective illness patterns are required if all serious infections are to be identified.

A baby who is functioning normally and who has no sign of being unwell on careful examination, apart from a fever, is not seriously ill despite the potential for it. Even if the baby has bacteriuria or bacteraemia, he or she is still not sick. At least 35% of babies with bacteraemia recover spontaneously[17] and it is likely that a similar number of babies with bacteriuria do the same.

Many studies have been done suggesting clinical signs and symptoms are not predictive of serious bacterial illness, though the endpoint used has been bacterial infection, not bacterial illness or sickness. Bacterial infection (bacteraemia and bacteriuria) cannot always be identified clinically, though serious bacterial invasive infection (or illness) can.[18,19]

Haematological and immunological

White cell count (WCC), band count or serum levels of acute-phase reactants such as C-reactive protein are often used to help in the identification of bacterial illness. However, there is little relevant work to suggest these markers are positive when careful clinical assessment shows no abnormality. When tested in the collaborative Baby Illness Research Project clinical signs were more predictive than laboratory markers.[1]

The laboratory markers are, however, very useful when either clinical signs are unreliable, e.g. when antibiotics are currently being given, or when the assessing doctor is inexperienced. They are also useful when the history is unreliable, e.g. when the caregiver is misleading or emotionally unavailable and so likely to be unaware of the baby's functioning.

Microbiological

Blood, urine, cerebrospinal fluid (CSF) and faeces collection will identify the 4–15% of febrile babies with bacterial infection. One still needs to identify serious viral infection by viral cultures of appropriate specimens or serology.

MANAGEMENT ISSUES

To effectively manage infective illness in young babies the main needs are to ensure:

1. the clinician is aware of the risk of serious illness;
2. the information the clinician is receiving is reliable;
3. the clinician knows the signs and symptoms associated with serious illness;
4. the caregivers can be taught the worrying signs and symptoms; and
5. reliable reassessment of the baby is possible as soon as the condition changes.

If these needs cannot be satisfied, then investigation and either admission to hospital or intramuscular antibiotics and review needs to be organized.

The first weeks of life

Traditionally newborn infections occurring whilst in maternity hospitals have been treated aggressively, because of the worry of fulminant group B streptococcal and Gram-negative sepsis. Investigation of all febrile neonates with blood cultures, urine microscopy and cultures, CSF examination and culture, full blood examination and C-reactive protein, and treatment with antibiotics until cultures are available is routine neonatal practice.[4] No definitive, recent study has looked at an alternative approach to term, well-looking, febrile babies in the maternity hospital. Early discharge from maternity hospital should not necessarily change the approach to the febrile baby in the first week of life. Obstetric risk factors associated with neonatal sepsis need to be considered as well as the functioning and appearance of the baby.

Obstetric risk factors

These include maternal sepsis, birth asphyxia and neonatal procedures. Of particular importance in the term baby are the following.

Prolonged rupture of membranes: There is a steady rise in risk of both chorioamnionitis and neonatal infection if the membranes are ruptured for longer than 18 h. There was a 5% incidence of sepsis in babies where the membranes had been ruptured for an average of 54 h.[20] The incidence of chorioamnionitis increases significantly after 18–24 h of ruptured membranes. Understandably, frequent vaginal examinations whilst membranes are ruptured is also associated with increased neonatal infection. Careful clinical evaluation and follow-up are necessary if there has been prolonged rupture of the membranes, though investigation or treatment is not generally commenced unless other infective risk markers are present. There is, however, a wide variety of opinion as to the best management.[21]

Maternal group B streptococcal (GBS) colonization: Between 10% and 30% of mothers are colonized with GBS and the incidence of neonatal GBS sepsis is usually between one and five per 1000 babies, with much higher attack rates (up to 70 per 1000) if risk factors are present, e.g. maternal fever, spontaneous preterm onset of labour, or prolonged rupture of the membranes.[22,23] Almost half (47%) of GBS infections occur following discharge from hospital.[24] These occur into the third month of life, though usually before 6 weeks if the mother is colonized with GBS. It is likely that late-onset GBS disease is not affected by the risk factors for early-onset disease.

Several studies have shown that giving intrapartum antibiotics to mothers who are GBS positive prevents neonatal sepsis, though many mothers will be treated unnecessarily.[22,23] Selective intrapartum chemoprophylaxis of GBS-positive mothers with risk factors present is becoming routine in the USA. Despite this, maternal antibiotics do not always prevent neonatal infection in the term baby when the mothers are febrile or the membranes have been ruptured for longer than 12 h.[25]

Maternal fever: Maternal fever prior to and during labour is associated with neonatal sepsis, whilst a decreased incidence of chorioamnionitis and neonatal sepsis has been associated with the increased use of antibiotics for febrile mothers in labour.[26]

Offensive liquor: Although difficult to quantify, offensive liquor may be a sign of chorioamnionitis and subsequent risk of invasive disease.

With the current trend to early discharge, the family doctor or community paediatrician may not have easy access to whether the obstetric risk factors for infection have been present. The younger the baby, the higher the risk of serious infective illness and the more cautious the clinician needs to be. Thus the approach for the baby in the first week should apply to babies up to 4 weeks of age.

Symptoms and signs in the first week of life

The main management difficulty in the first week of life is the uncertainty of whether the birth itself or any feeding difficulty is the cause of any symptoms or the result of sepsis. Birth asphyxia, poor feeding and hypoglycaemia can all mimic the signs of sepsis or, alternatively, be a result of sepsis.

Studies of clinical markers of sepsis in the first week confirm this difficulty, though the high-risk signs are those related to poor circulation (pallor, decreased perfusion, hypotension), CNS signs (irritability or lethargy) as well as abdominal distension, apnoea and tachycardia.[27] A combination of clinical and haematological markers are required to help identify those with serious bacterial infection.[27]

The following symptoms and signs are useful markers of possible infection and their presence indicates the need for further investigation:

1. Rectal temperature >38.0°C or axillary temperature >37.5°C.
2. Any of the following signs or symptoms:
   A. Poor arousal signs, i.e. drowsiness or decreased activity, poor tone, extended posture, weak cry
   B. Respiratory distress, i.e. intercostal recession, grunt, apnoea
   C. Generalized pallor or cold calves
   D. Poor feeding
   E. Unexplained jaundice
   F. Unidentified or petechial rash

Non-infective illness can cause any of the signs or symptoms in isolation, but if any occur in association with a fever, investigation and treatment for possible sepsis are necessary. The presence of any two without a fever also justifies investigation. The presence of drowsiness and pallor in association with fever is the most worrying combination of signs suggesting serious sepsis.

Consideration of maternal risk factors for sepsis is important and their presence in combination with any of the above symptoms and signs necessitates early investigation. The experienced clinician can consider withholding investigation in the first 24 h of the fever if:

1. the baby is functioning normally and there is no abnormality on examination apart from a low-grade fever (<38.5°C rectally);
2. the baby is breast-feeding and the mother has a fever and infection, e.g. mastitis or wound infection;
3. members of the family have low grade respiratory or gastrointestinal infections;
4. parents are reliable and access to adequate early follow-up is guaranteed.

When doubt exists readmission to hospital should be organized.

Management

Figure 13.1.1 is one possible management strategy within hospital, and a similar approach can be adopted with babies in the community in the first month of life.

Once a baby is at home in the first week, detailed 4–6-hourly review may not be practically possible and it is often difficult to ascertain whether obstetric risk factors have been present. Readmission to hospital is usually necessary and management as indicated in Figure 13.1.1 is most appropriate.

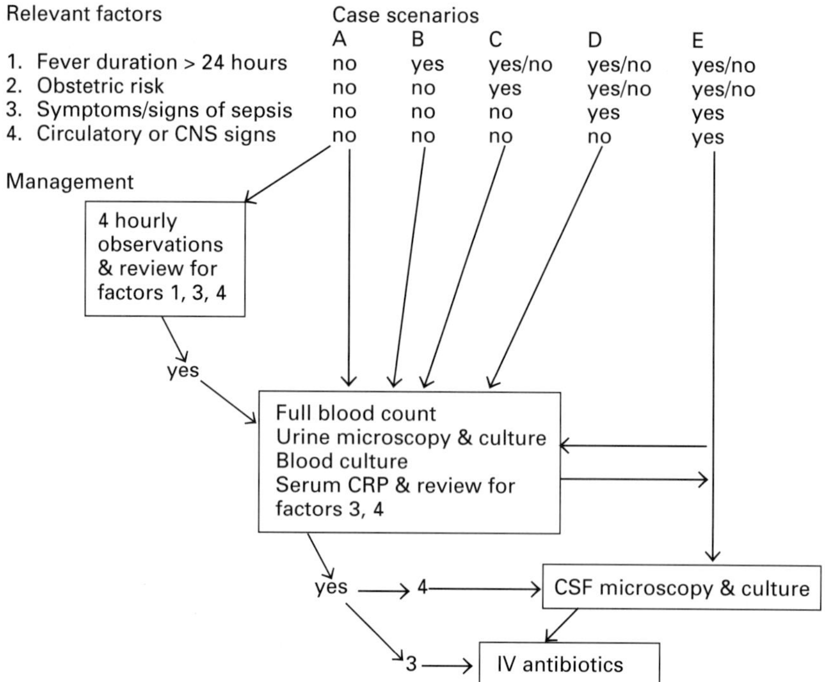

Fig. 13.1.1 Management of the term, febrile neonate in hospital.

Twenty-eight to ninety days

Symptoms and signs

The following clinical signs and symptoms have been proven to be associated with both infective and non-infective serious illness in early infancy.[19,28]

Poor arousal, decreased activity, decreased alertness: If the baby is less responsive than usual, not waking normally, not responding to normal environmental stimulation, including movement and sound, and is less active, then serious illness is more likely. The more drowsy the infant, the more likely is serious illness. Associated findings are often hypotonia with a hypotonic posture (extended arms, abducted but flexed hips) and a weak, whimpering cry.

Breathing difficulty: Serious respiratory infection is often associated with moderate to severe chest wall recession with intercostal and sternal recession. Tachypnoea has been proven to be a useful sign of pneumonia in older infants and children and also in respiratory distress in neonates. In young infants, recession in association with a moderately elevated respiratory rate is usual with pneumonia or more severe bronchiolitis. Tachypnoea without evidence of recession can be a consequence of fever or simply a high metabolic rate, as is the case with some very active (but very well) young infants. A fast respiratory rate whilst asleep (>60 breaths/min) is more predictive of a respiratory problem, though the average respiratory rate in well awake infants is 60 breaths/min when assessed with a stethoscope.[28] The most serious respiratory sign in young infants is that of central cyanosis or a respiratory grunt. A respiratory grunt may indicate increased compliance as in pneumonia, though may also be present with raised intracranial pressure, as in meningitis or in severe abdominal sepsis and abdominal distension.

Poor circulation: The sudden appearance of persistent, generalized pallor is an indication of circulatory compromise and, in the febrile baby, is suggestive of body tissue sepsis such as septicaemia associated with meningitis, pneumonia or pyelonephritis. Pallor can also occur transiently following a vomit or persistently with intussusception (which can also be associated with a febrile viral infection). Cold feet and cold hands are not predictive, though cold calves are a definite sign of circulatory compromise whether it be due to an infection or other causes of hypovolaemia. Skin mottling itself is more an indication of a relatively cold environment.

Decreased fluid intake: Taking less than 50% of the normal fluid intake over a 24 h period is an indication of increasing compromise and increasing difficulty in young infants suffering bronchiolitis or other infections. If breast-feeding mothers are asked to consider the duration of active sucking and the frequency of feeds then they have been found to give a reliable estimate of their babies' fluid intake compared to mothers of bottle-fed babies calculating the actual volume of milk ingested over a 24 h period.

Decreased urinary output: Once a baby's feeding is established (usually by the end of the first week) babies in their first 6 months pass urine on average 6 to 10 times per day. The passage of urine less than four times per day indicates decreased urine output, and is associated with more significant illness.

Overall picture: The combination of having a high temperature and being drowsy and pale was associated with a 75% risk of serious illness, including serious infection and serious surgical illness in a Melbourne population of infants.[19] The presence of any of the above findings on examination increased the risk of serious illness 10–15% compared to the finding being given on history alone.

If any of the above signs or symptoms are present in the young infant with a fever, admission to hospital and investigation for the cause of the infection is necessary.

Uncommon but high-risk signs of infective illness in early infancy are:

- Apnoea
- Petechial rash
- Tender lump on an extremity
- Asymmetrical movement of a limb
- Bulging fontanelle
- Convulsion

These all need investigation and treatment in hospital.

The well looking febrile young baby

Debate surrounds the management of the well looking and normally functioning, febrile baby under 90 days of age. Much of the debate has arisen because of the desire for uniform guidelines whatever the social situation, the experience of the clinician and the access to medical review.

Meta-analysis suggests that between 5% and 8% of febrile well looking infants under 3 months of age will have a bacteraemic illness, with up to 2% being due to bacterial enteritis, 2–3% being due to urinary tract infection and approximately 2% being due to bacteraemia.[5] Approximately 35% of young infants with a bacteraemia clear the bacteraemia spontaneously without antibiotics. The other 50–70% are at risk of developing more serious bacterial infection including meningitis. In the meta-analysis compiled by Baraff et al, five of 415 non-toxic febrile babies were found to have bacteraemia and one had bacterial meningitis.[5]

Table 13.1.1   Medical and psychosocial risk factors

Medical
1. Antibiotics in the previous 7 days
2. Temperature elevated for longer than 48 h
3. Low birth weight or prematurity
4. Doctor inexperience or uncertainty
5. Previous chronic illness or previous frequent hospitalization

Psychosocial
6. Uncertain parent reliability
7. Parents detached or emotionally unavailable
8. Lack of availability of medical follow-up
9. Parents socially disadvantaged

See Figure 13.1.2 for possible effect on management.

In situations where the baby is well and has a low-grade fever, of short duration, when there are no medical or social risk factors present (see Table 13.1.1), the baby comes from a family where upper respiratory tract infections are occurring, or where a maternal cause is suspected in a breast-feeding baby, experienced clinicians may hold off investigation. Adequate follow-up within 12–24 h and reliable parental observation need to be assured. Once the fever has been present for greater than 2 days in the baby over 4 weeks, or over 24 h in the first 4 weeks of life, investigation is necessary.

If medical or social risk factors are present, then the baby should be investigated, and either admitted to hospital or given an intramuscular dose of ceftriaxone, and follow-up arranged.[29-31] Which of the alternatives taken depends on the clinician and the risk factors involved. Suggested options are shown in Figure 13.1.2. Previous antibiotics and factors associated with any doubt regarding follow-up should necessitate admission. The ceftriaxone alternative may be useful for inexperienced clinicians.

If medical or social risk factors are not present, no investigation is necessary, and medical review can be organized for 6–24 h with phone call contact earlier if new symptoms occur. If urine can be collected without difficulty, then this should be carried out. Parents should be given a list of the relevant worrying symptons and signs. The shorter the duration of fever (or symptoms) the less predictable is the illness, and earlier review is necessary. If the fever has been

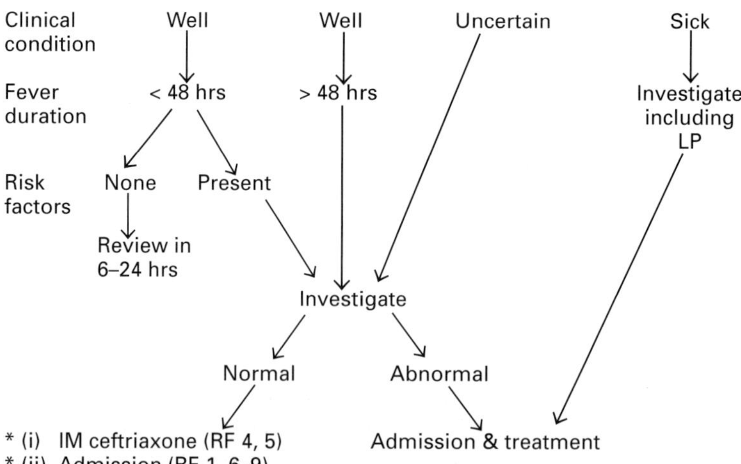

Fig. 13.1.2   Management of the febrile infant aged 28–90 days. *The possible alternative management strategies depend on the risk factors present. RF represents risk factors, with the number corresponding to those in Table 13.1.1.

present for longer than 48 h, but no other signs, symptoms or medical–social risk factors are present, then a urine microscopy and culture, full blood examination, blood culture and serum C-reactive protein are necessary. If the urine microscopy (nitrite and leucocyte esterase testing and Gram stain), WBC, band count and C-reactive protein are normal, then the alternatives are either ceftriaxone intramuscularly and review,[29] admission to hospital for observation, or review in 6–24 h or sooner if the clinical signs change.

Whenever antibiotics have been given in the previous 7 days prior to assessment, clinical signs and symptoms are unreliable and investigation will be necessary.

Investigations

First weeks (0–4 weeks)

The baby should usually be admitted to hospital and investigations performed as in Figure 13.1.1. Full blood examination, blood culture and urine microscopy should be performed in any baby febrile longer than 24 h or if they have any of the signs or symptoms detailed in Fig. 13.1.1. A lumbar puncture should be performed in any baby who is pale, less responsive than usual and whenever the clinician is worried about the possibility of meningitis. If the blood culture is subsequently found to be positive, then a lumbar puncture should be performed (if not done so already), because of the 20–30% risk of meningitis in septicaemic neonates.[32,33] Faeces microscopy and culture should be performed whenever there is diarrhoea or abdominal distension and chest X-ray should be performed whenever there is a cough, tachypnoea, intercostal recession or grunting respirations, apnoea or need for oxygen to maintain oxygen saturations above 92%.

C-reactive protein: Serum C-reactive protein is the single most predictive, commonly used laboratory marker of sepsis, though is still not reliable enough to determine management in isolation. The sensitivity of the C-reactive protein in neonatal intensive care with a population of term and preterm babies was found to be 70–74%, with a specificity of 72%.[34,35] It is more accurate after day 3 and will be elevated with significant birth trauma.

The peripheral blood white cell count (WCC): Various combinations of total WCC, immature forms or band count have been suggested as useful in identifying those febrile babies who do have bacterial infection, though these alone are not 100% sensitive.[4,27,35,36] A combination of clinical symptoms and signs in conjunction with haematological markers and serum C-reactive protein is the most sensitive identifier of babies with bacterial infection.

Infants aged 28–90 days

As previously indicated, investigations (urine microscopy and culture, blood culture, full blood count and serum C-reactive protein) are indicated in the febrile baby whenever:

1. significant symptoms and signs are present;
2. medical–social risk factors are present;
3. the fever does not settle within 48 h.

Serum C-reactive protein: The C-reactive protein is the best of the haematological or immunological markers of bacterial illness.[37–39] although does not replace clinical acumen. The sensitivity in bacterial meningitis was 80% compared to the sensitivity of clinical symptoms and signs being 100% and 70% respectively in infants and children with a median age of 6 months.[40] It is especially valuable when antibiotics have been given prior to the assessment. It is a marker of tissue damage and can be elevated in significant, life-threatening viral illness.

White cell count: Following over two decades of investigation, figures still vary widely for the predictability of haematological markers in the 1–3 month infant.[1,41,42] In general, a band count of >2000/mm³, a neutrophil count of >10 000/mm³ or a total WCC of > 20 000/mm³ is associated with a risk of bacterial infection of at least 30% though the sensitivity is also only 25–50%. If the haematological markers are within normal limits and the infant is clinically well, the risk of bacterial infection is 1.4% or lower.[5,29,43]

Urine analysis: The risk of a well febrile baby having a urinary tract infection (UTI) is approximately 2%, while if unwell the risk is up to 7.5%.[5,44] Ideally urine microscopy and culture should be performed on every febrile or symptomatic baby, though unfortunately a urine collected by bag is only useful if it is sterile. To diagnose a urinary tract infection a midstream 'catch', a catheter or suprapubic aspirate specimen is necessary. If the risk of a positive result is only 2%, then other factors including parental views need to be considered.[45]

Nitrite testing strips are only positive in 30–60% of urinary tract infections, while leucocyte esterase testing has a sensitivity of approximately 60%.[46] In one study, if both nitrite and leucocyte esterase testing strips were used in combination with a Gram stain on a suprapubic aspirate or catheter specimen of urine, 100% of UTIs were identified.[47] Group B streptococcal urinary antigen testing may also be worth performing when investigating for sepsis in early infancy when the community maternal carriage rate for this organism is high.

Lumbar puncture: This should always be performed in a febrile, pale, drowsy infant as part of the investigations. If previous antibiotics have recently been given, then it should also be undertaken prior to their recommencement or alteration.

Other indications for lumbar puncture, or consultation with a more experienced clinician, are apnoeic attacks, convulsions, alternating irritability and poor responsiveness, petechiae, coexistent septicaemia and UTI, and the presence of significant doubt.

Chest X-ray: In the absence of respiratory signs, febrile infants are unlikely to have any positive finding on a chest X-ray.[48]

Faeces microscopy and culture: This is only worth doing if diarrhoea, blood in the stool, abdominal distension or prolonged fever without symptoms is present.

Haematological and immunological markers of sepsis: Whenever a blood culture is taken, a full blood examination and serum C-reactive protein are worthwhile to avoid an unnecessary repeat venepuncture.

DANGEROUS DILEMMAS

Assessment of the young infant on antibiotics

In infants between 2 and 90 days of age, there are few indications for oral antibiotics. Oral antibiotics could be prescribed for mild to moderately infected eczema. Otitis media without major systemic features is likely to be viral, and if associated with significant systemic features full investigation and parenteral treatment is likely to be necessary. Urinary tract infection in early infancy should generally be treated with parenteral antibiotics. If, however, there is no fever associated with a bacteriuria with no systemic features of illness, oral antibiotics being given by a reliable care giver with close monitoring and follow-up is reasonable. Whenever there is a fever, lethargy, pallor or inactivity, the possibility of pyelonephritis exists and parenteral antibiotics should be used.

Thus it should only be rarely that one needs to assess a young infant who is already on antibiotics. Certainly, if antibiotics are being taken and the baby is sick or persistently febrile, the clinical assessment is unreliable and full investigation including a lumbar puncture is necessary.

The febrile, pale, slightly drowsy child

The differential diagnosis includes septicaemia with pyelonephritis, meningitis and pneumonia as well as intussusception.

The febrile infant who is vomiting in the first three months

The differential diagnosis includes gastroenteritis, viral infection with gastro-oesophageal reflux, UTI, meningitis, intussusception and pyloric stenosis.

The baby with symptoms for 4–8 h

The shorter the duration of illness the less predictable its outcome. Although many of these illnesses will be viral (in most studies 85–90%), the chance still exists of it being a fulminant bacterial infection. To discharge the patient without investigation is only possible if the child is well despite the fever, parents are reliable, the clinician is experienced, and access to medical follow-up within 4–8 h is possible.

Management guidelines

Guidelines for the young intern in an accident and emergency department need to be conservative and all encompassing,[3] whilst recommendations for experienced clinicians need to allow for their knowledge of the family, their ability to make future contact with the baby and their awareness of the current, local microbiological epidemiology.

Interestingly, inexperienced clinicians need to be the most cautious and investigate most often, whilst experienced clinicians may not investigate all infants, though are the most cautious in ensuring adequate, early follow-up.

REFERENCES

1 Hewson P H. Markers of serious illness in early infancy. MD thesis, University of Melbourne, Australia, 1988.
2 Klein J O, Schlesinger P C, Karasic R B. Management of the febrile infant three months of age or younger. In: Klein J O, Marcy S M, eds. Management of pediatric infectious disease in office practice. Pediatr Infect Dis 1984; 3: 75–81.
3 Pantall R H, Naber M, Lamar R, Dias J. Fever in the first six months of life. Clin Pediatr 1980; 19: 77–82.
4 Pearse R G, Roberton N R C. Infection in the newborn. In: Roberton N R C, ed. Textbook in neonatology. Edinburgh: Churchhill Livingstone, 1986.
5 Barraf I J, Auslund S A, Schrger D L, Steven M L. Probability of bacterial infections in febrile infants less than three months of age: a decision analysis. Pediatr Infect Dis J 1992; 11: 257–265.
6 Pomerance J J, Richardson J. Hyperpyrexia as a sign of intraventricular haemorrhage in the neonate. Am J Dis Child 1973; 126: 854–855.
7 Craig W S. The early detection of pyrexia in the newborn. Arch Dis Child 1963; 38: 29–39.

8 Sahib El-Radhi A, Carroll J E. Fever in paediatric practice. Oxford: Blackwell Scientific Publications, 1994.

9 Cheng T L, Partridge J C. Effect of bundling. Pediatrics 1993; 92: 238–240.

10 Bonadio W A,Hegenbarth M, Zachariason M. Correlating reported fever in young infants with subsequent temperature patterns and rate of serious bacterial infections. Pediatr Infect Dis 1990; 9: 158–160.

11 Morley C J, Hewson P H, Thornton A J, Cole T J. Axillary and rectal temperature measurents in infants. Arch Dis Child 1992; 67: 122–125.

12 Mayfield S R, Bahtia J, Nakumura K T. Temperature measurement in term and preterm infants. J Pediatr 1984; 104: 271–275.

13 Shann F, Mackenzie A. Axillary or rectal temperatures in children (letter). Lancet 1981; 3: 310.

14 Freed G L, Fraley J K Lack of agreement of tympanic membrane temperature assessments with conventional methods in a private practice setting. Pediatrics 1992; 89: 384–386.

15 McCarthy P l, Dolan T F. The serious implications of high fever in infants during their first three months. Clin Pediatr 1976; 15: 794–796.

16 Putto A, Ruuskanen O, Meurman O. Fever in respiratory virus infections. Am J Dis Child 1986; 140: 1159–1163.

17 Barraff L J, Lee S I. Fever without source: management of children 3 to 36 months of age. Pediatr Infect Dis J 1992; 11: 146–151.

18 Morley C J, Thornton A J, Cole T J, Hewson P H, Fowler M A. Baby check: a scoring system to grade the severity of acute systemic illness in babies under 6 months old. Arch Dis Child 1991; 66: 100–106.

19 Hewson P H, Gollan R A. A simple hospital triaging system for infants with acute illness. J Paediatr Chid Health 1995; 31: 29–32.

20 Guise J M, Duff P, Christian J S. Management of term patients with premature rupture membranes and unfavourable cervix. Am J Perinatol 1992; 9: 56–60.

21 Wiswell T E, Stoll B J, Tuggle J M. Management of asymptomatic term gestation neonates born to mothers treated with intrapartum antibiotics. Pediatr Infect Dis J 1990; 9: 826–831.

22 Garland S M, Fliegner J R. Group B streptococcus (GBS) and neonatal infections: the case for intrapartum chemoprophylaxis. Aust NZ J Obstet Gynecol 1991; 31: 119–122.

23 Yancey M K, Duff P. An analysis of the cost-effectiveness of selected protocols for the prevention of neonatal group B streptococcal infection. Obstet Gynecol 1994; 83: 367–371.

24 Dillon H C, Khare S, Gray B M. Group B streptococcal carriage and disease: a 6 year prospective study. J Pediatr 1987; 110: 31–36.

25 Ascher D P, Becker J A, Yoder B A et al. Failure of intrapartum antibiotics to prevent culture-proven neonatal group B streptococcal sepsis. J Perinatol 1993; 13: 212–216.

26 Romero R, Scioscia A L, Edberg S C, Hobbins J C. Use of parenteral antibiotic therapy to eradicate bacterial colonization of amniotic fluid in premature rupture of membranes. Obstet Gynecol 1986; 67: 15S.

27 Spector S A, Ticknor W, Grossman M. Study of usefulness of clinical and hematological findings in the diagnosis of neonatal bacterial infections. Clin Pediatr 1981; 20: 385–392.

28 Hewson P H, Humphries S M, Roberton D M, McNamara J M, Robinson M J. Markers of serious illness in infants under 6 months old presenting to a children's hospital. Arch Dis Child 1990; 65: 750–756.

29 Baker M D, Bell L M, Avner J R. Outpatient management without antibiotics of fever in selected infants. N Engl J Med 1993; 329: 1437–1441.

30 Fleisher G R, Rosenberg N, Vinci R et al. Intramuscular versus oral antibiotic therapy for the prevention of meningitis and other bacterial sequelae in young, febrile children at risk for occult bacteremia. J Pediatr 1994; 124: 504–512.

31 Long S S. Antibiotic therapy in febrile children: 'best laid schemes. . .'. J Pediatr 1994; 124: 585–588.

32 Vissar V E, Hall R T. Lumbar puncture in the evaluation of suspected neonatal sepsis. J Pediatr 1980; 96: 1063–1067.

33 Isaacs D, Barfield C, Grimwood K et al. Systemic bacterial and fungal infections in infants in Australian neonatal units. Med J Aust 1995; 162: 198–201.

34 Pourcyrous M, Bada H S, Korones S B, Barrett F F, Jennings W, Lockey T. Acute phase reactants in neonatal bacterial infection. J Perinatol 1991; 11: 319–325.

35 Russell G A B, Smyth A, Cooke R W I. Receiver operating characteristic curves for comparison of serial neutrophil band forms and C reactive protein in neonates at risk of infection. Arch Dis Child 1991; 67: 808–812.

36 Rodwell R L, Leslie A L, Tudehope D I. Early diagnosis of neonatal sepsis using a hematological scoring system. J Paediatr 1988; 112: 761–767.

37 Fasth A, Wadsworth C. C-reactive protein as a diagnostic tool excluding infection and differentiating between bacterial and viral infections: clinicians' opinion on usefulness and reliability of the CRP assay. In: Simons C, Wilkinson, eds. Diagnosis of infectious diseases: new aspects. New York: Schattauer, 1986.

38 McCarthy P L, Frank A L, Ablow R C, Masters S J, Dolan T F. C reactive protein test in the differentiation of bacterial and viral pneumonia. J Pediatr 1978; 92: 454–456.

39 Sabel K G, Hanson L A. The clinical usefulness of C reactive protein determinations in bacterial meningitis and septicemia in infancy. Acta Paediatr Scand 1974; 63: 381–385.

40 Lembo R M, Marchant C D. Acute phase reactants and risk of bacterial meningitis among febrile infants and children. Ann Emerg Med 1991; 20: 36–44.

41 Gregory J, Hey E. Blood neutrophil response to bacterial infection in the first month of life. Arch Dis Child 1972; 47: 747–753.

42 Roberts K B, Borzy M S. Fever in the first eight weeks of life. Johns Hopkins Med J 1977; 141: 9–13.

43 Barraff L J, Bass J W, Fleisher G R et al. Practice guidelines for the management of infants and children 0 to 36 months of age with fever without source. Ann Emerg Med 1993; 22: 1198–1210.

44 Crain E F, Gershel J C. Urinary tract infections in febrile infants younger than 8 weeks of age. Pediatrics 1990; 36: 363–367.

45 Kramer M S, Etezadi-Amoli J, Ciampi A et al. Parents' versus physicians' values for clinical outcomes in young febrile children. Pediatrics 1994; 93: 697–702.

46. Hoberman A, Wald E R, Reynolds E A, Penchansky L, Charron M. Pyuria and bacteruria in urine specimen obtained by catheter from young children with fever. J Pediatr 1994; 124: 513–519.

47 Lohr J A, Portilla M G, Geuder T G, Dunn M L, Dudley S M. Making a presumptive diagnosis of urinary tract infection by using a urinalysis performed in an on-site laboratory. J Pediatr 1993; 122: 22–25.

48 Crane E F, Bulas D, Bijur P E, Goldman H S. Is a chest radiograph necessary in the evaluation of every febrile infant less than 8 weeks of age? Pediatrics 1991; 88: 821–824.

DAY CARE

14.1. Approaches to the control of infections in child day care

14.1   Approaches to the control of infections in child day care

INTRODUCTION

There is a documented increased risk of infectious illness among children in child care, their family contacts and the staff caring for them. Children who attend group care (child care centres and preschools) suffer a greater number of episodes of upper respiratory and middle ear infections, pneumonia and gastroenteritis than children cared for at home.[1] They are also at increased risk of life-threatening infection caused by *Haemophilus influenzae* type b.[2] Conditions which commonly affect adult contacts include upper respiratory tract infections, hepatitis A, cytomegalovirus (CMV), enteric infections such as giardia, rotavirus and shigella, and skin infections and infestations.[3] There may also be an increased risk of complete or threatened miscarriage among child care workers; it has been postulated that infectious agents may be responsible.[4] A combination of strategies is required to reduce this burden of infectious diseases associated with child care (Fig. 14.1.1).

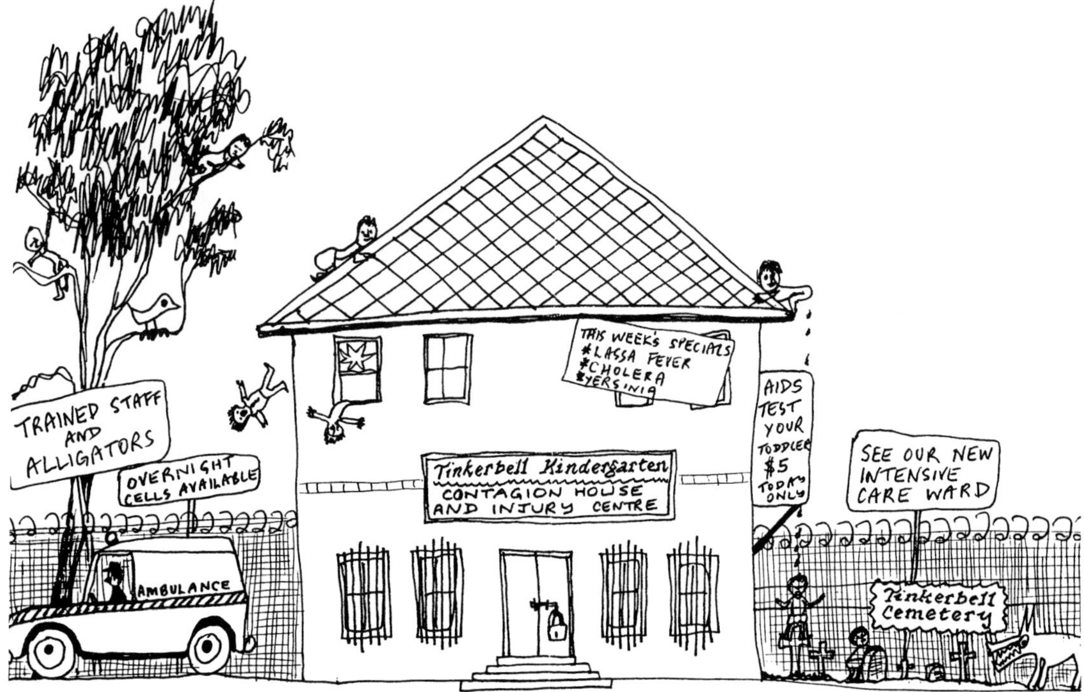

Fig. 14.1.1   'Day Care' by Dr Henry Kilham.

IMMUNIZATION OF CHILDREN

It is critically important for children attending child care to be up to date with their routine immunizations. Child care centres may provide an avenue by which public health authorities can monitor local immunization coverage. Moreover, directors of child care facilities should be reminded of their duty of care to protect infants in the centre by ensuring that they strongly encourage up-to-date immunization among the older children. Particular emphasis may be placed on the vaccines against *H. influenzae* type b and measles. Neither hepatitis B nor hepatitis A vaccines are recommended for routine use in children attending group care.

IMMUNIZATION OF STAFF

Protection of child care staff against occupationally acquired infections has received little emphasis. Adults working in child care should have completed primary vaccination and routinely recommended boosters of diphtheria and tetanus toxoids. Child care staff are probably at greater risk of childhood infections than paediatric hospital staff, so that it is advisable for child care workers who are unsure of their immune status to receive measles–mumps–rubella immunization. Influenza vaccination should be reserved for individuals at increased risk of serious complications of influenza; it is not routinely recommended for child care workers. The risk of carers acquiring hepatitis B at work appears negligible; in contrast, outbreaks of hepatitis A in child care centres cause great morbidity and lost time from work among child care employees.[5] A safe and effective inactivated hepatitis A vaccine is now available, and should be recommended for staff caring for children under 2 years of age, who are generally not toilet trained.

SPECIAL PRECAUTIONS FOR PREGNANT STAFF MEMBERS

If a child care worker is planning a pregnancy, it is strongly suggested that serological screening for immunity to rubella and CMV be carried out prior to conception. Individuals who are seronegative for rubella should be vaccinated and pregnancy delayed for 3 months. Those who are seronegative for CMV should be counselled regarding the small risk of primary maternal CMV infection causing damage to the fetus. Such individuals should be advised that attention to handwashing and not caring for children under 3 years of age can reduce the risk of CMV acquisition.[6]

HANDWASHING AND THE USE OF GLOVES

Human enteric bacteria[7] and viruses[8] are isolated readily from the hands of children and staff and from surfaces and toys in child care centres during gastroenteritis outbreaks. Pathogenic viruses including hepatitis A virus,[9] rotavirus,[10] rhinoviruses[11] and respiratory syncytial virus (RSV)[12] can survive on the hands for many minutes or hours. Hand contact appears to be important in the transmission of viral respiratory infections such as rhinovirus[13] and RSV[12] as well as diarrhoeal infections. Handwashing is the principal means of reducing this transmission. Nappy change areas must be located close to a handbasin. An intensive programme whereby carers washed hands after arrival at the centre, before handling food, and after using the toilet or changing children's nappies was shown to markedly reduce the incidence of diarrhoeal episodes among young children in child care centres.[14] Where a handbasin is not available, alcohol-based hand rinses, shown to reduce the bacterial skin flora,[15] should be used in the place of soap and running water. Handbasins must not be used for food or drink preparation, for rinsing soiled clothing or for cleaning potty chairs. Although staff may prefer to wear gloves when changing dirty nappies, their use is optional, and when worn must not replace handwashing. However, the use of gloves is recommended when blood spills occur, and for handling food, especially if any cuts or other open lesions are present on the hands.

MANAGEMENT OF EXPOSURE TO BLOOD AND BODY FLUIDS

If a child is brought to care with open cuts or sores which may ooze blood or serum, these should be covered with a waterproof bandage or dressing. If a child sustains a cut or abrasion during child care, first aid should be administered and the parents should be instructed about covering open skin lesions. The person giving first aid should wash hands with soap and running water as soon as possible.

If the hands or other skin surfaces are splashed with blood or body substances, the exposed parts should be washed immediately. If the eyes, mouth or nose are splashed, they should immediately be rinsed with running water for several minutes. Staff should be encouraged to report such incidents to their supervisor.

INDIVIDUAL-USE AND DISPOSABLE ITEMS

Most infections acquired in child care are spread from person to person. Although foodborne infections appear to be rare in this setting, acceptable standards for food preparation and handling, available from public health or local authority staff, must be adhered to. To minimize person-to-person transmission of infection, facilities require policies which prohibit children from sharing face cloths, brushes, combs, toothbrushes, sheets and pillow cases or other personal items. Staff should be instructed that a disposable tissue only should be used to wipe a child's nose and then discarded. Under no circumstances should a tissue, face cloth or towel be used on more than one child. The use of disposable paper towels for each child and staff member further reduces the chance of cross-infection resulting from contamination and reuse of fomites. However, if cloth towels are to be used, each person needs to use his or her own towel exclusively. Used paper towels and tissues should be discarded straight away into suitable plastic-lined containers. Enough rubbish bins should be provided and emptied before being allowed to overflow. There should be adequate spacing between adjacent cots or beds so that children cannot cough or breathe directly on one another.

NAPPY CHANGING, WASHING AND DISPOSAL

Carers are at greatest risk of acquiring diarrhoeal infections from toddlers and infants when changing their nappies (diapers).[16,17] The technique of nappy changing is critical in maintaining good hygiene in the child care setting. The use of disposable nappies has been shown to reduce faecal contamination of the child care environment.[18] If they are used, they should be placed into plastic-lined bins after use and suitable arrangements made for their separate collection and disposal by the local authority or a suitable waste disposal service. If cloth nappies are used, they should be washed as outlined below and not used for any other purpose. It may be safer to use a commercial nappy-washing service to minimize handling of potentially infectious nappies by child care staff.

It is suggested that gloves be worn when handling soiled nappies. Dirty nappies may be rinsed briefly in a sluice, but it is important to avoid splashing and spray of contaminated water onto the person handling the nappy or into the surrounding room. For the same reasons, wet nappies should be handled as little as possible.

If nappies are to be laundered within the centre, heavily soiled nappies should be briefly rinsed with the utmost care. All nappies should then be left overnight in a household bleach solution or other nappy sanitizer of the recommended strength prior to laundering. Care should be taken not to overload the soaking bucket or washing machine with soiled nappies.

CLEANING AND DISINFECTION

Contaminated fomites, surfaces, toys and utensils in the child care environment may also be vehicles for the spread of infection. Influenza viruses,[19] RSV,[12] rhino- and parainfluenza viruses[11] and CMV[20] may survive on non-porous objects for many hours. Rotavirus,[10] hepatitis A virus[21] and parasites such as Cryptosporidium[22] may remain viable for days or weeks outside the body.

Vigorous physical cleaning of toys and surfaces using a neutral detergent is generally all that is required to remove pathogens from contaminated articles. Disinfectants should have a supplementary role in the control of outbreaks of enteric infection, and should be chosen to suit the pathogen. For example, in-activation of rotavirus in faeces requires 95% ethanol or a phenolic disinfectant;[23] during an outbreak of Cryptosporidium, a quaternary ammonium disinfectant should be used.[24] Ideally, all surfaces and articles should be chosen for their ease of cleaning.

Nappy change areas should use a change mat which is non-absorbent and which can be cleaned easily after each use. If this is impractical, a covering such as paper towelling or a nappy should be placed on the change mat and disposed of after each use. Clothes, towels, soft toys and other fabric articles should be laundered regularly. Nappies and other items which are contaminated with urine, faeces or other body substances should be handled as little as possible, but preferably placed in bins for cleaning by a commercial laundry service. If these articles are laundered at the child care centre, they should be cold water sluiced with care to avoid splashing of potentially contaminated body substances, and machine washed in either hot or cold water using recommended detergents. Overloading the washing machine is to be avoided. Apart from nappies, there is no need to soak fabric articles in disinfectant or sanitizer prior to laundering.

SEPARATION OF CHILDREN IN NAPPIES FROM OLDER GROUPS

Most child care-related infections are more common in infants and toddlers than among older children. A study of bacterial contamination of the centre environment showed that the prevalence of faecal coliforms on hands, surfaces and in air samples was inversely related to the age of the children cared for in that room. Faecal contamination was greatest on the hands of infants and carers, and least on those of the older children.[25] A recent study has demonstrated the superiority of disposable nappies over cloth nappies in preventing faecal contamination of the child care environment.[18] It remains to be seen whether use of disposable nappies can reduce the incidence of diarrhoeal illness in child care centres.

Two prospective studies of risk factors for diarrhoeal illness found that centres with non-toilet-trained infants, and those in which food-handling staff also changed nappies, had higher diarrhoeal rates.[16,17] The risk of diarrhoeal illness in 3-year-old children who stayed in the same room as under-2-year-olds was 4.3 (95% CI, 2.1–9.0) times greater than the risk in those separated from the under-2-year-olds.[16] In common with other enteric infections, hepatitis A outbreaks are most likely to involve centres containing many children who are not yet toilet trained.[26]

Prevention of spread of enteric infections relies on ensuring that carers have not been involved in nappy changing prior to handling food on the same shift, that minimal contact occurs between children in nappies and older children, and that the same members of staff should not look after both age groups at the same time.

ACQUISITION OF INFECTION FROM PETS

Pets need not be excluded from the child care environment, and this is often not feasible in home-based care. It should be made clear that pets pose a small infection risk to children and staff. Enteric infections including Campylobacter[27] and Giardia[28] may be caught from dogs, cats, mice, birds, lizards and turtles. Birds and possibly cats may transmit *Chlamydia psittaci* to humans.[29] Tinea in children has been linked to cats, dogs, guinea-pigs, rabbits and mice.[30] Finally, infestation with parasites including Toxoplasma and Toxocara may in theory be acquired from sandpits contaminated with animal faeces. Prevention of such infections relies on adherence to the following hygienic principles: washing of hands after contact with pets; animals to be kept away from food preparation areas and food handlers not to touch pets; animals not to be fed uncooked meat or offal; sand pits to be covered when not in use; gloves to be worn when cleaning up animal excreta; pets to be immunized and wormed; and ill pets to receive immediate veterinary attention, and to be isolated from children and staff during treatment.

THE PLACE OF ANTIMICROBIALS IN OUTBREAK CONTROL

Antibacterial and antiviral agents

Antibiotics are routinely recommended for treatment of children attending child care who are suffering from bacterial infections where there is a significant chance of spread to contacts and treatment clearly benefits the individual child. Such conditions include bacterial conjunctivitis, streptococcal pharyngitis and the use of topical and/or oral antibiotics for impetigo. In other infections, use of antibiotics beyond a very early stage of the illness has no clear benefit for the patient, but may reduce the chance of transmission to contacts. This applies to Shigella infection, where use of antimicrobials forms but one aspect of case management or outbreak control[31,32] and in Campylobacter enteritis, in which erythromycin may be used to reduce the infectious period.[33] Administration of a 14-day course of erythromycin has also been recommended to reduce the infectious period in children with pertussis and may be given to susceptible child care contacts.[34] When a case of meningococcal or *Haemophilus influenzae* type b infection occurs in a child attending child care, there is a measurably increased risk to close contacts including child care contacts, and rifampicin prophylaxis may be warranted.[35] Prophylactic use of oral acyclovir was found useful in terminating outbreaks of primary herpes simplex infection in a child care centre,[36] although the agent is not approved in many countries for management of oral herpes simplex infection.

Treatment of giardiasis

The optimal approach to the use of antimicrobials during outbreaks of giardiasis in child care remains problematic. Asymptomatic Giardia infestation may be endemic in some child care centres. Giardiasis may be incidentally diagnosed in these children during diarrhoeal outbreaks caused by another, perhaps undetected, pathogen, and the outbreak falsely ascribed to Giardia. During proven Giardia outbreaks, symptomatic children may nonetheless have a negative faecal examination for Giardia, as a result of the inadequate sensitivity of routine diagnostic techniques for giardiasis. Furthermore, if an attempt is made to eradicate the parasite from the centre, it may well be reintroduced when new children enrol. One study found a prevalence of Giardia carriage of 10.5% in newly enrolled children.[37]

Because of these difficulties and the risk of adverse reactions, various approaches to antimicrobial therapy have been tried. These include: treatment of children in whose faeces Giardia is detected; treatment of all symptomatic children; or treatment of all children in an affected class. Steketee et al reported one child care centre which experienced three sequential Giardia epidemics, despite a 90–100% microbiological cure rate during each epidemic.[38] False negative faecal examinations and reintroduction of the parasite by new children were felt to be likely explanations for this series of events. Although the treatment of asymptomatic as well as symptomatic infected children appeared to reduce the prevalence of infestation,[37] it has been argued that treatment of asymptomatic Giardia carriers is not justifiable because of the possibility of adverse reactions and the lack of evidence that such treatment has any effect on an outbreak.[39]

THE PLACE OF IMMUNIZATION IN OUTBREAK CONTROL

Normal human immunoglobulin

In a limited number of viral infections, the intramuscular administration of normal human immunoglobulin may prevent disease in contacts if given prior to or soon after exposure. Immunoglobulin in a dose of 0.2 ml/kg may prevent measles infection if given within 6 days of contact. It is recommended for measles contacts who are under 9 months of age or the immunosuppressed. In a dose of 0.02 ml/kg, immunoglobulin may be used to prevent hepatitis A if used within 2 weeks of first contact. Mass administration of immunoglobulin has been used successfully to terminate hepatitis A outbreaks in child care centres.[40]

Vaccines

During measles outbreaks, either measles or measles–mumps–rubella vaccine is recommended for all susceptible contacts from 9 months of age (barring medical contraindications). Infants who are vaccinated against measles prior to 12 months of age should be revaccinated in 3 months time or after the age of 12 months (whichever is the later) to avoid interference by maternal antibody. There may also be a place for use of meningococcal, hepatitis A and pertussis-only vaccines, although they remain unproven under outbreak conditions. Advice on their use should be sought from local public health personnel.

EXCLUSION

It is generally agreed that children and employees should be excluded from the centre whilst infectious with a significant, acute illness. Children with mild illnesses, for example the common cold, or with chronic infections such as HIV, hepatitis B or CMV infection are generally not excluded.

Exclusion policies are time-honoured but have a number of major drawbacks. Parents may have difficulty in finding alternative care arrangements for mildly unwell children. As a result, they may be tempted to place the children in other centres, so increasing the chance of spread of the infection into the wider community. An alternative to exclusion may be sick care, discussed in a recent paper.[41] The childhood exanthemata are most infectious during the prodrome, before the illness is recognized and the child excluded. Persons with erythema infectiosum (fifth disease or slapped-cheek syndrome), caused by infection with parvovirus B19, are no longer infectious once the rash appears so that exclusion is generally not warranted.[42] There is evidence that exclusion of children with chickenpox has little effect on the course of an outbreak.[43,44] Recent studies suggest that children with rotavirus gastroenteritis are infectious for up to one week before onset of diarrhoea,[45] and respiratory transmission is also thought to occur.[46] Thus exclusion for some infections may be less effective than previously thought. Current exclusion guidelines can be found in Table 14.1.1.

Table 14.1.1   Guidelines for exclusion from day care

Condition	Exclusion of cases	Exclusion of contacts
Chickenpox	Exclude for at least 5 days after the spots first appear *and* until all blisters have formed scabs	Children with an immune deficiency should be excluded for their own protection. Otherwise not excluded (Pregnant women should seek medical advice)
Cold sores (herpes simplex)	Not excluded. Carers with cold sores should not look after babies younger than 2 months	Not excluded
Common cold	Not excluded	Not excluded
Conjunctivitis	Exclude until discharge from eyes has ceased	Not excluded
Cytomegalovirus (CMV)	Not excluded	Not excluded (Pregnant women should seek medical advice)
Diarrhoea (caused by campylobacter, cryptosporidium, rotavirus, shigella, salmonella and others; see also Giardia)	Exclude until diarrhoea has ceased (campylobacter and shigella may require antibiotic treatment; advice may be obtained from the public health authority)	Not excluded
Diphtheria	Exclude until two negative throat swabs, the last at least 72 h after stopping antibiotics	Exclude family/household contacts until cleared by public health authority
Erythema infectiosum (fifth disease)	Not excluded	Not excluded (Pregnant women should seek medical advice)
Giardia	Excluded until treatment given and diarrhoea has ceased	Not excluded (Stool testing suggested if contact has diarrhoea)

Table 14.1.1   *(contd)*

Condition	Exclusion of cases	Exclusion of contacts
Glandular fever	Not excluded	Not excluded
Haemophilus influenzae type b	Exclude until well	Not excluded (Contact public health authority regarding need for preventative antibiotics for family and child care contacts)
Hand, foot and mouth disease	Not excluded	Not excluded
Hepatitis A	Exclude for 7 days after onset of jaundice	Not excluded
Hepatitis B	Not excluded	Not excluded
Hepatitis C	Not excluded	Not excluded
Human immunodeficiency virus (HIV)	Not excluded unless another infection occurs which requires exclusion	Not excluded
Impetigo (school sores)	Exclude unless sores are covered with a waterproof dressing and antibiotic has been started	Not excluded
Influenza	During proven influenza epidemics, exclude on request of public health authority	Not excluded
Leprosy	Exclude until allowed to return by public health authority	Not excluded
Measles	Exclude for 4 days after the rash first appears	Immunized contacts not excluded
		Unimmunized contacts are to be immunized within 72 h of contact with a case
Meningitis, bacterial	Exclude until well	Not excluded (Contact public health authority regarding need for preventative antibiotics for family and child care contacts)
Meningococcal infection	Exclude until well	Not excluded (Contact public health authority regarding need for preventative antibiotics for family and child care contacts)
Mumps	Exclude for 9 days after symptoms first appear	Not excluded
Poliomyelitis	Exclude for at least 14 days after symptoms first appear	Not excluded
Ringworm (tinea), scabies, pediculosis (head lice), trachoma	Exclude until the day after treatment is started	Not excluded (It may be advisable for all household contacts to be treated at the same time as the case)
Roseola	Not excluded	Not excluded
Rubella	Exclude for 4 days after the rash appears	Not excluded (Pregnant women should seek medical advice)
Streptococcal infection and scarlet fever	Exclude until 24 h of antibiotics have been given	Not excluded
Tuberculosis	Exclude until allowed to return by public health authority	Not excluded (Household and child care contacts may need screening)
Typhoid and paratyphoid fever	Exclude until allowed to return by public health authority	Not excluded
Whooping cough (pertussis)	Exclude for 5 days of a 14-day course of erythromycin	A 14-day course of erythromycin should be considered for susceptible contacts

COHORTING OF INFECTIOUS CHILDREN

Cohorting of children during outbreaks has been examined with a view to reducing the need for exclusion. During Shigella outbreaks in child care, asymptomatic carrier children were successfully cohorted after initiation of specific antibiotic therapy until the organism was eradicated from the faeces.[31,32] The Centers for Disease Control and Prevention now recommend cohorting during convalescence in the management of Shigella outbreaks in child care.[47] Cohorting was used in a similar way during an outbreak of gastroenteritis caused by *Salmonella typhimurium*.[48]

EDUCATION, SURVEILLANCE AND REPORTING

Good infection control practices rely on knowledge of modes of spread of infection and of the importance of immunization and hygiene, in particular frequent handwashing. Child care workers need to be supported with formal in-service training and informal advice, which may be provided by infection control practitioners, clinical or public health personnel. Surveillance involving child care staff may result in early recognition of a problem in the centre and early seeking of medical advice,[49] and should be encouraged by public health staff and other medical advisers.

Medical practitioners seeing a patient with an infectious disease are strongly encouraged to ask about attendance in child care (in the case of a young child), about employment in child care or whether the person has had close contact with a child who attends child care. Any suspicion of multiple cases of illness in a centre should be communicated immediately to local public health staff. Public health authorities are responsible for control of infection in the community, and will devote resources to stop the spread of infection in a child care facility, often with the assistance of local medical staff. Thus public health personnel are reliant on medical practitioners to alert them to what may be the first indication of a significant outbreak in a child care centre.

REFERENCES

1 Ferson M J. Infections in day care. Curr Opinion Pediatr 1993; 5: 35–40.
2 Clements D A, Guise I A, MacInnes S J, Gilbert G L. Haemophilus influenzae type b infections in Victoria, Australia, 1985–1989. J Infect Dis 1992; 165 (Suppl 1): S33–34.
3 Reeves R R, Pickering L K. Impact of child day care on infectious diseases in adults. Infect Dis Clin N Amer 1992; 6: 239–250.
4 Göthe C-J, Hillert L. Spontaneous abortions and work in day nurseries. Acta Obstet Gynecol Scand 1992; 71: 284–292.
5 Hadler S C, Webster H M, Erben J J, Swanson J E, Maynard J E. Hepatitis A in day-care centers. N Engl J Med 1980; 302: 1222–1227.
6 Pass R F, Hutto C, Lyon M D, Cloud G. Increased rate of cytomegalovirus infection among day care centre workers. Pediatr Infect Dis J 1990; 9: 465–470.
7 Ekanem E E, DuPont H L, Pickering L K, Selwyn B J, Hawkins C M. Transmission dynamics of enteric bacteria in day-care centers. Am J Epidemiol 1983; 118: 562–572.
8 Wilde J, Van R, Pickering L, Eiden J, Yolken R. Detection of rotaviruses in the day care environment by reverse transcriptase polymerase chain reaction. J Infect Dis 1992; 166: 507–511.
9 Mbithi J N, Springthorpe V S, Boulet J R, Sattar S A. Survival of hepatitis A virus on human hands and its transfer on contact with animate and inanimate surfaces. J Clin Microbiol 1992; 30: 757–763.
10 Ansari S A, Sattar S A, Springthorpe V S, Wells G A, Tostowaryk W. Rotavirus survival on human hands and transfer of infectious virus to animate and nonporous inanimate surfaces. J Clin Microbiol 1988; 26: 1513–1518.
11 Ansari S A, Springthorpe V S, Sattar S A, Rivard S, Rahman M. Potential role of hands in the spread of respiratory viral infections: studies with human parainfluenza virus 3 and rhinovirus 14. J Clin Microbiol 1991; 29: 2115–2119.
12 Hall C B, Douglas R G, Geiman J M. Possible transmission by fomites of respiratory syncytial virus. J Infect Dis 1980; 141: 98–102.
13 Gwaltney J M, Moskalski P B, Hendley J O. Hand-to-hand transmission of rhinovirus colds. Ann Intern Med 1978; 88: 463–467.
14 Black R E, Dykes A C, Anderson K E et al. Handwashing to prevent diarrhea in day-care centers. Am J Epidemiol 1981; 113: 445–451.
15 Larson E L, Eke P I, Laughon B E. Efficacy of alcohol-based hand rinses under frequent-use conditions. Antimicrob Agents Chemother 1986; 30: 542–544.
16 Lemp G F, Woodward W E, Pickering L K, Sullivan P S, DuPont H L. The relationship of staff to the incidence of diarrhea in day-care centers. Am J Epidemiol 1984; 120: 750–758.

17 Sullivan P, Woodward W E, Pickering L K, DuPont H L. Longitudinal study of occurrence of diarrhoeal disease in day care centers. Am J Public Health 1984; 74: 987–991.

18 Van R, Wun C-C, Morrow A L, Pickering L K. The effect of diaper type and overclothing on fecal contamination in day-care centers. JAMA 1991; 265: 1840–1844.

19 Bean B, Moore B M, Sterner B, Peterson L R, Gerding D N, Balfour H H. Survival of influenza viruses on environmental surfaces. J Infect Dis 1982; 146: 47–51.

20 Hutto C, Little E A, Ricks R, Lee J D, Pass R F. Isolation of cytomegalovirus from toys and hands in a day care center. J Infect Dis 1986; 154: 527–530.

21 Hadler S C, McFarland L. Hepatitis in day care centers: epidemiology and prevention. Rev Infect Dis 1986; 8: 548–557.

22 Casemore D P. Epidemiological aspects of human cryptosporidiosis. Epidemiol Infect 1990; 104: 1–28.

23 Tan J A, Schnagle R D. Inactivation of a rotavirus by disinfectants. Med J Aust 1981; 1: 19–23.

24 Campbell I, Tzipori S. Effect of disinfectants on survival of cryptosporidium oocysts. Vet Rec 1982; 111: 414–415.

25 Petersen N J, Bressler G K. Design and modification of the day care environment. Rev Infect Dis 1986; 8: 618–621.

26 Hadler S C, Erben J J, Francis D P, Webster H M, Maynard J E. Risk factors for hepatitis A in day-care centers. J Infect Dis 1982; 145: 255–261.

27 Salfield N J, Pugh E J. Campylobacter enteritis in young children living in households with puppies. Br Med J 1987; 294: 21–22.

28 Swan J M, Thompson R C A. The prevalence of Giardia in dogs and cats in Perth, Western Australia. Aust Vet J 1986; 63: 110–112.

29 Studdert M J, Studdert V P, Wirth H J. Isolation of Chlamydia psittaci from cats with conjunctivitis. Aust Vet J 1981; 57: 515–517.

30 Zoophilic dermatophytes and their natural hosts in Western Australia. Med J Aust 1980; 2: 506–508.

31 Tauxe R V, Johnson K E, Boase J C, Helgerson S D, Blake P A. Control of day care shigellosis: a trial of convalescent day care in isolation. Am J Public Health 1986; 76: 627–630.

32 Hoffman R E, Shillam P J. The use of hygiene, cohorting, and antimicrobial therapy to control an outbreak of shigellosis. Am J Dis Child 1990; 144: 219–221.

33 Williams D, Schorling J, Barrett L J et al. Early treatment of Campylobacter jejuni enteritis. Antimicrob Agents Chemother 1989; 33: 248–250.

34 Bass J W. Pertussis (whooping cough). In: Donowitz L G (ed.). Infection control in the child care center and preschool. Baltimore: Williams & Wilkins, 1991; 220–226.

35 Isaacs D, Ferson M J, Gilbert G L, Grimwood K, Hogg G, McIntyre P. Chemoprophylaxis for Haemophilus and meningococcal infections. J Paediatr Child Health 1994; 30: 9–11.

36 Kuzushima K, Kudo T, Kido S et al. Prophylactic oral acyclovir in outbreaks of primary herpes simplex virus type 1 infection in a closed community. Pediatrics 1992; 89: 379–383.

37 Bartlett A V, Englender S J, Jarvis B A, Ludwig L, Carlson J F, Topping J P. Controlled trial of Giardia lamblia: control strategies in day care centers. Am J Public Health 1991; 81: 1001–1006.

38 Steketee R W, Reid S, Cheng T, Stoebig J S, Harrington R G, Davis J P. Recurrent outbreaks of giardiasis in a child day center, Wisconsin. Am J Public Health 1989; 79: 485–490.

39 Pickering L K, Morrow A L. Commentary [on 'Treatment of children with asymptomatic and nondiarrheal Giardia infection']. Pediatr Infect Dis J 1991; 10: 843–846.

40 Hadler S C, Erben J J, Matthews D, Starko K, Francis D P, Maynard J E. Effect of immunoglobulin on hepatitis A in day-care centers. JAMA 1983; 249: 48–53.

41 Ferson M J. Child care for mildly sick children. Aust J Public Health 1993; 17: 393–394.

42. Feder H M, Anderson I. Fifth disease: a brief review of infections in childhood, in adulthood, and in pregnancy. Arch Int Med 1989; 149: 2176–2178.

43 Ferson M J. Health and economic cost of chickenpox in child care. Med J Aust 1992; 156: 364.

44 Moore D A, Hopkins R S. Assessment of a school exclusion policy during a chickenpox outbreak. Am J Epidemiol 1991; 133: 1161–1167.

45 Pickering L K, Bartlett A V, Reves R R, Morrow A. Asymptomatic excretion of rotavirus before and after rotavirus diarrhea in children in day care centers. J Pediatr 1988; 112: 361–365.

46 Zheng B J, Chang R X, Ma G Z et al. Rotavirus infection of the oropharynx and respiratory tract in young children. J Med Virol 1991; 34: 29–37.

47 CDC. Shigellosis in child day care centers: Lexington—Fayette County, Kentucky, 1991. MMWR 1992; 41: 440–442.

48 Chorba T L, Meriwether R A, Jenkins B R, Gunn R A, MacCormack J N. Control of a non-foodborne outbreak of salmonellosis: day care in isolation. Am J Public Health 1987; 77: 979–981.

49 Davis J P, Pfeiffer J A. Surveillance of communicable diseases in child day care settings. Rev Infect Dis 1986; 8: 613–617.

CHAPTER 15

HUMAN IMMUNO DEFICIENCY VIRUS

15.1. Overview of HIV

15.1 Overview of HIV infection

INTRODUCTION

Immunodeficiency disorders were once rare conditions that only specialists in tertiary care facilities would see frequently. As a result of HIV-1, paediatricians throughout the world are increasingly required to recognize and treat children with profoundly impaired immunity. Women and children now constitute the fastest-growing groups of individuals newly infected with HIV in many industrialized nations. Unlike families of children with other life-threatening diseases, the parents are frequently themselves infected, ill and face discrimination rather than support from their communities. The care of such children involves a comprehensive, multidisciplinary approach which includes all affected family members.

EPIDEMIOLOGY

World-wide, more than 2.5 million people were estimated to have developed AIDS by mid-1993. Thirteen million adults and at least 1 million children were thought to be infected; 8 million of these infections had occurred in sub-Saharan Africa.[1] The epidemic is spreading rapidly in Asia. Infant and child mortality rates may increase by 30% above previously projected rates, as a direct consequence of perinatal HIV infection. By the end of the century, more than 5 million children under 15 years of age may be orphaned as a result of the premature death of their parents.

Vertical transmission from infected mothers to their infants will account for virtually all new infections in young children in the future. Perinatal transmission rates without intervention range from 14% to 39%, being higher in Africa than Europe or the USA.[2–5] In addition, a small proportion of children may be infected as the result of child sexual abuse.[6] Adolescents are at risk from unprotected sexual intercourse or use of contaminated needles. Several large studies confirm an extremely low risk of transmission through casual interactions amongst household contacts.[7–9] There has been one well-documented description of transmission from a child with AIDS to an unrelated 2-year-old in the same household. The mode of transmission was probably an unrecognized exposure of the 2-year-old's mucous membranes or excoriated skin to blood from nosebleeds or a laceration of the child with AIDS.[10] Rogers et al. documented lack of HIV transmission in seven individuals known to have bitten HIV-infected children.[11] There have been no reports of transmission in out-of-home child care settings or in school. Males and females are equally represented amongst children under 5 years old world-wide, although a higher proportion of older children are male in developed countries, because of blood-product acquired disease in haemophiliacs prior to the introduction of screening.

PATHOGENESIS

HIV-1 is a retrovirus, which means that it is able to transcribe its genetic material in a reverse direction, from RNA into DNA. Its only known natural host is man. The virion contains two copies of single-stranded RNA, encased by p24 antigen protein. This core is surrounded by an envelope, derived from the host cell plasma membrane during virus budding. It is a frail structure, unable to survive outside the body for more than a few seconds. Transmission therefore is confined to situations involving the exchange of bodily fluids:

- Across mucous membranes during sexual intercourse
- Directly into the circulation (through contaminated needles or transfusion of infected blood products)
- From an infected mother to her infant

Life cycle

It is worth understanding the HIV life cycle, as antiretroviral treatment is targeted at specific steps. The virus uses the CD4 receptor of T helper lymphocytes and macrophages as its target for binding to cells.[12] Following binding, HIV gains entry by simple fusion of the two membranes.[13,14] The virion core is released into the host cell cytoplasm, and uncoating occurs. Reverse transcription is catalysed by the HIV-1 enzyme, reverse transcriptase (RT). This yields a double-stranded 'proviral' DNA replica of the RNA genome. However, HIV-1 RT is error-prone and may produce several mis-incorporations per replication cycle, accounting for the rapid mutation rates observed *in vivo*. Some mutations may be lethal to the virus, but others may confer significant biological advantage. Under different selection pressures of humoral and cellular responses and drugs, this process may result in a heterogeneous population of viruses or 'swarm' of quasi-species in infected individuals.[15]

The proviral DNA is integrated into the host chromosomal DNA by another HIV-1 enzyme, integrase, and functions like a host cell gene. This constitutes a formidable obstacle to the eradication of HIV from infected individuals. Viral proteins are translated, cleaved by HIV-1 protease and assembled at the cell surface. The viral envelope glycoproteins are inserted across the host cell membrane, and budding of new virions occurs. A new round of infection ensues, either by release of mature virions to infect distant cells, or by direct interaction during budding of envelope proteins with a neighbouring CD4+ cell. Death of T cells results both from direct killing, for example during budding, and indirect mechanisms such as apoptosis, which is normally a physiological process of programmed cell death.[16]

Course of infection

The course of vertical HIV infection in children is similar to that seen in adults, but the length of the asymptomatic stage is frequently shorter. Acute infection may occur across a mucosal surface (such as by ingestion of contaminated maternal blood during delivery, or of breast milk postnatally) or parenterally (such as via a break in the integrity of the placental barrier). The acute mononucleosis-like illness experienced by 50–70% of adults is rarely detected in infants.

Following an initial burst of viral replication, there is wide dissemination of the virus, particularly to lymphoid tissue but also to other organs such as the thymus and central nervous system. Within 1–12 weeks antiviral immune responses develop, and coincide with a decrease in circulating virus burden.[17] Cellular immune responses in the form of cytotoxic T lymphocytes (CTLs) appear before a humoral antibody response.

A clinically asymptomatic period follows primary infection. In children, a bimodal pattern of disease progression has been observed, with one subset developing AIDS defining symptoms at a median of 5 months, and a second group who may develop symptoms from 1 to 12 years later.[3,18] In one study,[18] the median survival for the 'late progressors' was 8.4 years, which is shorter than the median survival now described in adults. With one notable exception,[19] it appears that virtually all infected children eventually develop disease.

No viral latency

Despite variable periods of clinical latency there is no period of viral latency. Throughout the course of infection, productively infected cells can be demonstrated in the lymphoid tissue and there is progressive destruction of CD4+ T cells. The extraordinary dynamics of this process have only recently been appreciated. An estimated 10^9 T cells are destroyed daily, and have to be replaced.[20] The virus is replicating at a rate of 300 or more life cycles per year. Every possible point mutation can be predicted to arise more than 10 000 times per day. No other infectious agent of man is known to be capable of such sustained, rapid turnover.

Late-stage disease in both adults and children is marked by a precipitous decline in CD4+ lymphocyte counts, profound impairment of the host's immunity and the risk of opportunistic infections and death.

PERINATAL TRANSMISSION

Perinatal or 'vertical' transmission encompasses transmission of virus from an infected mother to her child either prenatally, during delivery, or following delivery through breast-feeding. In non-breast-feeding populations, approximately 70% of transmission is thought to occur during delivery, but the precise mechanisms are not defined.

The majority of infants born to infected mothers are themselves uninfected (see Epidemiology section, above). Risk of transmission is higher with more advanced maternal disease, as evidenced by duration of infection, clinical status, lower CD4 counts, p24 antigenaemia, or higher levels of HIV DNA in peripheral blood.[2,21] Chorio-amnionitis, the presence of other sexually transmitted diseases and continued intravenous drug use in pregnancy have also been identified as risk factors.[22] Maternal vitamin A deficiency is associated with higher transmission rates.

Preliminary data suggest that higher maternal neutralizing antibody titres to HIV isolates may correlate with decreased transmission.[23]

Evidence for intrapartum transmission comes in part from observations in twins discordant for HIV infection. A multinational study of 115 sets of twins born to seropositive mothers demonstrated that transmission was more common to the first-born twin.[24] Thirty-five per cent of vaginally delivered and 16% of Caesarean-delivered first-born twins were infected, as opposed to 15% of vaginally delivered and 8% of Caesarean-delivered second-born twins. The first-born twin has more prolonged exposure to cervical and vaginal secretions, which have been shown to harbour infectious virus. The Caesarean-delivered second-born twin has virtually no contact with the birth canal. The 8% infection rate may represent a baseline for intrauterine transmission rate, although the baby's mucous membranes may be exposed to maternal blood during a Caesarean section.

The protective effect of Caesarean section is, at best, modest. A meta-analysis of 3202 deliveries found that transmission was 17% with Caesarean section and 21% with vaginal delivery.[25] A prospective, randomized trial of elective Caesarean versus vaginal delivery is in progress in Europe. The antiretroviral drug, zidovudine, has been shown to reduce the transmission rate, in a placebo-controlled study in the USA and France.[26] Zidovudine or placebo was given to mothers from the second trimester through delivery, and to the infants for 6 weeks after birth. The transmission rate for placebo recipients was 25.5%, compared to 8.3% for those randomized to zidovudine. To what extent this intervention can be abbreviated, and whether combinations of antiretroviral drugs may be more effective, are the subject of several current clinical trials.

The additional risk of transmission through breast-feeding, over and above in utero or peripartum transmission, appears to be around 14% (CI 7–22%).[27] Mathematical modelling has demonstrated that the benefits of breast-feeding outweigh the risks of transmission in countries in which safe water supplies and maintenance of sterility of bottle-feeding equipment cannot be guaranteed.[28] The current recommendation from the World Health Organization (WHO) is to encourage breast-feeding in countries 'where infectious diseases and malnutrition are the main causes of infant deaths and the infant mortality rate is high'.[29] In countries with relatively safe alternatives to breast-feeding, bottle-feeding is strongly encouraged.

In summary, what options are available to HIV-infected pregnant women to decrease the risk of transmission?

- Avoid breast feeding (if safe alternatives exist)
- Modify obstetric practices:
    - avoid scalp electrodes, fetal blood sampling
    - elective (pre-labour) Caesarean section?
    - virucidal cleansing of birth canal?
- therapeutic interventions:
    - antiretroviral therapy
    - correct maternal vitamin A deficiency
    - boost immune response of mother/baby?

No intervention can be offered unless the diagnosis of HIV infection is established before or during pregnancy. Unlinked anonymous testing in London has revealed that over 75% of HIV-infected women are unaware of their serostatus. Obstetricians and midwives play a crucial role in informing mothers of the advantages of being tested. When a mother is found to be infected, a coordinated plan involving paediatric and adult infectious disease teams must already be in place.

DIAGNOSIS

The aim of early diagnosis should ideally be to establish the infection status before a child becomes symptomatic, as the first clinical presentation may be with a rapidly fatal opportunistic infection. The diagnosis of HIV infection is normally established in adults by enzyme-linked immunosorbent assays (ELISA) for HIV-specific IgG antibodies, detectable within 4–24 weeks of initial infection.

For perinatally infected infants, these tests are of no diagnostic value beyond confirming the serological status of the mother. Virtually 100% of infants of infected mothers acquire IgG antibodies to HIV transplacentally. These passively acquired antibodies gradually wane, with a median time to disappearance of 10 months, although up to 2% of uninfected infants have detectable antibodies at 18 months.[2,3] Positive IgG tests are therefore only diagnostic of infection in children over the age of 18 months.

Hypogammaglobulinaemia, which is an occasional finding in HIV-infected children, may result in false negative tests.

Establishing the diagnosis in infants requires tests that directly detect the virus or its components. The three most widely accepted methods are virus culture, detection of HIV genetic material by polymerase chain reaction (PCR) and detection of serum p24 antigen by ELISA. Virus can be cultured from plasma, lymphocytes or whole blood in qualitative or quantitative assays. The requirement for special containment facilities and the labour-intensive nature of these assays which take 3–4 weeks to yield a result, makes them expensive and limits their availability.

PCR techniques are more rapid than culture, and provide a similar degree of sensitivity and specificity, approaching 100% by 2–3 months of age. Quality assurance procedures to rapidly detect contamination and false positive results in a PCR laboratory are mandatory.

p24 antigen detection is rapid and relatively cheap. The sensitivity has been considerably enhanced by the use of immune-complex disruption/dissociation (ICD p24) techniques, which free antigen from complexes with antibody.[30] However, the test is less sensitive than culture or PCR, and false positives may occur in the first few days of life if mothers are highly antigenaemic.[30] Despite the sensitivity of the direct tests for HIV, between 50% and 70% of children who subsequently prove to be infected have negative results in the first few days of life. This is suggestive of peripartum transmission with extremely low or absent circulating viral burden initially.[31] The need for follow-up samples to confirm an initial positive result or establish a negative diagnosis is apparent (see Table 15.1.1).

Detection of IgA-specific antibodies (which do not cross the placenta) offers promise, although this class of antibody is not usually produced earlier than

Table 15.1.1 Suggested follow-up for infants born to women who are known to be HIV-infected

Age	Action	Reason
24–48 hours	PCR, HIV culture,[a] p24 antigen[b]	Positive test(s) suggest in utero transmission, and carries higher risk of rapid disease progression
3–4 weeks	PCR, HIV culture,[a] p24 antigen[b]	Majority of infected infants will test negative initially but be positive now: suggests intrapartum transmission
	Start co-trimoxazole	PCP prophylaxis (should not be started at less than 3 weeks, but should be started by 8 weeks as PCP peak is between 10 and 20 weeks)
3–4 months	PCR, HIV culture[a], p24 antigen[b] and IgA	Will pick up >98% infected infants
5–6 months	Review infant and discuss results. If any tests positive or any clinical concern, repeat PCR, HIV culture,[a] p24 antigen[b] and IgA	If all three sets of tests are negative, and baby is clinically stable (particularly growth and development), child is almost certainly not infected and PCP prophylaxis can be stopped
12 months	Review. HIV antibody test	Median time to seroreversion is 10–11 months using ELISA
18 months	Review HIV antibody test	98% of uninfected children have seroreverted by now

In addition, all routine immunizations should be administered according to locally prevailing regimes with the substitution of inactivated for oral polio (see text for details).
[a] If available.
[b] Ideally, immune-complex dissociated (ICD) assays should be used, which are more sensitive than standard ELISA
At any time, a positive test result must be repeated (ideally with two assays on two samples) before telling care-giver that child is infected. If sufficient blood available, check T cell subsets (must include CD4+ absolute count and percentage) ± immunoglobulins.

2 months of age. IgM assays have not proved useful, due to the brevity and unpredictable duration of a detectable rise post partum.

Indirect laboratory parameters may also indicate HIV infection. Low CD4 counts and percentages taking into account the age-dependent normal range (Table 15.1.3) are suggestive but not diagnostic. Hypergammaglobulinaemia is a frequent finding by 3 months of age, but of poor positive predictive value since many uninfected infants of infected mothers have high levels of passively acquired IgG.[32] By 6 months of age, however, hypergammaglobulinaemia is a useful indicator, positive in 77% of infected and 3% of uninfected children.[33]

If culture, PCR and p24 antigen tests can be performed on three occasions in the first 3–4 months of life, ideally with an IgA assay on the final occasion, and all results are negative, it is highly likely that the infant is uninfected. If one or other of these tests are unavailable, an additional test at 6 months would be wise before telling parents the child is uninfected. It is extremely important that a positive test is confirmed, ideally by two different methods on two different samples.

CLINICAL

Infected infants are usually clinically normal during the newborn period. A bimodal pattern of disease progression has already been mentioned, with about a quarter progressing rapidly to AIDS within the first 12 months, and the remainder progressing more slowly. The early manifestations of disease in infants and children are varied and frequently non-specific. Persistent oral candidiasis and parotitis were found to be highly discriminatory for HIV infection in the European collaborative study while lymphadenopathy, hepatosplenomegaly, eczema, fever, rhinitis, otitis, and non-Gram-negative pneumonias were less specific.[33]

Damage to the developing immune system results in poor primary responses to common antigens, which may explain the increased incidence of bacterial infections. Children are also experiencing primary infections with opportunistic pathogens, resulting in more severe disease than in adults in whom opportunistic infections are usually due to reactivation.

As the CD4+ lymphocyte count declines and the immune system is progressively impaired, children develop symptoms that lie along a continuum from mild to life-threatening. The Centers for Disease Control (CDC) revised the classification of Paediatric HIV disease in 1994, dividing symptoms into four clinical categories: asymptomatic, mild, moderate and severe (Table 15.1.2), and three immunological categories (Table 15.1.3).[34]

There are geographic variations in clinical manifestations of AIDS, such as

Table 15.1.2   Centers for Disease Control 1994 revised classification system for HIV infection in children less than 13 years old

Category N: No Symptoms
Child has no signs or symptoms which are felt to be the result of HIV infection, or has only one of the conditions listed in category A below.

Category A: Mildly Symptomatic
Two or more of the conditions listed below but none of the conditions listed in categories B and C.

- Lymphadenopathy (>0.5 cm at >2 sites; bilateral = 1 site)
- Hepatomegaly
- Splenomegaly

Table 15.1.2 *(contd)*

- Dermatitis
- Parotitis
- Recurrent or persistent upper respiratory tract infections, including sinusitis or otitis media (4 or more episodes in a 12-month period)

Category B: Moderately Symptomatic
Symptomatic conditions occurring in a child which are not included among conditions listed in clinical category C and which are attributed to HIV infection.
Examples of conditions in clinical category B include, BUT ARE NOT LIMITED TO:

- Anaemia <8 g/dl or neutropenia <1000/mm^3 or thrombocytopenia <100 000/mm^3 persisting >30 days
- Bacterial meningitis, pneumonia, or sepsis (single episode)
- Candidiasis, oropharyngeal (thrush), persisting for >2 months in child >6 months of age
- Cardiomyopathy
- Cytomegalovirus infection with onset before 1 month of age
- Diarrhoea, recurrent or chronic
- Hepatitis
- Herpes simplex virus (HSV) stomatitis, recurrent (<2 episodes/year)
- Herpes zoster (shingles) involving at least two distinct episodes or more than one dermatome
- Leiomyosarcoma
- Lymphoid interstitial pneumonia or pulmonary lymphoid hyperplasia complex (LIP/PLH)
- Nephropathy
- Nocardiosis
- Persistent fever > 1 month
- Toxoplasmosis, onset before 1 month of age
- Varicella (persistent or complicated primary chickenpox)

Category C: Severely Symptomatic
Any condition listed in the 1987 surveillance case definition for AIDS, **with the exception of LIP**. The conditions in clinical category C are strongly associated with severe immunodeficiency, occur frequently in HIV-infected individuals, and cause serious morbidity or mortality.

- Serious bacterial infections, multiple or recurrent (any combination of at least two culture proven infections within a 2-year period, of the following types: septicaemia, pneumonia, meningitis, bone or joint infection, or abscess of an internal organ or body cavity: excludes otitis media, superficial skin or mucosal abcesses, and indwelling catheter related infections).
- Candidiasis, oesophageal or pulmonary
- Coccidioidomycosis, disseminated (at site other than or in addition to lungs or cervical or hilar lymph nodes)
- Cryptococcosis (extrapulmonary)
- Cryptosporidiosis or Isosporiasis with diarrhoea persisting 1 month
- Cytomegalovirus disease with onset of symptoms at age >1 month (at a site other than liver, spleen, or nodes)
- Encephalopathy (at least one of the following progressive findings present at least 2 months: (a) failure to attain or loss of developmental milestones or loss of intellectual ability, verified by standard developmental scale or neuropsychological tests; (b) impaired brain growth (acquired microcephaly demonstrated by head circumference measurements or brain atrophy demonstrated on CT or MRI); (c) acquired symmetric motor deficit manifested by two or more of the following: paresis, pathological reflexes, ataxia, or gait disturbance)
- Herpes simplex virus infection causing a mucocutaneous ulcer that persists longer than 1 month; or bronchitis, pneumonitis, or oesophagitis for any duration affecting a child > 1 month of age
- Histoplasmosis, disseminated (at site other than or in addition to lungs or cervical or hilar lymph nodes)
- Kaposi's sarcoma
- Lymphoma, primary, in brain
- Lymphoma, small, non-cleaved cell (Burkitt's), or immunoblastic or large cell lymphoma of B cell or unknown immunological phenotype
- *Mycobacterium tuberculosis*, disseminated or extrapulmonary
- *Mycobacterium*, other species or unidentified species, disseminated or extrapulmonary
- *Mycobacterium avium* complex or *M. kansasii*, disseminated (at site other than or in addition to lungs, skin, or cervical or hilar lymph nodes)
- *Pneumocystis carinii* pneumonia
- Progressive multifocal leukoencephalopathy
- Salmonella (non-typhoid) septicaemia, recurrent
- Toxoplasmosis of the brain with onset at age > 1 month
- Wasting syndrome (persistent weight loss (> 10% of baseline, or an infant who crosses 2 percentile lines or is below the 5th percentile and falling away from curve) which is unresponsive to oral alimentation) PLUS chronic diarrhoea OR fever for >30 days

Table 15.1.3   Centers for Disease Control 1994 revised classification system for HIV infection in children less than 13 years old: immunological categories based on age-specific CD4+ T lymphocyte counts and percentages of total lymphocytes

Immunological category	Age of child					
	<12 months		1–5 years		6–12 years	
	/µl	(%)	/µl	(%)	/µl	(%)
1. No evidence of immunosuppression	>1500	(>25)	>1000	(>25)	>500	(>25)
2. Moderate immunosuppression	750–1499	(15–25)	500–999	(15–25)	200–499	(15–25)
3. Severe immunosuppression	<750	(<15)	<500	(<15)	<200	(<15)

NB: Child is classified on basis of either the absolute count or the percentage. If both are available and are not concordant, the child should be classified into the more severe category. Initial and any subsequent changes in classification should be confirmed on two separate samples. A child should not be reclassified to a less severe category if subsequent CD4 determinations improve.

severe diarrhoeal disease and measles in sub-Saharan Africa, which make this classification less appropriate.[35] For adolescents, the revised classification system published by CDC in 1993 should be used.[36]

Pneumocystis carinii pneumonia (PCP)

Early in the HIV epidemic, *P. carinii* was noted to be a cause of pulmonary disease in young children with HIV despite apparently high CD4 counts. An early and frequently fatal peak is observed in infants around the age of 3 months who are presumably experiencing their primary infection. The presenting features of PCP are tachypnoea, dyspnoea, cough and fever.[37] The presentation may be insidious over a week or more rather than acute, and the chest may sound clear. Hypoxia is the hallmark of the disease. Radiologically PCP can present as a spectrum from almost no infiltrates to frank consolidation (Fig. 15.1.1). The diagnosis can frequently be established by sputum induction, but if this is negative and clinical suspicion is high, bronchoalveolar lavage is indicated.[38] Open lung biopsy is rarely necessary. Therapy should take into account which prophylactic regimen (if any) the child has broken through. The drug of choice remains trimethoprim/ sulphamethoxazole (TMP/SMX, 120 mg/kg per day i.e., 20 mg/kg per day TMP, in four divided doses i.v.). Only a documented serious allergic response (angioneurotic oedema, for example) should prompt alternative therapy with i.v. pentamidine or trimetrexate. Based on data from adult studies, adjunctive steroids are used for any child with an arterial oxygen tension of less than 70 mmHg.[39] It is important to look for other opportunistic pathogens, particularly tuberculosis and cytomegalovirus (CMV). If the BAL or buffy coat or urine are growing CMV, treatment with gancyclovir throughout the duration of steroid therapy should be considered, as fatal complications from this pathogen following initial response to treatment for PCP may occur. Surfactant treatment may be useful for children with PCP who develop adult respiratory distress syndrome.

Prophylaxis for PCP is a constantly evolving field. The current recommendations are that all children under the age of 12 months who are infected or indeterminate, and those with severe immunosuppression as defined by CD4+ lymphocyte counts (as shown in Table 15.1.3, but with an upper limit of 750 for children aged 12–24 months) should receive primary prophylaxis. Any child, regardless of CD4 count, with a history of PCP should receive secondary prophylaxis. The drug of choice in both situations is TMP/SMX (Table 15.1.4). Alternative

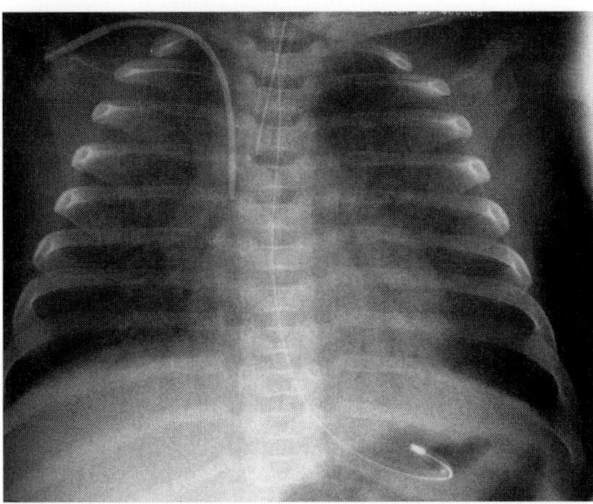

Fig. 15.1.1 *Pneumocystis carinii* pneumonia (PCP) in a 3 month old. Central venous catheter, endotracheal tube and nasogastric tube are seen. Diffuse bilateral ground-glass opacification, tending to confluence in right upper and both lower lobes. Air bronchograms are seen, which imply air space disease which is a late feature of disease. The earliest infiltrates are usually perihilar. The absence of pleural effusion or hilar adenopathy is typical. Less typical presentations include miliary, coin and nodular lesions, lobar consolidation, and cavitations. (With kind permission of Dr. Cathy Owens, St. Mary's Hospital, London.)

Table 15.1.4   Prophylaxis for *Pneumocystis carinii* pneumonia: suggested doses of trimethoprim/sulphamethoxasole (TMP/SMX), to be given once daily on three days per week (usually Monday, Wednesday and Friday). Dose is based on 900 mg/m^2 per dose of the two drugs (= 150 mg/m^2 per dose TMP)

Surface area (m^2)	Dose of TMP/SMX (mg)
< 0.25	120
0.25–0.39	240
0.40–0.49	360
0.50–0.75	480
0.76–1.0	720
> 1.0	960 (adult dose)

Alternatives for children with documented severe intolerance to co-trimoxazole:

Dapsone	2 mg/kg per day p.o.
Pentamidine	300 mg, regardless of age, once a month by nebulizer
Pentamidine	4 mg/kg, regardless of age, once a month, i.v.

regimens include aerosolized pentamidine for children old enough to comply with nebulized treatment, dapsone or intravenous pentamidine. Breakthroughs have been reported with all four regimens, but are least frequent with TMP/SMX.

Lymphocytic interstitial pneumonitis (LIP)

LIP is a chronic lung disorder of uncertain aetiology that affects up to 40–50% of vertically HIV-infected children.[40] It is less common in older children, haemophiliacs and adults. The disorder is characterized by a diffuse, interstitial, reticulonodular infiltrate on plain X-ray (see Fig. 15.1.2). If this is associated with larger nodules and hilar or mediastinal lymphadenopathy, it has been referred to as pulmonary lymphoid hyperplasia (PLH), which appears to represent one end of the continuum of this process. LIP is frequently accompanied by hepatosplenomegaly, generalized lymphadenopathy and parotitis, suggesting an exuberant activation of the reticuloendothelial system. These signs (including LIP) tend to

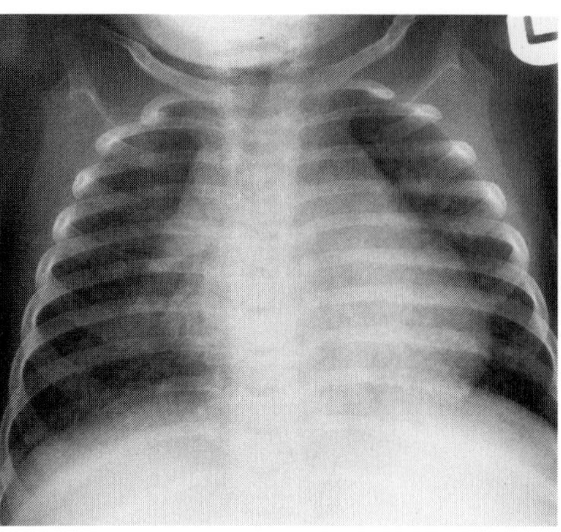

Fig. 15.1.2 Lymphoid interstitial pneumonitis (LIP), in the same child as in Fig. 15.1.1, now aged 9 months. Diffuse, well-circumscribed nodules distributed uniformly throughout both lung fields. May be associated with hilar adenopathy. A radiological spectrum is seen in LIP, ranging from fine linear interstitial infiltrates to large nodules that tend to confluence in the right middle and lingular lobes. (With kind permission of Dr Cathy Owens, St Mary's Hospital, London.)

wane with advancing disease. Clinically there is a wide spectrum of severity, from an asymptomatic individual in whom LIP is a purely radiological diagnosis to an individual with severely compromised exercise tolerance and oxygen dependency. A presumptive diagnosis may be made on the basis of suggestive X-ray changes which persist for months, are unresponsive to antimicrobial therapy and are not due to other specific infectious pathogens. *Pneumocystis carinii* pneumonia can coexist with LIP and any new onset of oxygen dependency should prompt an induced sputum examination and consideration of bronchoscopy to look for pneumocysts or trophozoites. A definitive diagnosis of LIP is made by lung biopsy, although this is rarely necessary. Characteristic findings are a diffuse lymphoid infiltration of the alveolar septa and peribronchiolar areas, with varying degrees of lymphoid aggregation which may show organization into early germinal centres. Both Epstein–Barr virus (EBV) DNA and HIV RNA have been identified by in situ hybridization in biopsies from children with LIP.[41] The precise aetiological role of either, and why LIP is less frequently seen in adults, is unclear. The fact that children may be experiencing a primary infection with EBV may be relevant.

Treatment for LIP is only indicated in the presence of hypoxia and shortness of breath. Overnight monitoring (which avoids movement artefacts) provides objective measurement of oxygen saturation. Oxygen dependency frequently resolves with oral steroids, used at high dose for at least 6 weeks to suppress the lymphocytic proliferation. Symptoms frequently return upon weaning steroids and the lowest maintenance dose must be sought. Zidovudine, anecdotally, may be beneficial, but controlled data are lacking. Bronchiectasis may complicate LIP, requiring physiotherapy and antibiotics for secondary bacterial infection.

Encephalopathy

Neurological problems occur frequently in symptomatic HIV-infected children, with estimates varying from 31% to 89% in different series.[42] HIV encephalopathy is rarely evident at birth but may present in infancy with signs such as delayed acquisition of a social smile, poor head control, or truncal hypotonia. Subsequently, progressive motor abnormalities such as spastic diplegia and oral motor dysfunction become apparent. Expressive language is frequently more affected than receptive language. Acquired microcephaly due to cerebral atrophy may be noted. Seizures are unusual in the absence of other complications, as HIV infection is predominantly a disease of white matter.

Computed tomographic (CT) scans are useful for demonstrating ventricular enlargement and cortical atrophy, or cerebral calcification which is seen particularly in the basal ganglia in association with vertically acquired HIV infection.

Magnetic resonance imaging (MRI) techniques are better than CT scans at delineating white matter abnormalities.

Failure to thrive

Growth failure is a specific marker of HIV disease progression and may become evident within the first few months of life. Decreased linear growth and weight gain are proportional initially, so that children do not appear wasted.

Growth failure may be a result of:

- Inadequate nutritional intake
  — suppressed appetite
  — oropharyngeal pathology (e.g. *Candida* or, less commonly, herpes simplex oesophagitis)
  — neurological disease, including HIV encephalopathy
- Malabsorption
  — HIV enteropathy
  — GI tract infections
  — bacterial pathogens: *Mycobacterium avium intracellulare*, *Salmonella*, *Shigella*
  — protozoal pathogens: cryptosporidiosis, giardiasis, isosporiasis, cyclosporiasis
  — viruses: rotavirus, enterovirus, cytomegalovirus
  — lactase deficiency
- Increased metabolic requirements
  — dysregulation of cytokines due to immune activation by HIV
- Endocrine abnormalities
  — hypothyroidism
  — adrenal insufficiency (e.g. with cytomegalovirus infection)
  — growth hormone deficiency (rare)

Children with oesophagitis may not complain of dysphagia; therefore a barium swallow or endoscopy is indicated in children with loss of appetite and weight loss.

Nutritional monitoring and dietary intervention should begin early, as malnutrition may enhance immunodeficiency. Deficiencies of iron, vitamin and other micronutrients should be considered. Providing sufficient calories and protein to maintain linear growth and weight gain is frequently difficult. A variety of calorically dense formulae and supplements should be available, to find one that the child will tolerate. Dietary advice should be sensitive to the family's ethnic and cultural constraints. Appetite stimulants such as cyproheptadine (Periactin), dronabinol (Marinol) or megestrol acetate (Megace) are worth considering, but rarely improve caloric intake more than 10–20%. If oral intake remains inadequate, tube-feeding may be necessary. However, nasogastric tubes may exacerbate sinusitis and upper airway infection, and gastrostomy sites may heal poorly and leak. Parenteral nutrition may therefore become necessary.

Other infectious complications

Bacteria

In addition to profound CD4+ T cell depletion, HIV infection causes an early dysregulation of B cell function in children. This results in recurrent serious bacterial infections. Otitis media, soft tissue infections, bacteraemia, pneumonia and sinusitis are the commonest presentations. If central venous catheter-associated infections are excluded, the commonest bacterial pathogens are the polysaccharide-encapsulated organisms, particularly *Streptococcus pneumoniae*.

Mycobacterial infections are of increasing concern. *Mycobacterium tuberculosis* may develop at any stage of HIV disease. The identification of strains multiply resistant to isoniazid, rifampicin and other drugs poses a serious threat to patients and their care givers.[43] Diagnosis is confounded by anergy in HIV-infected children: it is important to place a positive control (such as *Candida* antigens) when skin testing. Good-quality diagnostic specimens are essential. Gastric lavage was found to be more sensitive than bronchoalveolar lavage in one small series.[44] Guidelines for therapy have been prepared by the Advisory Council for the Elimination of Tuberculosis.[45] Isoniazid prophylaxis has been recommended for all HIV-infected children who are household or daycare contacts of adults with active TB.

Mycobacterium avium intracellulare (MAI) is a frequent opportunistic pathogen, at late stages of disease. It has been found in almost one in five children with advanced disease (CD4 < 50 cells/µl).[46] Presentation is typically with recurrent fevers, night sweats, abdominal pain, distension or diarrhoea, and weight loss. A diagnosis of systemic infection requires culture of the organisms from blood, as stool and respiratory isolates may only represent colonization. However, the majority of adults with such colonization eventually develop bacteraemia. Current therapy consists of at least three agents, which usually include a macrolide antibiotic (clarithromycin or azithromycin) and rifampicin or rifabutin, plus ciprofloxacin or clofazimine or ethambutol. The safety and toxicity of prophylactic rifabutin in children with CD4 counts less than 100 is being assessed.

Viruses

HIV-infected children are at risk of serious morbidity and mortality from a wide variety of viral pathogens. Of the herpes group, primary varicella can be associated with visceral dissemination and encephalitis.[47] Subsequent varicella zoster may recur with increasing frequency as the underlying immunodeficiency progresses, although it is seen at all stages of disease. Lesions may be atypical, with hyperkeratosis and increased pigmentation or hypopigmentation without obvious vesiculation.[48] They are usually painful. Chronic suppressive therapy with valacyclovir or foscarnet may be required. Herpes simplex virus has been associated with severe herpetic gingivo-stomatitis, oesophagitis and chronic labial infections. Cytomegalovirus (CMV) may cause retinitis, pneumonitis, enterocolitis, hepatitis and, more rarely, oesophagitis, pancreatitis or adrenal insufficiency.[49] It may be necessary to treat retinitis with a combination of gancyclovir and foscarnet in children who relapse on gancyclovir alone.[50]

Respiratory pathogens, particularly respiratory syncytial virus (RSV), influenza, parainfluenza and adenoviruses, may cause severe and even fatal pneumonitis and may be shed for prolonged periods, creating a significant dilemma in terms of patient isolation policies. PCP may be complicated by superinfection with any of these respiratory pathogens. Dual infection carries a very poor prognosis.

Measles is associated with a high incidence of pneumonitis in HIV-infected children and occasionally with encephalitis.

Hepatitis viruses A, B and C may be more fulminant, and B and C particularly can result in a chronic aggressive or frequently relapsing course. Maternal infection with HIV and HCV greatly increases the risk of transmission of HCV.

Protozoa

Toxoplasma gondii infections have been the subject of several case reports but the prevalence is much lower in children than in adults. Chronic suppressive therapy with daily pyrimethamine–sulphadiazine and folinic acid is recommended following treatment for active ocular or central nervous system toxoplasmosis.[51]

Cryptosporidial infection and other pathogens may cause intractable diarrhoea in some children, and there are few effective therapies.

Fungi

Of the fungal pathogens, *Candida albicans* is the most prevalent. Recurrent oropharyngeal candidiasis is seen in over 70% of children followed throughout their symptomatic stage of disease to death. *Candida* oesophagitis occurs in about 20%, diagnosed usually on clinical and radiological evidence. Disseminated candidiasis or fungaemias are rare, except in patients with chronic indwelling intravenous devices. For persistent or recurrent mucocutaneous candidiasis, chronic suppressive therapy is frequently required. Nystatin is virtually useless. If topical treatment with clotrimazole fails, oral ketoconazole or fluconazole is used. Resistance and breakthrough infections occur, which may require parenteral therapy with amphotericin B.[51] *Cryptococcus neoformans* is less prevalent than in adults but can cause meningitis with insidious onset of malaise and altered mental status in older children. Chronic suppressive therapy with oral fluconazole is required, following initial treatment.[51]

Other common clinical problems

Fluctuating elevations of hepatic transaminases are a frequent finding. Infectious causes other than HIV should be investigated, in particular the hepatitis viruses, CMV, EBV and MAI. Cryptosporidial infection of the biliary tree has been described. Many drugs that HIV-infected children receive may be implicated, in particular the rifamycins and antifungal azoles. Ceftriaxone and other antibiotics are implicated in biliary sludging.

Pancreatitis was an uncommon finding in children prior to the AIDS era. It can result from opportunistic infections such as CMV or more commonly as a side-effect of therapy, in particular as a dose-dependent toxicity of dideoxyinosine (ddI).[52,53] The precise mechanism is not well understood.

The commonest haematological abnormality is anaemia which, depending on definition and stage of disease and concomitant myelosuppressive drug exposure, is seen in up to 94% of children. Pure red cell aplasia has been occasionally described, associated with human parvovirus B19 infections.

Neutropenia is also common, and is the major dose-limiting toxicity to zidovudine therapy in infants. Side-effects of therapy are the commonest cause of neutropenia, but opportunistic infections with CMV and MAI may be implicated. In situations in which myelotoxic drugs are considered essential (such as zidovudine for encephalopathic children) granulocyte colony-stimulating factor can be used to maintain an absolute neutrophil count above 0.5×10^9 cells/l.

Thrombocytopenia may be the presenting complaint of HIV infection. It may be the result of direct effects of HIV or opportunistic infections of the bone marrow, autoimmune destruction, sequestration in the spleen, antiretroviral medication or rarely an artefact due to platelet clumping in ethylenediaminetetraacetic acid (EDTA)-anticoagulated samples. Depending on the aetiology, treatment with high-dose intravenous immunoglobulin (0.5–1.0 mg/kg per day i.v. daily for 3–5 days) may be effective.

Malignancies are less frequently observed in children compared to adults. As of December 1993, only 2% of the total 5210 children with AIDS reported to the CDC had malignancy as an AIDS-defining illness. Of these, 25 had Kaposi's sarcoma, 39 Burkitt's lymphoma (which is not normally associated with immuno-suppression), 20 had an immunoblastic lymphoma and 15 had primary CNS lymphoma. Clinically it can be impossible to differentiate between an EBV-driven polyclonal immunoproliferative response or lymphoma, and biopsy is essential in children presenting with new or asymmetric regional lymphadenopathy. An increased incidence of leiomyomas and leiomyosarcomas, which have also not previously been associated with immunodeficiency, has been reported.[54]

TREATMENT

Treatment recommendations for HIV disease are constantly evolving, as our understanding of the pathogenesis grows, and as the results of clinical trials become available. Table 15.1.5 summarizes the main components of therapy with some examples that are in use or are being evaluated in clinical trials at the present time.

Antiretroviral therapy: when to start?

If antiretroviral agents were developed that were capable of completely preventing viral replication, it would be rational to use these at the earliest possible stage of disease. The agents that are available at present are not capable of completely switching off viral replication, allowing subpopulations of virus to mutate, and drug-resistant strains to be selected. Benefits of early intervention must therefore be weighed against the cost, possible side-effects and limited duration of efficacy of these drugs. Current recommendations are to start treatment in children who have moderate or severe symptoms (Table 15.1.2) or a rapidly declining CD4 count (Table 15.1.3).[51] It is recognized that CD4 counts are an incomplete surrogate marker for disease progression in adults. Many centres caring for HIV-1-infected children report patients surviving for 5 years or more with less than 5% CD4+ lymphocytes. A low CD4 count therefore should not be a reason for therapeutic nihilism.

Table 15.1.5   Current treatment of paediatric HIV infection

Treatment category	Examples
Antiretroviral therapy aimed at molecular targets of HIV-1 life cycle (Both single agents and combinations are being studied.)	Reverse transcription • Nucleoside analogues (AZT, ddI, ddC, 3TC, d4T) • Non-nucleoside RT inhibitors (nevirapine) Protease (e.g. Merck, Abbott)
Prophylactic measures	• Prevention of mother–infant transmission • PCP prophylaxis • Intravenous immunoglobulin • MAI prophylaxis? • Immunizations (routine, pneumococcus, influenza) • For contacts of TB, VZV, measles
Treatment of opportunistic infections and chronic suppressive therapy	Infections • Candida species • Cytomegalovirus • Varicella zoster virus • Herpes zoster virus • Toxoplasmosis • Cryptococcosis Lymphoid interstitial pneumonitis
Supportive therapy	• Psychosocial support and family-based care • Nutritional interventions • Pain management • Palliative care

Other surrogate markers for disease progression (such as quantitative viral load assays) continue to be evaluated, but none are yet sufficiently validated to be used as sole criteria for starting treatment.

Antiretroviral therapy: what to use?

The only drugs widely used in children to date are reverse transcriptase inhibitors. Zidovudine (azidothymidine, AZT) has been shown to have clinical benefits in uncontrolled studies in symptomatic children.[55,56] Transient increases in age-adjusted CD4 counts and reductions in virus burden have also been noted. The most common side-effect is myelosuppenia (both anaemia and neutropenia). The incidence of haematological toxicity may be reduced by the use of lower doses of zidovudine than those which were originally evaluated. A trial comparing 360 with 720 mg/m^2 per day in minimally symptomatic children has shown no difference in outcome over a 3-year period of follow-up (AIDS Clinical Trial Group study number 128). Preliminary data from a study of 830 previously untreated, symptomatic children suggest that either ddI alone, or a combination of zidovudine and ddI, may be better tolerated and delay disease progression compared with zidovudine alone (ACTG 152). ddI is not myelosuppressive, has a sustained effect in maintaining CD4 counts, but does not penetrate the blood–brain barrier and may be associated with pancreatitis in 5–7% of recipients.[57] Retinal depigmentation has been reported in 5% of children but is non-sight threatening. Dideoxycytidine (ddC) is being studied in children in combination with zidovudine. Lamivudine (3-thiacytidine, 3TC) is another RT inhibitor that is showing considerable promise in combination with zidovudine.

Non-nucleotide RT inhibitors (nevirapine and α-apa for example) and new classes of drugs such as protease inhibitors are also entering clinical trials in children. Attacking the virus at more than one target in its life cycle may be a useful step toward the goal of shutting down replication, or generating mutants that are sufficiently crippled to inflict less damage on the immune system and prolong the period of clinical latency.

For children with HIV encephalopathy, zidovudine at high dose (720 mg/m^2 per day) is currently recommended. If neutropenia is a dose-limiting side-effect, granulocyte colony-stimulating factor can be effective, in doses as low as 1 μg/kg on alternate days.[58] Erythropoietin has been less predictable in trying to ameliorate zidovudine-induced anaemia.

In order to improve the outlook for HIV-infected children, as many as possible should receive treatment as part of carefully designed clinical trials. Ideally the decision to start antiretroviral therapy should be made in consultation with a physician experienced in managing children with HIV.[51] Information about clinical trials in Europe can be obtained through the Medical Research Council HIV Clinical Trials Centre ((0171) 380 9991/3). The Pediatric European Network for Treatment of AIDS (PENTA) studies are being coordinated through this centre. In the USA information is available by dialling 1-800-TRIALSA.

Antiretroviral treatment: when to change?

Indications for alternative therapy include intolerance to the initial drug(s) or clinical disease progression. The most widely accepted signs of disease progression that are felt to be attributable to HIV disease itself are growth failure or neurodevelopmental deterioration. It is important to document children's neuro-development regularly using standardized tests that enable deterioration to be picked up early.[57] Quantitative assays of virus burden may be useful, but, as with initiation of therapy, are not yet sufficiently validated to be used as sole criteria for change. Alternative drugs and combinations are under evaluation.

Intravenous gamma globulin

A double-blind study of 372 HIV-1-infected children compared intravenous immune globulin (IVIG) (400 mg/kg) every 28 days with placebo (0.1% albumin), over a median length of follow-up of 17 months. A reduction of bacterial infections and hospitalizations was observed for those children with CD4+ counts above 200 cells/mm^3 at entry.[59] Subsequent age-adjusted CD4+ slope analysis demonstrated a slowing of CD4+ count decline by 13.5 cells/month in the IVIG recipients.[60] The benefits, however, were not observed in children receiving trimethoprim–sulphamethoxazole for PCP prophylaxis, and were not found in another study of children with lower CD4+ counts. Children with significant recurrent bacterial infections, hypogammaglobulinaemia or documented poor functional antibody development may be candidates for IVIG 400 mg/kg every 28 days.[51]

Active and passive immunizations

All childhood immunizations are currently recommended, with the exception that inactivated poliovirus vaccine should be substituted for oral polio vaccine even after seroreversion, to prevent spread to immunodeficient family members.[51] In addition, pneumococcal vaccine is recommended at age 2 years, and influenza vaccine annually in symptomatic children (although the data supporting efficacy of the latter are lacking in this population). BCG is a subject of controversy: the WHO recommends that it should be given to asymptomatic children in areas of high prevalence. So far, there have been no reports of an upsurge in disseminated BCG in sub-Saharan Africa, but conversion rates to skin-test positivity are only 33–49%. In areas where measles outbreaks are frequent, antibody responses in HIV-infected children should be checked after MMR. If the response has been poor, a second MMR should be given. If the child fails to respond to a second dose, regular IVIG prophylaxis may be considered. Post exposure, normal human globulin (or IVIG) should be given to susceptible children.

Passive immunization is recommended for susceptible children with symptomatic HIV infection who are in contact with varicella zoster. Children receiving IVIG are considered susceptible if the last dose was greater than 2 weeks prior to exposure. Children with a documented past history of varicella or recurrent zoster need not be treated with varicella zoster immune globulin (VZIG). Administration of VZIG may prolong the incubation period to 28 days; therefore clinic visits should be postponed for this period.

Supportive therapy

Caring for a child with symptomatic HIV infection is a tremendous burden. In the context of perinatal transmission, this is compounded too frequently by illness in the parent, social isolation and feelings of guilt. An effective multidisciplinary team needs to find out what the major concerns are for each caregiver. These may be emotional, financial, legal, the need for more information about HIV, help in disclosing the diagnosis to the child, support regarding who else to tell, treatment issues for themselves or help with substance abuse problems. Appropriate community-based supportive services should be involved, always respecting the family's wishes regarding confidentiality. Families need active support and encouragement to maintain children in full-time normal education, as far as possible. There is no mandatory requirement in most countries to inform schools, but it is in the child's best interest if parents can at least let the head teacher or class teacher know.

Medical supportive care includes teaching parents to be alert for subtle signs of new illness and to seek help promptly. Fevers need to be evaluated carefully, with early intervention for treatable bacterial or opportunistic infections. Early nutritional intervention has been discussed above. Dental health and mouth care should be checked regularly.

Creative and aggressive attention to pain management is important. Pain is frequently associated with procedures, but also arises, for example, from infectious complications, side-effects of drugs, or from spasticity associated with central nervous system involvement. Palliative modes of care can begin to be introduced alongside active treatment, as end stages of disease become apparent. Always the child's quality of life must be carefully considered.

THE FUTURE

Numerous refinements of existing antiretroviral therapies in various combinations can be expected over the next few years. The role of new therapeutic strategies, in particular the use of immunomodulating therapies, and of gene therapy approaches which were beyond the scope of this review, will be investigated.

In the absence of a cure for infected individuals, prevention is of paramount importance. For perinatally acquired disease, lowering of transmission rates is now possible. Coordinated, family-based care with detection of infected mothers antenatally and appropriate intervention offers the only immediate hope of substantially reducing new cases in children.

REFERENCES

1 Quinn T. Population migration and the spread of types 1 and 2 human immunodeficiency viruses. Proc Natl Acad Sci USA 1994; 91: 2407–2414.
2 The European Collaborative Study. Risk factors for mother-to-child transmission of HIV-1. Lancet 1992; 339: 1007–1012.
3 Blanche S, Rouzioux C, Guihard Moscato M-L et al. A prospective study of infants born to women seropositive for human immunodeficiency virus type 1. N Engl J Med 1989; 320: 1643–1648.
4 Ryder R W, Nsa W, Hassig S E et al. Perinatal transmission of the human immunodeficiency virus type 1 to infants of seropositive women in Zaire. N Engl J Med 1989; 320: 1637–1642.
5 Lallemant M, Baillou A, Lallement-Coeur S et al. Maternal antibody response at delivery and perinatal transmission of human immunodeficiency virus type 1 in African women. Lancet 1994; 343: 1001–1005.
6 Gutman L T, St Claire K K, Weedy C et al. Human immunodeficiency virus transmission by child sexual abuse. AJDC 1991; 145: 137–141.
7 Friedland G H, Saltzman B R, Rogers M F et al. Lack of transmission of HTLV-III/LAV infection to household contacts of patients with AIDS or AIDS-related complex with oral candidiasis. N Engl J Med 1986; 314: 344–339.
8 Mann J M, Quinn T C, Francis H et al. Prevalence of HTLV-III/LAV in household contacts of patients with confirmed AIDS and controls in Kinshasa, Zaire. JAMA 1986; 256: 721–724.
9 Simonds R, Chanock S. Medical issues related to caring for human immunodeficiency virus-infected children in and out of the home. Pediatr Infect Dis J 1993; 12: 845–852.
10 Fitzgibbon J, Gaur S, Frenkel L, Laraque F, Edlin B, Dubin D. Transmission from one child to another of human immunodeficiency virus type 1 with a zidovudine-resistance mutation. N Engl J Med 1993; 329: 1835–1841.
11 Rogers M, White C, Sanders R et al. Lack of transmission of human immunodeficiency virus from infected children to their household contacts. Pediatrics 1990; 85: 210–214.
12 Dalgleish A, Beverley P, Clapham P, Crawford D, Greaves M, Weiss R. The CD4 (T4) antigen is an essential component of the receptor for the AIDS virus. Nature 1984; 312: 763–767.
13 Stein B, Gowda S, Lifson J, Penhallow R, Bensch K, Engleman E. pH-independent HIV entry into CD4-positive cells via virus envelope fusion to the plasma membrane. Cell 1987; 49: 659–668.

14 Dimitrov D, Golding H, Blumenthal R. Initial steps in HIV-1 envelope glycoprotein mediated cell fusion monitored by a new assay based on redistribution of fluorescence markers. AIDS Res Human Retroviruses 1991; 7: 799–805.

15 Meyerhans A, Cheynier R, Albert J et al. Temporal fluctuations in HIV quasispecies in vivo are not reflected by sequential HIV isolations. Cell 1989; 58: 901–910.

16 Finkel T, Tudor-Williams G, Banda N et al. Apoptosis occurs predominantly in bystander cells and not in productively infected cells of HIV- and SIV-infected lymph nodes. Nature Med 1995; 1: 129–134.

17 DeRossi A, Ometto L, Mammano F et al. Time course of antigenemia and seroconversion in infants with vertically acquired HIV-1 infection. AIDS 1993; 7: 1528–1529.

18 Byers B, Caldwell B, Oxytoby M. Pediatric Spectrum of Disease Project. Survival of children with perinatal HIV-infection: evidence for two distinct populations. Ninth International Conference on AIDS, Berlin, Germany, 1993: 91 (abstract WS-C10-6).

19 Bryson Y, Pang S, Wei L, Dickover R, Diagne A, Chen I. Clearance of HIV infection in a perinatally infected infant. N Engl J Med 1995; 332: 833–838.

20 Coffin J. HIV population dynamics in vivo: implications for genetic variation, pathogenesis, and therapy. Science 1995; 267: 483–489.

21 Blanche S, Mayaux M J, Rouzioux C et al. Relation of the course of HIV infection in children to the severity of the disease in their mothers at delivery. N Engl J Med 1994; 330: 308–312.

22 Nair P, Alger L, Hines S, et al. Maternal and neonatal characteristics associated with HIV infections in infants of seropositive women. J of AIDS 1993; 6: 298–302.

23 Scarlatti G, Leitner T, Hodara V et al. Neutralizing antibodies and viral characteristics in mother-to-child transmission of HIV-1. AIDS 1993; 7: S45–S48.

24 Duliege A-M, Amos C, Felton S et al. Birth order, delivery route, and concordance in the transmission of human immunodeficiency virus type 1 from mothers to twins. J Pediatr 1995; 126: 625–632.

25 Dunn D, Newell M, Mayaux M et al. Mode of delivery and vertical transmission of HIV-1: a review of prospective studies. J Acquir Immune Defic Syndr 1994; 7: 1064–1066.

26 Connor E, Sperling R, Gelber R et al. Reduction of maternal–infant transmission of human immunodeficiency virus type 1 with zidovudine treatment. N Engl J Med 1994; 331: 1173–1180.

27 Dunn D, Newell M, Ades E, Peckham C. Risk of human immunodeficiency virus type 1 transmission through breastfeeding. Lancet 1992; 340: 585–588.

28 Lederman S. Estimating infant mortality from human immunodeficiency virus and other causes in breast-feeding and bottle-feeding populations. Pediatrics 1992; 89: 290–296.

29 World Health Organization. Consensus statement from the WHO/Unicef consultation on HIV transmission and breast-feeding. Wkly Epidemiol Rec 1992; 67: 177–179.

30 Miles S, Balden E, Magpantay L et al. Rapid serologic testing with immune-complex-dissociated HIV p24 antigen for early detection of HIV infection in neonates. N Engl J Med 1993; 328: 297–302.

31 Bryson Y, Luzuriaga K, Sullivan J, Wara D. Proposed definition for in utero versus intrapartum transmission of HIV-1. N Engl J Med 1992; 327: 1246–1247.

32 Kline M, Hollinger F, Rosenblatt H, Bohannon B, Kozinetz C, Shearer W. Sensitivity, specificity and predictive value of physical examination, culture and other laboratory studies in the diagnosis during early infancy of vertically acquired human immunodeficiency virus infection. Pediatr Infect Dis J 1993; 12: 33–36.

33 The European Collaborative Study. Children born to women with HIV-1 infection: natural history and risk of transmission. Lancet 1991; 337: 253–260.

34 Centers for Disease Control. 1994 revised classification system for human immunodeficiency virus infection in children less than 13 years of age. MMWR 1994; 43 (No. RR-12): 1–10.

35 Belec L, Mbopi Keou F, Georges A. A case for the revision of the WHO clinical definition for African AIDS. AIDS 1992; 6: 880–881.

36 Centers for Disease Control. 1993 revised classification system for HIV infection and expanded surveillance case definition for AIDS among adolescents and adults. MMWR 1993; 41: 1–19.

37 Connor E, Bagarazzi M, McSherry G et al. Clinical and laboratory correlates of Pneumocystis carinii pneumonia in children infected with HIV. JAMA 1991; 265: 1693-1697.

38 Ognibene F P, Gill V J, Pizzo P A et al. Induced sputum to diagnose Pneumocystis carinii pneumonia in immunosuppressed pediatric patients. J Pediatr 1989; 115: 430–433.

39 The National Institutes of Health — University of California Expert Panel for Corticosteroids as Adjunctive Therapy for Pneumocystis Pneumonia. Consensus statement on the use of corticosteroids as adjunctive therapy for pneumocystis pneumonia in the acquired immunodeficiency syndrome. N Engl J Med 1990; 323: 1500–1504.

40. Connor E, Marquis J, Oleske J. Lymphoid interstitial pneumonitis. In: Pizzo P, Wilfert C, eds. The challenge of HIV infection in infants, children, and adolescents. Baltimore: Williams & Wilkins, 1991: 343–354.

41 Andiman W A, Martin K, Rubinstein A et al. Opportunistic lymphoproliferations associated with Epstein–Barr viral DNA in infants and children with AIDS. Lancet 1985; 2: 1390–1393.

42 Belman A L. Acquired immunodeficiency syndrome and the child's central nervous system. Pediatr Clin North Am 1992; 39: 691–714.

43 Khouri Y F, Mastrucci M T, Hutto C, Mitchell C D, Scott G B. Mycobacterium tuberculosis in children with human immunodeficiency virus type 1 infection. Pediatr Infect Dis J 1992; 11: 950–955.

44 Abadco D L, Steiner P. Gastric lavage is better than bronchoalveolar lavage for isolation of Mycobacterium tuberculosis in childhood pulmonary tuberculosis. Pediatr Infect Dis J 1992; 11: 735–738.

45 Centers for Disease Control. Initial therapy for tuberculosis in the era of multidrug resistance. Recommendations of the Advisory Council for the Elimination of Tuberculosis. MMWR 1993; 42: 1–8.

46 Lewis L L, Butler K M, Husson R N et al. Defining the population of human immunodeficiency virus-infected children at risk for Mycobacterium avium-intracellulare infection. J Pediatr 1992; 121: 677–683.

47 Jura E, Chadwick E G, Josephs S H et al. Varicella-zoster virus infections in children infected with human immunodeficiency virus. Pediatr Infect Dis J 1989; 8: 586–590.

48 Pahwa S, Biron K, Lim W et al. Continuous varicella-zoster infection associated with acyclovir resistance in a child with AIDS. JAMA 1988; 260: 2879–2882.

49 Hanson I, Kaplan S. Opportunistic infections. Semin Pediatr Infect Dis 1990; 1: 31–39.

50 Butler K M, De Smet M D, R.N. H et al. Treatment of aggressive cytomegalovirus retinitis with ganciclovir in combination with foscarnet in a child infected with human immunodeficiency virus. J Pediatr 1992; 120: 483–486.

51 Working Group on Antiretroviral Therapy: National Pediatric HIV Resource Center. Antiretroviral therapy and medical management of the human immunodeficiency virus-infected child. Pediatr Infect Dis J 1993; 12: 513–522.

52 Miller T L, Winter H S, Luginbuhl L M, Orav E J, McIntosh K. Pancreatitis in pediatric human immunodeficiency virus infection. J Pediatr 1992; 120: 223–227.

53 Butler K M, Venzon D, Henry N et al. Pancreatitis in human immunodeficiency virus-infected children receiving dideoxyinosine. Pediatrics 1993; 91: 747–751.

54 Mueller B U, Butler K M, Feuerstein I M et al. Smooth muscle tumors in children with human immunodeficiency virus infection. Pediatrics 1992; 90: 460–463.

55 Pizzo P A, Eddy J, Falloon J et al. Effect of continuous intravenous infusion of zidovudine (AZT) in children with symptomatic HIV infection. N Engl J Med 1988; 319: 889–896.

56 McKinney R E, Maha M A, Connor E M et al. A multicenter trial of oral zidovudine in children with advanced human immunodeficiency virus disease. N Engl J Med 1991; 324: 1018–1025.

57 Mueller B, Butler K, Stocker V et al. Clinical and pharmacokinetic evaluation of long-term therapy with didanosine in children with HIV infection. Pediatrics 1994; 94: 724–731.

58 Mueller B U, Jacobsen F, Butler K M, Husson R N, Lewis L L, Pizzo P A. Combination treatment with azidothymidine and granulocyte colony-stimulating factor in children with human immunodeficiency virus infection. J Pediatr 1992; 121: 797–802.

59 Mofenson L M, Moye J J, Bethel J, Hirschhorn R, Jordan C, Nugent R. Prophylactic intravenous immunoglobulin in HIV-infected children with CD4+ counts of $0.20 \times 10^9/L$ or more. Effect on viral, opportunistic, and bacterial infections. The National Institute of Child Health and Human Development Intravenous Immunoglobulin Clinical Trial Study Group. JAMA 1992; 268: 483–488.

60 Mofenson L M, Bethel J, Moye J J, Flyer P, Nugent R. Effect of intravenous immunoglobulin (IVIG) on CD4+ lymphocyte decline in HIV-infected children in a clinical trial of IVIG infection prophylaxis. The National Institute of Child Health and Human Development Intravenous Immunoglobulin Clinical Trial Study Group. J Acquir Immune Defic Syndr 1993; 6: 1103–1113.

CHAPTER 16

RECURRENT INFECTIONS

16.1. The child with recurrent infection

E. G. Davies   M. Sharland

16.1 The child with recurrent infection

INTRODUCTION

Immaturities in immune responsiveness and a limited repertoire of prior immunological experience combine to make childhood a time of frequent infections. This is particularly so in the first 4–5 years. The first and most important question when confronting the clinical problem of the child with recurrent infections is whether or not the nature, severity or frequency of the infections lie outside the boundaries of what one would expect as part of this immunodeficiency of immaturity. In other words, should the child be investigated? If the answer is yes then secondary questions will involve deciding on whether immunological or non-immunological factors are involved and, if the former, whether primary or secondary.

WHEN TO INVESTIGATE

The clinical approach should involve a careful history, noting numbers and types of infections, causative organisms, associated problems and a family history. Examination should include growth assessment, respiratory and ear, nose and throat (ENT) systems, a check for palpable lymphoid tissue and a check for possible syndromal associations.

The 'normal' childhood susceptibility to infections usually manifests as relatively mild respiratory illnesses[1] which are mostly of viral aetiology.[2] The frequency of such illnesses will depend on social factors such as number of siblings, attendance at school/nursery, and living conditions (e.g. overcrowding).[3] Their severity will be influenced by such factors as atmospheric pollution (including parental smoking) and the presence of a tendency to suffer virus-induced wheeze/asthma.

Bacterial complications of viral upper respiratory infections such as otitis media or lower respiratory tract infections can occur in normal children but if these are frequent (more than two episodes per winter season) an immunity problem should be considered.

Complicating bacterial lower respiratory infections can sometimes be difficult to distinguish from asthma on history alone, but the presence of fever, toxic appearance or the absence of wheeze on auscultation are all helpful signs of infection. Serious invasive bacterial diseases including meningitis, septicaemia, cellulitis, osteomyelitis/septic arthritis and severe pneumonia do occur in normal children. Many of these illnesses have a peak age of incidence in early childhood when immune responses are immature. Nevertheless, more than one episode in any one child should prompt further investigation.

Children with recurrent or persistent diarrhoea are often referred for investigation. In the history, care should be taken to rule out benign non-infectious

Table 16.1.1   Age-related susceptibility to infections in the absence of immune deficiency

Infection	Age of excess susceptibility
Disseminated herpes simplex virus infection	0–1 month
Group B streptococcal meningitis	0–3 months
Invasive salmonellosis (non-typhoidal)	0–6 months
Invasive *Haemophilus influenzae* type b disease	0–48 months

Table 16.1.2   When to investigate

1. Family history of immunodeficiency or other disorder
2. Single infection with an unusual/opportunistic organism
3. Single infection which is atypically severe or occurs at an atypical age
4. Recurrent minor bacterial infections, e.g. otitis media (>2 per year)
5. More than one episode of serious bacterial infection
6. Recurrent infections associated with severe allergy/autoimmune disorder

causes such as toddler diarrhoea. Episodes of diarrhoea may be associated with recurrent infections elsewhere in the body or with any antibiotic treatment administered. Recurrent or persistent gastrointestinal infections, particularly if followed by food intolerance and associated with failure to thrive, may indicate a serious problem such as severe combined immunodeficiency.

Age may be an important determinant in the decision to investigate. Thus, superficial candidal infection of the mouth or nappy area is a common and sometimes recurrent problem in the neonatal period, but at other ages, in the absence of other risk factors such as poor hygiene or recent antibiotic treatment, may merit investigation. Table 16.1.1 lists some other examples where age is relevant to host susceptibility.

Finally, the type of organism causing infections may be a clue to an underlying problem. Single episodes of opportunist infections, such as *Pneumocystis carinii* pneumonia or disseminated atypical mycobacterial infection, are highly suggestive of an underlying immune deficiency.

Table 16.1.2 summarizes the important points in distinguishing immunological immaturity from genuine immunodeficiency states.

NON-IMMUNOLOGICAL CAUSES OF RECURRENT INFECTIONS

Many systemic disorders can lead to a generalized increased susceptibility to infection. These include renal, hepatic, gastrointestinal and cardiorespiratory disorders. The precise mechanisms involved are often poorly understood, but will involve secondary immune dysfunction related to poor nutrition, metabolic disturbance, debility and stress. In diabetes mellitus, an additional factor is the increased tissue glucose level which predisposes to bacterial and fungal infections, which may occur at a number of sites. Sometimes treatments for these conditions, for example with corticosteroids and other immunosuppressive drugs, will exacerbate the problems.

The number of anatomical sites involved in recurrent infection may be a clue to the nature of the underlying cause. While occasionally immunodeficiency an disorder may present with recurrent infections at a single site (notably the respiratory tract) such infections are more likely to be associated with a non-immunological problem. For example, a common cause of recurrent sepsis confined to the skin is colonization with a virulent staphylococcus (which may also

Table 16.1.3   Recurrent infection at single anatomical sites due to non-immunological conditions

Site	Underlying condition	Keys to diagnosis
Lungs	Cystic fibrosis	Sweat Na^+ or Cl^-
	Primary ciliary dyskinesia	Ciliary beat studies and electron microscopy
	Recurrent aspiration	History, CXR, milk scan
	Bronchopulmonary dysplasia	History, CXR
Ears	Adenoidal hypertrophy	ENT assessment
	Primary ciliary dyskinesia	As above
Throat	Chronically infected tonsils	Clinical examination
Meningitis	Defect of coverings of the central nervous system	Clinical examination MRI scan
Urinary tract	Urological problem such as reflux or urethral valves	Radiological studies (see Ch. 26)
Skin	Eczema	Clinical examination
	Colonization with virulent strain of *Staphylococcus aureus*	Swabs from patient and family

affect other family members). Other examples of such disorders are shown in Table 16.1.3. It should be noted that recurrent urinary tract infections in the absence of infections at other sites are virtually never associated with immunodeficiency .

IMMUNOLOGICAL CAUSES OF RECURRENT INFECTIONS

The need to manage patients in an immunocompromised state is becoming increasingly common in paediatric practice.

Secondary immunodeficiency may result from cytotoxic and immunosuppressive (including steroid) therapy as well as HIV infection. Splenectomized patients, as well as those with sickle cell disease, are suspectible to invasive bacterial infection, particularly with encapsulated bacteria such as *Streptococcus pneumoniae*. These organisms also cause problems in patients with secondary immunoglobulin deficiency complicating protein-losing states such as nephrotic syndrome and protein-losing enteropathy. In most cases the cause of secondary immunodeficiency will be apparent from the history. HIV infection needs to be considered early in those children from a high-risk background but also in other cases as a diagnosis to be excluded when no other explanation for repeated or unusual infections can be found.

Primary immunodeficiency states can be classified into those predominantly affecting phagocytic cells; those producing defective humoral immunity; or those producing combined cell-mediated and humoral deficiency. Pure cell-mediated deficiencies are very unusual because of the close interrelationship between T cell and B cell responses — the nearest example is Di George syndrome. Other overlapping conditions affecting phagocytic and lymphocytic systems also occur.[4] Some disorders are part of syndromes which may be diagnosable from features other than the susceptibility to infection. Table 16.1.4 lists some of the more important primary immune deficiency states.[5]

In general terms it is often possible to predict the type of immunodeficiency (and thus the tests required) from the spectrum of infections suffered. The high-

Table 16.1.4 Important primary immunodeficiency disorders

Disorder	Main mode of inheritance (if known)	Particular features	Important tests
Humoral			
Selective IgA deficiency		Respiratory/GI infections and other invasive bacterial infections	Serum immunoglobulins + IgG subclasses
IgG subclass deficiency			Response to pneumococcal vaccine + other vaccines
Deficiency anti-carbohydrate responses			Salivary IgA
Transient hypogammaglobulinaemia		Usually < 3 years	As above
Agammaglobulinaemia (Bruton)	XL	'Pure' antibody deficiency	Serum Igs, B cell numbers
Common variable immunodeficiency (late onset hypogammaglobulinaemia)		Opportunistic infections as well as common bacterial infections Arthritis Autoimmune disorders	Serum Igs + IgG subclasses Response to vaccines Lymphocyte numbers and function
Hyper IgM syndrome	XL	Opportunistic infections	Serum Igs Lymphocyte function
Complement defects	Most AR	Bacterial infections, esp. meningococcal Autoimmune disorders.	Total haemolytic complement
Combined deficiencies			
SCID due to reticular dysgenesis	XL	Bacterial/fungal infections. Opportunistic infections. Chronic diarrhoea Failure to thrive.	Serum Igs Lymphocyte numbers and function Specific metabolite assays (ADA, PNP)
X-linked SCID	XL		
Autosomal SCID	AR		
Adenosine deaminase deficiency	AR		
Purine nucleoside phosphorylase deficiency	AR		
X-linked lymphoproliferative disorder	XL	Well until contract EB virus infection Then progressive combined immunodeficiency	EBV serology in patient (and mother). Demonstration of EBV genome in patient. Serum Igs, subclasses Lymphocyte function.
Syndromal			
Ataxia telangiectasia	AR	Ataxia usually by 2nd year Telangiectases usually appear after 3–4 years Bacterial and viral infections, malignancy	α-Fetoprotein DNA radiosensitivity
Wiskott Aldrich	XL	Bleeding Bacterial infections Malignancy	Platelet morphology Serum Igs Lymphocyte numbers and function
Chediak Higashi	AR	Partial oculocutaneous albinism Bacterial infections Lymphoproliferative disorders	FBC, white cell morphology.
Di George syndrome (Shprintzen's syndrome, velocardiofacial syndrome)	?	Cardiac defect, hypocalcaemia, abnormal facies, infections	CXR, lymphocyte numbers and function DNA studies (deletion on chromosome 22)

Table 16.1.4 (*contd*)

Disorder	Main mode of inheritance (if known)	Particular features	Important test
Neutrophil			
Congenital neutropenia	AR	Bacterial and fungal infections	FBC and bone marrow
Cyclic neutropenia	AD	Intermittent infections, esp. gingivostomatitis	Repeated FBCs
Chronic granulomatous disease	XL	Pneumonias Deep abscesses	NBT test
Leucocyte adhesion molecule deficiency	AR	Delayed cord separation Bacterial, fungal, and viral infections	Specific leucocyte monoclonal antibody studies
Hyper IgE syndrome	AR	Skin infections. Cold abscesses Pneumonias and pneumatoceles	Serum IgE
Neutrophil chemotactic defects		Bacterial infection Delayed wound healing	Neutrophil chemotaxis

Key: AD = Autosomal Dominant; AR = Autosomal Recessive; XL = X-linked

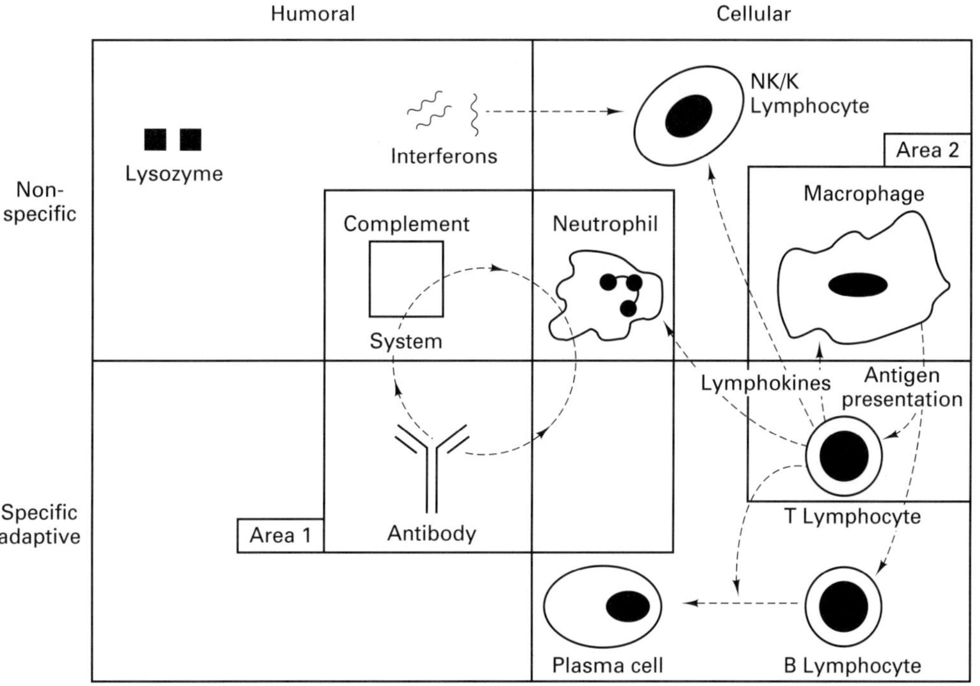

Fig. 16.1.1 Compartments of the immune system.

lighted areas in Figure 16.1.1 are useful in this respect. Area 1 comprises the triad of antibody, complement and neutrophil, which is particularly important in the handling of pyogenic bacteria. Deficiency in any of these components results in problems with this group of organisms though subtle differences in the particular types of bacteria occur, depending on which component is affected. Thus in

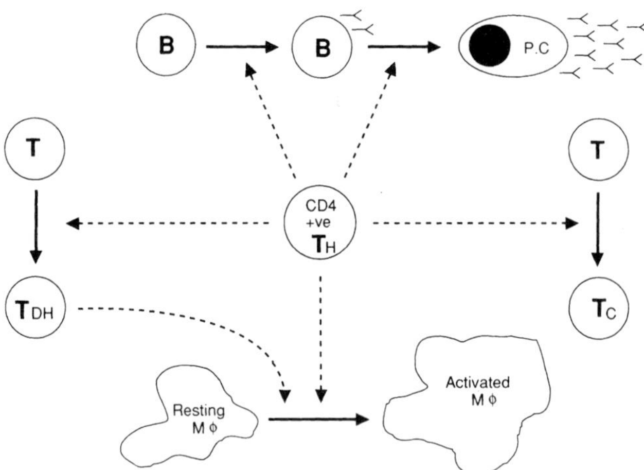

Fig. 16.1.2 Central role of CD4+ ve (helper) T cell in specific immune responses.

neutrophil disorders, staphylococcal infections predominate, with Gram-negative (including *Pseudomonas* and *Serratia* species) and fungal infections also occurring. In pure humoral deficiencies streptococcal, *Haemophilus* and *Moraxella* infections tend to predominate, while in late-component complement deficiencies the problems are restricted to the handling of neisserial species. An exception to the 'bacterial rule' for Area 1 disorders is that in pure antibody deficiency states there is an increased susceptibility to *Giardia lamblia* infection and to enteroviral infections, the latter sometimes running a chronic progressive course affecting nervous and muscular tissue. Children with predominantly antibody deficiency states, but with a cell-mediated component (hyper IgM syndrome, common variable immmunodeficiency) will have a wider range of susceptibilities.

Area 2 in Figure 16.1.1 comprises the cell-mediated immune system. Figure 16.1.2 shows the central role of the T cell and particularly the CD4-positive helper/inducer cell, and illustrates how defective function in this system can result in susceptibility to a wide range of microbes. Impairment of T cell regulation of B cell development and function results in poor antibody responses and thus a susceptibility to bacterial infection. Impaired generation and function of cytotoxic T cells (Tc) leads to problems in handling viruses and other intracellular pathogens. Failure of production of immunity-enhancing cytokines and generation of delayed hypersensitivity T cells (Tdh) results in failure of macrophage activation, with impaired killing of intracellular organisms such as mycobacteria and *Salmonella* species. Children with cell-mediated immunodeficiency will therefore suffer recurrent infections with a wide variety of common and opportunistic pathogens.

SPECIFIC DEFECTS OF IMMUNITY: HOW TO TEST FOR THEM

Though books outlining immunological tests in children are available,[6] complex and/or unusual tests are best performed after discussion with the laboratory.

Neutrophil tests

Full blood counts will reveal neutropenia which may be continuous or cyclical in nature. To diagnose the latter, a series of counts (twice weekly for up to 4 weeks) may be needed to detect the characteristic cycling of neutrophils, which occurs with a periodicity of around 21 days in cyclic neutropenia. Since this condition is often inherited as a dominant trait, performing counts on the parents may also be helpful. Non-cycling neutropenia may be due to either failure of production or excessive destruction. A bone marrow examination usually helps distinguish these.

Neutrophil function tests are performed when the clinical picture suggests neutrophil disorder but the total neutrophil count is not sufficiently low to explain the problems. A great variety of functional tests are available, many on a research basis. The important aspects of neutrophil activity to study when investigating recurrent infections are chemotaxis, phagocytosis and bacterial killing. Neutrophil chemotaxis is measured in the laboratory as the distance migrated by neutrophils (usually through a millipore filter) in response to a chemotactic stimulus in a given time when compared to controls. Unfortunately, test results are not always easily reproducible and the values obtained may vary considerably from assay to assay both for normals and patients. Defective chemotaxis is found in patients with Schwachmann's syndrome, in leucocyte adhesion molecule disorders and in the hyper IgE syndrome. It can also be found as an isolated finding in the absence of any other demonstrable abnormality.

Phagocytic defects can be measured directly by looking at the uptake of labelled opsonized particles or bacteria by neutrophils, either by direct counting under a microscopic or by a flow cytometric method. Primary defects of phagocytosis are unusual unless associated with cytoskeletal abnormalities in the neutrophil (as in Chediak–Higashi syndrome) but secondary abnormalities of phagocytosis may occur, for example, in stressed newborns.

Defects of bacterial killing are an important group of neutrophil disorders. The classical disorder resulting in this finding is chronic granulomatous disease (CGD), in which there is failure of the normal oxidative burst after phagocytosis. The typical clinical picture of a child with CGD is one of recurrent deep abscesses usually caused by staphylococci and/or fungi and there is often hepatospleno-megaly due to accumulation in the reticuloendothelial system of cellular debris which cannot be adequately digested. Bactericidal tests are the most direct means of assessing these disorders and involve measuring the killing of ingested organisms (usually staphylococci) by neutrophils. This is defective in CGD and also in other less well-defined neutrophil killing disorders, including those in which the NBT test (see below) is normal. The best screening test for CGD is the nitroblue tetrazolium (NBT) slide reduction test. In this test, incubation of neutrophils on a microscope slide with NBT should result in uptake of the NBT and its reduction in the phagolysosome to form a brown/black dense deposit in the cells. Using appropriate stimuli, almost all neutrophils on the slides should produce this reductive change, whereas in CGD none will do so. The test can also be used as a method of detecting carriers, in whom approximately 50% of the neutrophils (depending on ionization) reduce NBT. More sophisticated tests looking at the defect in the cytochrome system can then be undertaken for confirmation of the diagnosis.

A commonly used screening test for neutrophil function disorders is the mea-surement of luminol-enhanced chemiluminescence. A sensitive photomultiplier measures photons emitted during the oxidative burst that follows phagocytosis. This allows quantitative indirect assessment of the efficiency of phagocytosis and of the oxidative metabolism, which is most important in bacterial killing. Chemiluminescence is not generated by cells from patients with CGD.

Generalized disorders of immune function can present with staphylococcal infection producing a picture characteristic of neutrophil function disorder. Leucocyte adhesion molecule deficiency states[7] are disorders of expression of a related group of surface molecules on leucocytes which have a dimeric structure, including a common β subunit. These molecules include leucocyte function antigen 1 (LFA 1), and Mac 1 (the type 3 complement receptor, CR3). Deficiency is associated with profound defects of immune function, including neutrophil chemotaxis and phagocytosis as well as specific lymphocyte responses, especially cytotoxic mechanisms. In its severe form this condition leads to susceptibility to a wide variety of pathogens, but it often presents initially with pyogenic bacterial infections associated with the neutrophil dysfunction component. Characteristically there is also a history of delayed separation of the umbilical cord. A moderate form associated with some expression of the molecules has also been described. Diagnosis of this condition can be made by demonstrating the absence of surface markers on lymphocytes and neutrophils using monoclonal antibodies against the relevant surface antigens (CD11 and CD18).

In hyper IgE syndrome (Job's syndrome)[8] there is a marked susceptibility to bacterial infections, particularly staphylococci, resulting in 'cold' abscesses, and pneumonias leading to pneumatocele formation. It has been postulated[9] that the basic defect is a T cell-regulatory defect resulting in imbalance in the cytokines controlling B cell function, which drives the immune system to produce excessive amounts of IgE. This is associated with failure of neutrophil function, especially chemotaxis. The best way of diagnosing this problem is to measure the circulating IgE level, which is often extremely high (>2000 IU/L in under-5-year-olds or >5000 IU/L in over-5-year-olds).

Complement tests

Complement deficiencies are relatively rare.[10] They are associated with a tendency to autoimmune disorders such as systemic lupus erythematosus or other unusual disorders and also with a tendency to bacterial infections. The central component in the complement system is C3; its cleavage product C3bi is deposited on the bacterial surface and acts as a powerful opsonin. Congenital deficiencies of C3 have been described but, more commonly, persistently low C3 levels are due to secondary (consumptive) deficiency associated with autoimmune disease. The result is a marked tendency to pyogenic bacterial infection with a wide variety of organisms, including staphylococci and encapsulated bacteria.

C3 is cleaved either through alternate-pathway antibody-independent activation or by the antibody-dependent classical pathway involving factors C1, 4 and 2. Defects of alternate pathway factors result in recurrent infections and their elucidation requires the involvement of a specialist laboratory to measure the individual factors. Defects in the early classical pathway factors result in a tendency to relatively minor bacterial infections in early childhood. Often this susceptibility does not persist into adulthood, though a marked susceptibility to autoimmune disease does.

Deficiencies in the later complement components, C5 to C9, result in defective handling of infection with neisserial species, notably meningococcus and gonococcus. Typically, these patients get recurrent meningococcal infection and any child with more than one episode should be investigated. Defects when found usually involve congenital deficiency of a single factor which breaks the cascade. The screening test for complement deficiencies from C1 to C9 is the total haemolytic complement test (CH50); which involves measuring lysis of antibody-coated sheep red cells in the presence of test serum as a source of complement. If lysis fails to occur, a factor is missing in the cascade and then further, more sophisticated tests of individual components are required. Deficiencies are more common in certain parts of the world, notably Japan and the Middle East. It is not generally considered worth investigating children after single episodes of meningococcal disease.

Antibody tests

Antibody is an important factor in the opsonization of bacteria. Deficiency states most commonly present with bacterial infections of the upper and lower respiratory tract. Measurement of immunoglobulin levels is generally straightforward and available in most laboratories. If deficiency is suspected then not only should the major classes of IgG, IgA and IgM be measured but also IgG subclass levels. Care is needed in the interpretation of levels, which are highly age dependent, and laboratories regularly measuring paediatric samples should quote age-related normal ranges.

Major deficiencies in the main immunoglobulin classes are therefore relatively easily diagnosed. When low levels of IgG occur, consideration should be given to whether this might be secondary through protein loss, but otherwise it will be due to a failure of production. Transient hypogammaglobulinaemia may produce remarkably low levels in the first few years of life. Otherwise very low levels indicate one of the major primary deficiency states: Bruton's X-linked agammaglobulinaemia (XLA), common variable hypogammaglobulinaemia or immunoglobulin deficiency with hyper IgM. Circulating B cells are absent or only present in very low numbers in XLA and so their enumeration may be helpful in confirming the diagnosis. The genes for both XLA and hyper IgM syndrome have been identified and so genetic confirmation of the diagnosis can be achieved. Less profound immunoglobulin deficiency states are more common than the major disorders. Selective IgA deficiency is the most common. This may be associated with disturbances of IgG subclass levels, especially deficiency of IgG_2. Both IgA and IgG_2 subclass deficiency may be either partial or complete. Partial deficiencies are often transient, being present only over the first few years of life but nevertheless associated with considerable morbidity. Complete deficiencies are more likely to be permanent. It has become increasingly apparent in recent years that in children with minor immunoglobulin disturbances there is a poor correlation between susceptibility to infection and the actual levels of immunoglobulins and subclasses. Tests of functional antibody are more predictive.[11] These include measurements of IgM, and of isohaemagglutinin antibodies against the major blood group antigens (which should be present from about 9 months of age in all except blood group AB individuals). Antibody responses can also be measured to common vaccine antigens such as tetanus toxoid, *Haemophilus influenzae* type b antigen and polio virus. The most discriminating tests have been found to be those looking at anti-carbohydrate antibodies, usually those against pneumococcal polysaccharides.[12] This can be done before and after challenge with pneumococcal polysaccharide vaccine (e.g. Pneumovax). Using these techniques it can be shown that a small number of individuals may have recurrent bacterial infections due to antibody deficiency but with normal immunoglobulin levels. Conversely, some children with deficiencies in IgG subclasses may produce normal antibody responses. These functional antibody tests should therefore be used routinely as part of the assessment of humoral immunity in children with recurrent infections. It should, however, be remembered that children under 2 years of age do not respond reliably to pure polysaccharide antigens, such as Pneumovax, and care is therefore needed in interpreting results below this age.

Tests of cell-mediated immunity

The simplest and sometimes most revealing test of cell-mediated immunity in severe forms of combined immunodeficiency is the differential white blood cell count. A majority of children with severe combined immunodeficiency disease (SCID) are lymphopenic, with counts persistently below $2.8 \times 10^9/L$ and often much more profoundly depressed.[13] Chest radiograph may also be helpful, revealing an absence of the normal thymic shadow in the major disorders affecting T cell ontogeny.

Further enumeration of lymphocyte subsets reveals total T cell numbers and the functional subsets using monoclonal antibodies against surface antigens. This is usually done automatically by a fluorescent cell sorter which counts the cells stained with fluorescent antibody and relates it to the size of the cells. In most cases of SCID, circulating cells bearing any of the common T cell markers are present only in very low numbers or absent. In SCID, marker analysis shows one of two patterns: either B cells are present (often in high numbers) in so-called B-SCID or they are absent. The former type is usually inherited in X-linked fashion, the latter as an autosomal recessive disorder. In partial deficiency states T cells may be present in normal or low numbers and interpretation of the results may be difficult. Functional studies of cell-mediated immunity are important in diagnosing those disorders in which T cells are present but non-functional. The most commonly used test is the PHA (phytohaemagglutinin) response, in which lymphocytes are stimulated with this T cell-specific mitogen and the response measured as uptake of [^{3}H]thymidine. Other mitogens or antigens can be used in a similar way, the latter being more useful in more subtle (partial) deficiency states. 'In vivo' tests of cell-mediated immunity can also be used, usually by injecting small quantities of common antigens to which the child is very likely to have been exposed (such as candida, streptococcal, tetanus toxoid) by the intradermal route and looking for a delayed hypersensitivity reaction. Pre-prepared multi-antigen kits are available for this purpose.

Tests for syndromes which include immunodeficiency

A number of immunodeficiencies are associated with syndromes (Table 16.1.4). In these cases specific diagnostic tests, either genetic, biochemical or haematological, may be available. This does not preclude the need for immune function testing since the immunodeficiency component of some of these syndromes is variably expressed (e.g. in ataxia telangiectasia) and management will depend on identifying its presence and severity.

PREVENTION OF INFECTIONS IN IMMUNODEFICIENCY STATES

General

Cases of major immunodeficiency should ideally be managed under the supervision of a specialist centre. A balance needs to be struck between exposure to potentially serious infections and allowing the child to follow as normal a lifestyle as possible. The position of this balance will depend on the severity of the condition. Thus in SCID, children should normally be kept in protective isolation facilities until definitive treatment such as bone marrow transplantation can be undertaken. In other cases, prophylaxis with antibiotics and/or immunoglobulin often allows unrestricted activity. Immunization with 'live' vaccines is contraindicated in those with a cell-mediated component to their deficiency and in major antibody deficiency states but not in the other disorders.

Particular care is needed in preventing the development of chickenpox and measles in children with compromised cell-mediated immunity. Postexposure prophylaxis with immunoglobulin is indicated and early hospitalization and aggressive treatment should these diseases develop.

Antimicrobial prophylaxis

Penicillin prophylaxis is used in sickle cell disorders and protein-losing states to prevent pneumococcal disease and in complement deficiencies to prevent meningococcal disease. For antibody deficiency states not severe enough to require immunoglobulin replacement, daily co-trimoxazole remains the treatment of choice, in a dose of 12mg/kg per day in one or two doses. This is also used for neutrophil disorders such as chronic granulomatous disease. For other neutrophil disorders flucloxacillin is effective. Antifungal treatment in the form of non-absorbable agents should be used for patients with neutrophil or cell-mediated disorders. The use of systemic antifungals such as flucanozole or the broader-spectrum itraconazole is still under evaluation. In cell-mediated deficiency states prophylaxis against *Pneumocystis carinii* is vital. Co-trimoxazole is the agent of choice and although used thrice weekly in other circumstances it is generally used daily in primary immunodeficiency disorders because these children also need protection against bacterial infections. Acyclovir can also be used prophylactically, but only in those with the most severe deficiencies or in individuals with a previous history of herpetic disease.

Intravenous immunoglobulin (IVIG)

This should only be used in cases where failure of antibody production has been demonstrated. In such cases the benefits are great and fully justify the high cost and disruption to the child's life.

Normally between 200 and 500 mg/kg weight is administered 2–4 weekly with the aim of keeping the trough IgG level in the mid–normal age-related range. Recently, there have been major advances in facilitating home therapy with IVIG or using subcutaneous infusion of immunoglobulins.

Care should be taken in giving IVIG to children with complete IgA deficiency since anaphylaxis can occur, triggered by the small amounts of IgA present in most IVIG preparations.

Cytokines

Potential new therapies for immunodeficiency have emerged with the generation of recombinant forms of cytokines and growth factors. In many instances their role has not been fully established. Recombinant human granulocyte colony-stimulating factor has been shown to be of benefit in congenital agranulocytosis,[14] while in chronic granulomatous disease interferon γ is of benefit to some patients.[15]

Therapies for correcting the disorder

Bone marrow transplantation, enzyme replacement (in adenosine deaminase-deficient SCID) and somatic gene therapy all offer the potential of cure for the more serious disorders.

REFERENCES

1 Rosenblatt R A, Cherlin D C, Schneeweiss R, Hart L G. The content of ambulatory medical care in the United States: an interspecialty comparison. N Engl J Med 1983; 309: 892.
2 Denny F W, Denny M D, Clyde W A Jr. Acute lower respiratory tract infections in nonhospitalized children. J Pediatr 1988; 108: 635–646.
3 Colley J R T. The epidemiology of respiratory tract infections in childhood. In: Recent advances in paediatrics 5. Edinburgh, Churchill Livingstone, 1976.
4 Davies E G. Immunodeficiency. In: McIntosh N, Campbell A, eds. Forfar & Arniel, Textbook of Paediatrics, 4th edn. Edinburgh: Churchill Livingstone, 1991.
5 Rosen F S, Wedgewood R J, Eibl M. Primary immunodeficiency diseases. Report of a World Health Organization Scientific Group. Clin Immunol Immunopathol 1986; 40: 166–196.

6 Watson J G, Bird A G. Handbook of immunological investigations in children. London: Wright, 1990.

7 Fischer A, Losowska-Grospierre B, Anderson D C et al. Leukocyte adhesion deficiency: molecular basis and functional consequences. Immunodef Rev 1988; 1: 39.

8 Davis S D, Schaller J, Wedgewood R J. Job's syndrome: recurrent 'cold' staphylococcal abscesses. Lancet 1966; i: 1013.

9 Hill H R. Modulation of host defences with interferon-γ in paediatrics. J Infect Dis 1993; 167 (Suppl 1): S23.

10 Hauptman G. Frequency of complement deficiencies in man, disease associations and chromosome assignment of complement genes and linkage groups: a summary of the data from the literature. Complement 1989; 6: 74.

11 Gross S, Blaiss M, Herrod G. Role of immunoglobulin subclasses and specific antibody determinations in the evaluation of recurrent infection in children. J Pediatr 1992; 121: 516.

12 Sanders L A M, Rijkers G T, Kuis W et al. Defective antipneumococcal polysaccharide antibody response in children with recurrent respiratory tract infections. J Allergy Clin Immunol 1993; 91: 110.

13 Hague R A, Rassam S, Morgan G, Cant A J. Early diagnosis of severe combined immunodeficiency syndrome. Arch Dis Child 1994; 70: 260.

14 Welte K, Zeidler C, Reiter A et al. Differential effects of granulocyte–macrophage and granulocyte colony stimulating factor in children with severe congenital neutropenia. Blood 1990; 75: 1056.

15 The International CGD Cooperative Study Group. A controlled trial of interferon gamma to prevent infection in chronic granulomatous disease. N Engl J Med 1991; 324: 509.

CHAPTER 17

IMMUNE COMPROMISE

17.1. Opportunistic infections in the immunocompromised

M. Sharland   E. G. Davies

17.1 Opportunistic infections in the immunocompromised

INTRODUCTION

A combination of therapeutic advances and changing disease prevalence (Table 17.1.1) has produced a marked increase in the numbers of children seen with significant immunocompromise.[1] The 10 general principles of caring for a child with immunocompromise are:

1. Minimal symptoms and signs are important.
2. All fevers must be fully evaluated.
3. Invasive investigations are often required.
4. Start empirical treatment early.
5. Modify empirical treatment if symptoms persist.
6. Consider opportunistic and rare organisms.
7. Remember resistant organisms.
8. Common infections may present in atypical forms.
9. Most infections are predictable and treatable.
10. Follow protocols.

With these principles in mind, knowledge of the underlying immune deficit does allow prediction of the commoner opportunistic infections, and guides initial management.

Table 17.1.1   Causes of increase in number of immunocompromised patients

Increased organ and bone marrow transplantation
Intensified chemotherapy in haematology/oncology
Increased prevalence of HIV infection
Wider therapeutic use of immunosuppressive drugs
Improved survival of children with congenital and acquired immunodeficiencies

PREDICTION OF INFECTION BY IMMUNE DEFECT

Neutrophil defects

- Neutropenia (below 1000/µl)
- Caused by cytotoxic chemotherapy
- Bacterial — Staphylococci, Gram negatives
- Fungal — *Candida, Aspergillus*

Neutrophil function defect

- Caused by congenital disorders
- Bacterial — *Staphylococcus* (skin/sinopulmonary)
- Gram negatives, mycobacteria
- Fungal — *Candida, Aspergillus*

Altered cell-mediated immunity (CMI)

- Caused by congenital immunodeficiencies, immunosuppressive drugs, radiation, malignancies, and HIV infection
- Bacterial — Gram-negative infections, mycobacteria, *Listeria*, *Nocardia*, *Legionella*, *Mycoplasma*
- Viral — herpes (CMV, EBV, HSV, VZV), respiratory (adeno, parainfluenza, RSV), and enteric (rota, adeno)
- Fungal — *Candida*, *Aspergillus*, *Cryptococcus*, *Pneumocystis*
- Protozoal — *Toxoplasma*, *Cryptosporidium*

Humoral and complement deficits

- Caused by congenital deficiency, BMT, HIV infection, asplenia, excess immunoglobulin losses (e.g. nephrotic syndrome)
- Bacterial — encapsulated organisms, Gram negatives, meningococcus and gonococcus (with terminal complement abnormalities)
- Viral — chronic CNS enterovirus (with X-linked agammaglobulinaemia)
- Fungal — *Pneumocystis*, *Aspergillus* (rare)

MANAGEMENT OF SPECIFIC CLINICAL PROBLEMS

Fever

Aetiology

Fever over 38°C is an extremely important sign in immunocompromised children, particularly those most at risk from septicaemia (children with neutropenia, HIV infection, and humoral deficits).

In neutropenic cancer patients, bacterial infections account for about three-quarters of all documented infections, although the fever may be unexplained in 60–70% of cases.[2] The depth and duration of neutropenia are very important, with neutropenia <100/µl or for longer than 7 days associated with more serious Gram-negative and fungal infections. There has been a shift towards Gram-positive infections in the last 20 years, probably associated with increasing use of central venous catheters (CVCs) and changing antibiotic policies.[3] The commonest Gram-positive organism isolated is the coagulase-negative *Staphylococcus epidermidis*, but *Staphylococcus aureus* and *Streptococcus* species are also seen. Aerobic Gram-negative infections, caused by *Pseudomonas aeruginosa*, *Klebsiella*, *Enterobacter* species and other Enterobacteriacae are of particular concern because of their association with the rapid onset of fulminant endotoxic shock.

Management

Examination of the febrile neutropenic child should particularly focus on the mouth (*Candida*/herpes), teeth (gingivitis), ears and sinuses (*Aspergillus*), the skin (ecthyma gangrenosum) and perineal region (anaerobes), the chest with early chest X-ray (CXR), and any central venous catheter (CVC) (exit site or tunnel infection).

Empiric broad-spectrum antibiotics should be started immediately after peripheral and central (if CVC present) blood cultures have been taken. Local policies vary, but the traditional combination is an antipseudomonal β-lactam (e.g. piperacillin, azlocillin) and an aminoglycoside (e.g. gentamicin, amikacin). Because of aminoglycoside toxicity, monotherapy with an antipseudomonal cephalosporin (e.g. ceftazidime) or a carbipenem (e.g. imipenem) is increasingly used.[2] Although *Staphylococcus epidermidis* is a common cause of bacteraemia, its relatively low pathogenicity allows time for appropriate antibiotics (e.g. vancomycin, teicoplanin) to be added after a positive culture result. Prolonged fever, the development of localized clinical disease, or identification of an organism often requires postempiric alteration of the antibiotic regime. The high risk of acute disseminated candidosis (fungaemia, with cutaneous lesions), chronic disseminated candidosis (hepatosplenic disease, with persistent fever), and sinopulmonary aspergillosis means that early empiric use of systemic antifungals (amphotericin B) is recommended (e.g. amphotericin B: test dose 0.1 mg/kg — maximum 1 mg initially, followed by 0.5–1 mg/kg per day; infuse as single dose over 4–6 h).[4]

In distinction to the febrile neutropenic cancer patient, children with impaired humoral immunity (e.g. HIV infection, nephrotic syndrome and sickle cell disease) have a high incidence of infection with encapsulated organisms (*Streptococcus pneumoniae*, *Haemophilus influenzae*). The same principles of early empiric treatment apply, due to the pathogenicity of these organisms. A broad-spectrum β-lactam (e.g. cefotaxime, ceftriaxone) is often used.[5]

Pulmonary infections

Aetiology

There is unfortunately a poor correlation between the clinical and radiological picture, and the pathological diagnosis in pneumonia in the immunocompromised child. Non-infectious processes also need to be considered. Likely infections can generally be predicted from appearances on CXR (Table 17.1.2), but considerable variation in presentation exists.

Pneumonia due to *Pneumocystis carinii* (PCP) needs to be considered in virtually all children with compromised cell-mediated immunity presenting with respiratory disease. Clinically the child may have a low-grade fever, cough and breathlessness. The onset is usually over a few days, but may be slower or more fulminant. The child is often hypoxic. Although diffuse patchy infiltrates are classically seen, the CXR may be normal, or demonstrate pneumatoceles.[6] In an infant the diagnosis may be made from a nasopharyngeal aspirate specimen, or from an induced sputum in some older children.[7] For children between these ages, specimens need to be obtained by bronchoscopy and bronchoalveolar lavage (BAL).[8] The diagnosis is usually confirmed by silver stain or immunofluorescence of lavage fluid for the cysts, although PCR is available in some centres. The treatment of PCP is with high-dose intravenous co-trimoxazole for 2–3 weeks (trimethoprim 20 mg — sulphamethoxazole 100 mg/kg per day oral/i.v. in three divided doses for 14–21 days) and methylprednisolone.

The role of CMV in lower respiratory disease varies with the type of immunocompromise. One to two months after bone marrow transplant (BMT) a severe pneumonitis due to CMV may develop, particularly if both recipient and donor are CMV IgG positive. Both the virus and an abnormal host response to the

Table 17.1.2 Typical radiological appearances of opportunistic infections

Diffuse/interstitial	Viral: CMV, adeno, parainfluenza, measles, RSV, VZV Parasitic: *Toxoplasma*, Bacterial: mycobacteria, *Legionella*, *Mycoplasma*, *Chlamydia*, *Nocardia* Fungal: Pneumocystis, *Aspergillus*, *Candida*, Zygomycetes
Localized/lobar	*S. pneumoniae*, Gram negatives, *H. influenzae*, *S. aureus* *Nocardia*, *M. tuberculosis*, *Legionella* *Aspergillus*
Nodules/abscesses	*Aspergillus* *Nocardia*

virus appear to be involved in the pathogenesis of this condition, with a high mortality.[9] In children with AIDS, lung disease may develop as part of disseminated CMV infection, usually in children with rapidly progressing disease. The virus is occasionally detected in BAL fluid from children with HIV and PCP, where it may not have a pathogenic role. CMV PCR may detect viraemia earlier than standard early antigen rapid tests.

Management

The general principles of treatment are to start empiric therapy early with broad-spectrum antibiotics, depending on the patient group and CXR appearances. An early decision should be made about bronchoscopy and BAL. In the ill child empiric therapy with intravenous co-trimoxazole and erythromycin/azithromycin should be considered, with the early use of amphotericin B. Lung biopsy should be undertaken if there is no clinical improvement on the above therapies.

Gastrointestinal infections

Aetiology

Oral mucositis may be due to either *Candida* or herpes simplex virus (HSV), while necrotizing gingivitis suggests anaerobic infection. Dysphagia and retrosternal pain due to oesophagitis can be caused by *Candida*, HSV or CMV, and may require endoscopic biopsy for confirmation. Abdominal pain, distension and occasionally bleeding may indicate necrotizing colitis (typhilitis) which occurs in neutropenic patients,[10] or CMV colitis in children with altered CMI. Persistent diarrhoea may be caused by a variety of organisms (Table 17.1.3). Perianal pain and localized tenderness can be caused by staphylococci, Gram negatives, anaerobes and enterococci. Perianal inflammation is a late sign.

Management

It is important to swab children with oral mucositis, and treat with an oral antifungal (e.g. amphotericin lozenges) or acyclovir if HSV is suspected. Persistent diarrhoea should be treated on the organism identified, and endoscopic biopsy may be required. Empiric courses of metronidazole for possible *Giardia* infections are often useful. Typhilitis can be managed with aggressive broad-spectrum antibiotic and supportive therapy, with occasional surgical intervention. Perirectal disease requires combination treatment (e.g. ceftazidime, vancomycin and metronidazole).

Table 17.1.3   Causes of diarrhoea in the immunosuppressed child

Viruses	Adenoviruses, rotavirus, CMV
Bacteria	*Campylobacter, Salmonella,* mycobacteria (tuberculosis and atypical)
Protozoa	Cryptosporidia, *Isospora, Giardia,* microsporidia
Toxins	*Clostridium difficile*

Neurological infections

Aetiology

Central nervous system infections are surprisingly rare in immunocompromised children. The signs are often subtle, with headache, altered level of consciousness and focal neurology the most important. A low threshold for cranial CT scan and lumbar puncture is required.

Meningitis in children with reduced CMI may be caused by *Cryptococcus neoformans,* a fungus that is blood-spread from a respiratory focus, and produces a mild CSF pleocytosis. Although Indian ink stains may be positive in over 50% of cases, a latex agglutination test is very reliable on CSF and plasma. *Listeria monocytogenes*, Gram negatives and *Candida* species also occur. The low CSF white count in neutropenic patients with meningitis needs to be remembered.

Encephalitis may be caused by enteroviral infections in children with X-linked agammaglobulinaemia. Herpes simplex, CMV and a subacute measles encephalitis are also more common in children with altered CMI. Focal lesions on cranial CT scan raise the possibility of toxoplasmosis, when the lesions are often ring shaped, found in the white matter, and usually enhance with contrast. Serology and magnetic resonance imaging can help in diagnosis, but differentiation from other pathology (e.g. lymphoma) may require a brain biopsy, if there is no improvement following empiric treatment. *Aspergillus* CNS infections may spread from frontal sinuses. The CT scan appearances may be focal or diffuse, and serology and CSF cultures are often not helpful. *Nocardia asteroides* may also present with focal CNS lesions.

Management

Cryptococcal infection requires prolonged combination therapy with amphotericin B, and 5-flucytosine, with fluconazole maintenance therapy. Third-generation cephalosporins are not suitable for *Listeria* infections, which respond to ampicillin and an aminoglycoside. In children with a diffuse encephalitis, herpes simplex polymerase chain reaction (PCR) of the CSF is useful, and early empiric therapy with acyclovir and amphotericin B should be considered. Focal lesions are often empirically treated with a trial of pyramethamine and sulphadiazine for toxoplasmosis.

Skin disease

Aetiology

Disseminated *Pseudomonas* infection produces a necrotic rash (ecthyma gangrenosum) in severely neutropenic patients. The most important rash in immunosuppressed children is caused by either varicella zoster or herpes simplex. Chickenpox can be lethal in any child with reduced CMI. The risk is particularly high if the absolute lymphocyte count is $< 500/\mu l$.[11] Visceral dissemination with pneumonitis, hepatitis and encephalitis occurs. Death is due to respiratory failure and secondary infections. Herpes zoster is usually more severe in immunosuppressed children, but systemic spread is rare. Disseminated herpes simplex virus infection is rare, but can occur from an untreated primary lesion. In children with reduced CMI, superficial chronic fungal infections and molluscum contagiosum can be persistent, and difficult to treat.

Management

All children at risk should be identified, and treated with varicella zoster immunoglobulin (VZIG) within 3–5 days of a chickenpox contact. If a rash appears, intravenous acyclovir in a dose of 1500 mg/m² per day should be given. Primary herpes simplex virus lesions should be rapidly diagnosed by culture, electron microscopy or immunofluorescence. Oral acyclovir is often successful, but failure of oral therapy should prompt the early use of intravenous acyclovir.

PREVENTION OF INFECTIONS

Prevention of serious infections begins with education of the child and their family about immunocompromise. This includes advice about the importance of fever, minor symptoms, chickenpox and measles contacts, and immunizations.

Table 17.1.4 Possible disease prevention strategies

Infection	Prevention
Influenza	Influenza vaccine
Pneumococcal disease	Pneumococcal vaccine
	Oral penicillin
Oral herpes simplex	Oral acyclovir
Pneumocystis carinii	Co-trimoxazole/dapsone
	Pentamidine
Oral *Candida*	Oral antifungals
Neutropenic septicaemia	Oral antibiotics
Systemic fungal disease	Prophylactic fluconazole/amphotericin
Disseminated CMV	Ganciclovir
Varicella zoster/measles	Postexposure immunoglobulin

Rapid access to specialist advice needs to be available. In severely immuno-suppressed children (e.g. post-BMT), nosocomial infections may be acquired from food (Gram negatives), water (*Pseudomonas*) and air (*Aspergillus*). Bone marrow transplantation is therefore usually carried out with protective isolation by high-efficiency particulate air (HEPA) filtration, reverse barrier nursing, and specialist advice for a clean diet and water supply. Other preventive measures that may be considered are listed in Table 17.1.4.

Early use of empiric therapy, combined with improved methods of diagnosing opportunistic infections has led to an improved outcome for the immuno-suppressed child. As increasing numbers of affected children are living longer, the development of microbial drug resistance will produce major challenges.

REFERENCES

1 Davies E G. Immunodeficiency. In: Campbell A G M, McIntosh N, eds. Forfar and Arneil's textbook of paediatrics, 4th edn. Edinburgh: Churchill Livingstone, 1992: pp 1299–1330.
2 Pizzo P A, Hathorn J W, Hiemenz J W et al. A randomised trial comparing ceftazidime alone with combination antibiotic therapy in cancer patients with fever and neutropenia. N Engl J Med 1986; 315: 552–558.
3 Weinberger M, Pizzo P A. The evaluation and management of neutropenic patients with unexplained fever. In: Patrick C C, ed. Infections in immunocompromised infants and children, 1st edn. Edinburgh: Churchill Livingstone, 1992: pp 335–356.
4 EORTC International antimicrobial therapy cooperative group. Empirical antifungal therapy in febrile neutropenic patients. Am J Med 1989; 86: 668–672.
5 The National Institute of Child Health and Human Development Intravenous Immunoglobulin Study Group. Intravenous immunoglobulin for the prevention of bacterial infections in children with symptomatic HIV infection. N Engl J Med 1991; 325: 73–80.
6 Berdon W E, Mellins R B, Abramson S J. Pediatric HIV infection in its second decade: the changing pattern of lung involvement. Radiol Clin North Am 1993; 31: 453–463.
7 Gibb D M, Davison C F, Holland F J. Pneumocystis carinii pneumonia in vertically acquired HIV infection in the British Isles. Arch Dis Child 1994; 70: 241–244.
8 Abadco D L, Amaro-Galvez R, Rao M et al. Experience with flexible fibreoptic bronchoscopy with bronchoalveolar lavage as a diagnostic tool in children with AIDS. Am J Dis Child 1992; 146: 1056–1059.
9 Meyers J D, Flourney N, Thomas E D. Risk factors for cytomegalovirus infection after human marrow transplantation. J Infect Dis 1986; 153: 478–488.
10 Kocoskis S A. Other disease of the small intestine and colon. In: Wyllie R, Hyams J S, eds. Pediatric gastrointestinal disease: pathophysiology, diagnosis, management. Philadelphia: Saunders, 1992; pp 815–832.
11 Feldman S, Lott L. Varicella in children with cancer: impact of antiviral therapy and prophylaxis. Pediatrics 1987; 80: 465.

CHAPTER 18

IMMUNIZATION

18.1 Immunization: diphtheria, tetanus, pertussis, polio, BCG, MMR, varicella, influenza, meningococcal, pneumococcal

INTRODUCTION

Immunization is one of the most cost effective of all public health measures. Each year, millions of children worldwide receive vaccines to protect them from diseases such as measles, tetanus, diphtheria and poliomyelitis which were highly prevalent prior to the introduction of immunization. Now in many countries, these diseases are rare.

Recently, the availability of vaccines for the prevention of hepatitis A and B, *Haemophilus influenzae* type b disease (Hib) and varicella has greatly extended the scope for immunization. New vaccines for other important childhood infections such as rotaviral and respiratory syncytial viral (RSV) infection are under clinical trial. Improved technology is contributing to the development of vaccines which incorporate multiple antigens (e.g. diphtheria, tetanus, pertussis, hepatitis B, Hib), and vaccines which are more immunogenic and more temperature stable. Single-dose, slow-release vaccines are also being developed.

IMMUNITY, VACCINES AND VACCINE-PREVENTABLE DISEASES

There are a number of specific and non-specific mechanisms by which the body prevents infection. Specific immunity may be provoked by infection or by immunization. Specific immunity has both antibody-mediated (B lymphocyte-dependent) and cell-mediated (T lymphocyte-dependent) components. The two components are closely related to each other.[1] Specific antibody and cell-mediated immune responses vary in magnitude and quality in different infections. The very young infant is capable of responding to a number of antigens but to a lesser level than an adult. This is the reason for providing booster doses of some vaccines later in childhood.

Infants and children under the age of 2 years respond poorly to polysaccharide antigens which are T cell independent (e.g. pneumococcal and meningococcal vaccines). They respond well to tetanus toxoid, hepatitis B vaccine and polio-myelitis vaccines which are T cell dependent.

Conjugation of the polysaccharide antigen of Hib to protein makes it a T cell-dependent antigen and markedly improves its immunogenicity in young children. Passively transferred maternally derived IgG antibodies provide the neonate with some protection against diphtheria, tetanus, measles, poliomyelitis and rubella. This protection falls off rapidly in the first 6 months of life but may suppress the infant's response to some inactivated vaccines in the first weeks and to live measles vaccine for the first 9–12 months of life.

Vaccines are used to provoke active, specific immunity. They may contain whole inactivated organisms (e.g. whole cell pertussis vaccine, hepatitis A vaccine), live attenuated or temperature-modified organisms (e.g. measles vaccine, live influenza vaccines), subunits of organisms (e.g. subunit influenza vaccines), immunogenic polysaccharides (e.g. Hib vaccine) or other surface components, altered toxins (e.g. diphtheria toxoid), combination of the latter (e.g. acellular pertussis vaccines) or antigens prepared by using recombinant technology (e.g. hepatitis B vaccine).

The selection of vaccines to be included in a childhood immunization programme depends upon the incidence of infection in the geographical area, the availability of safe, cost-effective vaccines for the diseases and of resources to fund the programme. It is important that programmes are planned with a knowledge of disease burden and age-specific attack rates so the most appropriate and cost-effective programme can be delivered.[2] Decisions must be made about the benefits of universal or targeted vaccination programmes. For example, vaccination of all children (universal) for measles, poliomyelitis, tetanus, diphtheria and pertussis is appropriate worldwide, whereas vaccination for Japanese B encephalitis is appropriate for children in Japan.

Passive immunization, using pooled or specific immunoglobulins, is also important in some clinical situations (e.g. tetanus immunoglobulin for management of tetanus-prone wounds, pooled immunoglobulin for short-term prophylaxis of hepatitis A), but this form of protection is only temporary.

DIPHTHERIA

Diphtheria is acquired through personal contact; the incubation period is generally 2–5 days. Diphtheria may affect the tonsils, pharynx, larynx and nose. In some communities the organism may cause skin lesions similar to impetigo. Subclinical infection is common and asymptomatic carriage sometimes occurs. The toxin may cause local inflammation and necrosis with respiratory obstruction. It also causes motor and sensory nerve palsies and myocarditis. The case fatality rate is 5–10%. In the preimmunization era, diphtheria usually occurred in children under the age of 10 years.

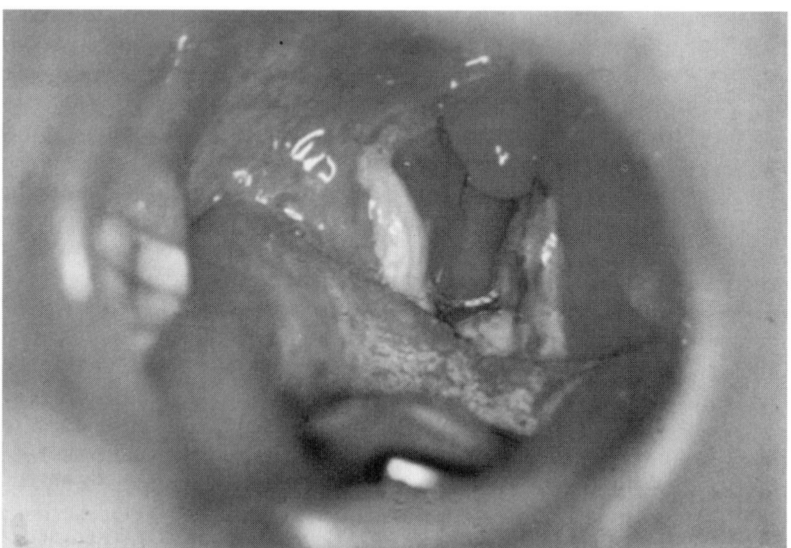

Fig. 18.1.1   Diphtheria. Adherent grey membrane. See also colour plate.

Antitoxin (antibody to toxin) may be acquired from natural infection or immunization. Antitoxin levels between 0.01 and 0.09 IU/ml are considered sufficient to protect against disease. Antitoxin can pass through the placenta and provides passive immunity to the newborn during the first few months of life.[3]

All toxigenic strains of *Corynebacterium diphtheriae* produce the same toxin. When this toxin is treated with formaldehyde and heated, it is converted to a toxoid which retains immunogenicity but is unable to bind to cells and act as an enzyme. When used as a vaccine the toxoid is usually adsorbed onto an adjuvant (e.g. aluminium phosphate or hydroxide) to increase its immunogenicity.

Immunization with toxoid commenced in the 1930s in developed countries and more recently in developing countries. Schedules and vaccine strengths vary.[4] Vaccines prepared for use in older children and adults usually have a lower dose of toxoid; this lessens the possibility of reactions at the injection site. Each region's choice of schedule depends on the epidemiology of diphtheria. The need for booster doses occurs when opportunities for natural boosting by exposure to infection are low. Vaccine-induced immunity wanes with time and does so more rapidly than immunity induced by tetanus vaccine. A primary course of three doses of vaccine, commencing at the age of 1 or 2 months and given at 1- or 2-monthly intervals, is recommended in both developed and developing countries. In developed countries this may be followed by one or two booster doses in the preschool-aged child, usually in the second and fifth years of life. Immunity in adults varies according to the epidemiology of the disease and the proportion of a community who are vaccine immune. Where there has been a long period since the initiation of mass vaccination, adults, especially those over the age of 40 years, may have low levels of immunity, with only 40–50% being protected. For this reason some countries recommend booster doses at the age of 15 years and then either every 10 years or whenever tetanus toxoid is indicated. However, not all authorities agree that booster doses are necessary in adults.[4]

In the 1980s small outbreaks of diphtheria were reported in Sweden, Germany and Portugal. In the former Soviet Union, diphtheria started to increase in the 1980s and almost 4000 cases were reported in 1992. Many of these outbreaks involved adolescents and adults.[3]

Diphtheria vaccine is usually given in combination with tetanus or tetanus and pertussis vaccines and reactions to the combined vaccine are usually due to the pertussis component. Rarely, diphtheria vaccine may cause transient fever, headache, malaise and local reactions at the injection site. Local reactions occur more frequently where the preparation used for primary immunization of infants contains higher doses of toxoid.[4]

In cases of suspected clinical diphtheria, antitoxin prepared from horse serum should be given immediately with appropriate precautions.

TETANUS

Tetanus is a severe, often fatal disease caused by the toxin produced by the anaerobic bacterium *Clostridium tetani*. Tetanus spores may contaminate wounds or the umbilicus in the newborn. Tetanus can occur even after apparently trivial wounds but is more likely with compound fractures, wounds contaminated with soil, wounds containing foreign bodies, especially wood splinters, and wounds with extensive tissue damage, including burns.

The incubation period is usually 4–21 days, with the possibility that the disease will be more severe if the incubation is short. Muscle rigidity and spasms

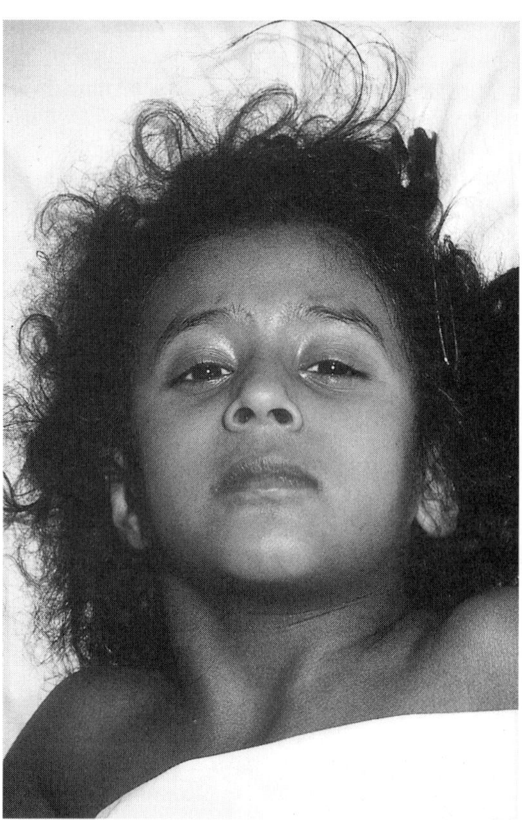

Fig. 18.1.2 Tetanus. Unimmunized 7-year-old who developed tetanus 2 weeks after having her ears pierced in a local market.

occur and death results from respiratory failure, hypertension, hypotension or cardiac arrhythmia.

Tetanus toxin can be inactivated by formaldehyde to produce tetanus toxoid which, when adsorbed with aluminium salts (aluminium hydroxide or phosphate) to increase its antigenicity, is an excellent immunizing agent. Tetanus toxoid may be used as a monovalent vaccine or as a component of tetanus–diphtheria or diphtheria–tetanus–pertussis (DTP) vaccines. The vaccine stimulates the production of antitoxin, an IgG antibody which crosses the placenta and protects the newborn from neonatal tetanus. Immunization does not prevent infection but provides antitoxin to neutralize toxin produced in an infected wound. Immunity to tetanus toxin is only produced by immunization. Patients with clinical tetanus do not become immune and should be immunized. Opinion varies about the minimum protective level of antitoxin because serological tests such as enzyme-linked immunosorbent assay (ELISA) do not always equate with the neutralization method. An antitoxin level of 0.01 IU/ml serum is considered protective using the neutralization method; with other methods 0.1 IU/ml is considered safe.[5]

In the older child or adult, three doses of tetanus toxoid given at convenient intervals, or optimally at intervals of 1–2 months and 6–12 months, induce excellent antitoxin levels. One dose, however, gives little if any protection. The duration of protection after three doses is at least 5 years. Protection for a further 10 years should be provided after a fourth dose and 20 years after a fifth dose in adults.[5] Some authorities suggest no further doses for those who have received five doses as adults.

Immunization of infants with three doses of DTP vaccine will provide tetanus immunity for 1–3 years. It may be convenient to consider three doses of tetanus toxoid received as an infant as equivalent to two doses in an older child or adult.[5] A fourth dose in the second year of life should protect for a further 5 years and a fifth dose given at school entry (fifth year of life) should provide immunity for another 10 years. An additional dose at 15–18 years should protect for a further 20 years.[5]

In developing countries, pregnant women should be immunized with two or three doses of vaccine or given a booster dose if previously immunized.[5] Maternal immunization dramatically reduces the death rate from neonatal tetanus. Best results are obtained when immunization is commenced as early as possible in the pregnancy. There is no evidence of risk to the fetus from immunizing pregnant women. In 1992, only 43% of pregnant women in developing countries had received at least two doses of tetanus toxoid (EPI Information System 1993).

Significant reactions to tetanus toxoid are rare. Mild discomfort at the injection site is frequent and may recur about 10 days after the injection. Occasionally headache, lethargy, malaise, myalgia and fever may occur. Acute anaphylaxis, urticaria and peripheral neuropathy are reported.[5] Too frequent administration of tetanus vaccine may provoke local or generalized hypersensitivity reactions. The need for further doses should be carefully assessed if an individual has previously had a severe reaction to tetanus vaccine.[6]

Individuals who have sustained a tetanus-prone wound can be given passive protection with tetanus immunoglobulin. The indications for use of tetanus immunoglobulin depend upon the vaccination status of the patient and the severity of the wound.[7]

PERTUSSIS

Pertussis is caused by the Gram-negative coccobacillus *Bordetella pertussis*.[8] Transferred maternal antibody does not provide useful protection for the neonate. Neither natural infection nor immunization provides lifelong immunity.[9]

Several types of vaccine are now produced. These can be described as whole cell vaccines, endotoxin-depleted whole cell vaccines, or acellular vaccines. Acellular vaccines may contain one or more of the following components: filamentous haemagglutinin (FHA), pertussis toxin (PT, also known as lymphocytosis-promoting factor, which is inactivated to a toxoid), a 69 kDa outer membrane protein (pertactin, Pn) and agglutinogens of at least two types (fimbriae (Fim) types 2 and 3).[8–10]

Whole cell vaccines were developed in the 1930s and are available in most countries. Acellular vaccines have been approved in Japan for use in primary immunization and in North America for booster doses. Acellular vaccines have a lower reactogenicity than whole cell vaccines. Serological studies show that acellular vaccines have good immunogenicity. The results of efficacy trials with acellular vaccines will be available soon. It is likely that acellular vaccines will then be licensed worldwide. Whole cell and acellular vaccines may be combined with diphtheria and tetanus toxoids. Some manufacturers are preparing combinations of these vaccines with Hib and hepatitis B vaccines.

The efficacy of immunization with whole cell vaccines is beyond doubt. Even though complete protection from disease occurs in only about 80% of vaccinees, protection from severe disease is high (95%).[11] Duration of protection is relatively short and is related to the number of doses of vaccine a child has received and the time since the last dose.[12,13] The protection rate falls to 50% after 5 years and almost zero after 12 years.[13,14] When pertussis occurs in vaccinated children it is usually mild, of short duration, and uncomplicated.

The efficacy of pertussis immunization was demonstrated when vaccine uptake fell in the 1970s in the UK, Sweden and Japan. These countries subsequently sustained major epidemics which were only interrupted by the reinstitution of vaccination programmes.

Very high uptake is necessary for good community protection. Even when there is high uptake, transmission may not be interrupted. Most countries with childhood immunization programmes continue to have small outbreaks of pertussis. This is because the organism continues to circulate in vaccinated communities. Once immunization rates reach 95%, serious pertussis infection should become uncommon.

Primary immunization requires three doses of vaccine. This may be commenced from the age of 1 month (it may be less effective if given earlier as there is evidence of reduced efficacy if given in the first 2 weeks of life). The interval between doses is arbitrary but is usually 1 or 2 months. The objective is to complete the primary course early to give protection to young infants who are most likely to develop complications from the disease. Opinion varies about the benefit of booster doses. Most developed countries give a booster dose in the second year of life and some give a fifth dose at school entry.[9] Some countries (e.g. the USA) do not recommend using pertussis vaccine after the age of 7 years;[15] other countries (e.g. the UK) put no upper age limit on the use of the vaccine. The value of booster doses for adolescents and adults is currently under consideration.

Because at least three doses are required to promote immunity, vaccination cannot be used to contain an outbreak.

Adverse reactions to pertussis vaccine

Pertussis vaccine causes mild to moderate systemic and local side-effects and is responsible for most reactions to trivalent DTP vaccine.[16] There is slight variation in the incidence of side-effects according to the composition of the whole cell vaccine. Using the whole cell vaccine, about 50% of children will have swelling or redness at the injection site, 20% will become febrile and about 30% will cry or be irritable; these reactions are self-limited and should last about 24–48 h. A very few children will have more significant reactions: convulsions in 0.05%, hypotonic, hyporesponsive episodes (possibly due to small amounts of endotoxin in the vaccine) in 0.05% and high-pitched unusual screaming in 0.1%.[16] No long-term adverse effects have been seen after these reactions.[17]

Previously there was concern that pertussis vaccine might cause acute neurological illness. The National Childhood Encephalopathy Study (NCES) was set up in the UK to investigate this possibility and there have been a series of reviews of this and other studies.[18,19] Even now, the data are insufficient to allow a definite statement that pertussis vaccine does or does not cause neurological illness.

The US Institute of Medicine report concluded that pertussis vaccine was very rarely associated with encephalopathy (0.0–10.5 cases per million vaccinations) or with febrile seizures.[19] It is possible that it may very rarely cause or provoke encephalopathy and that this may extremely rarely lead to permanent neurological impairment. The vaccine does not cause infantile spasms, sudden infant death syndrome or epilepsy.[19] The vaccine has a two or three times greater risk of provoking a febrile convulsion in children with a family history of convulsions (in a first-degree relative) but the risk of neurological damage in these children is extremely low.[20] If a febrile convulsion occurs after a dose of pertussis vaccine, appropriate measures to prevent fever should be used with further doses.

The side-effects of pertussis vaccine can be reduced significantly by the routine use of paracetamol (15 mg/kg per dose) just prior to the vaccination and for three or four further doses at approximately 4-hourly intervals.[21,22] This is recommended routinely in some countries.

Contraindications

Contraindications to the use of pertussis vaccine have been reviewed in many countries recently and have been liberalized.[15,23,24] Misinterpretation of the contraindications often occurs; this contributes to poor uptake in some areas, disadvantages children and allows outbreaks to occur.

Children with contraindications fall into two groups: (1) those who have active or progressive neurological disease; and (2) those who have had a severe, possibly life-threatening reaction to a previous dose. Children with stable neurological disease including controlled epilepsy and children with a family history of epilepsy or neurological disease may be immunized with the usual precautions.

Children who have developed encephalopathy within 7 days of a dose of vaccine, or an immediate, severe allergic or anaphylactic reaction, have absolute contraindications to further doses. However, the following reactions, once thought to be contraindications, should be considered relative, and each case should be reviewed, as many children who have these reactions can be given further doses without incident: a convulsion within 3 days; persistent inconsolable screaming for three or more hours; collapse or shock-like state (hypotonic hyporesponsive episode) within 48 h, a temperature of 40.5°C or more, unexplained by other causes, within 48 h; or a severe local reaction. Local reactions are often due to subcutaneous rather than intramuscular injection of the vaccine.

POLIOMYELITIS

Poliomyelitis occurs following gastrointestinal infection by one of the three types of poliovirus (1, 2 and 3).[25] The disease remains endemic in some developing countries. The World Health Organization aims to eradicate poliomyelitis globally by the year 2000. Polio has recently been eliminated in the Americas and is almost eradicated in many developed countries, although, from time to time, outbreaks occur in small unvaccinated or under-vaccinated communities.[26] The benefits of a programme aimed at eradication rather than elimination lie in the fact that once a disease is eradicated worldwide (e.g. smallpox) routine immunization is no longer required.

Several types of vaccine are produced for immunization against poliomyelitis.[25,26] The first vaccine to be approved was the injectable inactivated preparation developed by Salk (IPV) in 1955 and containing all three strains of virus. Recently, an improved formulation (enhanced potency inactivated poliovaccine, eIPV) has become available. Live oral poliovaccine (Sabin type, OPV) was introduced in 1961, and is prepared as a trivalent (types 1, 2 and 3) or monovalent vaccine. Many developed countries use only OPV, a few use IPV; developing countries may prefer inactivated vaccine if experience with OPV has resulted in poor seroconversion. Poor seroconversion rates are thought to be due to interference with the 'take' of the oral vaccine in the gastrointestinal tract by maternal antibodies, overgrowth of one vaccine strain (usually type 2), concurrent viral infection or diarrhoea.[25] OPV is preferred by WHO; it is cheaper and has the advantage of spreading to, and immunizing, unvaccinated contacts. Inactivated vaccine has no risk of causing paralysis but is less effective in preventing spread of wild virus.

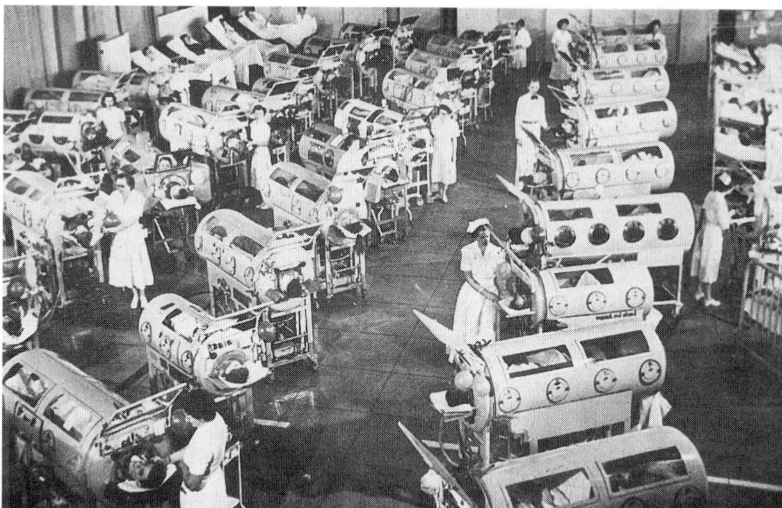

Fig. 18.1.3 Poliomyelitis. Patients in iron lungs (respirators) after contracting paralytic poliomyelitis in the 1950s epidemic in the USA.

Live vaccine very occasionally causes vaccine-associated paralysis.[25] One case is reported for approximately every three million doses of OPV distributed. The risk of paralysis is slightly greater after first doses, in adults than children, and in contacts than recipients. Paralysis is very unlikely to occur in healthy vaccinated contacts but the need for handwashing for contacts of recently vaccinated infants and children should be indicated. Healthy unvaccinated parents or caregivers should be vaccinated prior to or at the same time as an infant receiving OPV.

A primary course of three doses of OPV is usually given at 1- or 2-monthly intervals and may be commenced at the age of 1 or 2 months. Children receiving OPV are usually given a booster dose at school entry and a further booster dose is often recommended at age 15–18 years in developed countries where there are few opportunities for boosting by exposure to natural infection. Inactivated vaccine is effective if given in the first month of life; it may be given in a two- or three-dose course depending on the vaccine used and the circumstances. In Scandinavia and The Netherlands, six doses of IPV are usually given by the age of 15 years. Sequential schedules using one or more doses of IPV followed by OPV are used successfully in some countries and may partly overcome the risk of vaccine-associated disease, which now comprise about 50% of the number of cases in countries such as the USA where mass vaccination has eliminated the wild disease. It has been suggested, however, that these sequential schedules may promote reversion of the vaccine virus to neurovirulence.[27]

Contraindications

OPV must not be given to persons likely to have immune deficiency, including those on high dose corticosteroids (2 mg/kg per day of prednisolone for more than 1 week) or other immunosuppressant drugs, recent general radiation therapy, or malignant conditions of the reticuloendothelial system such as leukaemia, lymphoma or Hodgkin's disease. It is not given during acute or febrile illness (temperature greater than 38°C) or when illness causes vomiting or diarrhoea. OPV should be avoided in pregnancy although adverse effects on the fetus have not been reported. OPV should not be given to household contacts of immuno-suppressed persons. IPV may be given in pregnancy and to household contacts of immunosuppressed persons. IPV may also be given to immunosuppressed individuals who may require additional doses to provoke an adequate response. OPV has not proved harmful to asymptomatic HIV-infected children but IPV is usually preferred as household contacts are often HIV positive.

Both OPV and IPV may contain trace amounts of antibiotics such as neomycin. Their use is contraindicated only in cases of extreme hypersensitivity. Recent administration of immunoglobulin is not a contraindication to OPV although vaccine efficacy may be reduced. OPV or IPV may be administered at the same time as other vaccines in the infant schedule. OPV cannot be given with oral typhoid vaccine. Poliovaccines are effective in the management of outbreaks.

Care should be taken to store these vaccines according to the manufacturers' instructions. OPV deteriorates rapidly on exposure to heat and sunlight.

BCG VACCINE

BCG vaccine contains a suspension of live attenuated *Mycobacterium bovis*.[28] It is derived from the attenuated strain named bacille Calmette–Guérin in 1921 after its developers who worked at the Pasteur Institute. There is now wide antigenic variation among the BCG strains produced by different manufacturers. Reports of differing efficacy may relate to the heterogeneity of the recipients as well as to the differences in the vaccines.[29] There is no good explanation for these variations in protective efficacy (ranging from 0 to 80%). Most trials have shown that the vaccine protects against haematogenous spread of the organism and the development of meningeal disease better than pulmonary disease. There is no evidence that BCG reduces the risk of becoming infected with *M. tuberculosis*.

Vaccination is recommended by the WHO as one of the most important ways of protecting against illness. Almost 200 countries use the vaccine routinely or officially recommend it. Some developed countries (e.g. the USA, Australia) no longer recommend mass vaccination. Most developing countries have a high incidence of infection which is increasing as a result of HIV. These countries usually offer BCG soon after birth. Some developed countries offer BCG only to high-risk neonates, others continue with universal infant or adolescent vaccination or selective vaccination of non-immune adolescents. The increased incidence of multiply drug-resistant organisms in migrants to developed countries and in persons with HIV is important and may indicate need for immunization of their contacts including health care workers. It is of interest that a prospective trial of childhood immunization in Malawi found BCG to be protective against leprosy but not tuberculosis.[30]

Intradermal vaccination is recommended. Multiple puncture is an alternative; it is not recommended by WHO; neither is the use of a jet injector.[28]

Different preparations are available for intradermal and percutaneous use. BCG vaccine should only be given by staff who have been trained in the procedure. Subcutaneous vaccination may reduce vaccine efficacy. The skin over the lower deltoid is usually used. A small red papule forms at the injection site. This heals in about 6 weeks with minimal scarring. The local lymph nodes may become swollen. Abscesses, severe local reactions and disseminated infection are rare. These may be treated with antituberculosis drugs. Anaphylactoid reactions have been reported.

BCG provokes a specific cell-mediated immune response. There is no satisfactory in vitro test to measure this response. Immunity usually develops about 6 weeks after vaccination. The presence of vaccine-induced delayed hypersensitivity may be measured by the Mantoux test. There appears to be no correlation between protective effect and Mantoux conversion. The presence of a scar at the injection site may help in confirming immunization has been given.

Contraindications

BCG is contraindicated in individuals who are tuberculin positive; patients who are immunocompromised by HIV infection, other diseases or drugs; individuals with a high risk of HIV infection but whose status is unknown; individuals with generalized septic skin disease, or significant fever. BCG can cause fatal tuberculosis in immunocompromised patients. BCG is not used in pregnancy but has not been shown to cause fetal damage.

MMR VACCINE (MEASLES–MUMPS–RUBELLA VACCINE)

Live attenuated vaccines for the prevention of measles have been used since the 1960s.[31] Countries which have adopted mass infant vaccination have experienced very large reductions in the incidence of disease but have not yet eliminated the infection. This is due to the high degree of communicability of the virus, to the presence of clusters of unvaccinated individuals, and to the occurrence of primary and secondary vaccine failures.

In developing countries some children acquire measles before the age of 9 months, when vaccination is recommended. Vaccination at an earlier age has been tried but is not recommended at present by WHO. Seroconversion rates are affected by the presence of placentally transmitted antibody which seems to be lost more rapidly by children in developing countries.[31] In developed countries good seroconversion rates (95%) occur when the vaccine is given from the age of 12 months onwards. Many countries now give a second dose at school entry (aged about 5 years) or adolescence (aged 10–16 years). The second dose is aimed to protect primary and secondary vaccine failures. High uptake of the first dose is most important.

A number of different vaccine strains are available in Europe, Russia, Asia and North America. They have similar side-effects and contraindications. The vaccine may be available as a monovalent, a bivalent (measles–mumps), trivalent (measles–mumps–rubella) or quadrivalent (measles–mumps–rubella–varicella) preparation.

Side-effects from the measles component predominate with the MMR combination (see below).

Mumps

Several different live attenuated mumps vaccines are available. They differ slightly in their incidence of side-effects. The Urabe Am9 strain causes occasional meningoencephalitis (one in 11 000).[32] For this reason the Jeryl Lynn strain is presently preferred although it may be less immunogenic and provide less protection in its present dosage. Many developed countries now include mumps vaccine in the infant schedule. This has resulted in rapid decreases in the incidence of infection. Side-effects are generally mild (see below).

Rubella

Live attenuated rubella vaccines have been available since the late 1960s. The RA 27/3 strain is now most frequently used. The main objective is to prevent congenital infection. For this reason some countries targeted their rubella vaccination programmes at adolescent girls and women.[33] Most countries now advocate universal infant vaccination and targeted vaccination of non-immune adolescents and women. Where vaccination has been introduced, the incidence of congenital infection has gradually fallen to very low levels.

MMR Vaccine

This vaccine contains a mixture of the three live attenuated vaccines (measles, mumps and rubella) in a set dosage combination. Seroconversion rates have been shown to be equally as good as when the monovalent preparations are used, and side-effects are not potentiated.

Fever, malaise and measles-like rash may occur about 7 days after the immunization and last for 2 or 3 days. Fever is the most frequent side-effect and febrile convulsions have been reported in 0.1% of vaccines. Parotid swelling occurs in about 1% and meningoencephalitis in one in a million (with the Jeryl Lynn strain). Thrombocytopenia, joint pain and swelling are occasionally associated with the rubella component. Joint involvement is more frequent in post-pubertal recipients. The rubella component has not been shown to adversely affect the fetus. Severe neurological reactions to measles or rubella vaccine are extremely rare (one in a million) and not proved to be causally associated with the vaccines.

Parents should be given advice about the management of fever after the vaccination and informed that vaccinees are not infectious.

Contraindications

The vaccine is contraindicated for children who are immunosuppressed due to radiation or other therapy or disease. Measles vaccine is recommended for HIV-infected children, who have not responded adversely to the vaccine. The measles component of the vaccine is cultured in chick fibroblasts and its use has been said to be contraindicated in individuals who have severe anaphylactic reaction to egg. Recent experience with the vaccine indicates that it can usually be given safely to severely egg allergic children provided this is done under close observation (in an emergency room or hospital short-stay admission) and with adrenaline ready for injection.[34,35] The vaccine is contraindicated in children with allergies to neomycin. It should be deferred in children who have an acute febrile illness, in children who have received another live vaccine within 3 weeks, and in pregnancy.

The measles component of the vaccine is unstable on exposure to heat and rapidly loses potency if heated after reconstitution. Measles (or MMR) vaccine may be used to prevent measles in a non-immune contact and may be effective if given within 72 h of the contact. Mumps and rubella vaccines are not similarly effective after contact.

Pooled human immunoglobulin may also be used to prevent or modify measles during the incubation period. Immunoglobulin is effective as a prophylactic for rubella but does not significantly protect the fetus. It is not useful in preventing mumps.

VARICELLA

Live attenuated varicella vaccines have been developed from the Oka strain first isolated 20 years ago in Japan.[33] There are several commercial preparations. Vaccines are approved for use in Japan, several European countries and the USA. The vaccines are safe and effective but not completely protective.[36] Some strains are less heat stable than others and have to be stored as the freeze dried preparation at –20°C and used promptly after reconstitution. One manufacturer recommends a single dose for healthy children and two doses, 4–8 weeks apart, for healthy adolescents and immunosuppressed children. Protective efficacy is reasonably high in normal children but some vaccinated children get mild disease after exposure to natural infection. The duration of protection is not yet known as vaccinees have only been followed for about 10 years.

Side-effects are low in healthy children; they include reactions at the injection site, fever and varicella type rash (1–2%) which is usually mild.[33] General reactions are more frequent in immunosuppressed individuals and occur in about 12% and up to 40% of leukaemic subjects. About 40% of leukaemic patients develop a rash after the first dose and in 4% this is severe enough to warrant the use of acyclovir. It appears that the incidence of zoster is lower after vaccination than after natural infection.

The vaccine has been recommended for use in preventing varicella in immuno-compromised children and in children with malignant disease who are in re-mission or on maintenance (not induction) chemotherapy. It could also be used for susceptible health care workers, family members of immunocompromised patients and other adults in high-risk occupational situations. It is necessary to look carefully at the likely cost–benefit in a given population before recom-mending routine infant vaccination.[36] If routine vaccination is adopted it will be important to encourage high uptake so that the age of infection in the un-vaccinated part of the population is not shifted into older age groups in whom varicella is usually more severe.

INFLUENZA

A number of different influenza vaccines are produced commercially worldwide; these include both inactivated and temperature-modified live preparations.[37] The vaccines most often used in developed countries at present are inactivated polyvalent subunit vaccines which are reformulated on an annual basis to include the strains (usually three) most likely to prevail in the current winter season.

Some countries recommend annual vaccination for children with chronic cardiac, pulmonary, renal and metabolic disorders, including those with asthma, cystic fibrosis and immune deficiency or malignancy.[23,38] It is also recommended in the USA for children and teenagers who are receiving long-term aspirin therapy and who may be at risk of developing Reye's syndrome after influenza.[38] However, there is no evidence that annual vaccination reduces the cumulative risk of infection in children or that it benefits significantly either those who are severely compromised (e.g. children with HIV infection) or those who are not (e.g. asthmatics or some children with cystic fibrosis). Vaccination of high-risk children is indicated in a year when a major outbreak or a new strain is anti-cipated and may reduce the need for hospital admission. It may also be indi-cated for children in a season when additional compromise is anticipated, e.g. surgery, bone marrow or organ transplantation. Vaccination of household con-tacts of children who are about to receive transplants should be considered. Some institutions also offer vaccination to staff in transplant units to help reduce transmission to patients. Serological studies have shown that immunocom-promised children often respond to vaccination but at a lower level than con-trols. There are no recent studies of the efficacy of influenza vaccines in high-risk children. A clinical study, in 1971, of children with acute lymphoblastic leu-kaemia suggested some protection.[39] Children (or adults) who are vaccinated on an annual basis have only short-term protection and ultimately acquire infection.[40]

Immunocompromised children and children vaccinated for the first time require two doses separated by an interval of 4 or more weeks.

Pain at the injection site, fever (more common in children under 5 years of age), malaise and myalgia are the usual side-effects.

Immediate allergic reactions occur extremely rarely and in some instances may be due to the presence of very small amounts of egg protein. In 1976 an influenza vaccine (swine strain) produced in the USA caused an increased frequency of Guillain–Barré syndrome but this has not been seen subsequently. The fact that subunit vaccines are reformulated on an annual basis means that particular attention is needed in reporting any unexpected side-effects promptly.

Influenza vaccine is contraindicated in individuals who have anaphylactic hypersensitivity to egg.[38]

MENINGOCOCCAL VACCINE

Neisseria meningitidis is the commonest cause of bacterial meningitis in children in some countries. Vaccines to protect against serogroups A, C, Y, N and W-135 are available. No vaccine is licensed yet for protection against group B strains, which are usually the most prevalent infection in developed countries.[41] Currently available vaccines give only short-term protection and are less effective in children under the age of 2 years. They have an important role in controlling outbreaks of group A or group C disease. More immunogenic conjugated vaccines are likely to be available soon and may be suitable to combine into multivalent preparations. Several group B vaccines are presently under trial or being evaluated.

The current vaccines are given as a single dose and children as young as 6 months old may be immunized. A second dose is recommended 3 months later for children under 18 months old. The vaccine should be repeated after 2–3 years in subjects who remain at risk.

Vaccination is indicated for control of appropriate outbreaks, for travellers or residents in the areas of the world where epidemics of group A or C disease are frequent (e.g. the 'meningitis belt' of Africa), children with inherited defects of properdin or complement, or functional or anatomical asplenia, and pilgrims attending the annual Hajj. It is indicated, together with chemoprophylaxis, for close contacts of an index case caused by one of the strains represented in the vaccine.

Local reactions are mild and infrequent. Fever occurs in approximately 2% of young children but significant general reactions are rare.

Contraindications

These include previous severe reactions to phenol or meningococcal polysaccharide. The vaccine is not recommended in pregnancy. It should be deferred during a severe febrile illness.

PNEUMOCOCCAL VACCINE

Streptococcus pneumoniae is a major cause of pneumonia, meningitis and otitis media.[37] The incidence of invasive infection is high in developing countries and some indigenous groups (e.g. Australian Aboriginal and Papua New Guinea children).

Vaccines have been developed using pneumococcal capsular antigens. The most recent vaccine contains polysaccharides from the 23 most prevalent capsular types in the USA. However, vaccines containing the six or seven most frequent pathogens in children are currently being developed into more immunogenic conjugated preparations which ultimately may be able to be combined with other bacterial vaccines (e.g. Hib).

Vaccination with the pneumococcal polysaccharide vaccine is indicated in individuals with functional or anatomical asplenia, including sickle cell disease, patients at increased risk of pneumococcal disease (e.g. patients with HIV infection, nephrotic syndrome) and patients with CSF leaks.[42]

Booster doses should be given every 5 years to those at highest risk (e.g. individuals with asplenia, sickle cell disease and nephrotic syndrome). Many authorities recommend continuous penicillin prophylaxis in addition to vaccination for high-risk groups.

The vaccine may cause mild to moderate reactions at the injection site and fever.

Contraindications

Contraindications include anaphylaxis after a previous dose and pregnancy. Local reactions may be more frequent if revaccination is given within 3 years.

IMMUNIZATION SCHEDULES, DELIVERY AND COMPLIANCE

Immunization schedules vary considerably from country to country. They need to be easy to deliver and timed to provide protection prior to exposure. Simple schedules are more likely to be delivered effectively. When DTP, Hib, hepatitis B, poliomyelitis and MMR are included in the infant schedule there is often difficulty delivering all the doses on time. The availability of multi-dose vaccines will help. Vaccines may be inadvertently lowered in potency by exposure to high temperature or inappropriate freezing. This is frequently overlooked. Greater attention needs to be paid to maintaining the cold chain, particularly in transit and at the point of delivery.

Many countries experience difficulty in achieving high compliance. The UK has improved compliance recently and the USA has increased its rate of immunizations delivered on time (rate of age-appropriate immunization). Compliance is often better in developing than in developed countries. The measures most likely to improve compliance will vary with the community. Improving access to services, keeping costs low, dispelling myths about the vaccines, educating both professionals and public, identifying risk groups and having school entry requirements may help with compliance. A thorough understanding of the schedule and of the true contraindications (as distinct from the perceived contraindications) for each vaccine is extremely important for all those who provide children's health care. Having available a list of misconceptions about the contraindications may be helpful.[15,23,43] In the UK, immunization uptake in a district is directly related to the general practitioner's knowledge and attitude to immunization. It is likely that the primary health care provider's attitude is also important in other countries. We should be continually educating and motivating the vaccinators. We should also be using every health care encounter as an opportunity to take a full immunization history and give vaccines which are due. Only by improving compliance can we expect to attain the goal of a world free from vaccine preventable diseases.

REFERENCES

1 Ada G L. The immunological principles of vaccination. Lancet 1990; 335: 523–526.
2 Anderson R M, May R M. Immunisation and herd immunity. Lancet 1990; 335: 641–645.
3 Galazka A M. Diphtheria. In: The immunological basis for immunization, Module 2. World Health Organization, Geneva 1993.12. Expanded Programme on Immunization, 1990.
4 Mortimer E A. Diphtheria toxoid. In: Plotkin S A, Mortimer E A (eds). Vaccines, 1st edn. Philadelphia: Saunders, 1988.
5 Galazka A M. Tetanus. In: The immunological basis for immunization, Module 3. World Health Organization, Geneva 1993.13. Expanded Programme on Immunization.
6 Wassilak S G F, Orenstein W A. Tetanus. In: Plotkin S A, Mortimer E A (eds). Vaccines. 1st edn. Philadelphia: Saunders, 1988.
7 Centers for Disease Control. Update on adult immunization: recommendations of the Advisory Committee on Immunization Practices (ACIP). MMWR 1991; 40 (No. RR-12): 17–19.
8 Moxon E R, Rappuoli R. Haemophilus influenzae infections and whooping cough. Lancet 1990; 335: 1324–1329.
9 Galazka A M. Pertussis. In: The immunological basis for immunization, Module 4. World Health Organization, Geneva 1993.14. Expanded Programme on Immunization.
10 Centers for Disease Control. Pertussis vaccination: acellular pertussis vaccine for reinforcing and booster use — supplementary ACIP statement. Recommendations of the Immunization Practices Advisory Committee (ACIP). MMWR 1992; 41 (No. RR-1): 1–10.
11 Onrato I M, Wassilak S G, Meade B. Efficacy of whole-cell pertussis vaccine in preschool children in the United States. JAMA 1992; 267: 2745–2749.
12 Cherry J D, Brunell P A, Golden G S, Karzon D T. Report of the task force on pertussis and pertussis immunization. Pediatrics 1988; 81 (Suppl): 955–984.
13 Lambert H. Epidemiology of a small pertussis outbreak in Kent County, Michigan. Public Health Rep 1965; 80: 365–369.
14 Jenkinson D. Duration of effectiveness of pertussis vaccine: evidence from a 10 year community study. Br Med J 1988; 296: 612–614.
15 Centers for Disease Control and Prevention. General Recommendations on Immunization: recommendations of the Advisory Committee on Immunization Practices (ACIP). MMWR 1994; 43 (No. RR-1): 1–38.
16 Cody C L, Baraff L J, Cherry J D et al. Nature and rates of adverse reactions associated with DTP and DT immunisations in infants and children. Pediatrics 1981; 68: 650–660.
17 Barraff L J, Shields W D et al. Infants and children with convulsions and hypotonic–hyporesponsive episodes following diphtheria–tetanus–pertussis immunization: follow-up evaluation. Pediatrics 1988; 81: 789–794.
18 Miller D, Madge N, Diamond J et al. Pertussis immunisation and serious acute neurological illness in children. Br Med J 1993; 307: 1171–1176.
19 Stratton K R, Howe C H, Johnston R B Jr. DTP vaccine and chronic nervous system dysfunction: a new analysis. Washington, DC: Institute of Medicine, National Academy of Sciences, National Academy Press, 1994.
20 Centers for Disease Control and Prevention Advisory Committee on Immunization Practices (ACIP). Pertussis immunization: family history of convulsions and use of antipyretics — supplementary ACIP statement. MMWR 1987; 36: 281–282.
21 Ipp M M, Gold R, Greenberg S et al. Acetaminophen prophylaxis of adverse reactions following vaccination of infants with diphtheria–pertussis–tetanus toxoids and polio vaccine. Pediatr Infect Dis 1987; 6: 721–725.
22 Lewis K, Cherry J D, Sachs M H et al. The effect of prophylactic acetaminophen administration on reactions to DTP vaccination. Am J Dis Child 1988; 142: 62–65.
23 Department of Health Welsh Office, Scottish Office Home and Health Department, DHSS (Northern Ireland). Immunisation against infectious disease. London: HMSO, 1992: pp 1–222.
24 Report of the Committee on Infectious Diseases, 22nd edn. G Peter et al, eds. American Academy of Pediatrics, 1991.
25 Robertson S E. Poliomyelitis. In: The immunological basis for immunization, Module 6. World Health Organization, Geneva, 1993.16. Expanded Programme on Immunization.
26 Hull H F, Ward N A, Hull B P et al. Paralytic poliomyelitis: seasoned strategies, disappearing disease. Lancet 1994; 343: 1331–1337.

27 Ogra P L, Faden H S, Abraham R et al. Effect of prior immunity on the shedding of virulent revertant virus in feces after oral administration with live attenuated poliovirus vaccines. J Infect Dis 1991; 164: 191–194.

28 Milstein J. Tuberculosis. In: The immunological basis for immunization, Module 5. World Health Organization, Geneva, 1993.15. Expanded Programme on Immunization.

29 Fine P E M, Rodrigues L C. Mycobacterial diseases. Lancet 1990; 335: 1016–1020.

30 Ponnighaus J M, Fine P E M et al. Efficacy of BCG vaccine against leprosy and tuberculosis in northern Malawi. Lancet 1992; 339: 636–639.

31 Cutts F T. Measles. In: The immunological basis for immunization, Module 7. World Health Organization, Geneva 1993:17. Expanded Programme on Immunization.

32 Miller E, Goldacre M et al. Risk of aseptic meningitis after measles, mumps, and rubella vaccine in UK children. Lancet 1993; 341: 979–982.

33 Isaacs D, Menser M. Measles, mumps, rubella, and varicella. Lancet 1990; 335: 1384–1387.

34 Kemp A, Van Asperen P, Mukhi A. Measles immunisation in children with clinical reactions to egg protein. Am J Dis Child 1990; 144: 33–35.

35 Beck S A, Williams L W et al. Egg hypersensitivity and measles/mumps/rubella vaccine administration. Pediatrics 1991; 88: 913–917.

36 Watson B A, Starr S E. Varicella vaccine for healthy children. Lancet 1994; 343: 928–929.

37 Shann F. Pneumococcus and influenza. Lancet 1990; 335: 848–901.

38 Centers for Disease Control. Prevention and control of influenza: recommendations of the Advisory Committee on Immunization Practices (ACIP). MMWR 1992; 42 (No. RR-9): 1–17.

39 Brown A E, Steinherz P G, Miller D T et al. Immunization against influenza in children with cancer: results of a three dose trial. J Infect Dis 1992; 145: 126.

40 Hoskins T W, Davies J R et al. Assessment of inactivated influenza-A vaccine after three outbreaks of influenza at Christ's Hospital. Lancet 1979; i: 33–35.

41 Lepow M L. Meningococcal vaccines. In: Plotkin S A, Mortimer E A, eds. Vaccines. 1st edn. Philadelphia: Saunders, 1988.

42 Centers for Disease Control and Prevention. Recommendations of the Advisory Committee on Immunization Practices (ACIP): Use of vaccines and immune globulins in persons with altered immunocompetence. MMWR 1993; 42 (No. RR-5): 1–18.

43 Peter G. Childhood immunizations. N Engl J Med 1992; 327: 1794–1799.

18.2 *Haemophilus influenzae* type b

INTRODUCTION

The advent of routine immunization against *Haemophilus influenzae* type b (Hib) in developed countries has been a major triumph in disease control. Even where vaccine uptake has been only moderate (50–75%), dramatic declines have been observed in the incidence of serious Hib infections such as meningitis and epiglottitis. This suggests that vaccination has a significant effect on both individual and herd immunity and it raises the possibility that Hib disease can be eradicated.

THE ORGANISM

H. influenzae is a Gram-negative coccobacillus which is classified into six serotypes (a–f) on the basis of differences in its polysaccharide capsule. Unencapsulated variants are defined non-typeable.

EPIDEMIOLOGY

Only humans are infected by *H. influenzae*. Type b is the most virulent serotype and was responsible for the great majority of serious *Haemophilus* disease prior to the widespread use of Hib conjugate vaccines. Hib is a major cause of meningitis, the predominant cause of epiglottitis and a leading cause of pneumonia, cellulitis and septic arthritis in young children. Non-encapsulated *H. influenzae* are responsible for otitis media much more commonly than Hib, and cause most neonatal *H. influenzae* disease. Neonatal infection occurs more commonly in infants compromised by prematurity or congenital abnormality. Most invasive Hib infections are seen in early childhood, 90% of cases being between 4 months and 4 years of age.[1] The incidence of disease peaks between 6 and 11 months of age after infants lose the protection afforded by transplacental antibody and breast-feeding. Important risk factors include day care attendance of greater than 20 h per week and the presence of older siblings in the household. Epidemiological surveillance during the 1980s in industrialized countries revealed that invasive Hib disease was more common than previously thought.[1,2] It occurred at a yearly rate of between 30 and 100 cases per 100 000 in children aged less than 5 years.[1–3] Hib meningitis affected between 1 : 300 and 1 : 900 children. Aboriginal populations of Australia, Canada and the USA were more commonly afflicted, deprivation (with attendant overcrowding and malnutrition) being the unifying risk factor predisposing to disease in these diverse ethnic groups. In developing countries Hib disease occurs at an earlier age, with the majority of cases in those under 1 year of age.[3]

In most Western countries the epidemiology of serious *Haemophilus* infections changed dramatically within 2 years of the introduction of efficacious vaccines.[4] Declines in excess of 80% in the overall rate of invasive *H. influenzae* disease, whether type b or not, have occurred. Vaccination has also had a significant impact on the carriage of Hib in the nasopharynx.[5] Carriage of the organism by unvaccinated older siblings of vaccine recipients is also lower,[5] suggesting that the vaccine effect of decreasing colonization has in turn diminished transmission. There is no evidence that the nasopharynx is being repopulated by non-type b *H. influenzae* of similar virulence to Hib; no change in the incidence of non-type b *H. influenzae* invasive infection has been observed.

PATHOGENESIS AND PATHOLOGY

H. influenzae is a commensal of the human upper respiratory tract. Carriage is common in childhood, and generally produces no ill-effect; the maximal rate is about 10% in the preschool-age group. Invasive disease occurs following translocation through the nasopharynx by the organism into the bloodstream and subsequent invasion of tissues such as the meninges to cause meningitis, or of synovial membranes of joints to cause septic arthritis. It is probable that most serious infection transpires within a few days of nasopharyngeal colonization. Direct local invasion of tissues such as the epiglottis and lung may also occur. The major determinant of virulence is the organism's polysaccharide capsule which consists of polyribosylribitol phosphate (PRP).[6]

Immunity

The seminal work of Fothergill and Wright showed that the incidence of Hib disease was inversely related to the capacity of blood to kill the organism.[7] Later it became clear that serum antibody (IgG) to the type b capsular polysaccharide PRP is a major protective factor against serious infection.[8] The production of IgG_2 is particularly important. However, it takes some years for children to be able to produce antibody, so young children bear the brunt of disease.

Invasive infection in infants less than 1 year of age usually does not induce protective immunity. Without immunization, most children acquire natural immunity to Hib by 5 years of age, either through the immunostimulation of Hib carriage in the nasopharynx or because cross-reactive antigens contained in other bacteria colonizing either the upper respiratory or gastrointestinal tracts induce antibodies against PRP and other antigen.

Spread

Hib is believed to be spread by close contact with respiratory secretions. Shared handkerchiefs in the day care setting have also been implicated.

CLINICAL FEATURES

Meningitis makes up about two-thirds of proven invasive Hib infections in most countries. Epiglottitis accounts for a variable proportion from negligible up to 40% of cases. Proven Hib pneumonia represents only a few per cent of cases. However, it occurs much more frequently than the isolation rate from blood culture would suggest. Before routine vaccination against Hib, it was second only to pneumococcus as a cause of bacterial pneumonia in young children. Cellulitis and bone/joint infections each contribute about 5% of cases.

Signs and symptoms of these infectious syndromes are covered elsewhere in this book.

Diagnosis

Appropriate samples such as blood or cerebrospinal fluid should be collected prior to antibiotics being given in order to perform Gram stain and culture. If antibiotics have been given, latex agglutination becomes particularly useful; this test is less helpful when performed on urine because false positive (such as when Hib vaccine has recently been given) and false negative results are not uncommon.

If cultures are negative, the measurement of serum antibody to PRP on acute and convalescent samples can be done in reference centres. However, if no rise is seen in an infant < 2 years, Hib infection is not ruled out because the immune system may not have matured enough to respond.

The accurate typing of *H. influenzae* isolates in vaccine recipients is especially important as incorrect assignment as Hib could adversely effect vaccine uptake.

Treatment

A third-generation cephalosporin like ceftriaxone or cefotaxime is preferred for the treatment of invasive infections like meningitis. Cefuroxime is not recommended as it is associated with delayed sterilization of the CSF and greater neurological sequelae. Between 15% and 20% of isolates are ampicillin resistant. Resistance to chloramphenicol is uncommon but increasing. As a result, most clinicians no longer consider dual therapy with these antibiotics as first-line.

Chemoprophylaxis with rifampicin is given to the index case and also to all other family members and close contacts if there is another unimmunized sibling in the household of preschool age. In the UK a combination of vaccination and chemoprophylaxis is recommended for children in a nursery or playgroup if two cases occur within months of each other. Even one infected child should stimulate efforts to vaccinate contacts.

Prevention

A key objective of vaccine development was to hasten the onset of protective immunity. Pure polysaccharides like PRP are poorly immunogenic, particularly in infancy.[8] Effective Hib vaccines consisting of purified polysaccharide PRP were first used in the 1970s but these only protected children older than 2 years. Conjugate vaccines were developed whereby PRP or an oligosaccharide derivative is covalently linked (either directly or by a spacer molecule) to a protein such as tetanus toxoid (PRP-T), diphtheria toxoid (PRP-D), a non-toxic mutant of diphtheria toxin (HbOC) or a group B meningococcus outer membrane protein (PRP-OMP). The carbohydrate antigen is thereby invested with T cell dependency, becoming immunogenic in infancy and able to prime for a later anamnestic response. These conjugate vaccines have been extensively evaluated in trials, shown to be both safe and highly protective and are licensed for routine use in many developed and developing countries. A three-dose course is given in the first 6 months after birth. The child is thereby primed for a boosting response to later exposure to the Hib organism, cross-reactive antigen, or the polysaccharide PRP vaccine. The carrier protein given alone does not boost.

PRP-OMP stands out as being able to induce a detectable serum antibody response after only one dose in infancy. The immunogenicity of the other three Hib conjugate vaccines can be heightened by priming with the carrier protein contained in the triple diphtheria–tetanus–pertussis (DTP) vaccine. If infants are given one or more doses of DTP before the first dose of conjugate vaccine, a greater antibody response occurs such that, in the case of PRP-T, efficacy (disease prevention) is achieved, at least in the short term.

A commonly expressed concern is that vaccination in infancy will merely postpone the age at which invasive disease occurs. However, immune responses to polysaccharide-encapsulated pathogens mature during early childhood and there is increasing evidence that a three-dose course of Hib conjugate vaccine in early infancy results in long-term protection irrespective of whether a booster dose is given in the second year of life. Furthermore, it has been shown that preschool-aged children who become colonized by Hib achieve much higher concentrations of antibody against PRP if they were immunized in infancy.[9]

There are several at-risk groups, including asplenics, premature infants, and children with sickle cell disease or HIV infection in whom the efficacy of vaccination has not been formally addressed. Even so, they should be offered vaccine as there is evidence of immunogenicity, albeit reduced. Booster doses may be appropriate and their use can be guided by the results of anti-PRP antibody estimation.

VACCINE FAILURES

Invasive *H. influenzae* disease is rare in immunized children, and when it occurs it is as likely to be caused by another serotype or non-typeable *H. influenzae* as by Hib. Such cases, whether caused by type b or not, commonly have an underlying medical condition such as prematurity, chromosomal abnormality, or immunoglobulin deficiency, especially IgG_2; baseline investigation of their immunological competence is therefore indicated, including antibody response to Hib infection, total immunoglobulins and IgG subclass estimation. Consideration should be given to revaccination against Hib as well as vaccination against other encapsulated bacteria such as meningococcus and pneumococcus.

THE FUTURE

Since Hib only infects humans, it may be possible to eradicate this organism. Vaccination reduces carriage as well as transmission, although studies are awaited of whether the number of secondary cases from each primary case is diminished below 1, the prerequisite for elimination. Although that may be possible in industrialized countries, the larger hurdle to eradication is whether an expensive vaccine can be implemented widely enough in resource-poor countries.

REFERENCES

1 Booy R, Hodgson S A, Slack M P E, Anderson E C, Mayon-White R T, Moxon E R. Invasive *Haemophilus influenzae* type b disease in the Oxford region (1985–91). Arch Dis Child 1993; 69: 225–229.
2 Wenger J D, Hightower A W, Facklam R R, Gaventas, Broome C V and the Bacterial Meningitis Study Group. Bacterial meningitis in the United States, 1986: report of a multistate surveillance study. J Infect Dis 1990; 162: 1316–1323.
3 Bijlmer H A. World-wide epidemiology of *Haemophilus influenzae* meningitis: industrialised versus non-industrialised countries. Vaccine 1991; 9: S5–S9.
4 Peltola H, Kilpi T, Antilla M. Rapid disappearance of *Haemophilus influenzae* type b meningitis after routine childhood immunisation with conjugate vaccines. Lancet 1992; 340: 592–59.

5 Barbour M L, Mayon-White R T, Coles C, Crook D W M, Moxon E R. The impact of conjugate vaccine on carriage of *Haemophilus influenzae* type b. J Infect Dis 1995; 171: 93–98.

6 Moxon E R, Vaughan K A. The type b capsular polysaccharide as a virulence determinant of *Haemophilus influenzae*; studies using clinical isolates and laboratory transformants.
J Infect Dis 1981; 143: 517–534.

7 Fothergill L D, Wright J. Influenzal meningitis: relation of age incidence to the bactericidal power of blood against the causal organism. J Immunol 1933; 24: 273–284.

8 Anderson P, Johnston R, Smith D H. Human serum activities against *Haemophilus influenzae* type b. J Clin Invest 1972; 51: 31–38.

9 Barbour M L, Booy R, Crook D W M et al. Haemophilus *influenzae* type b carriage and immunity 4 years after receiving the *Haemophilus influenzae* oligosaccharide–CRM197 (HbOC) conjugate vaccine. Pediatr Infect Dis J 1993; 12: 478–484.

18.3 Immunization: hepatitis A and hepatitis B vaccines

HEPATITIS A

Introduction

Hepatitis A virus (HAV) is an RNA enterovirus of the picornavirus family. Approximately 50% of children under age 6 years with hepatitis A are asymptomatic and many of the remainder have mild symptoms often not recognized as being due to hepatitis A.[1] The infection resolves with a fatality rate of less than 1% and no chronic sequelae. Transmission is via the faecal/oral route or rarely parenterally and there is no known carrier state. Prevention of faecal contamination of food, water and other sources, frequent handwashing and the avoidance of sharing of personal objects are important in interrupting transmission.

Epidemiology

The prevalence of HAV appears to be decreasing in some countries previously highly endemic for the infection, for example in Europe and Asia, but not in others, particularly Africa. Paradoxically, HAV transmission occurs in older age groups as endemicity decreases with improved standards of sanitation and hygiene, and the reported rate of clinical hepatitis A can actually increase due to a shift in the average age of infection to an age when clinical illness is more frequent.[2]

Various risk factors for HAV infection have been identified and these are shown in Table 18.3.1. These risk factors have a bearing on whom should be considered for vaccine.

Table 18.3.1   Risk factors for hepatitis B virus infection

Overcrowding, poor hygiene, poor sanitation
Large family size
Institutions for developmentally disabled, military facilities, prisons
Homosexual men
Day care attendance/workers in day care centre
Travel to endemic area

Immunology

The antigenicity of strains of HAV from many sources has been found to be strongly conserved. Although the immune response to HAV may involve both cytotoxic T cells and antibody-secreting cells of the B lineage, any individual who has antibodies detectable by the standard HAVAB (Abbott Laboratories) competitive inhibition immunoassay, with or without immunization, is likely to be protected. Although prophylactically administered immunoglobulin results in barely detectable levels of anti-HAV antibodies in comparison with the level produced by infection, these low levels still afford protection. Passive immunization with immunoglobulin completely suppresses or markedly attenuates clinical hepatitis A but the rate of infection remains unchanged compared with controls.

Passive immunization

Short-term pre-exposure protection against hepatitis A is afforded by the administration of 0.02–0.04 ml/kg (2 ml for adults) i.m. of normal human immunoglobulin if the anticipated exposure is less than 2 months. For protection up to 6 months a dose of 0.06 ml/kg (5 ml for adults) is given. With longer-term residence in an endemic area seroconversion is likely to occur under cover of immunoglobulin and the anti-HAV status can be checked at regular intervals to ascertain the need for further immunoglobulin.

Postexposure administration of immunoglobulin is indicated in certain circumstances. For the household contact, 0.01–0.02 ml/kg of immunoglobulin is given without waiting for the anti-HAV status and this applies also for those in close personal contact with a case. If hepatitis A occurs in an attendee, parents of a child or employee of a day care centre, 0.02 ml/kg of immunoglobulin should be given to all employees and children within 2 weeks of the exposure. For casual contacts outside day care centres, prophylaxis is not required. Infected infants and children can return to day care 2 weeks after the onset of symptoms. Postexposure immunoglobulin is not recommended in schools, preschools and institutions for custodial care unless an institutional or classroom outbreak is identified or unless there is regular and close contact with the case. It is not recommended for workers in hospitals, offices or factories.

Active immunization

The two major currently available formalin-inactivated hepatitis A vaccines are the SmithKline HM175 derived vaccine and the Merck CR326F' derived vaccine. They are both highly immunogenic and safe in children,[3,4] although there is little information concerning very young infants. These vaccines are also highly protective. Werzberger et al[4] performed a study of 1037 healthy seronegative children aged 2–16 years in a Hasidic Jewish community in upstate New York using the Merck CR326F' vaccine, which conferred 100% protection after one dose. Innis et al[3] studied 40 119 Thai children aged 1–16 years given the SmithKline HM175 vaccine. Following two doses at 0 and 1 month, protective efficacy was 94%. There appears no doubt that safe, immunogenic and effective hepatitis A vaccines are available. The question is, who needs them?

Recommendations for the use of hepatitis A vaccines

Certain groups are at risk for HAV infection (see Table 18.3.1) but almost one-third of reported cases have no identifiable source of their infection.[5] As standards of hygiene and sanitation improve, children come into first contact with HAV at an increasing age, leaving more adults susceptible. The major public health problem with hepatitis A occurs in developing countries, Eastern Europe and the Middle East, with high levels of viral circulation and large cohorts of susceptible older children and adults. In such countries the eventual objective should be to integrate hepatitis A vaccine into routine universal childhood immunization schedules.

For those persons living in areas where hepatitis A is not highly endemic, hepatitis A vaccine should be used selectively. For travellers to endemic areas, including children, active immunization should be offered as an alternative to passive immunization unless the travel is at short notice, regardless of the anticipated length of stay. Those with occupational risk such as health care workers, those working with the intellectually disabled and workers in day care centres should be offered active immunization, as should non-immune homosexuals.

Various schedules have been assessed and it appears that the initial doses at 0 and 1 or 2 months should be followed up by a booster at 6–12 months, with the duration of protection calculated to be at least 10 years. It is possible that a two-dose schedule will be appropriate for the Merck product, and in fact single-dose inactivated vaccines are under development.

In haemodialysis patients and in those with an impaired immune system, adequate antibody titres may not be obtained after the primary immunization course and such patients may therefore require administration of additional doses of vaccine.

Inactivated hepatitis A vaccine may be administered simultaneously with hepatitis B vaccine with no interference in the immune response to either antigen. The contraindications to hepatitis A vaccine are hypersensitivity to any component of the vaccine or the presence of a severe febrile infection. Vaccination cannot yet be recommended to replace passively administered immunoglobulin for postexposure prophylaxis, although larger doses of vaccine may achieve this. However, results from studies with one inactivated hepatitis A vaccine indicate that both passive and active immunoprophylaxis can be administered at the same time, but the active immune response to the vaccine is approximately one-half that measured when vaccine alone is administered.[6]

New hepatitis A vaccines are under development, for example, a live attenuated vaccine and an inactivated virosome hepatitis A vaccine. Combined hepatitis A/hepatitis B vaccines are also under development.

HEPATITIS B

Introduction

Hepatitis B vaccines have been available for longer than hepatitis A vaccines but the same question needs to be asked, i.e. who needs them? Groups at high risk of contracting hepatitis B are obvious candidates but there is an argument which supports universal immunization as an alternative to or as a follow-on from targeted immunization. Indeed the USA has adopted a policy of universal infant immunization, as have Israel, Italy and New Zealand. The UK has not adopted such a policy but like many countries offers hepatitis B vaccine to high-risk groups. By preventing hepatitis B virus (HBV) infection, hepatitis B vaccination also prevents chronic hepatitis and hepatocellular carcinoma resulting from HBV, and by extension also prevents hepatitis D infection.

Immunogenicity of hepatitis B vaccine

Krugman et al[7] produced a vaccine containing hepatitis B surface antigen (HBsAg) purified from the plasma of asymptomatic viral carriers. Efficacy trials of plasma-derived hepatitis B vaccine showed that over 90% of persons in all age groups under 60 years, including infants, had high antibody titres of anti-hepatitis B surface antibody (anti-HBs) after three doses of vaccine.[8,9] Age is an important factor influencing the response to vaccine, with younger vaccinees, including newborn infants, having the highest rates of seroconversion. Yeast-recombinant hepatitis B vaccines were licensed in the USA in 1986. Both plasma-derived and yeast-recombinant hepatitis B vaccines are used extensively worldwide.

Clinical and epidemiological considerations

Young infants who become infected with HBV have a high likelihood of becoming HBV carriers, with no acute clinical manifestations, while older subjects are less likely to become carriers but are more likely to have acute clinical manifestations.

There are two well-recognized patterns of transmission of hepatitis B, namely vertical and horizontal. Vertical transmission occurs from an HBsAg-positive mother to her baby around the time of birth (or occasionally in utero) and is more likely if the mother is also hepatitis B e antigen (HBeAg) positive. It is common in some areas of high endemicity such as Southeast Asia (with a high relative frequency of HBeAg positivity in carrier mothers), where the total HBV carriage attributable to perinatal transmission is between 30% and 50%. In contrast, this rate is only 10–20% in tropical Africa (with a low relative frequency of HBeAg positivity in carrier mothers). Horizontal transmission, i.e., transmission occurring without apparent parenteral, sexual or perinatal exposure, occurs in areas of intermediate endemicity and high endemicity such as tropical Africa. It is a direct result of a large number of HBsAg carrier children and occurs predominantly within families in children at a young age. Sexual contact among adults is the primary route of HBV transmission in areas of low HBV endemicity.

Protective efficacy of hepatitis B vaccine

Recombinant hepatitis B vaccines are 90–95% effective in preventing infection when administered to newborn infants of HBsAg-positive mothers with or without hepatitis B immunoglobulin (HBIG). In The Gambia, infant immunization was 84% and 94% effective against infection and chronic carriage, respectively, regardless of the HBeAg status of the mother.[10] Vaccine fails to elicit an antibody response in up to 10% of subjects, especially in adults, which is major histocompatibility complex-associated and inherited in a dominant fashion.[11]

Risk groups for hepatitis B

Certain groups are at particular risk for contracting hepatitis B (Table 18.3.2). It follows that hepatitis B vaccination should be targeted at these groups. Although horizontal transmission of hepatitis B has been demonstrated in New Zealand schools,[12,13] a study by Burgess et al[14] found that there was no evidence of horizontal transmission of hepatitis B between high-risk and low-risk urban Australian school children despite many years of potential contact. This raises the question of whether or not low-risk children need to be vaccinated against hepatitis B.

Focal programmes targeted for selective vaccination of high-risk groups in areas of low hepatitis B endemicity (which characterizes the majority of current programmes in Western countries) have no relevance to the requirements for control in areas of intermediate and high endemicity, and nothing short of large-scale immunization of infants in the latter areas can be expected to reduce appreciably the incidence of HBV infection and the prevalence of the HBV persistent carrier state.[15] The World Health Organization has recommended that hepatitis B vaccine be added to BCG, triple antigen, polio and measles vaccines provided through the Expanded Programme on Immunization. A multivalent combined hepatitis B/triple-antigen vaccine is under development.

Table 18.3.2   Risk groups for hepatitis B

1. Vertical transmission — babies born to carrier mothers and babies born into ethnic groups with high carrier rates
2. Horizontal transmission
    (a) Households — seronegative household contacts of carrier, children of chronic carriers or contact with patients with acute hepatitis B
    (b) Institutions — seronegative intellectually disabled persons in institutions, prisoners
    (c) Intravenous drug users
    (d) Sexual — sexual partners of chronic carriers and patients with acute hepatitis, homosexuals with multiple sexual partners
    (e) Health care workers
    (f) Persons receiving multiple transfusions or haemodialysis

Immunization schedules

There are two widely available recombinant DNA HBV vaccines: the SmithKline product and the Merck product. The standard schedule is for vaccinations at 0, 1 and 6 months, 1 ml for adults and children over the age of 10 years, and 0.5 ml for neonates and for children less than 10 years. For more immediate protection with the SmithKline product a 0-, 1- and 2- month schedule may be followed with a booster at 12 months. The timing of a booster dose after the primary course is uncertain but appears to be some time between 5 and 10 years later. It is possible, however, that booster doses will not be recommended other than for those at continuing high risk.

A number of side-effects have been reported to be associated with hepatitis B vaccination in adults and children, ranging from nausea and malaise to more severe neurological, dermatological and other effects. The most worrying are Guillain–Barré syndrome, erythema nodosum and polyarthritis. No serious side-effects of the vaccine have been reported for preterm or full-term infants. In general, however, minor side-effects are rare, and major side-effects are extremely rare. Transient surface antigenaemia is a frequent occurrence in newborn infants and the presence of this serological marker alone in the postvaccination period should not be attributed to HBV infection unless confirmed by other tests.

Currently, low-dose regimens cannot be recommended and, despite the robustness of the hepatitis B vaccine, it should be stored at the recommended temperature and not frozen.

Hepatitis B immunoglobulin

Other than the use of HBIG for immunoprophylaxis in the newborn period to infants of HBsAg-positive mothers, HBIG is also used at the time of accidental exposure to potentially HBV-infected blood, for example a needle-stick injury. It may be administered at the same time but at a different site to hepatitis B vaccine and does not interfere with the immune response to the vaccine. If the recipient is non-immune or their status is unknown and the source is HBsAg positive or status unknown then the recipient should receive HBIG immediately in addition to a course af active immunization (see Table 18.3.3). HBIG is also used to delay or prevent recurrent HBV infection after liver transplantation.

Table 18.3.3 Hepatitis B virus postexposure recommendations

Type of exposure	Hepatitis B immunoglobulin		Vaccine	
Perinatal	100 IU i.m.	Within 12 h of birth	0.5 ml i.m.	Within 7 days,[a] repeat at 1 and 6 months
Percutaneous	400 IU i.m.	Single dose within 24 h	1.0 ml i.m.[b]	Within 7 days,[a] repeat at 1 and 6 months
Sexual	400 IU i.m.	Within 14 days of sexual contact	1.0 ml	Within 7 days,[a] repeat at 1 and 6 months

[a] The first dose can be given at the same time as the hepatitis B immunoglobulin dose but should be administered at a separate site.
[b] For persons under 10 years of age, use 0.5 ml dose recommended by the manufacturers.

Vaccine-induced escape-mutant HBV

Carman et al[16] described a replicating, infectious hepatitis B virus that has mutated so that it is no longer susceptible to neutralizing immunity. It seems likely that the region in which the mutation occurs is an important epitope of HBV, to which vaccine-induced neutralizing antibody binds, and that viruses lacking this epitope are therefore not neutralized by antibody of this specificity.

Until the epidemiological and clinical significance of these viruses is determined, a change in the current hepatitis B vaccine is not indicated. Vaccines based on the pre-S region of HBV may circumvent infection by the currently identified S gene escape mutants. Pre-S type vaccines may also be useful in immunizing non-responders to conventional vaccines.

Hepatitis B vaccine is less immunogenic in preterm infants.[17] If the mother is not a hepatitis B carrier, hepatitis B vaccination should be delayed until the preterm infant reaches a body weight of 2000 g. If the mother is a hepatitis B carrier, vaccine and HBIG should be given and the infant evaluated later regarding the need for a fourth dose.[17]

Human immunodeficiency virus (HIV) infection and the need for hepatitis B vaccination

As infants and children infected with HIV may be at increased risk of HBV infection through perinatal exposure to HBV, exposure to HBV-infected household contacts and exposure to blood products, special mention should be made of the role of hepatitis B vaccination in this group. Hepatitis B vaccine is poorly immunogenic in symptomatic HIV-infected children and a schedule consisting of twice the recommended dose or booster doses may be necessary.[18] Children with protective antibody titres will need to be monitored to establish the duration of detectable antibody. The accepted protective level of anti-HBs antibody is 10 mIU/ml.

REFERENCES

1 Hadler S, Webster H, Erben J et al. Hepatitis A in day-care centers: a communitywide assessment. N Engl J Med 1980; 302: 1222–1227.
2 Shapiro C, Margolis H. Worldwide epidemiology of hepatitis A virus infection. J Hepatol 1993; 18 (Suppl 2): S11–S14.
3 Innis B, Snitbhan R, Kunasol P et al. Protection against hepatitis A by an inactivated vaccine. JAMA 1994; 271: 1328–1334.
4 Werzberger A, Mensch B, Kuter B et al. A controlled trial of a formalin-inactivated hepatitis A vaccine in healthy children. N Engl J Med 1992; 327: 453–457.
5 Margolis H, Shapiro C. Considerations for the development of recommendations for the use of hepatitis A vaccine. J Hepatol 1993; 18 (Suppl 2): S56–S60.
6 Leentvaar-Kuijpers A, Continho R, Brulein V, Safary A. Simultaneous passive and active immunization against hepatitis A. Vaccine 1992; 10 (Suppl 1): S138–S141.
7 Krugman S, Giles J, Hamond J. Viral hepatitis, type B (MS–2) strain: studies on active immunization. JAMA 1971; 217: 41.
8 Szmuness W, Stevens C, Harley E et al. Hepatitis B vaccine: demonstration of efficacy in a controlled clinical trial in a high-risk population in the United States. N Engl J Med 1980; 303: 833–841.
9 Szmuness W, Stevens C, Zang E, Harley E, Kellner A. A controlled trial of the efficacy of the hepatitis B vaccine ('Heptavax'): a final report. Hepatology 1981; 1: 377–385.
10 Fortuin M, Chotard J, Jack A et al. Efficacy of hepatitis B vaccine in the Gambian expanded programme on immunisation. Lancet 1993; 341: 1129–1131.
11 Kruskall M, Alper C, Awdeh Z, Yunis E, Marcus-Bagley D. The immune response to hepatitis B vaccine in humans: inheritance patterns in families. J Exp Med 1992; 175: 495–502.
12 Milne A, Allwood G, Moyes C et al. Prevalence of hepatitis B infections in a multiracial New Zealand community. NZ Med J 1985; 98: 529–532.
13 Milne A, Moyes C. Hepatitis B carriage in children. NZ Med J 1983; 96: 238–241.
14 Burgess M, McIntosh E, Allars H, Kenrick K. Hepatitis B in urban Australian schoolchildren: no evidence of horizontal transmission between high risk and low risk groups. Med J Aust 1993; 159: 315–319.
15 Maynard J, Kane M, Hadler S. Global control of hepatitis B through vaccination: role of hepatitis B vaccine in the Expanded Programme on Immunization. Rev Infect Dis 1989; 2 (Suppl 3): S574–S578.
16 Carman W, Zanetti A, Karayiannis P et al. Vaccine-induced escape mutant hepatitis B virus. Lancet 1990; 326: 325–329.

17 Lau Y. Hepatitis B vaccination in preterm infants. Pediatr Infect Dis J 1994; 13: 243.
18 Diamant E, Schechter C, Hodes D, Peters V. Immunogenicity of hepatitis B vaccine in human immunodeficiency virus-infected children. Pediatr Infect Dis 1993; 12: 877–878.

CHAPTER 19

INFECTIONS IN TRAVELLERS

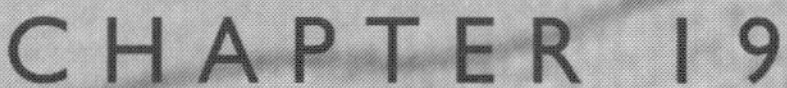

19.1. Infections in travellers: prevention and treatment

C. R. J. C. Newton   M. C. Steinhoff

19.1 Infections in travellers: prevention and treatment

INTRODUCTION

Infections, accidents (especially those involving motor vehicles) and exposure to extremes of temperature are the major risks to the health of children travelling abroad. Since infections are particularly common in children travelling to hot and temperate climates, this chapter provides succinct advice about the common infections acquired in these areas. Detailed discussion of these infections are available in standard sources.[1-7]

PREPARATION FOR TRAVEL

Pre-travel advice depends upon the age of the child, itinerary, duration and mode of travel, type of accommodation and access to medical facilities while abroad. The diseases to which a child may be exposed during travel can be determined.[7,8] Children travelling to tropical areas should be seen at least a month prior to departure, to ensure that all the necessary immunizations can be given. A dental examination is advisable if the journey is longer than 2 weeks.

Immunizations

Routine childhood immunizations (see Ch. 18.1) should be completed before travel. The schedule can be started earlier and the intervals can be shortened, to complete primary immunizations before departure (see Table 19.1.1). Further details of the vaccines against meningococcal disease, typhoid, rabies, hepatitis A and B, Japanese B encephalitis and yellow fever are discussed in the text. Tuberculosis is common in most developing countries, so a skin test and a BCG vaccine may be required (see Ch. 18.1). Cholera vaccine is no longer recommended for travellers since it provides limited protection of short duration, and no country requires it for entry (17). (New oral cholera vaccines are being developed, but are not available yet). Proof of vaccination should be carried by the travellers, to prevent obligatory vaccines being readministered, often under unhygienic conditions.

Medications

A medical kit should be assembled prior to departure (see Table 19.1.2 for a list of a basic kit). The contents will vary according to the destination and the time spent in foreign parts. A more extensive kit will be needed if the child has limited access to medical facilities; in particular a suture kit, ointments for burns and equipment for intravenous fluid administration, including blood transfusion, should be considered for long journeys. Potential blood donors can be identified by typing the blood group and performing a viral screen of the people travelling with the child.

Table 19.1.1   Recommendations for travellers to developing countries

Preventive measures[a]	Length of travel[b]			Comments
	Brief (<2 weeks)	Intermediate (2 weeks to 3 months)	Long-term residential (>3 months)	
Immunization				
Review and complete age-appropriate childhood schedule	+	+	+	See Chapter 18.1
H. influenzae type b	+	+	+	Any of three vaccines can be used in infants 2 months or older (see Ch. 18.2)
OPV	+	+	+	Can be started at birth with an extra newborn dose. Interval can be shortened to 4 weeks
DPT	+	+	+	1st dose may be given at 4 weeks, next two doses at intervals of 4 weeks and fourth dose 6 months after third dose
Measles	±	+	+	Extra dose given if first dose given at 6–11 months old
Hepatitis A	+	+	+	See text
Hepatitis B	±	±	+	Routine in USA
Yellow fever	+	+	+	For endemic areas
Typhoid	–	±	+	Indicated for travellers who will consume food at non-tourist facilities
Meningococcus	±	±	±	
Rabies	–	±	+	
Japanese B encephalitis	–	±	+	
Tuberculosis skin test (PPD)	±	+	+	
Chemoprophylaxis for malaria	+	+	+	

Adapted from Peter.[1]
[a] See text for details of endemic areas, dosage and schedules.
[b] '+', recommended; '±', consider; '–', not recommended.

Table 19.1.2   Medical kit

First aid kit	Plasters, sterile gauze pads, tape, sterile cotton, small scissors, tweezers, eye dropper
Equipment	Thermometers (two in case of breakage), sterile syringes and needles
Skin medications	Antiseptics (povidone iodine), antifungals (clotrimazole or nystatin), soothing lotions for sunburn. Hydrocortisone creams should be rarely used
Analgesics	Paracetamol, acetaminophen or ibufopen
Antihistamines	Diphenhydramine
Antibiotics	Erythromycin or trimethoprim–sulphamethoxazole
Motion sickness	Dimenhydrinate
Gastrointestinal medication	Oral rehydration fluid and loperamide
Ophthalmic	Sulphacetamide solution or erythromycin ointment
Ear medications	Antibiotic/antifungal combinations
Special requirements	Medication for specific diseases, e.g. epilepsy; or susceptibilities, e.g. allergy kit
Water purification	Water purification system, tablets
Infant	Feeding formulas, materials to clean and sterilize bottles
Personal protection	Sunscreen, insect repellents, mosquito net, car seats or seat belts

TRAVELLING

Food substances, mosquitoes and blood products are the main sources of serious infections in child travellers.

Water and food

Children should be given fluids that have been boiled and allowed to cool (fluids sterilized with tablets are less palatable to children). Infants should be breast-fed for as long as possible. Older children can quickly learn which water in the household is safe to drink and which water to avoid. Carbonated beverages and bottled water opened under observation are usually safe. The source of dairy products should be ascertained, since pasteurization processes in developing countries are often limited. Uncooked food, especially the childhood favourites, ice cream, sweets, desserts, salads and all items from street vendors, should be regarded with suspicion. Meat needs to be cooked thoroughly since the larval stages of worms may resist high temperatures. Cooked foods should be eaten while still warm and not reheated. Special attention should be given to the washing of eating utensils.

Insect and animal bites

Protecting children from insect bites is not only important for the prevention of serious mosquito-borne diseases, but also prevents minor skin lesions which may become infected. Most mosquitoes bite in the evening or at night. Appropriate clothing reduces the amount of skin exposed. Insect repellents are important: the most effective contains *N,N*-dimethyl-*m*-toluamide (DEET) in a 35% concentration. However, DEET should be used sparingly, since it can cause skin rashes and, if large quantities are absorbed, may induce seizures and neurological damage.[9] Bed nets, especially those impregnated with permethrin, are very effective in preventing bites from mosquitoes and other insects. All travellers to malarial areas should sleep under a bed net every night. Burning coils and soaps can be useful adjuncts, but do not replace the protection afforded by the above measures. Children should avoid contact with domestic animals, since they may be a source of worm infestations or rabies. Likewise children should not be allowed to touch insects, reptiles and aquatic animals, all of which can cause painful stings or bites — wounds that easily become infected.

Other considerations

In warm climates, cool, loose clothing worn during the day helps prevent heat rash and fungal infections. Wet nappies should be changed quickly. Footwear reduces the chance of worm infestation from the soil and prevents cuts, which easily become infected. Swimming in chlorinated pools or the sea is generally safe, but fresh water should be avoided and if unavoidable the children should keep their heads above the water to avoid oral ingestion of organisms. Anyone caring for the children or preparing their food should be free of infection and infestations and wash their hands frequently.

MALARIA

Malaria is a febrile illness caused by *Plasmodium* parasites which have been transmitted by a bite from an infected *Anopheles* mosquito. Four species infect humans (*P. falciparum*, *P. ovale*, *P. vivax* and *P. malariae*), but *P. falciparum* is the most serious, as it can cause rapidly progressive life-threatening disease, and the spread of drug-resistant strains has complicated treatment.

Prevention

The most important measure in preventing malaria is to avoid being bitten by the mosquitoes (see above). Chemoprophylaxis does not guarantee protection and the drugs may be difficult to administer to children. Ensuring that children are under bed nets early in the evening is mandatory.

The following factors need to be considered when choosing drugs for prevention and treatment of malaria:

1. The areas that the child will visit. The susceptibility of parasites to antimalarials varies considerably and the spread of chloroquine and sulphonamide-resistant falciparum parasites have limited the usefulness of these drugs in some areas. Up-to-date information should be obtained from national information centres.
2. A history of allergy or adverse reactions to antimalarial drugs, in particular sulphonamides.
3. Duration of stay in malarious areas, since some drugs are unsuitable for prolonged use, e.g. mefloquine.
4. Medical facilities available in the areas visited, as initial treatment may need to be started in the absence of diagnostic facilities.

    Table 19.1.3 lists the main antimalarial drugs, some of which may not be available in all countries. The unpalatable taste of the drugs used for prophylaxis may be masked by jam or honey.

Diagnosis

Malaria is often wrongly diagnosed during its early stages.[10] It should be suspected in any child who is travelling or has travelled in a malarial area within the last 3 months (and considered up to 3 years later) and who develops a fever associated with influenza-like symptoms, gastrointestinal disturbances or anaemia. Appropriately stained thick or thin blood films (Giemsa or Wright stains) confirm the diagnosis, and determine the species and the degree of parasitaemia, all of which influence management. New fluorescent tests are being developed. Films repeated every 6–12 h over a period of 48 h may be required to detect an infection. If the index of suspicion is high, presumptive treatment should be started immediately.

Severe falciparum malaria

Any child with falciparum malaria, who develops seizures, impairment of consciousness, respiratory distress, a rapidly dropping haemoglobin or has more than 5% of their red cells infected should be regarded as having severe malaria and treated with parenteral therapy (Table 19.1.3). The level of hydration needs to be assessed, but over-zealous fluid replacement should be avoided, as this may precipitate pulmonary oedema. Hypoglycaemia is common and should be detected with 4–6-hourly blood glucose estimations. Blood transfusions may be required for rapidly dropping haemoglobin levels or high parasitaemia. Exchange transfusion may be useful in children with hyperparasitaemia (>10%). Other adjunct therapies have not been adequately tested in children. Parenteral therapy should be continued for at least 24 h; oral therapy can be started when the child tolerates it. The regimen should be at least 5 days, although it can be shortened with the administration of a pyrimethamine/sulphadoxine combination. Malaria contracted in South East Asia may require more than 10 days of quinine and a course of clindamycin to eradicate the infection. Artemisinin and related compounds (artemether and artesunate) are effective against multi-resistant strains and are available in some South East Asian countries, but not elsewhere.

Table 19.1.3 Antimalarial drugs

Generic name	Formulation	Dose	Adverse effects
Prevention			
Chloroquine phosphate	500 mg salt (300 mg base) tablets Syrup: 50 mg base/5 ml	5 mg/kg base once weekly	Occasional: gastrointestinal upsets, headache, dizziness, blurred vision and pruritus Severe toxicity with overdose. May interfere with antibody response to human diploid rabies vaccine
Proguanil	100 mg tablets	3 mg/kg daily	Occasional: gastrointestinal upsets and mouth ulcers
Mefloquine	250 mg tablets	4 mg/kg weekly 15–19 kg ¼ tab 20–30 kg ½ tab 31–45 kg ¾ tab >45 kg 1 tab	Limited experience in children Frequent: gastrointestinal upset, bad dreams Rare: seizures
Presumptive treatment or treatment for non-severe malaria			
Pyrimethamine/ sulphadoxine	25 mg/ 500 mg tablets	Single dose 5–10 kg: ½ tab 11–20 kg: 1 tab 21–30 kg: 1½ tab 31–45 kg: 2 tab >45 kg: 3 tab	Occasional: gastrointestinal upsets and folate deficiency. Rare: Severe cutaneous reactions C/I infants < 2 months sulphonamide sensitivity
Mefloquine	250 mg tablets	20 mg base/kg in two divided doses, 6–8 h apart	See above
Halofantrine	250 mg tablets syrup	8 mg/kg 8-hourly for three doses, repeat regimen a week later	Occasional: gastrointestinal upsets, cough, rash Rare: cardiovascular toxicity, especially if used with mefloquine
Treatment for severe malaria			
Quinine dihydrochloride	300 or 500 mg/ml ampoules (122 mg = 100 mg base)	Loading dose of 15–20 mg/kg over 4 h, then 10 mg base/kg 12-hourly i.v.	Higher loading dose and more frequent administration are recommended in malaria contracted in SE Asia
Quinine sulphate	125 mg or 300 mg tablets (121 mg = 100 mg base)	10 mg base/kg 8-hourly p.o.	Well tolerated in children[10] Uncommon: tinnitus, vomiting, hypoglycaemia, cardiac arrhythmias,[11] neurotoxicity
Quinidine gluconate	Various formulations (230 mg = 200 mg base)	10 mg base/kg loading dose in normal saline over 1 h, followed by a continuous infusion 0.02 mg/kg per minute	Well tolerated in children[10]
Treatment of non-falciparum malaria			
Chloroquine phosphate	Same as above	10 mg/kg, 5 mg/kg 6 h later, followed by 5 mg/kg daily for two further doses	See above
Primaquine phosphate	5 or 7.5 mg tablets	0.3 mg/kg daily for 14 days (for eradication)	Frequently: diarrhoea and vomiting Haemolysis in G6PD-deficient individuals

Non-falciparum malaria

The other forms of malaria rarely present as life-threatening disease, although *P. vivax* is occasionally associated with splenic rupture or severe anaemia, and prolonged exposure to *P. malariae* with nephrotic syndrome. *P. vivax*, *P. ovale* and *P. malariae* are treated with chloroquine sulphate, except the chloroquine-resistant strains of *P. vivax* from Oceania which should be treated with other antimalarial drugs (Table 19.1.3). Primaquine phosphate is required to eradicate the *P. vivax* and *P. ovale* hypnozoites from the liver, but glucose 6-phosphate dehydrogenase deficiency should be excluded in susceptible groups before administering this drug, as it can precipitate severe haemolysis.

DIARRHOEAL DISEASE

Infectious gastroenteritis is very common both in travellers and long-term expatriate residents of developing countries. Up to 40% of European children developed acute diarrhoea during a 2-week trip to developing countries, particularly if they were less than 2 years old or travelled to India or North Africa.[11]

Causes

The most common cause of acute childhood diarrhoea worldwide is probably rotavirus, with the enterotoxigenic *Escherichia coli* (ETEC), *Campylobacter, Shigella* species, giardiasis, amoebiasis and rarely *Vibrio cholerae* accounting for most of the remaining disease (see Ch. 3.1). These organisms are usually acquired through faecally contaminated food and drink.

Children with diarrhoeal episodes should be offered clear fluids frequently, preferably oral rehydration fluids (see Ch. 3.1), which can be obtained in most regions. Loperamide reduces gut motility and inhibits gut fluid secretion and may be useful during actual travel but only in children >2 years.[12]

Antibiotic therapy

Most episodes of acute diarrhoea do not require antibiotic therapy, but the following situations should prompt antimicrobials:[13] (1) blood in stool (bacillary dysentery) which may be caused by *Shigella* and should be treated with trimethoprim–sulphamethoxazole for 3 days or furazolidone for 5 days depending on the local antibiotic sensitivity pattern; (2) profuse watery diarrhoea with rapid dehydration suggests cholera, which should be treated with a single dose of doxycycline, even in young children (a single dose does not stain teeth). Trimethoprim–sulphamethoxazole or furazolidone may also be used.

Diagnosis

Microbiological facilities for the diagnosis of prolonged or severe diarrhoea are often unavailable or unreliable in many developing regions, but if available stool microscopy may be useful. The presence of white cells suggest an invasive rather than toxigenic or viral organisms. Experienced microscopists can identify *Giardia species* or amoeba cysts — findings which provide a diagnosis with specific treatments (see Ch. 3.1). However, most therapy will be empirical.

Prevention

There are few vaccines (typhoid and cholera) that can prevent diarrhoeal disease, hence the most important preventive measures are careful attention to the child's food and drink (see above). Most authorities do not recommend cholera vaccine since the risk to travellers is low and the current vaccines have limited efficacy.[4,5] However, the new cholera toxin vaccine does provide limited protection against ETEC diarrhoea.[14] Prophylactic antibiotics are not recommended for child travellers.[15,16]

TYPHOID FEVER

Typhoid fever is a septicaemic illness in young children, who generally present with high fever, with or without diarrhoea, abdominal pain, headache, lethargy and cough. Examination may show splenomegaly, and even Rose spots, pink abdominal macules, but children can have no signs. Typhoid is an important differential diagnosis in a child with high, spiking fever recently returned from an endemic area in whom malaria has been excluded. Treatment is with IV cefotaxime or oral ciprofloxacin until sensitivities are available, because of increasing resistance.

This infection is difficult to avoid in regions of Latin America, Asia and Africa where typhoid fever is endemic. The recent emergence of *Salmonella* strains with multiple antibiotic resistance underscores the necessity for careful monitoring of the children's food and drink, and for immunization.

Three vaccines to prevent typhoid fever are now available. An oral typhoid vaccine with attenuated *S. typhi* is available for children older than 6 years of age. A capsule is taken with liquid 1 hour before meals on alternate days for 4 doses. Rare side effects include nausea, vomiting and rash, and efficacy is 60–90% in endemic areas. Re-immunization is recommended every 5 years for continuing exposure. (A liquid preparation was shown to be effective and safe in 1–5 year old children in Chile, but is not yet available.)

A new injectable vaccine consisting of the *S. typhi* Vi polysaccharide has been licensed for children 2 years and older. A single dose is associated with minimal side-effects, and provides 60 to 80% protection in endemic regions. Re-immunization every 2 years is recommended if exposure continues. See chapter 22 for treatment of typhoid.

MENINGOCOCCAL VACCINE

This vaccine is recommended for travellers to regions with endemic or epidemic meningococcal disease such as the sub-Saharan African meningitis belt, and Mecca during the Hajj. Vaccines incorporating capsular polysaccharides of meningococcal groups A, C, Y and W-135 are available, but there is no vaccine for meningococcal type B. The vaccine has high efficacy against type A meningococcal disease in infants as young as 3 months, and against type C in infants older than 24 months of age. Local and systemic reactions to the vaccine are rare. A single subcutaneous dose of 0.5 ml is recommended for protection.[1]

VIRAL INFECTIONS

The risk of exposure to hepatitis viruses A and B is greater in tropical countries than in temperate zones. Hepatitis A and B viruses are endemic in developing regions and are the most common vaccine-preventable illnesses in travellers; children may acquire either virus by direct contact with playmates.

Hepatitis B virus infection may be acquired through child-to-child transmission or through contact with infected body fluids. If hepatitis B immunization is not routine, the child should receive a full course (0, 1 month, 2–12 months) of hepatitis B vaccine before departure.

Hepatitis A virus is contracted from faecally contaminated food or water, or by child-to-child transmission. A vaccine consisting of inactivated hepatitis A virus is now available. For 2–18 year old children, two doses one month apart are required for primary immunization, with a booster at 6–12 months. The vaccine has been shown to be 94% effective with rare side-effects (see Ch. 18.3). Immunoglobulin G is highly effective and may be used in infants less than 2 years of age for passive protection against hepatitis A infection.

Hepatitis E is a water-borne virus which causes epidemics in Asia, Africa and Latin America. There is no vaccine for hepatitis E, and immunoglobulin prepared in North America or Europe is not protective. Prevention is by avoidance of faecally contaminated water and food.

Rabies

Rabies vaccination should be considered in children travelling in endemic areas (Central and South America, most of tropical Africa and Asia) particularly if they are likely to be exposed to domestic animals. Human diploid cell vaccine (HDCV) is recommended but other non-HDCV vaccines which are commonly available should not be used for pre-exposure prophylaxis (because of neurological complications). HDCV vaccine is often available at embassies in developing countries. The dose and schedule for pre-exposure and postexposure prophylaxis are the same as for adults;[4] for pre-exposure, three doses (1.0 ml) of HDCV intramuscularly or 0.1 ml intradermally (cheaper, but less effective) on days 0, 7 and 28. The vaccine may not be protective if the child is taking chloroquine or in young infants. A bite or scratch from a domestic or wild animal should be quickly and thoroughly washed with soap and water. If the animal is suspected of carrying rabies (usually dogs), rabies immune globulin (RIG) (20 IU/kg) is given to unvaccinated children, followed by a five-dose course of post-exposure prophylaxis: 0.1 ml i.m. on days 0, 3, 7, 14 and 28. Children who have received pre-exposure immunization should receive a further two doses of 0.1 ml i.m. on days 0 and 3 after exposure, and do not require RIG. Tetanus prophylaxis should also be considered after such an injury. HDCV vaccine is highly effective and all reported failures of HDCV vaccine in North America have been associated with lapses in wound care procedures, failure to use RIG or inadequate immunization.

Dengue fever

Dengue is caused by a mosquito-borne flavivirus and is a common illness of travellers and residents in the Caribbean, Central and South America, Southern Asia and the Pacific. Most episodes of primary dengue infection in young children occur as a mild febrile illness and are probably managed as an upper respiratory tract infection. Older children will often have a classic dengue illness with abrupt onset of fever, accompanied by headache, retro-orbital pain with eye movement, myalgia, arthralgia and a transient blanching macular rash. The fever may be biphasic with a reappearance at 7–10 days. Leucopenia is common, but platelet counts remain normal.

Some children will develop the dengue haemorrhagic fever–dengue shock syndrome (DHF-DSS) on the second to fifth day of illness, manifested by petechiae, ecchymoses and bleeding from venepuncture sites. Thrombocytopenia and bleeding is a cardinal sign of DHF, and DSS is diagnosed if the child becomes hypotensive or has a narrow (<20 mmHg) pulse pressure. The DHF-DSS syndrome is characterized by activation of the complement and haemostatic systems, and by increased vascular permeability.

Therapy for dengue fever is supportive. If DHF-DSS is suspected the child should be hospitalized and carefully managed with fluids for the shock and given blood transfusions if necessary. The period of shock usually lasts 48 h or less.

Although dengue vaccines are in development, none is available at present. Prevention is based on reducing exposure to *Aedes aegypti* mosquitoes (see section on insect and animal bites).

Japanese B encephalitis

Although the attack rate of this virus for travellers is said to be low, families who plan to spend more than a couple of weeks in rural rice-growing areas of the Indian subcontinent, Southeast Asia, China, Korea and Taiwan should consider receiving the new vaccine. Most cases of this mosquito-borne illness are asymptomatic, but the development of disease has a 30% risk of death or neurological sequelae. A killed virus vaccine is produced by Biken and distributed by Connaught. Three doses are required for immunization, and an efficacy of greater than 90% has been demonstrated in the endemic areas of Thailand.

Yellow fever

The mosquito-borne yellow fever virus is endemic in tropical Africa and Latin America, but not in Asia or the Pacific. The attenuated live yellow fever virus vaccine is required for travel to endemic regions, and has high efficacy and low incidence of local reactions. A single subcutaneous dose of 0.5 ml is recommended, with a booster every 10 years. The vaccine should not be given to infants < 9 months (who have an increased risk of encephalitis), persons with anaphylactic reactions to eggs, or those who are immunosuppressed.

LYMPHATIC FILARIASIS

Filaria are acquired from *Culex*, *Anopheles* and *Aedes* species mosquito bites in the endemic regions of Asia, Africa and South America. There is no multiplication of filaria in the host, so the extreme forms of disease with signs of lymphatic obstruction are seen only after prolonged exposure. Acute lymphatic inflammation may occur after months of constant exposure and tropical pulmonary eosinophilia (a syndrome characterized by chronic cough often with wheezing at night, with miliary mottling on chest X-ray and striking eosinophilia) may develop. Both syndromes respond to diethylcarbamazine. Prevention is by avoiding mosquito bites.

LEISHMANIA

Leishmaniasis is a group of infections caused by protozoa transmitted by sand flies. The clinical disease varies according to the protozoan species and the host's immune status; the cutaneous and visceral (kala-azar) forms are common. Treatment with antimony compounds is not uniformly effective,[2] and there are no vaccines. Measures to prevent sand fly bites are similar to those against mosquitoes.

WORM INFESTATIONS

Worm infestation is common in temperate and tropical countries. The risk of exposure can be reduced by avoiding contact with faecally contaminated soil and infested water. The symptoms and treatment of the most common worms are presented in Table 19.1.4. Eosinophilia is suggestive of helminth infections.

Schistosomiasis

Schistosomiasis is common throughout most of the tropical world; the species varies with geographical location. It is prevented by avoiding contact with infected water. Transient pruritic, purpuric rashes occur after initial exposure; thereafter a non-specific febrile illness develops (usually 3–12 weeks after

Table 19.1.4 Diagnosis and treatment of common worm infestations

Worm	Presentation	Diagnostic test	Treatment
Ascaris (*Ascaris lumbricoides*)	Usually asymptomatic. Transient pneumonitis. Intestinal obstruction. Peritonitis.	Ova in stool.	Mebendazole Pyrantel pamoate Albendazole
Pinworm, threadworm (*Enterobius vermicularis*)	Pruritus ani or vulvae. Rarely vaginitis, salpingitis or peritonitis.	Application of transparent adhesive tape to perianal skin.	Mebendazole Pyrantel pamoate
Trichinosis (*Trichinella sp.*)	Gastrointestinal symptoms, muscle pain, facial oedema and neurological symptoms.	Muscle biopsy for confirmation.	Mebendazole Thiabendazole Corticosteroids for the invasion of tissues
Hookworm Infections (*Necator americanus, Ancylostoma sp.*)	Pruritic papules, pneumonitis, gastrointestinal symptoms, iron deficiency anaemia, oedema.	Ova in stool.	Mebendazole Albendazole Pyrantel pamoate
Whip worm (*Trichuris trichiura*)	Usually asymptomatic. Gastrointestinal symptoms, rectal prolapse.	Eggs in stool.	Mebendazole Albendazole
Strongyloidiasis (*Strongyloides stercoralis*)	Usually asymptomatic, may cause pneumonitis, gastrointestinal symptoms or malabsorption. Overwhelming infection in immunocompromised hosts.	Repeated stool samples for larvae. String test or duodenal aspirate has better yield.	Thiabendazole
Cutaneous larva migrans (*Ancylostoma sp.*)	Red papules, followed by intensely pruritic serpiginous tracts.	None required, biopsy rarely indicated.	Self-limiting Treatment not usually required Larva can be killed with ethyl chloride spray or thiabendazole
Toxocariasis (*Toxocara canis* or *T. catis*)	Low-grade fever, hepatomegaly, pneumonitis, general ill-health. Loss of vision leading to strabismus, encephalitis.	Usually presumptive, rarely serological or tissue biopsy.	Diethylcarbamazine Thiabendazole
Trichostrongylus	Usually asymptomatic.	Eggs in the stool.	Thiabendazole Pyrantel pamoate

infection). *Schistosoma mansoni* and *S. japonicum* cause mucoid bloody diarrhoea, often accompanied by tender hepatomegaly, while *S. haematobium* causes dysuria, urgency, and terminal and gross haematuria. The diagnosis is confirmed by finding eggs in stool or concentrated mid-morning urine samples, although several specimens may need to be examined. Rectal biopsy may be necessary for *S. mansoni* or *S. japonicum*. Praziquantel is the drug of choice for all species. Oxamniquine as a single dose may be used for *S. mansoni* and a 2-week course of metrifonate for *S. haematobium*.

Cysticercosis

Cysticercosis is the presence of larval cysts of the pork tapeworm (*Taenia solium*), acquired by the ingestion of tape worm eggs, usually from food or beverages contaminated with faeces of someone with the adult tapeworm. The cysts may develop in any organ, but 60% of cases have brain cysts. Albendazole or praziquantel are effective therapy, although treatment is not always indicated. Instruction in personal hygiene and testing for egg secretion of the family's food handlers are practical approaches to family prevention.

Hydatid disease

Cystic hydatid disease is caused by the larval stage of *Echinococcus granulosus*, which are ingested as eggs, usually from dog faeces. Liver, lung, muscle, bone and brain are the most common sites of the cysts, which will sometimes require surgery. Albendazole is the recommended therapeutic drug. Prevention consists of chemotherapy of pet dogs and denying access of dogs to viscera.

OTHER DISEASES

Skin infections are common in travellers. Most are superficial bacterial or fungal infections which should be treated promptly since the infections tend to spread rapidly and lead to abscess formation. Ectoparasites, e.g. *Sarcoptes scabies* and lice are also common, and furuncular lesions caused by larval myiasis (tombu or bot flies) can be avoided by not leaving clothes to dry on the ground and ironing all clothes, including under-garments. Skin lesions often occur as part of worm infestations (e.g. Guinea worm disease) and tropical diseases. Eye infections are also common. Most are bacterial, but in some areas other causes are also common e.g. onchocerciasis in West Africa.

Other diseases such as trypanosomiasis and leprosy present with characteristic features, months to years after exposure. The management of these and other tropical diseases are described in excellent texts on tropical paediatrics.[2,3]

REFERENCES

1 Peter G (ed). Red book: report of the Committee on Infectious Diseases, 23rd edn. Elk Grove Village, IL: American Academy of Pediatrics, 1994.
2 Stanfield P, Brueton M, Chan M, Parrin M, Waterson T (eds). In: Diseases of children in the subtropics and tropics, 4th edn. London: Edward Arnold 1991.
3 Hendickse R G, Barr D G D, Matthews T S (eds). Paediatrics in the tropics. Oxford: Blackwell Scientific Publications, 1991.
4 Barry M. Medical considerations for international travel with infants and older children. Infect Dis Clin North Am 1992; 6: 389–404.
5 Preblud S R, Tsai T F, Brink E W, Nahlen B L, Parsonnet J. International travel and the child younger than two years: I. Recommendations for immunization. Pediatr Infect Dis J 1989; 8: 416–425.
6 Nahlen B L, Parsonnet J, Preblud S et al. International travel and the child younger than two years: II. Recommendations for prevention of travellers' diarrhoea and malaria chemoprophylaxis. Pediatr Infect Dis J 1989; 8: 735.
7 International travel and health: vaccination requirements and health advice. Geneva: World Health Organization, 1995.
8 Wilson M E. A world guide to infections: diseases, distribution, diagnosis. New York: Oxford University Press, 1991.
9 Roland E H, Jan J E, Rigg J M. Toxic encephalopathy in a child after brief exposure to insect repellents. Can Med Assoc J 1985; 132: 155–156.
10 McCaslin R I, Pikis A, Rodriguez W J. Pediatric Plasmodium falciparum malaria: a ten year experience from Washington, DC. Pediatr Infect Dis J 1994; 13: 709–715.
11 Pitzinger B, Steffen R, Tschopp A. Incidence and clinical features of traveller's diarrhoea in infants and children. Pediatr Infect Dis J 1991; 10: 719–723.
12 Diarrhoeal Disease Study Group. Loperamide in acute diarrhea in childhood: results of a double blind, placebo-controlled multicentre clinical trial. Br Med J 1984; 289: 1263.
13 DuPont H L, Ericsson C D. Prevention and treatment of traveller's diarrhoea. N Engl J Med 1993; 328: 1821–1827.
14 Peltola H, Siitonen A, Kyronseppa H et al. Prevention of travellers' diarrhoea by oral B-subunit/whole cell cholera vaccine. Lancet 1991; 338: 1285–1289.
15 Johnson P C, DuPont H L, Ericsson C D. Chemoprophylaxis and chemotherapy of travellers' diarrhoea in children. Pediatr Infect Dis 1985; 4: 620–621.
16 Reves R R, Johnson P C, Ericsson C D et al. A cost-effectiveness comparison of the use of antimicrobial agents for treatment or prophylaxis of travellers' diarrhoea. Arch Intern Med 1988; 148: 2421–2427.
17 *International Travel and Health 1995. Vaccination Requirements and Health Advice,* WHO, Geneva, 1995.

APPENDIX

Dosages of antihelminthics

Mebendazole	100 mg b.d. for 3 days, except for pinworm infection (100 mg one dose only) Not recommended for children < 2 years
Pyrantel palmoate	11 mg/kg one dose
Albendazole	Ascaris, hookworm and trichuriasis 400 mg single dose. Strongyloidiasis and taeniasis, 400 mg daily × 3 days, may need to be repeated 3 weeks later
Thiabendazole	25 mg/kg b.d. for 2 days (most worm infections), but for toxocariasis the course is 5 days
Diethylcarbamazine	3 mg/kg t.d.s. for 21 days for *Toxocara* sp.
Praziquantel	20 mg/kg b.d. for 1 day, except for *S. japonicum* same dose t.d.s.
Oxamniquine	10 mg/kg b.d. for 1 day
Metrifonate	10 mg/kg t.d.s. for 2 weeks

Dosage of antibiotics used in this chapter

Clindamycin HCl hydrate	3–6 mg/kg per day q.i.d.
Doxycline hyclate	6 mg/kg as a single dose for chlorea
Furazolidine	7.5 mg/kg/day q.i.d.
Trimethoprim–sulphamethoxazole	4 mg/kg of trimethoprim b.d.

ANTIBIOTIC ALLERGY

20.1. Allergic reactions to antibiotics

20.1   Allergic reactions to antibiotics

An adverse drug reaction may be defined as any undesirable and unintentional response that occurs at appropriate doses of a drug given for the therapeutic benefit of the patient. More than 90% of adverse drug reactions are non-immunologically mediated, leaving only 6–10% with an allergic or immunologically mediated basis.[1] Antibiotics, especially the penicillins and sulphonamides, account for a large proportion of allergic drug reactions. Although American figures suggest that 5% of adults in the USA may be allergic to one or more drugs, as many as 15% believe that they are, and therefore are frequently denied treatment with an indicated drug as well as providing their physicians with an added problem.[2]

RISK FACTORS

Risk factors for the clinical expression of antibiotic allergy include previous exposure (which may have been non-therapeutic, e.g. in utero, food products), age — with the greatest risk between ages 20 and 49 and a lower risk for children or the elderly — and route of administration, with allergic reactions to penicillin occurring more frequently following parenteral than oral administration.[3]

CLASSIFICATION

Allergic reactions to antibiotics can generally be classified according to the immunopathological reactions proposed by Gell and Coombs.[4] However, a more clinically useful classification may be that of Levine, who proposed classifying adverse reactions to penicillin according to their time of onset (Table 20.1.1).[5]

IS THIS REALLY AN ANTIBIOTIC ALLERGY?

The diagnosis of antibiotic allergy is almost never clear-cut. When a physician is faced with a possible drug reaction, it is often not clear whether the symptoms are due to the patient's underlying condition or to the treatment. For example, a rash may be caused by the underlying infection or by an antibiotic allergy. Rashes are the commonest manifestations of drug allergy and can take almost any form, including urticaria, maculopapular or morbilliform eruptions, erythema multiforme, photosensitivity and fixed eruptions. The most severe drug-related cutaneous reactions are exfoliative dermatitis and vesiculobullous eruptions such as Stevens–Johnson syndrome and toxic epidermal necrolysis (Lyell's syndrome).

Table 20.1.1 Classification of allergic reactions based on their time of onset

Reaction type	Onset	Clinical reactions
Immediate	0–1 h	Anaphylaxis Hypotension Laryngeal oedema Urticaria/angioedema Wheezing
Accelerated	1–72 h	Urticaria/angioedema Laryngeal oedema Wheezing
Late	>72 h	Morbilliform rash Interstitial nephritis Haemolytic anaemia Neutropenia Thrombocytopenia Serum sickness Drug fever Stevens–Johnson syndrome Exfoliative dermatitis

Trimethoprim–sulphamethoxazole is most commonly associated with allergic skin reactions, causing a rash in 5.9% of recipients in one large study, followed by ampicillin, which caused a skin reaction in 5.2%.[6] Urticaria may occur alone or as part of a serum sickness reaction. Almost any drug can be involved, but in children the penicillins are the most common cause. However, urticaria and maculopapular rashes may also occur as a result of viral infections, and an antibiotic may be wrongly implicated as the cause of the rash. Stevens–Johnson syndrome and Lyell's syndrome are usually regarded as more severe drug reactions in which drugs are causally related in approximately 40% of cases,[7] with sulphonamides and penicillins being the most frequently associated antibiotics. However, infectious agents alone may produce similar skin reactions with drug-induced toxic epidermal necrolysis and staphylococcal scalded skin syndrome being clinically indistinguishable. Kawasaki disease must also be considered in the differential diagnosis of Stevens–Johnson syndrome.

The history of the events surrounding the onset of the adverse reaction is often most important in making the diagnosis. The historical analysis of a possible antibiotic allergy should include:

1. Clinical classification of the reaction.
2. Immunopathological classification of the reaction.
3. Compilation of a complete list of possible causes.
4. Consideration of the known propensities of the possible drugs to cause such a reaction.
5. Proximity of the onset of therapy to the onset of the reaction and previous exposure to the drug: in general, primary immune responses take several days to lead to a clinical reaction and medications in use over long periods are less likely to be a problem than recently introduced agents.

LABORATORY DIAGNOSIS

There is no single test for antibiotic allergy. A basic problem in diagnosing antibiotic allergy by immunological methods is the fact that most antibiotics are not complete antigens but rather haptenic metabolites of the parent drug, coupled with a carrier tissue protein and, except for penicillin, immunoreactive drug metabolites have rarely been identified.

IDENTIFICATION OF PATIENTS AT RISK

Penicillin

To be clinically useful, a test should be rapid, specific, sensitive and safe. At present, skin testing is the only immunodiagnostic method which satisfies these criteria and effectively identifies nearly all patients at risk for an allergic reaction caused by IgE antibodies.[9] Immediate hypersensitivity skin testing is therefore of definite value in assessing hypersensitivity to certain antibiotics, primarily penicillin. It should be realised that most non-pruritic maculopapular rashes will not be predicted by skin testing as they are not caused by IgE antibodies. Approximately 95% of penicillin molecules which become conjugated to carriers and thus become immunoreactive antigens are in the penicilloyl configuration.[10] The remaining 5% of conjugates are in a variety of forms, collectively referred to as minor determinants. Skin testing for penicillin allergy should be done with penicilloyl poly-L-lysine (PPL, marketed as Pre-Pen, Kremers-urban, Milwaukee, WI) and penicillin G (Pen G), giving a 95% sensitivity. Skin testing can provoke a systemic reaction, but such reactions are rare and usually not severe.[7]

Radioallergosorbent (RAST) tests are less sensitive and less informative than skin testing to penicillin allergens, take longer to complete and are expensive. Most important, a negative test is of little value because marked clinical sensitivity may still be present in RAST-negative patients. In general, RAST tests should only be used in patients who cannot be skin-tested. RAST assays for serum IgE to cephalosporins, sulphonamides, trimethoprim[11] and other antimicrobials have been reported, but at present have limited availability. Skin testing can identify patients who have a history of allergic reactions to penicillin, but who are no longer sensitive and can thus be treated with the antibiotic of choice when a penicillin is indicated. There is, however, a risk of resensitization which varies from less than 1% to 10% according to route of administration.[12,13]

Reactions to penicillin in history-positive, skin test-negative patients do occur, but the risk is very slight, with mild allergic reactions occurring in 1–3% and anaphylaxis in < 0.1%.

Other β-lactam antibiotics

Semi-synthetic penicillins such as ticarcillin and piperacillin contain the same nucleus as penicillin G, hence sensitivity to these antibiotics can be assessed by skin testing to penicillin. Cephalosporins share a common β-lactam ring with the penicillins and early retrospective studies reported that patients with a history of penicillin allergy were up to eight times more likely to have an allergic reaction when given a cephalosporin than those without a history of penicillin allergy.[14,15] However, a positive history of penicillin allergy was confirmed by skin testing in only 25% of cases. The degree of clinical cross-reactivity of cephalosporins with penicillins remains unresolved but is proving much lower than was previously thought, with an adverse reaction rate of 3–7% for cephalosporins in patients with positive histories of penicillin allergy.[16] The predictive value of skin testing to cephalosporins themselves has not been adequately determined. Monobactams such as aztreonam may be safely administered to penicillin-allergic subjects but carbapenems such as imipenem represent a significant risk to penicillin-allergic patients and should be withheld from penicillin skin test-positive patients.

ANTIBIOTIC REACTIONS FREQUENTLY ENCOUNTERED IN CHILDREN

Penicillin

Penicillin is the most common cause of serious allergic drug reactions in children as in adults. The vast majority of penicillin-allergic individuals will be identified by testing with PPL and Pen G. Skin testing should be done by an experienced person in a place where appropriate emergency equipment is available, since the skin test itself can cause anaphylaxis in patients with extreme penicillin allergy. A history of penicillin allergy does not necessarily imply that a patient is actually sensitive. In a group of children aged 9 months to 14 years with a historical diagnosis of penicillin allergy, only 10% exhibited a positive reaction to both major and minor penicillin determinants.[17] Skin testing was more commonly positive in patients with systemic anaphylaxis or urticaria within 24 h of penicillin administration and who were tested within 1 year of their reaction.

Patients having a maculopapular rash (common in children) usually have a negative penicillin skin test. If the skin tests are positive, the patient should be considered allergic to penicillin. If the skin tests are negative, the results weigh against penicillin allergy but *do not rule it out*. These patients should be challenged cautiously and under controlled conditions with penicillin if they need this antibiotic. Oral challenge is considered safest. If a penicillin must be given to a patient with proven penicillin allergy then desensitization is necessary. This process involves administering gradually increasing amounts of drug over a short period of time whilst controlling any allergic reactions with subcutaneous adrenaline as necessary.

Most experience has been with penicillin desensitization and there are various protocols for the oral, subcutaneous and intravenous routes. The intravenous route offers better control than the subcutaneous route and is probably preferable (Table 20.1.2). Similar procedures may be used for desensitization to other antibiotics. A general principle is to start the desensitization procedure with 1/10 000 of the final dose (e.g. if the final dose of penicillin G is to be 1 g every 6 h then you start with 0.1 mg which can be given as a 1 ml aliquot of a solution of 1 mg penicillin G in 10 ml of normal saline).

Table 20.1.2   Protocol for intravenous desensitization of penicillin-allergic patients

Step[a]	Penicillin G (mg in 10 ml saline)[b]	Volume given (ml)	Dose given (mg)
1	1	1	0.1
2	1	2	0.2
3	1	4	0.4
4	1	8	0.8
5	10	1	1
6	10	2	2
7	10	4	4
8	10	8	8
9	100	1	10
10	100	2	20
11	100	4	40
12	100	8	80
13	1000	1	100
14	1000	2	200
15	1000	4	400
16	1000	8	800
17	1000	10	1000

[a] Interval between doses 15 min.
[b] For the more dilute concentrations of penicillin G it is useful to dilute 1 gram of the antibiotic in 1 litre of normal saline, giving a concentration of 1 mg/ml.

Ampicillin

A maculopapular rash due to ampicillin is one of the most common cutaneous adverse drug reactions, occurring in 5–10% of children.[18] When ampicillin is administered to patients with infectious mononucleosis, the incidence of rash increases dramatically and in one study reached 100%.[19] Several investigations have attempted to determine whether the rash in this setting is an allergic response to ampicillin or the result of a two stage process in which Epstein–Barr virus (EBV) initiates a biological response and causes an immunological reaction that results in a rash when ampicillin is administered.

The biological mechanisms of the EBV–ampicillin interaction are not completely understood but the consensus at present is that an IgE-mediated mechanism is not involved and that children with ampicillin rash are highly unlikely to develop an immediate or accelerated reaction following penicillin or ampicillin therapy in the future.[20] Urticarial eruptions due to ampicillin, on the other hand, are more likely to be on an allergic basis and subsequent administration of penicillin or ampicillin in such patients may induce a severe allergic reaction.[21]

Vancomycin

The use of vancomycin in hospital settings is increasing because of the rising incidence of infections caused by methicillin-resistant staphylococci. The most common adverse effect of vancomycin is the 'red-man' syndrome,[22] a constellation of signs and symptoms characterized by pruritis, erythema and flushing of the upper body, angioedema and rarely cardiovascular depression. This is an example of a pseudo-allergic drug reaction, as the vancomycin acts directly on mast cells and basophils to cause the release of histamine. The rate of infusion is believed to be the most important risk factor for this reaction.[23]

Multiple antibiotic sensitivity

When there is a history of antibiotic allergy, the usual advice given is to use an alternative drug. However, there are some patients who develop allergic reactions to more than one antibiotic, i.e. multiple antibiotic sensitivity (MAS). In a review of MAS in a paediatric population,[24] the most commonly implicated drugs were the β-lactam antibiotics, closely followed by the sulphonamides. A history of atopic disease was common in patients with MAS. Rashes were the most commonly encountered reactions, with urticaria being the most frequent of these. The structures of the drugs involved are quite diverse, as are the clinical patterns of the reactions, suggesting that MAS is not simply a consequence of the atopic predisposition to form IgE antibodies, but may also depend on other aspects of the host immune response.

CONCLUSIONS

1. Avoid the use of antibiotics associated with prior reactions when an alternative antibiotic of equal efficacy can be found.
2. Immunodiagnostic tests are at present only readily available for IgE-mediated penicillin allergy. Negative skin tests indicate that the risk of a life-threatening reaction to penicillin is negligible. Positive skin tests indicate a high risk of an immediate or accelerated allergic reaction.
3. The maculopapular rash associated with ampicillin is not IgE-mediated and future administration of ampicillin or penicillin does not imply an increased risk of an immediate reaction. This does not apply to an urticarial rash secondary to ampicillin.
4. The best treatment for any kind of drug reaction is to discontinue the drug

promptly and to warn about future exposure to the same drug and cross-reacting drugs.

5. Desensitization is necessary in patients who are allergic to an antibiotic and who *must* be given that antibiotic in the absence of an appropriate alternative. If penicillin or a cross-reacting β-lactam antibiotic is required, administration of the drug should be carried out using an acute desensitization protocol, which substantially reduces the risk of a serious allergic reaction. Desensitization for antibiotics other than penicillin follows similar principles but is still an unproven therapy.

REFERENCES

1 Boston Collaborative Drug Surveillance Program. Drug-induced anaphylaxis: a cooperative study. JAMA 1973; 224: 613–615.
2 De Swarte R D. Drug allergy: problems and strategies. J Allergy Clin Immunol 1984; 74: 209–332.
3 Sullivan T J, Yecies L D, Shatz G S, Parker C W, Wedner H J. Desensitization of patients allergic to penicillin using orally-administered beta-lactam antibiotics. J Allergy Clin Immunol 1982; 69: 275–282.
4 Gell P G H, Coombs R R A. Classification of allergic reactions responsible for clinical hypersensitivity and disease. In: Gell P G H, Coombs R R A, Lachmann P J, eds. Clinical aspects of immunology. Philadelphia: Davis, 1968: pp 575–596.
5 Levine B B. Immunologic mechanisms of penicillin allergy: a haptenic model system for the study of allergic diseases of man. N Engl J Med 1966; 275: 1115–1125.
6 Arndt K A, Jick H. Rates of cutaneous reactions to drugs: a report from the Boston Collaborative Drug Surveillance Program. JAMA 1976; 235: 918.
7 Bottiger L E, Strandberg J, Westerholm B. Drug-induced febrile mucocutaneous syndrome with survey of the literature. Acta Med Scand 1975; 198: 229.
8 Sullivan T J. Drug allergy. In: Middleton E, Reed C E, Ellis E F, Adkinson N F, Yunginger J W, eds. Allergy: principles and practice. St Louis: C V Mosby, 1988: pp 1523–1530.
9 Sullivan T J , Wedner H J, Shatz G S, Yecies L D, Parker C W. Skin testing to detect penicillin allergy. J Allergy Clin Immunol 1981; 68: 171–180.
10 Parker C W. Practical aspects of diagnosis and treatment of patients who are hypersensitive to drugs. In: Samter M, ed. Hypersensitivity to drugs. New York: Pergamon Press, 1972: p 307.
11 Harle D G, Baldo B A, Smal M A, Van Nunen S. An immuno assay for the detection of IgE antibodies to trimethoprim in the sera of allergic patients. Clin Allergy 1987; 17: 209–216.
12 Parker P J, Parinello J T, Condemi J J, Rosenfoed S I. Penicillin resensitization among hospitalised patients. J Allergy Clin Immunol 1991; 88: 213–217.
13 Mendelson L M, Ressler C, Rosen J P, Selcon J E. Routine elective penicillin allergy skin testing in children and adolescents: study of sensitization. J Allergy Clin Immunol 1984; 73: 70–81.
14 Anderson J A. Cross-sensitizing to cephalosporins in patients allergic to penicillin. Pediatr Infect Dis 1986; 5: 557–561.
15 Thoburn R, Johnson J E III, Cluff L E. Studies on the epidemiology of adverse drug reactions. IV. The relationship of cephalothin and penicillin allergy. JAMA 1966; 198: 345–348.
16 Saxon A, Beal G N, Rohr A S, Adelman D C. Immediate hypersensitivity reactions to beta-lactam antibiotics. Ann Intern Med 1987; 107: 204–216.
17 Bierman C W, Van Arsdel P P Jr. Penicillin allergy in children: the role of immunologic tests in its diagnosis. J Allergy 1969; 43: 267–271.
18 Kerns D L, Shira J E, Sumio G, Summers R J, Schwab J A, Plunket D C. Ampicillin rash in children. Am J Dis Child 1973; 125: 187–190.
19 Patel B M. Skin rash with infectious mononucleosis and ampicillin. Pediatrics 1967; 40: 910–911.
20 Haverkos H W, Amsel Z, Drotman D P. Adverse virus–drug interactions. Rev Infect Dis 1991; 13: 697–704.
21 Bierman C W, Pierson W E, Zeitz S J, Hoffman L S, Van Arsdel P P. Reactions associated with ampicillin therapy. JAMA 1972; 220: 1098–1100.

22 Garrelts J C, Peterie J D. Vancomycin and the 'red-man's syndrome'. N Engl J Med 1985; 312: 245.
23 Polk R E, Healy D P, Schwartz L B, Rock D T, Garson M L, Roller K. Vancomycin and the red-man syndrome: pharmacodynamics of histamine release. J Infect Dis 1988; 157: 502–507.
24 Kamada M M, Twarog G, Leung D Y M. Multiple antibiotic sensitivity in a pediatric population. Allergy Proc 1991 12: 347–351.

CHAPTER 21

TROPICAL

21.1. Infectious diseases in developing countries

21.1 Infectious diseases in developing countries

INTRODUCTION

The burden of disease in children of developing countries is mainly infectious diseases, and the chief causes of morbidity and mortality are common conditions like malaria, diarrhoeal diseases, acute respiratory infections, malnutrition and now AIDS. Paediatrics is greatly influenced by the site of practice, probably more by economic factors than by geography or climate. In other words, paediatrics in the developing world is above all a medicine of poverty, in both the sense that we treat patients from *poor* families and have *poor* resources for the task. These countries have high childhood mortality, high fertility, low income (gross national product or GNP per capita), extremely limited resources available for health, and a high prevalence of childhood infectious diseases.

Medical discussion in developing countries tends to be dominated by Western textbooks and technology, and even 'tropical' books tend to discuss issues in an idealized context which bears little relation to the reality of crowded and chaotic children's wards. Consequently, this discussion will attempt to reflect the reality of paediatric practice at district or provincial hospitals, primarily in Africa, with limited nursing care, drug supplies and laboratory facilities. For good clinical practice in this context, it is essential to adopt a critical attitude to the clinical data and be painstaking about accurate diagnoses. This is an arduous task in view of late presentations of disease, polypharmacy, and laboratory results which are often unavailable or inaccurate. Deficient primary care medicine in many developing countries has resulted in an emphasis on diagnostic algorithms, scoring systems, uniform case management, essential drugs and training courses for health workers. This attention is welcome, but the approaches adopted may be inappropriate if they ignore local knowledge, 'bedside' supervision and clinical judgement.

Another key feature of paediatric practice in developing countries is variability, which unduly complicates the task of generalizing about infectious diseases. Despite these differences between developing countries, uniformity of approach (and rhetoric) dominates discussions of case management and health care by WHO, UNICEF and other donor agencies. The need for local solutions to site-specific problems needs to be continually reinforced.[1]

Although written from a clinical perspective, this chapter also seeks to give a community perspective and deal with preventive child health programmes, instead of limiting discussion to the hospital context.

HUMAN IMMUNODEFICIENCY VIRUS INFECTION

Epidemiology

The HIV epidemic has transformed the face of paediatrics in Africa, and Asia will soon follow. The prognosis of clinical presentations such as malnutrition, chronic diarrhoea, pneumonia, and tuberculosis is clouded by the spectre of HIV, and hospitals are overwhelmed with cases. In Africa, unlike America, paediatric AIDS accounts for as many as 15–20% of all AIDS cases. However, this may not be reflected in paediatric mortality rates in hospital, which are often as high as 10–15% of admissions in Africa, because HIV cases tend to be chronically ill and go home for traditional remedies if not responding to 'Western' treatment. In any case, most childhood deaths in Africa have always taken place outside hospital.

Over the next decade it is estimated that 2.7 million children worldwide will die and an additional 5.5 million children may be orphaned because of AIDS.[2] This is particularly disheartening because many developing countries have made substantial progress in improving child health over recent decades by means of more widespread use of immunizations, oral rehydration solutions, antibiotics and antimalarials as well as improved living standards. But high rates of perinatal HIV transmission are threatening much of the progress in child survival in developing countries over recent decades.

HIV infection is also causing profound disruption of families due to death or disease of parents and the resulting decline in socioeconomic status. Of particular concern is the increasing number of children orphaned by AIDS. They have traditionally been relocated within the extended family network, but this is becoming overwhelmed by the large numbers of children needing care, particularly infants needing to be breast-fed. Even uninfected infants of HIV-positive (HIV+) mothers fare badly, because sick mothers cannot breast-feed and care adequately for their infants. In addition, the lack of effective therapy for HIV creates distrust in the health care system, and increases vulnerability of cases to unverified claims of cures by traditional or unscrupulous practitioners.

Transmission

The median rate of mother-to-child (vertical) transmission of HIV-1 is 24–29% (range 13–40%), with the higher rates tending to be from the developing world.[2] For unknown reasons, HIV-2 has a considerably lower rate of vertical transmission. It is the mother's viral load which seems to correlate best with the risk of transmission which is highest in the early and late stages of infection. Most perinatal transmission seems to occur around the time of delivery so prolonged exposure to the birth canal during labour and delivery could be an important risk factor for vertical transmission.[3] Consequently, an intervention trial of vaginal irrigation with an antiseptic during labour and delivery was carried out in Malawi by the Johns Hopkins University project; this failed to affect transmission, but documented by PCR a transmission rate of approximately 27% at birth.

Since 30% of mothers are HIV-infected in Blantyre, Malawi, it means that around 10% of all births are infected by mother-to-infant transmission either at birth or from breast-feeding. Low vitamin A levels in mothers was associated with higher transmission, so is being investigated by an intervention trial.[4] Zidovudine treatment in pregnancy reduces vertical transmission, but is too expensive for African countries.[5] Although lowering vertical transmission is an important objective, it may not accomplish much if the mother dies before the uninfected infant is able to survive without her. An important issue is whether the higher risk of vertical transmission of HIV in developing countries is due to breast-feeding. Analysis of five studies showed that when the mother was infected prenatally, the additional risk of transmission through breast-feeding, over and above transmission in utero or during delivery, was 14% (95% CI 7–22%).[6] Preliminary evidence from follow-up studies in Africa using PCR suggest the additional risk from breast-feeding may be as low as 8%. Since breast-feeding offers considerable protection against infant deaths from infectious diseases, it is still recommended in developing countries with high infant mortality from infectious diseases, despite the additional risk of HIV transmission. This is vital, because infants of poor families who are deprived of breast milk almost never survive in Africa and artificial feeding is not a viable option.

Blood transfusion for severe anaemia is another important risk factor for HIV transmission. This mode of transmission accounted for up to 15% of cases in a study from Zaire[7] and, unlike haemophiliacs in developed countries, is still an important mode of transmission in areas of Africa which transfuse without enzyme-linked immunosorbent assay (ELISA) screening. The emergence of chloroquine resistance has increased the risk of severe malarial anaemia, which occurs mainly in children under 2 years who present acutely in congestive heart failure, so decreasing the rate of blood transfusion in this context is very difficult.[8,9] Nevertheless, there is still a tendency to overuse blood transfusions for chronic anaemias, which can only be countered by establishing accurate diagnoses of the cause of anaemia based on blood films.

Clinical features

WHO has proposed a clinical case definition of paediatric AIDS where diagnostic resources are limited, requiring two major and two minor signs in the absence of other known causes of immunosuppression. The major signs are weight loss or slow growth, chronic diarrhoea and persistent fever. The minor signs include lymphadenopathy, candidiasis, recurrent infections, persistent cough, dermatitis and confirmed maternal HIV infection. This case definition has been criticized as designed for epidemiological surveillance but inadequate clinically due to a low positive predictive value (38%). It also ignores important historical data about the health of parents or siblings, TB contacts and whether the child is still breast-fed, which play an important part in clinical decision-making.

The mean birth weight of infants of HIV+ mothers averages about 100 g lower than for seronegative (HIV−) mothers, and there is no difference in birthweight between infected and uninfected (seroreverted) infants of HIV+ mothers. However, infected infants falter in growth from as early as 4 months of age.

A striking feature of paediatric HIV infection is that children under 6 months of age have a poor prognosis. This is partly due to *Pneumocystis carinii* pneumonia (PCP) in infancy, but at this age any AIDS-related complication has a shorter survival time. Table 21.1.1 is modified from the New York State Medicaid study of 789 AIDS children, demonstrating the importance of age and HIV-

Table 21.1.1 Gradient of severity of paediatric HIV complications and recommended treatment categories

	Treatment category[a]
Level 1 complications	
[HIV infection itself]	3
Impetigo/atopic dermatitis/eczema	1
Upper respiratory tract infection	1
Malaria (anaemia, cerebral, uncomplicated)	1
Intestinal helminths/giardiasis	1
Molluscum contagiosum	1
Congenital syphilis	1
Congenital toxoplasmosis	2
Asthma/bronchospasm	1
Urinary tract infection/cystitis	1
Cutaneous cellulitis/abscess	1
Gastroenteritis/dysentery	1

Table 21.1.1 (*contd*)

	Treatment category[a]
Level 1 complications (*contd*)	
Dental/periodontal infection	1
Dermatomycosis	1
Sinusitis/otitis media	1
Mucocutaneous candidiasis	1
Herpes stomatitis	4
Hepatosplenomegaly/lymphadenopathy/parotitis	3
Lymphoid interstitial pneumonitis	1
Level 2 complications	
Lobar/atypical (non-opportunistic) pneumonia	1
Thrombocytopenia	3
Anaemia/neutropenia	2
Varicella/measles (may be haemorrhagic)	1
Unspecified hepatitis	2
Chronic herpes zoster	4
RSV bronchiolitis/pneumonia	1
Bronchiectasis	2
Persistent diarrhoea/abdominal distension	2
Bone and joint infection	2
Pyelonephritis	2
Visceral abscess	2
Pulmonary tuberculosis > 2 years	1
< 2 years	2
Septicaemia	1
Meningitis	2
Gram-negative pneumonia/empyema	2
Chronic herpes simplex	4
Encephalitis (? herpes)	3
Pericardial effusion	2
Primary/secondary seizures	2
Cryptosporidiosis	3
Isosporiasis	1
Malabsorption	3
Fever of unknown origin	2
Level 3 complications	
Failure to thrive/wasting and stunting	2
Dementia/encephalopathy	3
Miliary tuberculosis	2
Tuberculous meningitis	2
Cardiomyopathy/myocarditis	2
Chronic renal disease (nephritis/nephrosis)	4
Cryptococcal meningitis	4
P. carinii pneumonia	2
Measles croup/pneumonia	2
Candida oesophagitis	2
Central nervous system abscess	2
Protozoal encephalitis	4
Progressive multifocal leukoencephalopathy	3
Atypical mycobacterial infection	3
Renal/respiratory failure	4
Kwashiorkor/protein-energy malnutrition	1 (oedema), 2 (wasting)
Disseminated toxoplasmosis/CMV/herpes/mycosis	4
Malignant tumours	4

[a] Treatment categories:
1. Give standard treatment, and expect resolution.
2. Give (inexpensive) standard treatment, but of transient or dubious value.
3. No effective specific treatment is available.
4. Effective specific treatment is too expensive, so give only symptomatic or palliative treatment and allow home.

related complications for prognosis, since the level 1 complications presented at a median age of 22 months and survived 66 months, compared to 7 and 9 months respectively for level 3.[10]

In Blantyre, Malawi, where at least 30% of antenatal mothers are HIV+, the common presentations of HIV infection that we recognize in hospitalized children under 2 years are:

1. Interstitial pneumonia in well-nourished infants of 3–9 months, often with marked tachypnoea and frothy sputum, but no wheezes or crackles in the chest, and usually no hepatosplenomegaly or lymphadenopathy (probable PCP).
2. Extreme failure to thrive at around a year of age, with severe wasting and stunting (usually weighing 4–6 kg).
3. Marasmus or marasmic kwashiorkor in a breast-fed child.
4. An increase in serious bacterial infections in infancy, particularly meningitis and pneumonia.

But uninfected infants of ill mothers with AIDS, who are not producing enough breast milk, may also present with malnutrition. Unfortunately, it is not possible to be sure that they are uninfected, until the ELISA test reverts to negative by about 12 months of age. In a study of 519 admissions to the nutrition ward,[11] we found that HIV infection was associated with marasmus and marasmic kwashiorkor, but not with kwashiorkor (which accounted for 38.5% of admissions). Compared to seronegative cases of malnutrition, HIV+ cases were more likely to be still breast-fed, to be both wasted and stunted, and to have sick parents. Surprisingly, a history of persistent diarrhoea, and the presence of oral thrush and lymphadenopathy were not significantly different between HIV+ and HIV– cases. Although hepatosplenomegaly was more common in HIV+ malnutrition, it was still less common than in well-nourished controls, in whom hepatosplenomegaly was related to endemic malaria.

The developing central nervous system (CNS) of children is unusually susceptible to HIV infection, and encephalopathy is common in both developing and developed countries. The usual clinical manifestations are neurodevelopmental delay, particularly gross motor retardation, microcephaly, seizures and subtle changes in muscle tone. HIV encephalopathy is less recognized in the developing world, possibly because affected infants die before severe neurological manifestations develop, or are missed because developmental assessment is not done. Non-suppurative parotitis, pericardial effusion, myocarditis, pericarditis and chronic dermatitis are other helpful diagnostic features of HIV. In high prevalence regions, virtually any unusual clinical presentation needs to have HIV excluded, since an unusual HIV picture is more likely than a rare disease with typical features. However, there is still considerable resistance to HIV testing from many quarters.

Opportunistic infections

Although the incidence and course of infections such as malaria, respiratory syncytial virus (RSV) and rotavirus do not seem to be worsened by HIV, bacterial infections with non-typhoidal salmonella, pneumococci and other common bacteria are more common in HIV+ cases. But the pattern of opportunistic infections is characterized by unusual organisms such as cryptococcus, pneumocystis, cryptosporidium, toxoplasmosis, isosporiasis, histoplasmosis, coccidiomycosis as well as more usual organisms like candida and herpes (see Table 21.1.1). Unfortunately, most of these organisms are difficult to document, and some also occur with (HIV-negative) malnutrition. Indeed, the already difficult microbiological diagnosis of opportunistic infections in the developing country context is made even more difficult by atypical presentations due to immunosuppression. Although HIV-related bacterial infections are usually treatable in developed countries, this is not so obviously the case in the developing world, where bacterial sepsis is far more common, and fulminant or late presentations with a high mortality are common.

Although common enteric pathogens are isolated equally from HIV+ and HIV– children with diarrhoea, the risk of progression to persistent diarrhoea is five to six times greater in HIV+ infants, and two to four times greater in seronegative infants of infected mothers, compared to controls. But the usual story in HIV+ children is of diarrhoea on and off, so they also have a two-fold risk of recurrent episodes of diarrhoea and an overall 11-fold increased risk of mortality from diarrhoeal disease. The usual enteric organisms associated with HIV are *Cryptosporidium*, microsporidia, *Isospora belli* and cytomegalovirus (CMV), but possibly also astrovirus, calicivirus, *Blastocystis hominis*, atypical mycobacteria and adenovirus.[12] Mucosal damage has also been documented in HIV infection.[13]

A recent postmortem study of 77 HIV+ children under 8 years (median age 17 months) in Ivory Coast, West Africa found pyogenic pneumonia in 45%, CMV in 26%, viral pneumonia in 16%, *Pneumocystis* (PCP) in 13%, purulent meningitis in 14%, acute enteritis in 13%, cerebral malaria in 4%, and tuberculosis or lymphocytic interstitial pneumonia (LIP) in only 1%.[14] Notably, PCP accounted for 31% of the infant deaths in the study and was under-diagnosed, whereas TB was uncommon yet was grossly over-diagnosed clinically. This is crucial data and refutes the conventional wisdom that PCP is rare and TB very common in HIV+ African children. The new diagnostic techniques for PCP and TB need to be employed to confirm these findings.

Ethical considerations

The treatment of HIV+ children under 2 years of age presents a real dilemma in the hospital context in high prevalence regions. The general experience in Africa is that those presenting with HIV-related disease at this age do poorly and do not benefit, or only very transiently, from treatment. There seem to be two radically different points of view to this issue. Where one lies between these two poles may of course depend on local conditions, such as the health resources available and HIV prevalence, but it is clear that these decisions should not be made by armchair ethicists with no clinical experience of the problem.

On the one hand, it is argued that HIV status should not affect treatment decisions, so all malnourished children should receive high-energy milk, suspected TB cases should be given the standard TB drugs, etc., without regard to HIV status. In this view, children with HIV should not be discharged once the diagnosis and poor prognosis is established, because it is inhumane and the hospital has a responsibility to the community to care for dying children. As a corollary, some argue against even testing for HIV.

The opposing viewpoint, to which I subscribe, is that hospitals with such limited resources need to select patients who are likely to benefit from treatment. Scientific medicine depends upon accurate diagnoses which determine the appropriate management, so we need to know which children are HIV+, and more importantly which are negative. If the wards are overcrowded with hopeless cases then those who might potentially benefit will not do so. There seems little point in watching malnourished HIV+ cases slowly deteriorate in hospital, while consuming expensive milk, drugs and nursing care from which others could benefit.

Clinicians in developing countries need to consider carefully what complications associated with HIV are worth treating. For example, acute bacterial infections in young children with AIDS should be treated with antibiotics, although probably not with ceftriaxone or other expensive antibiotics (if these are even available). Tuberculosis only responds to standard treatment regimes (SHRZ) in children over 2 years of age, and in any case is grossly over-diagnosed. Cryptococcal meningitis and malignant tumours are not worth treating, other than symptomatically. Table 21.1.1 is a crude attempt to approach this issue by grading complications into treatment categories. Obviously, antiretroviral agents, immunoglobulins, etc., are not justifiable in the 'Third World' context, where per capita drug budgets are often less than $1 (US) per annum. There is a real risk of bankrupting drug budgets by inappropriate prescribing of expensive antiretroviral or antimicrobial drugs, following the pattern of practice in developed countries. Decisions not to treat are difficult and unpleasant, but should not be avoided.

Finally, the Western emphasis in ethical discussions on patient autonomy and detailed informed consent is not appropriate. This is not meant to justify authoritarian or paternalistic attitudes. Although illiterate mothers are confused by too much scientific information, they do not hesitate to 'vote with their feet' when they see no benefit from staying in hospital. Perhaps we need to explore new paradigms of ethical thinking for developing countries, such as ones based on the more familiar concepts of barter or exchange of favours.

ACUTE RESPIRATORY INFECTIONS

Acute respiratory infections (ARI) are frequently cited as causing 30% of childhood deaths in the developing world, mainly from bacterial pneumonia. Community data from 10 developing countries[15] found marked variability in the incidence of ARI, with 6.6–14.3 episodes per child year, including 0.1–3.0 for lower respiratory tract infections (LRTI). But there are serious problems with the accuracy of epidemiological data on ARI, particularly the case definition of 'pneumonia'. High rates of 'pneumonia' have been reported using WHO criteria based on respiratory rates (fast breathing), but there is considerable doubt about the reliability of such 'diagnoses'.[16] There are similar problems with mortality data due to the unreliability of verbal postmortems in infancy and confusion of the mode of dying with cause of death. These problems were avoided by Gambian studies, which found an incidence rate of only 0.45 episodes of LRTI (0.17 for radiologically proved pneumonia) per child year in a rural community cohort and ARI mortality of 9% of all childhood deaths in hospital and 12% in the community. In a 3-year prospective hospital study,[8] the principal diagnosis in 16.7% of 9584 admissions was an acute lower respiratory tract infection (ALRTI), 65% of which were probable bacterial pneumonia with a 15% case fatality rate. Thus, the main message is to be sceptical of ARI epidemiological data and look closely at how pneumonia was diagnosed.

Microbiology

There are a number of important differences in the microbiology of pneumonia between industrialized and developing countries. An obvious difference is the generalization that viruses (atypical pneumonias) tend to predominate in the former and bacteria (lobar pneumonias) in the latter. Indeed, lung aspirate studies from developing countries have isolated a bacterial cause in over 60% of selected cases. Although the commonest bacteria are *Streptococcus pneumoniae* and *Haemophilus influenzae*, there is striking variability in serotypes, with non-typeable strains of invasive *Haemophilus* isolates varying from 31% in The Gambia[17] compared to only 6% in the UK.[18] However, it is important to emphasize the difficulty of establishing the cause of pneumonia in children, particularly in the developing world, and that antigen tests on blood and urine may give misleading results.[19]

Bacterial colonization of the nasopharynx is another important difference between developed and developing countries. Carriage of *S. pneumoniae* and *H. influenzae* in healthy children occurs at a much earlier age and in a much higher proportion of children in developing countries than in Western countries[20] — hence the younger age of onset of diseases such as meningitis and pneumonia, which were 6 and 14 months (medians) respectively in a Gambian hospital setting.[8] However, nasopharyngeal bacterial carriage does not necessarily increase susceptibility to LRTI,[20] and is certainly not an indication for antibiotic therapy. Indeed, indiscriminate use of antibiotics may lead to the emergence of resistance, which is a particular concern for developing countries because alternatives to penicillin, co-trimoxazole and chloramphenicol are prohibitively expensive for available drug budgets.

The BOSTID studies[15] identified viruses in about 30–40% of ARI episodes, including RSV (15–20%), parainfluenza (7–10%), influenza (5%) and adenovirus (2–4%). Some studies have reported a high frequency of mixed viral and bacterial infections, particularly in association with RSV. This could be seen to justify antibiotic use in viral infections to prevent secondary bacterial infections, except that there are good studies showing this to be ineffective.[21] The BOSTID studies also established risk factors for respiratory infections, including low birth weight, malnutrition, lack of breast-feeding, vitamin A deficiency, crowding and indoor air pollution (from cooking smoke and passive smoking).

A final difference worth noting about the epidemiology of ARI in the developing world is the relative uncommonness of infectious croup (excluding measles), and epiglottitis in many areas of the developing world. In a 3-year Gambian hospital study,[8] for example, there were only 24 cases (0.25%) of croup, and no cases of epiglottitis despite *H. influenzae* meningitis and pneumonia being common. This low incidence of epiglottitis and severe croup in many parts of the tropics seems to be more a function of temperature than rainfall or humidity, but remains ill understood.

The ARI programme

WHO has developed an intervention programme to reduce ARI morbidity and mortality by improved case management using an algorithm. In essence, m*ild pneumonia* is diagnosed by fast breathing (respiratory rate > 60 at 0–2 months, > 50 at 2–12 months and > 40 at 1–4 years) and treated as an outpatient with co-trimoxazole. *Severe pneumonia* is based on chest indrawing and is treated in hospital with procaine penicillin. *Very severe pneumonia* is recognized by the presence of danger signs (e.g. not able to drink, abnormally drowsy, seizures, malnutrition) and is treated in hospital with chloramphenicol. Many research studies have shown reduced mortality from pneumonia using some components of WHO case management.[22,23] The difficulty with these studies is that the rate of antibiotic use in control groups is not given, so they may only show that better access to antibiotics for sick children in poor countries lowers mortality from bacterial pneumonia.

The ARI programme has run into problems. Studies from Malawi[24] and The Gambia[25] have found an overlap between malaria and pneumonia which the case management algorithm does not differentiate. Even worse is the fact that, in the Gambian study, 77.6% of URTI cases fulfilled the WHO criteria for pneumonia. Fever, grunting, cyanosis and toxicity are not considered by the algorithm, yet are clearly relevant in the clinical context. Although locally developed standard *treatment* protocols have greatly improved practice, universal *diagnostic* algorithms do not work and are no substitute for clinical experience.

The high sensitivity and specificity of respiratory rate for predicting pneumonia in research studies does not translate into the everyday reality of clinical practice at health facilities in the developing world, where practical difficulties are encountered in counting respiratory rate (invariably dismissed as inadequate training) and in following the algorithm. In a health facility survey in Papua New Guinea, we found that health workers were better at diagnosing pneumonia clinically than by following the protocol.[16] What is needed is to build upon the clinical judgement of health workers in recognizing sick children with pneumonia. Rather than finding the right algorithm or flow sheet, the real challenge is to ensure proper on-site supervision of health workers.

Although there are problems with the ARI programme's approach to clinical medicine, it is only fair to acknowledge the importance of vital signs such as respiratory rate (preferably with repeated measurements over time) in assessing children with cough and fever. In addition, the ARI programme has been instrumental in focusing attention on the microbiology of pneumonia in developing countries. Probably the main benefit of an effective ARI programme is improved supply of antibiotics to health facilities for sick children. Certainly, in regions where antibiotics are readily accessible, such as the Philippines, it proved difficult to show any impact of an expensive research-run ARI programme. But it is an impossible task to design a universal programme for such variable conditions, when one country gives antibiotics to over 90% of ARI cases at health facilities and another to less than 5%. Clearly, the emphasis needs to be on adapting to local conditions and building on clinical experience of health workers.

DIARRHOEAL DISEASES

Epidemiology

Reviews of the global epidemiology of diarrhoeal diseases give estimates of the mean incidence in children under 5 years old of 2.6–3.5 episodes per child per year, with the highest incidence in 6–12 month olds.[26,27] But much higher attack rates of 5–12 episodes per child per year have been reported from developing countries, with peak age-specific rates of up to 19 in the poorest areas. In terms of mortality, 276 WHO/CDD surveys from 60 developing countries found a median mortality of 6.5 per thousand children per year. In sub-Saharan Africa, the median mortality was higher at 10.6 per thousand, but the range was 3.1 to 54.9.[28]

The three most significant causative organisms in the developing world are rotavirus, *Shigella* and enterotoxigenic *E. coli* (ETEC).[29] However, no organism is isolated from around 30% of diarrhoeal cases and, conversely, 10% or more of apparently healthy children also harbour organisms. *Campylobacter*, enteropathogenic *E. coli* (EPEC), *Salmonella*, *Cryptosporidium* and *Giardia* are other frequently isolated organisms from children with and without diarrhoea. The advent of specific nucleotide (DNA or RNA) probes based on virulence-associated genes has transformed the diagnostic capability of research laboratories. Although they are not available for routine clinical testing, they have altered our understanding of *E. coli* diarrhoea. There have also been two recent large epidemics of diarrhoea in developing countries, caused by a new organism, *Vibrio cholera* 0139 (Bengal) in Asia and by *Shigella dysenteriae* type 1 in southern Africa.

The terminology of diarrhoea differentiates a*cute*, *persistent* and *chronic*. But these research definitions are often blurred in clinical practice, because the history is often vague, and symptoms recurrent or intermittent. The severity of acute diarrhoea is assessed by degree of associated dehydration. *Dysentery* refers to the presence of blood and mucus in the stool (or *inflammatory* if there are leucocytes on microscopy). Persistent diarrhoea is an episode that begins acutely with at least three loose stools daily for 14 days whereas in chronic diarrhoea the duration is at least 1 month. Persistent diarrhoea is also strongly associated with malnutrition, and often ceases shortly after admission to hospital with the administration of hygienic and appropriate feeds. Chronic diarrhoea tends to be associated with conditions such as coeliac disease or hereditary syndromes in the developed world, but is more associated with AIDS, giardiasis, malnutrition and a contaminated environment in the developing world.

Acute diarrhoea

The assessment of hydration is dealt with in standard texts, so we shall only highlight some important points for developing countries. A shortcoming of diarrhoeal case management protocols is that they ignore factors such as age of the child, quality of child care, whether still breast-fed, distance from health facility, compliance with Western health care (e.g. immunization status), and even time of day, which are frequently relevant to decision-making about management. Thus, the mildly dehydrated 12-month-old breast-fed child of a competent mother seen at a morning clinic may be sent home with oral rehydration salt (ORS), whereas a similarly dehydrated child with different characteristics might be admitted.

The earliest physical sign of dehydration is diminished peripheral circulation, which can be assessed by the time for capillary refilling (return of colour after blanching the fingernail bed). Mild dehydration corresponds to capillary refilling times of > 1.5 s and severe dehydration to > 3 s.[30] However, like any physical sign, it should not be taken in isolation but needs to be used in conjunction with the other classical signs of dehydration. Capillary return, sunken eyes and dry mouth are particularly useful signs in marasmus or kwashiorkor, when the skin elasticity is unreliable.

The principal acute complications other than dehydration are acidosis, hypokalaemia and hypoglycaemia. Clinically relevant hypo- or hypernatraemia is uncommon except in the context of herbal poisoning or use of an erroneous rehydration solution. In metabolic acidosis, an elevated serum anion gap (normally 8–12 mmol/l) points to the presence of unmeasured ions, such as ketones, lactate, protein, phosphate, salicylates or renal failure acids, whereas in acidosis caused by stool losses of bicarbonate there is hyperchloraemia without an elevated anion gap. The acidosis of severe diarrhoea with dehydration is more profound than would be expected from stool losses of bicarbonate because of the superimposition of lactic acidosis and renal failure, so there is an increased serum anion gap and normal chloride.

Hypokalaemia is more common with malnutrition and acidosis, and is manifested by hypotonia and abdominal distension during recovery, but is less likely if ORS with 20 mmol/l of K^+ is used, rather than home-based salt–sugar solutions. Hypoglycaemia complicated 4.5% of diarrhoeal admissions in a Bangladeshi study, particularly in shigellosis and cholera, but had a 43% mortality.[31] Hypoglycaemic diarrhoea cases were more acute, had more prolonged fasting, and had a hormonal picture of depletion of liver glycogen and failure of gluconeogenesis (elevated glucagon, adrenaline and lactate, with low C-peptides), but malnutrition was not a risk factor.

There is still a tendency for overuse of intravenous rehydration where this is available. On the other hand, the decreased need for intravenous therapy for rehydration has reduced the number of health workers experienced in inserting intravenous needles or cannulas, so intravenous access may be more of a problem.

Although the nasogastric and peritoneal routes have been used for rehydration, they are unsatisfactory for some situations such as shock or persistent vomiting, but the intraosseous route (tibia) is advantageous and can also be used for blood transfusions and drug administration. Rapid rehydration with Ringer's lactate 100 ml/kg over 4 h has proved a simple, safe and effective regime for severe dehydration, but there is no substitute for careful monitoring of fluid administration and hydration status. Older children with cholera may have very high purging rates, requiring very large volumes of rehydration fluids (> 10 l per day).

Most dehydrated children can be rehydrated orally, if mothers can be encouraged to get them to drink. Of course, dehydrated children are thirsty so will drink ORS if offered, whereas refusal to drink it because of taste usually indicates the child is not dehydrated. There has been considerable interest in newer formulations, such as cereal-based or hypo-osmolar ORS. A meta-analysis of 15 studies indicated no advantage of rice-based ORS over standard glucose-based ORS for childhood diarrhoea, provided early feeding is introduced once dehydration has been corrected. Nevertheless, many recent studies have documented definite advantages for cereal- and particularly rice-based solutions.

The current WHO estimate (1993) for global access to ORS is 75%, compared to 51% for the actual use, but the documented use of ORS was only 26.4% (range 0–53) from the 276 WHO/CDD studies in 60 countries.[28,32] Surveys have also documented a median use of other medicines (mostly unnecessarily) of 48.3% (range 7.4–71.0) and of 'traditional' medicines in 21.3% (range 2.1–69.1). Unfortunately, in southern Africa, these herbal remedies for diarrhoea can result in severe acidosis in infants, with a high mortality. Although diarrhoeal disease programmes have tended to concentrate their attention on dehydration, it is now clear that more prolonged illness without dehydration, although less common than acute diarrhoea, is more strongly associated with malnutrition and death.

Persistent diarrhoea

There is considerable evidence from the developing world that apparently healthy individuals often have abnormalities of small bowel structure and function. Instead of the normal finger-shaped villi on small bowel biopsy, there are leaves, ridges or convoluted villi with hypercellularity of the lamina propria, and also abnormalities of intestinal absorption/permeability and small bowel bacterial overgrowth. This syndrome of subclinical malabsorption or 'tropical enteropathy' affects 30–50% of the population in tropical areas and may also affect Western expatriates in whom the changes revert to 'normal' upon return home.[33] The likely explanation of these changes is small intestinal mucosal damage as a result of over-exposure to enteric pathogens in a contaminated environment.

Although the significance of the mucosal changes in tropical enteropathy is uncertain, they may contribute to persistent diarrhoea and malnutrition, since a Gambian study[34] attributed 40% of growth faltering to changes in intestinal permeability. Evidence is emerging that acute episodes of diarrhoea become persistent due to factors in the host, so it may be that the capacity of the intestine to regenerate is reduced after acute infection in these children, leading to persistent symptoms. Prolonged damage to the small intestinal mucosa is central to the persistence of diarrhoea, and may be due to cell-mediated immune damage. Although cow's milk protein sensitivity is the commonest cause of persistent diarrhoea following acute gastroenteritis in Western countries, persistent diarrhoea in developing countries is not the same disease as intractable diarrhoea of infancy or postenteritis syndromes in developed countries.

The epidemiology of persistent diarrhoea reveals marked variability between regions. In studies mainly from Asia and Latin America, persistent diarrhoea accounts for about 3–23% of all diarrhoeal episodes and 45% (range 23–62) of all diarrhoea-related deaths.[35,36] The highest mortality rates tend to be from sub-Saharan Africa, but the highest burden of disease is from Latin American urban slums. For example, a Brazilian study[37] reported a mean annual incidence of 11 episodes of diarrhoea (of which 11% were persistent), and a prevalence of 82 days (41 days of persistent) for children under 5 years. A community study in North India[38] had case fatality rates for acute watery diarrhoea of 0.6%, for dysentery of 4.3% and for non-dysenteric persistent diarrhoea of 11.9%. Other risk factors for severe disease were: age under 12 months, low socioeconomic status, poor personal and domestic hygiene, lack of breast-feeding, delayed cutaneous hypersensitivity responses to antigens (anergy), low birth weight, and possibly also antibiotic use and vitamin A or zinc deficiency.

A consensus seems to be emerging that no particular organism is associated with persistent diarrhoea, but frequent reinfections with enteropathogens commonly found in that community (rather than persisting infection) is the main reason for the prolonged illness.[34] Some organisms have been associated with persistent diarrhoea, such as *Cryptosporidium*, giardiasis, and diffuse entero-adherent *E. coli* (DAEC) and enteroaggregative *E. coli* (EAggEC), although not in every study. Notably, the initial enthusiasm for EAggEC as a cause of persistent diarrhoea has waned, leaving doubts about its pathogenicity. There are no clinical or laboratory features of acute diarrhoea that are strongly predictive of persistence.[39]

Diet is the mainstay of management of persistent diarrhoea. Antibiotics were initially thought to be effective (gentamicin, metronidazole) but have now been shown not to reduce stool output. However, specific treatment of *Shigella*, giardiasis and amoebiasis may shorten a particular episode and a recent Bangladeshi trial of cotrimoxazole for persistent diarrhoea showed reduced duration (6.0 vs 8.3d), higher recovery rate and prevention of nosocomial infection.[61] Vitamins, particularly vitamin A, and micronutrients, especially zinc, are indicated. Other drugs such as bismuth subsalicylate, antimotility drugs and cholestyramine are not recommended. Dietary management of persistent diarrhoea seems to vary greatly between regions, but tends to use local weaning foods with yoghurt, soya beans, lentils or chicken and a low-lactose diet. If persistent diarrhoea is associated with malnutrition, then the standard graded milk regime for kwashiorkor is usually satisfactory and simple. It seems unlikely that cow's milk protein sensitivity enteropathy is a common cause of persistent diarrhoea in the developing world, as it is in Western countries, since cow's milk powder, which is readily available for nutritional rehabilitation, gives better results than a maize-based diet.

Control of diarrhoeal diseases

The World Health Organization has developed a programme for control of diarrhoeal diseases (CDD).[32] The current priorities of the programme are: (1) health worker training in case management; (2) breast-feeding promotion and improved weaning practices; (3) management of persistent diarrhoea and dysentery; and (4) use of rice-based and low-osmolality ORS. Other priority interventions are immunizations, improved water supply and sanitation facilities, and promotion of personal and domestic hygiene. The main components of the breast-feeding promotion are exclusive breast-feeding for the first 4–6 months of life, prolonged breast-feeding into the second year of life, and lactation management training for health workers to support breast-feeding mothers and deal with problems. Other priority preventive measures include improved weaning foods (e.g. germination or fermentation of cereals), supplementation of micronutrients such as vitamin A and zinc, and research into vaccines (e.g. rotavirus, cholera, *Shigella* and ETEC).

Young children are even more exposed to a contaminated environment than adults, so it is not surprising that the features of tropical enteropathy syndrome are acquired in early childhood in communities in the developing world. This contamination is a particular risk in the weaning period and the rainy season, affecting drinking water and wet foods such as cereal gruels and cow's milk. The current view on water supply is that quantity is more important than quality.[40] Water quantity reflects water used for hygiene to prevent water-washed diseases, whereas water quality relates more to water-borne transmission. Although one would expect improved hygiene to reduce the rate of diarrhoea, this has not yet been convincingly demonstrated. The difficulty of documenting benefit from hygiene interventions may be related to the S-shaped curve relationship between the degree of contamination and health benefit from hygiene interventions, so they are unlikely to be effective in a grossly contaminated environment (bottom of the curve) but may have an impact higher up on the curve.

A final important controversy concerns the interactions of diarrhoea and malnutrition, which has traditionally been conceived as a vicious cycle. But the impact of diarrhoea on malnutrition has been questioned recently due to catch-up growth.[41] The answer probably depends on the context. In hospital one sees many cases of malnutrition precipitated by diarrhoea, but this probably occurs in very few cases of diarrhoea. From a community perspective, the majority of diarrhoeal cases have no impact on nutritional status, or only a transient one due to convalescent catch-up growth. But the important issue underlying this controversy is the contribution of infection (diarrhoea) versus diet (food supply) in causing childhood malnutrition. In other words, should donor agencies fund food distribution or diarrhoeal control measures? Once again, there is no universal answer to this question, which should be decided on local evidence of cost-effectiveness and feasibility.

MALARIA

Falciparum malaria is a major cause of morbidity and mortality in developing countries. In The Gambia, severe malaria accounted for about a quarter of all paediatric hospital admissions, with a 15% case-fatality rate.[8,9] The main manifestations of severe malaria in children are, of course, cerebral malaria and severe anaemia. The median ages for these complications differ, with cerebral malaria occurring at an average older age (42 months) than severe anaemia (23 months). The interval between symptom onset and death is short, averaging less than 3 days. Unlike adults, renal failure, pulmonary oedema, shock, jaundice and DIC are uncommon in childhood malaria. Similarly the classical malaria paroxysm of 'cold shivers → burning heat → drenching sweats' is infrequently encountered in childhood falciparum malaria, which more typically involves irregular fevers due to asynchronous infections.

Malaria is a disease of paradoxes. The first paradox, which is too readily forgotten in the hospital context, is that parasites are not synonymous with disease. For example, if we could study prospectively 1000 children bitten by an infectious mosquito, we might find 400 asymptomatic infections, 200 cases of clinical malaria, 12 cases of severe malaria and two deaths.[42,43] Not only do many apparently healthy children have parasitaemia, but also peripheral blood parasitaemia does not reflect total parasitaemia due to infected red cells cytoadhering and sequestering in the microvasculature. These factors complicate the diagnosis of malarial disease based on the presence of parasites on thick blood film. This is further complicated by gross inaccuracies in thick film results in practice (as opposed to research studies), due to factors such as dirty glass slides, too thick smears, contaminated stains and (especially) inexperienced or lazy microscopists. This can be improved by proper supervision and checking results, but the development of a dipstick test is a promising approach,[44] although cost is the major constraint to this antigen-capture assay.

Yet another paradox is the relationship between intensity of transmission and clinical disease. For example, transmission is high in the Solomon Islands and low in The Gambia, yet severe disease is much more prevalent in the latter. It seems as though progression to severe disease is determined early in the course of an infection by genetic or immunological characteristics, such as protective immunity, sickle cell trait, tumour necrosis factor (TNF)-suppressor genes, and HLA antigens in the host; and sporozoite dose, virulence factors or drug sensitivity in the parasite.[45]

The incidence of clinical attacks in African children is estimated at one to five attacks per year, but with marked seasonal variations. For example, over two-thirds of malarial illness and death occurs in a 4-month rainy season in The Gambia, but parasite prevalence and density show relatively little variation during the year.[8,42,43] Moreover, cerebral malaria in some parts of Africa is occurring in older children due to delayed exposure and late development of immunity because of shortened rainy seasons, prolonged drought, urbanization, etc. The promise of an effective vaccine could have a dramatic effect on mortality and morbidity in Africa, and should be given priority in view of the problems of drug-resistant malaria. The Columbian SPf66 vaccine was only 31% effective in Tanzania,[46] and was ineffective in The Gambia,[62] but will hopefully lead on to better vaccines.

Cerebral malaria

Cerebral malaria has been defined as unrousable coma not attributable to any other cause in a patient with falciparum malaria. The level of consciousness is of course confounded by convulsions and the postictal state, so coma must persist for 30 min after a convulsion for a diagnosis of cerebral malaria. The coma score is assessed by responses to rubbing knuckles on the sternum and placing firm pressure on the thumbnail bed. A simple coma score for clinical use is:

0 *no response* or decerebrate/decorticate or opisthotonic postures
1 *non-specific* response (e.g. moans or moves)
2 *withdraws* the limb
3 *localizes* the painful stimulus
4 responds and *cries, but relapses* into coma
5 *normal* or fully conscious

Unrousable coma means unable to localize pain (coma score 0–2), which is used as a research criterion for cerebral malaria, but is not a useful clinical definition because it excludes too many children with persisting coma who obviously have cerebral malaria. So a more useful definition is any abnormal state of consciousness which persists without other explanation. This has important therapeutic implications, since a diagnosis of cerebral malaria implies quinine treatment rather than sulphadoxine–pyrimethamine. But the main differential diagnosis is febrile convulsions associated with malaria, so the duration as well as the depth of coma are crucial.

The pathophysiology of cerebral malaria is yet another paradox, in that the mechanism of coma is still unclear. The classical hypothesis is that sequestration of infected erythrocytes in the cerebral microcirculation causes multifocal abnormalities of blood flow resulting in hypoxaemia, acidosis, hypoglycaemia and other metabolic derangements. An alternative hypothesis is the cytokine theory, that TNF, interleukin 1 (IL-1) and other mediators released in response to malaria pigment in macrophages may be over-produced due to genetic factors in the host and cause brain dysfunction through generation of nitric oxide.[47] Undoubtedly, cerebral malaria is the result of the interplay of many factors, including sequestration with impaired cerebral microcirculation, cytokines and other mediators of inflammation, genetic predisposition of the host, and probably unknown factors in the parasite. These are likely to be clarified by scientific studies over the next decade, since this is a productive area of research.

Cerebral malaria has a mortality of around 15% and causes neurological sequelae in about 9% of survivors in Africa, but with considerable variability between regions (e.g. it tends to be less common and severe in children from Asian, Pacific and Latin American countries). The main clinical features of severe encephalopathy are hypoglycaemia, status epilepticus and lactic acidosis. The hypoglycaemia is usually in the range of 1.6–2.2 mmol/l, is related to impaired host gluconeogenesis, and is a marker of severe disease, so correction does not improve the conscious level. Kenyan studies[48,49] have underlined the importance of brain swelling and ischaemia in cerebral malaria, and suggested considering delaying lumbar puncture until the child regains consciousness to avoid the danger of herniation. The importance of lactic acidosis-induced respiratory distress as a prognostic feature of severe malaria has also been documented.[63]

The drug of choice for severe falciparum malaria is quinine 20 mg/kg loading and 10 mg/kg every 12 h for 5 days, but changing to oral as soon as feasible. Another option is to change to oral sulphadoxine–pyrimethamine, so the child can complete treatment and be discharged sooner. Quinine can be given over 2 h by infusion or by intramuscular injection provided it is diluted to 60 mg/ml. Artemether, from the traditional Chinese remedy *qinghaousu*, is being studied in several countries for severe malaria, and is rapid acting and at least as effective as standard treatment. Mefloquine is an effective oral drug, but still too expensive for routine use. Concern has been raised about cardiotoxicity of halofantrine, which has caused Q–T prolongation and heart block in adults.

In terms of other medications in cerebral malaria, control of recurrent or prolonged convulsions is an important objective. Prophylactic phenobarbitone has been tried with variable results, but a selective approach to phenobarbitone in a dose of 15 mg/kg per day is warranted (in spite of concerns about deepening coma) if initial management with paraldehyde 0.2 ml/kg i.m. (or rectal diazepam 0.4 mg/kg) fails to control convulsions. It is important to ensure, as with meningitis cases, that intravenous fluids do not flow too fast, due to the risk of inappropriate ADH secretion, water intoxication and worsening cerebral oedema. Steroids are not indicated in cerebral malaria, and mannitol infusions and iron chelation (desferrioxamine)[50] are still experimental.

Severe anaemia

The mechanisms of anaemia are (1) haemolysis and (2) defective production. Red cell destruction occurs both intravascularly and by sequestration of parasitized cells in the spleen and other parts of the microcirculation. Despite frequently positive direct Coombs antiglobulin tests, immune destruction of red cells is thought not to play an important role in the anaemia. There appears to be random destruction by activated macrophages in the reticuloendothelial microcirculation, and the haemoglobin may continue to drop for several weeks after parasite clearance. Dyserythropoietic changes in the marrow with a relatively poor reticulocyte response to the anaemia, elevated plasma ferritin levels and sequestration of iron in the reticuloendothelial system with low serum iron have been described in malarial anaemia.

Severe anaemia accounted for 11% of paediatric admissions in The Gambia with a 10% case fatality.[8] For unknown reasons, the emergence of chloroquine resistance resulted in a substantial increase in severe anaemia cases. The majority of hospital cases present in heart failure due to an abrupt drop in haemoglobin, requiring *prompt* blood transfusion. The severity of cardiovascular compromise and age of the child are more important than the actual haemoglobin level, but decisions to transfuse are unfortunately usually made exclusively on haemoglobin level, often by nursing staff. The need for transfusion can be confirmed on blood film by heavy parasitaemia and lack of reticulocyte response. On the other hand, in a child with malaria pigment, with few or no parasites and many reticulocytes and nucleated red cells (marrow response) but without overt cardiac failure, it may be possible to hold off on transfusion, since rapid clinical improvement can usually be expected within 24 h. Excessive transfusion is a great risk, particularly in infants, so it is important to monitor volumes, give packed cells where possible and limit transfusions to 10–15 ml/kg over not less than 4 h.

MENINGITIS AND SEPSIS

Sepsis

The evaluation of a child with fever in the developing world is a challenge. The potential diagnosis may vary from a self-limited viral infection to a potentially life-threatening disease like malaria, pneumonia or meningitis, and the primary health care worker assessing the child is likely to be inadequately trained and have no laboratory tests available. Table 21.1.2 outlines the terminology of the spectrum of septic illnesses. In industrialized countries, occult bacteraemia has been reported in 2.5–12% of febrile episodes (> 39°C) in children aged 3–36 months, with pneumococcus (66%) and *Haemophilus influenzae* type b (Hib, 20%), accounting for most bacteraemias. It has proved difficult to identify such children, so many resort to empirical antibiotic treatment for those at risk, but a number of common risk factors have been identified such as young age (6–18 months), clinical observations (irritable, poor peripheral perfusion, tachypnoea), leucocytosis (> 15×10^9/l, especially with neutrophilia and left shift) and pyuria (> 10/HPF).

Data from the developing world have shown a prevalence of bacteraemia in febrile children without a focus of 9–12%, rising to as high as 20% in infancy.

Table 21.1.2 Terminology of the septic process

1. Systemic inflammatory response syndrome	Encompasses all the stages of infection (not only bacterial) from sepsis to death
2. Occult bacteraemia	Febrile episode without a focus or toxicity, but with bacteria isolated from blood culture
3. Sepsis	A systemic response to a possible infection with changes in vital signs (temperature, tachycardia, tachypnoea, toxicity)
4. Sepsis syndrome	Altered organ perfusion (mental status changes, oliguria, cyanosis)
5. Septic shock: refractory	Hypotension or poor peripheral circulation (slow capillary refill); persists for an hour in spite of treatment
6. Multiple organ dysfunction syndrome	Any combination of renal, hepatic, CNS, haematology or respiratory system dysfunction (e.g. adult RDS, DIC)

The progression through these stages is typically rapid in children (e.g. Gram-negative septicaemia), but may vary from insidious (typhoid) or subtle (malnutrition) to fulminant (meningococcaemia).

Although malaria does not increase the risk of bacteraemia, the presence of parasites is likely to mislead clinicians. The bacteraemia tends to be short-lived, since the organism is usually cleared promptly by the monocyte–macrophage system after opsonization by antibody and complement. The organisms isolated tend to be similar to those in Western countries, except that some have found *Staphylococcus aureus*, *Klebsiella* and particularly *Salmonella* species to be more common.[51,52] The median age of *Salmonella* sepsis has tended to be older (20 months in The Gambia and 75 months in Rwanda), but this is mainly due to *S. typhi*, which accounted for 11/21 Gambian isolates typed and 47/83 in Rwanda. Typhoid fever as a clinical syndrome is uncommon in children under 5 years, but *S. typhi* bacteraemia in endemic areas is not uncommon at this age with a non-specific clinical picture or even no symptoms. This milder clinical picture in young children may be due to less cytokine response since there are less prominent intestinal lesions in Peyer's patches.[53] Salmonellosis is also associated with schistosomiasis and may be more common with malarial anaemia.

Meningitis

Neonatal meningitis has a uniformly bad prognosis in developing countries, with very high mortality and sequelae rates. Unlike the developed world, group B streptococcus is rare outside intensive care nurseries in cities, but pneumococci and coliforms predominate, including *Salmonella* and *Klebsiella*. In a 3-year prospective Gambian study,[8] out of a total of 292 meningitis admissions (Table 21.1.3) there were 72 cases (25%) aged 0–2 months with a 40% case fatality. The organisms identified in this age group were: pneumococcus (22), Hib (14), coliforms, including *Salmonella* (14), other streptococci (4) and unknown (18). The poor outcome in this age group is related to the prolonged period it takes to eradicate the organism from the CSF due to ventriculitis, and sometimes to multi-resistant organisms. The use of intrathecal antibiotics, very expensive antibiotics and intensive care have not substantially altered the poor prognosis, although they may decrease mortality and increase morbidity in survivors. In summary, it is not a high-priority area for aggressive treatment, so practices such as routine lumbar puncture in neonatal sepsis and use of intravenous fluids in neonatal meningitis are questionable.

Although the same organisms (Hib, pneumococci and meningococci) cause meningitis after the neonatal period in developed and developing countries, the median ages are much younger in the latter. In industrialized countries, a recent meta-analysis of 19 prospective follow-up studies reported a mean mortality of 4.8% (Hib 3.8%, meningococcal 7.5% and pneumococcal 15.3%) and sequelae rate of 16.4%.[54] This compares to hospital case fatality rates in developing countries of 20–30% (Table 21.1.3) and 40–50% sequelae or post-discharge mortality rates.[55] The higher mortality rates in the developing world are due to late presentations, younger age and suboptimal management. Indeed, in some settings such as Papua New Guinea many patients abscond before completing treatment. Clinical risk factors for poor outcome on admission are coma, seizures, grossly purulent CSF and symptoms for more than 3 days before admission, particularly if the diagnosis was missed initially. Control of seizures is important, and some authors have recommended prophylactic phenobarbitone for all children under 2 years with meningitis. Since seizures occur in only 30–50% of cases, selective use of phenobarbitone is probably preferable, with intramuscular paraldehyde or rectal diazepam for first-line seizure control, as in cerebral malaria.

There is still controversy about lumbar punctures (LP), namely, their routine use in febrile convulsions or cerebral malaria and the risk of cerebral herniation

Table 21.1.3 Meningitis in The Gambia, West Africa

Causative organism	Cases (n (%))	Mortality (%)	Major sequelae[a] (% of survivors)
Haemophilus influenzae	107 (37)	24	12
Pneumococcal	80 (27)	53	24
No organism (bacterial)	50 (17)	28	14
Gram-negative coliforms	20 (7)	65	40
Meningococcal	8 (3)	13	14
Tuberculous	7 (2)	43	25
Other Gram-positive	5 (2)	40	33
Presumed viral	7 (2)	–	
Secondary cases[b]	8 (3)	–	
Ages of cases (months)			
< 6	161 (55)	36	15
6–11	66 (23)	33	20
12–23	27 (9)	41	25
24–47	16 (5.5)	44	22
48–71	10 (3.5)	30	14
⩾ 72	12 (4)	17	10
Total	292 (100)	35.3%	16.4%

[a] Obvious in hospital without audiometry.
[b] (E.g. meningomyeloceles, dural sinus thromboses.)

or coning. In developing countries, delayed or missed diagnosis of meningitis in infants causes more morbidity than LP-related herniation, so early diagnosis and a high index of suspicion for meningitis are important.[56] Nevertheless, coning does occur in both severe meningitis and cerebral malaria, and may be associated with LP. It is rare, however, in infants with an open fontanelle and in children with only mild to moderate illness. It may well be that coning is a marker of severity of disease, so children who herniate would die with or without an LP in a developing country context without intensive care. The experienced clinician rarely needs an LP to differentiate meningitis from cerebral malaria, but fear of doing an LP by junior staff could worsen the problems of misdiagnosis and polypharmacy (e.g. the practice of quinine, penicillin and chloramphenicol for all febrile convulsions). Although the priority remains on doing LPs to make accurate specific diagnoses, paediatricians should be aware that unresponsive coma, focal neurological signs, pupillary abnormalities and decerebrate/decorticate posturing are strong reasons to postpone the LP and start treatment. But rather than setting blanket policies on LPs, there is no substitute for proper clinical supervision of health workers and decision-making based on local circumstances. When CSF is collected, rapid diagnostic tests such as latex particle agglutination are quite sensitive and specific for the three common organisms.[57]

Despite good evidence that chloramphenicol alone is a satisfactory antibiotic regime in developing countries[58] (unless there is widespread resistance), the practice of combining penicillin and chloramphenicol (usually for the full course) persists in many countries. But of greater concern is the use of erroneous drug dosages in children and intravenous fluids at excessive rates, when there are no infusion pumps or cannulas for intermittent drug dosages without infusions. In the chaotic children's wards in developing countries, with limited nursing care and microbiology, a cheap and simple regime for meningitis such as chloramphenicol (intramuscular followed by oral) without intravenous fluids has distinct advantages.[59] The convenience of using ceftriaxone 100 mg/kg i.m. once daily for 7 days is attractive in selected cases if it is affordable, but it has not yet been shown to improve outcomes compared to conventional regimes in the developing world. Significant resistance of meningitis organisms to penicillin has emerged in many developing countries and, unlike for pneumonia has necessitated a change in empirical therapy. Thus, in Malawi we have reverted to initial therapy with penicillin and chloramphenicol for meningitis.

The high incidence, mortality and morbidity of acute bacterial meningitis in the developing world means that prevention is a high priority. Rifampicin prophylaxis of household contacts is not recommended for developing countries, due to the high cost and concerns about drug resistance against TB. Even in meningococcal epidemics, now that resistance to inexpensive sulphonamides is widespread, mass vaccination — although unavailable for group B — is the preferred option.[60] The new protein polysaccharide-conjugated vaccines against the three common meningitis organisms have been or are being developed, and the success of immunization programmes (EPI) in developing countries makes this approach particularly attractive. But the early age of onset of pneumococcal and Hib meningitis means that up to 15–20% of cases would occur before infants were fully immunized, unless it were also given to pregnant mothers. As these new vaccines become available it is important to make them available to developing countries, since they are likely to be cost-effective interventions.

CONCLUSION

The appalling disparities in child mortality and burden of disease between rich and poor countries are unacceptable. Most of us would like to ignore this problem, because it makes us feel uncomfortable. Some argue that it is really the countries' own problem, and they must be left to improve things without outside meddling. At the other extreme are the so-called 'do-gooders' whose well-intentioned actions are laudable, but often end in bitter cynicism when faced with the reality of the Third World. Many African countries like Malawi and The Gambia are caught in a trap (demographic, economic, ecological and health), from which they cannot escape without help. But we cannot extricate them alone either, so it involves a collaborative effort.

This issue can no longer be left to politicians, development specialists and the World Bank, for it concerns us as health professionals. There is general agreement that aid programmes are not producing the desired results. It is a truism that aid programmes rob the poor of rich countries for the rich of poor countries, promote foreign policy and trade objectives of donor countries, and lead to corruption in recipients. There are no easy solutions, but we need to adopt a new paradigm for aid to the developing world, one oriented to humanitarian concerns instead of political considerations. This does not necessarily imply more money for aid, but rather more effective use of aid funds in a different structure. It is essential that health professionals and their organizations become involved in this venture, and wrest the agenda away from conventional donor agencies, be they multilateral, bilateral or non-governmental.

REFERENCES

1 Taylor C E, Ramalingaswami V. Reducing mortality in children under five: a continuing priority. In: Jamison D T, Mosley W H, Measham A R, Bobadilla J-L, eds. Disease control priorities in developing countries. Oxford: Oxford University Press, 1993: Appendix B, p 728.
2 Quinn T C, Ruff A, Halsey N. Pediatric acquired immunodeficiency syndrome: special considerations for developing nations. Pediatr Infect Dis J 1992; 11: 558–568.

3 Goeddert J J, Duliege A M, Amos C I et al. High risk of HIV-1 infection for first-born twins. Lancet 1991; 338: 1471–1475.

4 Bridbord K, Willoughby A. Vitamin A and mother-to-child HIV-1 transmission. Lancet 1994; 343: 1585–1586.

5 Connor E M, Sperling R S, Gelber R et al. Reduction of maternal–infant transmission of human immunodeficiency virus type 1 with zidovudine treatment. N Engl J Med 1994; 331: 1173–1180.

6 Dunn D T, Newell M L, Ades A E, Peckham C S. Risk of human immunodeficiency virus type 1 transmission through breastfeeding. Lancet 1992; 340: 585–588.

7 Greenberg A E, Nguyen-Dinh P, Mann J M, Kabote N et al. The association between malaria, blood transfusion, and HIV seropositivity in a pediatric population in Kinshasa, Zaire. JAMA 1988; 259: 545–549.

8 Brewster D R, Greenwood B M. Seasonal variation of paediatric diseases in The Gambia, west Africa. Ann Trop Paediatr 1993; 13: 133–146.

9 Brewster D R. Blood transfusions for severe anaemia in African children. Lancet 1992; 340: 917.

10 Turner B J, Denison M, Eppes S C, Houchens R, Fanning T, Markson L E. Survival experience of 789 children with the acquired immunodeficiency syndrome. Pediatr Infect Dis J 1993; 12: 310–320.

11 Brewster D R, Legett S. HIV infection and protein-energy malnutrition in Malawian children. Presented at the 3rd Commonwealth Conference on Diarrhoea and Malnutrition, Hong Kong, 11–14 November, 1994.

12 Grohmann G S, Glass R I, Pereira H G et al. Enteric viruses and diarrhoea in HIV-infected patients. N Engl J Med 1993; 329: 14–20.

13 Mathan M M, Griffin G E, Miller A et al. Ultrastructure of the jejunal mucosa in human immunodeficiency virus infection. J Pathol 1990; 161: 119–127.

14 Lucas S B, Hounnou A, Koffi K, Beaumel A, Andoh A, De Cock K M. The pathology of paediatric HIV infection in Cote D'Ivoire. J Pathol 1993; 170: 342A (Abstract).

15 Selwyn B J. The epidemiology of acute respiratory tract infection in young children: comparison of findings from several developing countries. Coordinated Data Group of BOSTID Researchers. Rev Infect Dis 1990; 12 Suppl 8: S870–S888.

16 Brewster D R, Pyakalya T, Hiawalyer G, O'Connell D L. Evaluation of the ARI Programme: a health facility survey in Simbu, Papua New Guinea. PNG Med J 1993; 36: 285–296.

17 Wall R A, Corrah P T, Mabey D C, Greenwood B M. The etiology of lobar pneumonia in the Gambia. Bull World Health Org 1986; 64: 553–558.

18 Falla T J, Dobson S R M, Crook D W M et al. Population-based study of non-typable Haemophilus influenzae invasive disease in children and neonates. Lancet 1993; 341: 851–854.

19 Isaacs D. Problems in determining the etiology of community-acquired childhood pneumonia. Pediatr Infect Dis J 1989; 8: 143–148.

20 Montgomery J M, Lehmann D, Smith T et al. Bacterial colonization of the upper respiratory tract and its association with acute lower respiratory tract infections in Highland children of Papua New Guinea. Rev Infect Dis 1990; 12 (Suppl 8): S1006–S1016.

21 Gadomski A M. Potential interventions for preventing pneumonia among young children: lack of effect of antibiotic treatment for upper respiratory infections. Pediatr Infect Dis J 1993; 12: 115–120.

22 Sazawal S, Black R E. Meta-analysis of intervention trials on case-management of pneumonia in community settings. Lancet 1992; 340: 528–533.

23 Mulholland E K, Simoes E A, Costales M O, McGrath E J, Manalac E M, Gove S. Standardized diagnosis of pneumonia in developing countries. Pediatr Infect Dis J 1992; 11: 77–81.

24 Redd S C, Bloland P B, Kazembe P N, Patrick E, Tembenu R, Campbell C C. Usefulness of clinical case-definitions in guiding therapy for African children with malaria or pneumonia. Lancet 1992; 340: 1140–1143.

25 O'Dempsey T J D, McCardle T F, Laurence B E, Lamont A C, Todd J E, Greenwood B M. Overlap in the clinical features of pneumonia and malaria in African children. Trans R Soc Trop Med Hyg 1993; 87: 662–665.

26 Bern C, Martines J, De Zoysa I, Glass R I. The magnitude of the global problem of diarrhoeal disease: a ten-year update. Bull World Health Org 1992; 70: 705–714.

27 Claeson M, Merson M H. Global progress in the control of diarrheal diseases. Pediatr Infect Dis J 1990; 9: 345–355.

28 Martines J, Phillips M, Feachem R G. Diarrheal diseases. In: Jamison D T, Mosley W H, Measham AR, Bobadilla J-L, eds. Disease control priorities in developing countries, Oxford: Oxford University Press, 1993: pp 91–116.

29 Huilan S, Zhen L G, Mathan M M et al. Etiology of acute diarrhoea among children in developing countries: a multicentre study in five countries. Bull World Health Org 1991; 69: 549–555.

30 Saavedra J M, Harris G D, Li S, Finberg L. Capillary refilling (skin turgor) in the assessment of dehydration. Am J Dis Child 1991; 145: 296–298.

31 Bennish M L, Azad A K, Rahman O, Phillips R E. Hypoglycemia during diarrhea in childhood: prevalence, pathophysiology, and outcome. N Engl J Med 1990; 322: 1357–1363.

32 Programme for Control of Diarrhoeal Diseases: Ninth Programme Report 1992–1993. Geneva: WHO/CDD/94.46, 1994: 1–107.

33 Baker S J, Mathan V I. Tropical enteropathy and tropical sprue. Am J Clin Nutr 1972; 25: 1047–1055.

34 Lunn P G, Northrop Clewes C A, Downes R M. Intestinal permeability, mucosal injury, and growth faltering in Gambian infants. Lancet 1991; 338: 907–910.

35 Victora C G, Huttly S R A, Fuchs S C et al. International differences in clinical patterns of diarrhoeal deaths: a comparison of children from Brazil, Senegal, Bangladesh, and India. J Diarrhoeal Dis Res 1993; 11: 25–29.

36 Black R E. Persistent diarrhea in children in developing countries. Pediatr Infect Dis J 1993; 12: 751–761.

37 Schorling J B, Wanke C A, Schorling S K, McAuliffe J F, de Souza M A, Guerrant R L. A prospective study of persistent diarrhea among children in an urban Brazilian slum: patterns of occurrence and etiologic agents. Am J Epid 1990; 132: 144–156.

38 Bhandari N, Bhan M K, Sazawal S. Mortality associated with acute watery diarrhea, dysentery and persistent diarrhea in rural north India. Acta Paediatr 1992; 81 (Suppl 381): 3–6.

39 Lima A A, Guerrant R L. Persistent diarrhea in children: epidemiology, risk factors, pathophysiology, nutritional impact, and management. Epidemiol Rev 1992; 14: 222–242.

40 Esrey S A, Potash J B, Roberts L, Shiff C. Effects of improved water supply and sanitation on ascariasis, diarrhoea, dracunculiasis, hookworm infection, schistosomiasis, and trachoma. Bull World Health Org 1991; 69: 609–621.

41 Briend A. Is diarrhoea a major cause of malnutrition among the under-fives in developing countries? A review of available evidence. Eur J Clin Nutr 1990; 44: 611–628.

42 Marsh K. Malaria: a neglected disease? Parasitology 1992; 104 (Suppl): S53–S69.

43 Greenwood B M, Marsh K, Snow R W. Why do some African children develop severe malaria? Parasitology Today 1991; 7: 277–281.

44 Beadle C, Long G W, Weiss W R et al. Diagnosis of malaria by detection of Plasmodium falciparum HRP-2 antigen with a rapid dipstick antigen-capture assay. Lancet 1993; 343: 564–568.

45 Hill A V, Allsopp C E, Kwiatkowski D et al. Common west African HLA antigens are associated with protection from severe malaria. Nature 1991; 352: 595–600.

46 Alonso P L, Smith T, Armstrong Schellenberg J R M et al. Randomised trial of SPf66 vaccine against Plasmodium falciparum malaria in children in southern Tanzania. Lancet 1994; 344: 1175–1181.

47 Grau G E, de Kossodo S, Clark I A et al. Pathophysiology of cerebral malaria. Parasitology Today 1994; 10: 408–414.

48 Newton C R, Peshu N, Kendall B et al. Brain swelling and ischaemia in Kenyans with cerebral malaria. Arch Dis Child 1994; 70: 281–287.

49 Newton C R, Kirkham F J, Winstanley P A et al. Intracranial pressure in African children with cerebral malaria. Lancet 1991; 337: 573–576.

50 Gordeuk V, Thuma P, Brittenham G et al. Effect of iron chelation therapy on recovery from deep coma in children with cerebral malaria. N Engl J Med 1992; 327: 1473–1477.

51 Akpede G O, Sykes R M. Malaria with bacteraemia in acutely febrile preschool children without localizing signs: coincidence or association/complication? J Trop Med Hyg 1993; 96: 146–150.

52 Lepage P, Bogaerts J, van Goethem C et al. Community-acquired bacteraemia in African children. Lancet 1987; i: 1458–1461.

53 Mahle W T, Levine M M. Salmonella typhi infection in children younger than five years of age. Pediatr Infect Dis J 1993; 12: 627–631.

54 Baraff L J, Lee S I, Schriger D L. Outcomes of bacterial meningitis in children: a meta-analysis. Pediatr Infect Dis J 1993; 12: 389–393.

55 Salih M A. Childhood acute bacterial meningitis in the Sudan: an epidemiological, clinical and laboratory study. Scand J Infect Dis Suppl 1990; 66: 1–103.

56 Akpede G O, Sykes R M. Convulsions with fever as a presenting feature of bacterial

meningitis among preschool children in developing countries. Dev Med Child Neurol 1992; 34: 524–529.

57 Cuevas L E, Hart C A, Mughogho G. Latex particle agglutination tests as an adjunct to the diagnosis of bacterial meningitis: a study from Malawi. Ann Trop Med Parasitol 1989; 83: 375–379.

58 Shann F, Barker J, Poore P. Chloramphenicol alone versus chloramphenicol plus penicillin for bacterial meningitis in children. Lancet 1985; ii: 681–685.

59 Shann F, Linnemann V, Mackenzie A, Barker J, Gratten M, Crinis M. Absorption of chloramphenicol sodium succinate after intramuscular administration in children. N Engl J Med 1985; 7: 410–414.

60 Greenwood B M. Selective primary health care: strategies for control of disease in the developing world. XIII. Acute bacterial meningitis. Rev Infect Dis 1984; 6: 374–389.

61 Alam N H, Bardhan P K, Haider R, Malahanabis D. Trimethoprim-sulphamethoxazole in the treatment of persistent diarrhoea: a double-blind placebo-controlled trial. Arch Dis Child 1995; 72: 483–486.

62 D'Alessandro U, Leach A, Drakely C J et al. Efficacy trial of malaria vaccine SPf66 in Gambian infants. Lancet 1995; 346: 462–467.

63 Marsh K, Forster D, Wariuri C et al. Indicators of life-threatening malaria in African children. N Engl J Med 1995; 332: 1399–1404.

ANTIMICROBIAL AGENTS

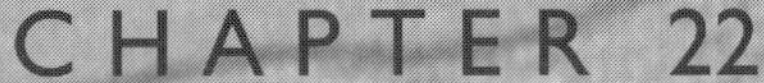

22.1. Antimicrobial agents, incorporating tables of doses of common antimicrobial agents

22.1 Antimicrobial agents, incorporating tables of doses of common antimicrobial agents

The choice of an appropriate antimicrobial agent is dependent upon many factors which should be considered by the attending physician. These factors include:

1. The disease itself — the natural history, likely aetiology or aetiologies, severity of illness, historical and/or published experience with a particular antimicrobial or group of antimicrobials.
2. The causative organism, if known — predictable antimicrobial resistance, local antimicrobial resistance patterns, new developments in antimicrobial resistance, site of infection, historical or published experience with the antimicrobial against the organism.
3. Suitability of the antimicrobial for the site of the infection — different antibiotics with similar spectrum of antimicrobial activity may have very different pharmacokinetics restricting their use in some infections, e.g. different cephalosporins, even those of the same 'generation', have differing penetration into the cerebrospinal fluid, affecting their suitability for the treatment of meningitis.
4. Individual patient factors — known or suspected allergic reactions, concurrent illnesses, coexisting system impairment, e.g. impaired renal or hepatic function, presence of organic central nervous system disease.
5. Concurrent or previous drugs — known or suspected drug interactions and side-effects.
6. Degree of immune suppression of the patient.
7. Appropriate route of delivery of an antimicrobial agent — appropriateness of oral therapy versus the various forms of parenteral delivery for the patient and the severity of illness.
8. Side-effects of the antimicrobial chosen — all antimicrobials have side-effects of varying acceptability and severity. The clinical circumstances, and individual patient and the family must be considered.
9. Need to monitor drug concentration — if monitoring is required, usually to ensure a therapeutic concentration is reached or minimize toxicity, then the practical availability, and cost, of drug monitoring needs to be considered.
10. Cost of the antimicrobial — either to the issuing organization or to the patient, which may depend upon the indication for which the antimicrobial is being prescribed.
11. Availability of the antimicrobial — which is dependent upon the national formulary and restrictions, and local antimicrobial policies.
12. Local physician experience and acceptance by the general public of a particular antimicrobial.

The choice of agent, and choice of regimen, in paediatric practice involves additional factors:

1. Does the antimicrobial have real or potential side-effects peculiar to the paediatric age group?
2. Is the route of delivery acceptable, and practical, for the patient and for the person administering the chosen agent?
3. Are any of the potential side-effects going to interfere with effective delivery of the antimicrobial agent, or even cause the person administering the agent to cease giving the treatment?
4. Is the calculated dose reasonable in view of the usual adult dose? For some antimicrobials the paediatric daily dose when calculated purely as a drug dose per weight conversion becomes disproportionately excessive when compared to the usual adult daily dose if relative body weights are considered, and toxicity from the antimicrobial is a real risk. Do not exceed the daily adult dose.

The table of common antimicrobial agents in this chapter is a guide only. In all circumstances the antimicrobial agents listed, and the suggested dosages, must be considered with regard to local experience and prescribing regulations, found in various local prescribing guides, national formularies, and packaging information inserts. The prescriber is therefore advised to check all dosages carefully. Not all the antimicrobials listed have been approved for use, and particularly paediatric use, in all countries. Seeking local advice from medical microbiologists or infectious diseases physicians is strongly advised.

There is insufficient space for the table of doses to include all information for the correct prescription and administration of agents. A brief summary of the antimicrobial agent groups is given for each section, with mention of some of the more common side-effects, and some of the more common or most important drug interactions. Additionally, some individual antibiotics have specific comments listed that may be useful. However, this table cannot be considered the definitive guide to antimicrobial prescribing. There is much more about each anti-microbial agent that the prescribing physician needs to know than can be included here, and the package insert information, approved product information and local and national formularies should be consulted.

Although great care has been taken with the final information supplied, and presentation, prescribing information and recommendations, errors may have occurred which have not been detected in the final format. Also prescribing information, recommendations, precautions and contraindications will change as medical knowledge and experience continue to advance.

Table 22.1.1   Table of doses of common antimicrobial agents

Please note that the table of common antimicrobials is not suitable for calculating the dosage of antimicrobials for newborns and infants less than 3 months of age. Due to the different pharmacokinetics in this age group, specialized advice regarding doses in the newborn group should be sought.

Penicillins

The penicillins are widely used β-lactam antibiotics. Generally they are relatively safe except for their most important side-effect of hypersensitivity, which can manifest in various clinical reactions, the most severe of which is anaphylactic shock. The prescribing physician should always carefully enquire into the past drug history and reactions. Encephalopathy has occurred with the use of some penicillins, usually in association with very high doses, or high doses in renal failure. Penicillins should not be administered intrathecally. Other adverse effects have been described and usually affect the renal, hepatic, gastrointestinal and haematological systems. The penicillins have varying susceptibilities to β-lactamases, of which there are many types. Some of the penicillins, e.g. amoxycillin, ticarcillin and piperacillin, have been formulated in combination with β-lactamase inhibitors to expand their spectrum of antibacterial activity. Some brief notes are provided here but the physician is advised to seek more detailed information regarding specific bacteria. Some organisms such as *Neisseria gonorrhoeae* have varying susceptibility to the penicillins, which may be geographically relatively specific. Other bacteria which were uniformly susceptible to the penicillins have developed strains with increasing resistance to penicillins, and often other antimicrobial agents as well which must be monitored with care and prescribing practices modified appropriately if these organisms are suspected. These bacteria include *Streptococcus pneumoniae*, *Neisseria meningitidis* and several *Enterococcus* species. If these strains are suspected or diagnosed, it would be advisable to seek advice regarding therapy. None of the penicillins have reliable clinical activity against methicillin-resistant *Staphylococcus aureus* (MRSA) or methicillin-resistant coagulase-negative staphylococci.

Antimicrobial	Route	Usual dose (mild to moderate infection)	Maximal dose (severe infection)	Usual daily maximal adult dose	Comments
Ampicillin	p.o., i.m., i.v.	50–100 mg/kg per day divided into four doses	200–300 mg/kg per day divided into four to six doses	12 g	Some Gram-positive and Gram-negative activity, but inactivated by common β-lactamases. NB: Maculopapular rashes common in glandular fever, lymphocytic leukaemia, some drugs, and human immuno-deficiency virus infection.
Amoxycillin	p.o., i.m., i.v.	25–50 mg/kg per day divided into three doses	100–300 mg/kg per day divided into three to four doses	6–12 g	As above for ampicillin. Better oral absorption than ampicillin.
Amoxycillin/ Clavulanic acid N.B: Dose calculated on amoxycillin component	p.o., i.v.	25–50 mg/kg per day divided into three doses	100 mg/kg per day divided into four doses	4 g	Amoxycillin combined with the β-lactamase inhibitor clavulanic acid to extend spectrum. See notes above for ampicillin and amoxycillin. NB: Cholestatic hepatitis reported.
Benzylpenicillin (Penicillin G, crystalline)	i.m., i.v.	60–120 mg/kg per day (100 000–200 000 U) divided into four doses	180–300 mg/kg per day (300 000–500 000 U) divided into four to six doses	14.4 g (24 million U)	Narrow spectrum, mainly against Gram-positive organisms, but still treatment of choice for many infections. Inactivated by common β-lactamases.
Phenoxymethyl penicillin (Penicillin V)	p.o.	25–50 mg/kg per day divided into three to four doses	Not appropriate	1–2 g	Similar spectrum to, but less active than, benzylpenicillin (penicillin G). NB: Oral absorption is variable, therefore phenoxymethyl-penicillin should not be used for serious infections.
Procaine penicillin	i.m. only	25–50 mg/kg per day (25 000–50 000 U) once daily or divided into two doses	Not appropriate	2.4–4.8 g	Formulation of benzylpenicillin (penicillin G) with procaine. NB: Contraindicated in procaine allergy.
(Flu)cloxacillin	p.o., i.m., i.v.	50–100 mg/kg per day divided into four doses	150–200 mg/kg per day divided into four to six doses	12 g	Antistaphylococcal penicillins not inactivated by staphylococcal penicillinase. Flucloxacillin has more reliable oral absorption. Similar doses are used for oxacillin and nafcillin; check product information. NB: Hepatitis and cholestatic jaundice have been reported with flucloxacillin.
Piperacillin	i.m., i.v.	100–150 mg/kg per day divided into four to six doses	200–300 mg/kg per day divided into four to six doses	18–24 g	Antipseudomonal penicillin with broader anti-Gram-negative spectrum compared with ampicillin. NB: Note sodium content, especially in high doses.

Antimicrobial	Route	Usual dose (mild to moderate infection)	Maximal dose (severe infection)	Usual daily maximal adult dose	Comments
Ticarcillin	i.v.	100–200 mg/kg per day divided into four to six doses	200–300 mg/kg per day divided into four to six doses	24 g	As above for piperacillin. Doses up to 400 mg/kg per day i.v. divided into six doses have been recommended for cystic fibrosis.
Ticarcillin/ Clavulanic acid NB: Dose calculated on ticarcillin component	i.v.	100–200 mg/kg per day divided into four to six doses	200–300 mg/kg per day divided into four to six doses	18 g	Ticarcillin combined with the β-lactamase inhibitor clavulanic acid to extend spectrum. NB: Cholestatic hepatitis reported with amoxycillin–clavulanic acid.

Cephalosporins and related β-lactams

The cephalosporins are also widely used β-lactam antibiotics and also are considered relatively safe except for their most serious side-effect of hypersensitivity. Estimates vary, but about 3–10% of patients hypersensitive to penicillins will also exhibit cross-reacting allergy to the cephalosporins, emphasizing the need for a careful history of drug reactions. Effects on blood coagulation, due to a variety of mechanisms, have been noted with several cephalosporins. Other adverse effects are similar to those of the penicillins as well. The different cephalosporins have varying susceptibilities to different β-lactamases. This is broadly represented by the groups or 'generation' they are divided into. First-generation cephalosporins, as a group, have more anti-Gram-positive activity than the second generation, which has more than the third. Conversely, the higher number correlates with increased anti-Gram-negative activity, as resistance to β-lactamase increases. However, within a generation, the antimicrobial activity of individual agents may vary quite significantly clinically, so it must not be assumed that all the cephalosporins within a generation are interchangeable. This also applies when considering the different pharmacokinetics of agents. None of the cephalosporins have yet been found to be clinically effective against enterococci, MRSA or methicillin-resistant coagulase-negative staphylococci. Some of the Enterobacteriaceae and other Gram-negative bacilli produce 'inducible' β-lactamase and resistance to the cephalosporin may develop during therapy. More recently some strains of Enterobacteriaceae, especially *Klebsiella* species and *Escherichia coli*, have developed 'extended spectrum' β-lactamases, making them resistant to the third-generation cephalosporins. Parallel to the development of resistance to penicillin, some strains of *Streptococcus pneumoniae* have also developed resistance to cefotaxime. Seek advice regarding optimal therapy for infections caused by highly resistant bacteria. The anti-anaerobic activity of different cephalosporins is variable.

Aztreonam is a monocyclic β-lactam, or 'monobactam'. It is similar to the cephalosporins but due to its different structure, the incidence of cross-reacting allergy in patients hypersensitive to the penicillins is thought to be less. It has broad anti-Gram-negative activity against 'aerobes', including against *Pseudomonas aeruginosa*, but it is not active against Gram-positive bacteria or anaerobes. Some of the strains of Gram-negative bacilli with increasing resistance to the cephalosporins also have increased resistance to aztreonam.

Imipenem is a carbapenem β-lactam. It is formulated with cilastatin, a dipeptidase inhibitor, to prevent its renal metabolism. Hypersensitivity is again an important side-effect, and it is important to ascertain whether there is any patient history of hypersensitivity to either the penicillins or cephalosporins. Another important side-effect is neurotoxicity, including seizures, which has an increased incidence at higher doses, in renal failure, and in pre-existing central nervous system disorders. Imipenem has a very broad spectrum of activity against both many Gram-negative and Gram-positive microorganisms, including anaerobes. It does not have reliable clinical activity against MRSA or methicillin-resistant coagulase-negative staphylococci.

Antimicrobial	Route	Usual dose (mild to moderate infection)	Maximal dose (severe infection)	Usual daily maximal adult dose	Comments
Cefaclor (second generation)	p.o.	20–50 mg/kg per day divided into two to four doses	Inappropriate	1.5–2 g	Activity against *Haemophilus influenzae*. NB: Serum sickness-like reactions have been reported.
Cefotaxime (third generation)	i.m., i.v.	100–150 mg/kg per day divided into three to four doses	150–225 mg/kg per day divided into three to four doses	6–12 g	Used for the therapy of meningitis.

Antimicrobial	Route	Usual dose (mild to moderate infection)	Maximal dose (severe infection)	Usual daily maximal adult dose	Comments
Cefoxitin (second generation, a cephamycin)	i.m., i.v.	50–100 mg/kg per day divided into three to four doses	80–160 mg/kg per day divided into four doses	12 g	Clinically significant activity against anaerobes.
Ceftazidime (third generation)	i.v.	75–100 mg/kg per day divided into three doses	100–150 mg/kg per day divided into three doses	6 g	Clinically significant activity against *Pseudomonas*.
Ceftriaxone (third generation)	i.m., i.v.	50–75 mg/kg given once daily or divided into two doses	80–100 mg/kg given once daily or divided into two doses	2–4 g	Used for the therapy of meningitis. Long half-life. NB: (1) Precipitates of calcium ceftriaxone, which may be symptomatic or mistaken for gallstones, may form in the gall-bladder. NB: (2) May displace bilirubin from serum albumin, therefore some authorities advise that it not be used in neonates.
Cefuroxime axetil (second generation)	p.o.	30–40 mg/kg per day divided into three doses OR 125 mg twice daily (up to 250 mg twice daily if over 2 years of age if necessary in otitis media)	Inappropriate	1 g	
Cefuroxime (second generation)	i.m., i.v.	60–100 mg/kg per day divided into three to four doses	100–240 mg/kg per day divided into three to four doses	6 g	Highest doses of 200–240 mg/kg per day are used in meningitis. Cefotaxime or ceftriaxone are more active in the cerebrospinal fluid, therefore use of cefuroxime for meningitis is decreasing.
Cephalexin (first generation)	p.o.	25–50 mg/kg per day divided into four doses	Not appropriate	4 g	Doses of up to 75–100 mg/kg per day have been recommended for therapy of otitis media.
Cephalothin (first generation)	i.m., i.v.	40–100 mg/kg per day divided into four doses	100–160 mg/kg per day divided into four to six doses	12 g	
Cephamandole (second generation)	i.m., i.v.	50–100 mg/kg per day divided into three to four doses	100–150 mg/kg per day divided into four to six doses	12 g	Anti-Gram-positive activity similar to first-generation cephalosporins.
Cephazolin (first generation)	i.m., i.v.	25–50 mg/kg per day divided into three to four doses	100 mg/kg per day divided into four doses	6 g	
Aztreonam (monobactam)	i.v.	90 mg/kg per day divided into three doses	120 mg/kg per day divided into four doses	8 g	For severe infections in patients 2 years of age or older, up to 200 mg/kg per day divided into four doses has been recommended.
Imipenem/ cilastatin NB: Dose calculated on imipenem content	i.v.	Does not apply	60 mg/kg per day divided into four doses	2–4 g	

Aminoglycosides

The most important side-effects of the aminoglycosides are ototoxicity and nephrotoxicity. Other side-effects include neuromuscular blockade. Toxicity is often dose related, including duration of therapy and repeated courses of aminoglycosides, and is aggravated by pre-existing renal impairment. Serum/plasma levels should be monitored. Twice-daily and single-daily dosing regimens are available for use in adults but there is limited experience in paediatric patients at this stage. Amikacin, gentamicin, netilmicin and tobramycin are active against a wide spectrum of aerobic Gram-negative bacteria, including *Pseudomonas aeruginosa*, and some Gram-positive organisms, but are inactive against anaerobes. Activity against streptococci and enterococci is poor, but the aminoglycosides are used in endocarditis regimens for their synergistic effect with other antimicrobial agents. Recently some strains of enterococci have developed high-level resistance to the aminoglycosides, limiting therapeutic options in severe infections such as endocarditis.

Antimicrobial	Route	Usual dose (mild to moderate infection)	Maximal dose (severe infection)	Usual daily maximal adult dose	Comments
Amikacin	i.m., i.v.	Usually not appropriate	15–22.5 mg/kg per day divided into two to three doses	15 mg/kg per day (maximum 1.5 g per day)	Most stable of the aminoglycosides to inactivating enzymes.
Gentamicin	i.m., i.v.	Usually not appropriate	3–7.5 mg/kg per day divided into three doses	3–5 mg/kg per day	The higher-range mg/kg per day dosage recommendations generally are for the younger age group. For patients aged 10–12 years or older consider using the lower range doses as for adults.
Netilmicin	i.m, i.v.	Usually not appropriate	4–7.5 mg/kg per day divided into three doses	4–7.5 mg/kg per day	
Tobramycin	i.m., i.v.	Usually not appropriate	3–7.5 mg/kg per day divided into three doses	3–5 mg/kg per day	

Clindamycin and macrolides

Clindamycin is a lincosamide antibiotic but is often grouped with the macrolides, as here, because of the many similarities between the two groups. Clindamycin has a wide variety of side-effects affecting the gastrointestinal system, most notably antibiotic-associated diarrhoea, including pseudomembranous colitis. It has activity against many Gram-positive aerobes, and a wide spectrum of anaerobes, both Gram-positive and Gram-negative.

The macrolides have a wide variety of side-effects, most frequently affecting the gastrointestinal system, but others include adverse hepatic reactions, hearing loss and cardiotoxicity. Drug interactions must be checked for the macrolides, including some combinations that have been associated with hazardous arrhythmias. Their antimicrobial spectrum includes some Gram-positive aerobes, some Gram-negative aerobes, some anaerobes, and many of the more 'unusual' bacteria such as *Bordetella*, *Chlamydia*, *Legionella* and some mycoplasmas. The newer agents generally have fewer gastrointestinal side-effects than erythromycin. For the newer agents consult with a medical microbiologist or infectious diseases specialist for the appropriate dosages.

Antimicrobial	Route	Usual dose (mild to moderate infection)	Maximal dose (severe infection)	Usual daily maximal adult dose	Comments
Clindamycin	p.o., i.m., i.v.	15–25 mg/kg per day divided into three to four doses	25–40 mg/kg per day divided into three to four doses	2.7 g (even up to 4.8 g has been recommended)	NB: Some regimens recommend that in severe infections children be given no less than 300 mg per day regardless of weight.
Erythromycin	p.o, i.v.	20–50 mg/kg per day divided into three to four doses	25–50 mg/kg per day divided into four doses	4 g	NB: Very important to check product information for appropriate route of admini-stration and formulation used, as product recommendations vary according to formulation.

Antimicrobial	Route	Usual dose (mild to moderate infection)	Maximal dose (severe infection)	Usual daily maximal adult dose	Comments
Azithromycin	p.o.	Check local product advice	Check local product advice	500 mg	Greater activity against Gram-negative bacteria, especially *Haemophilus*, but reduced against some Gram positives.
Clarithromycin	p.o.	Check local product advice	Check local product advice	1 g	Spectrum of activity includes many mycobacteria, including *Mycobacterium avium-intracellulare*.
Roxithromycin	p.o.	Check local product advice	Check local product advice	300 mg	

Tetracyclines

The use of tetracyclines in paediatric patients is limited because they bind to calcium (see table). Gastrointestinal, dermatological and neurological side-effects also occur, among others, and tetracyclines may exacerbate renal failure. They have a broad spectrum of activity, including brucella, chlamydia, mycoplasma, rickettsiae and some of the spirochaetes.

Antimicrobial	Route	Usual dose (mild to moderate infection)	Maximal dose (severe infection)	Usual daily maximal adult dose	Comments
Tetracycline	p.o, i.v. (see comments)	20–50 mg/kg per day p.o. divided into four doses	For severe infection and intravenous administration check product information as product formulations and recommended dosages vary	2 g	NB: Contraindicated in young children, as tetracyclines are deposited in growing bones and teeth. Minimum recommended ages before tetracyclines should be used vary from over 8 years, to 12 years of age, therefore check local prescribing formulary. Can be used in patients with renal impairment.
Doxycycline	p.o.	2–4 mg/kg once daily or divided into two doses	Usually not appropriate	100–200 mg	NB: (1) See comment for tetracycline. NB: (2) Dose for the first day of therapy may be larger than for subsequent days, therefore see product information.

Nalidixic acid and quinolones

Nalidixic acid is mainly used for uncomplicated urinary tract infections. It has less antimicrobial activity than the newer agents. Ciprofloxacin is a fluoroquinolone with activity against a wide range of aerobic Gram-negative bacteria, including *Pseudomonas aeruginosa*, some Gram-positive bacteria, some of the more unusual bacteria and mycobacteria. It has little clinical anti-anaerobic activity. Due to the production of arthropathy in experimental immature animals ciprofloxacin is not recommended for use in prepubertal children. Side-effects include those afffecting the gastrointestinal and central nervous systems. Drug interactions must be reviewed before quinolones are prescribed.

Antimicrobial	Route	Usual dose (mild to moderate infection)	Maximal dose (severe infection)	Usual daily maximal adult dose	Comments
Nalidixic acid	p.o.	50 mg/kg per day divided into four doses reduced to 30 mg/kg per day divided into four doses for prolonged therapy	Not appropriate	2 g reduced to 1 g for prolonged therapy	NB: Not to be used in infants younger than 3 months of age.
Ciprofloxacin	p.o., i.v.	Not appropriate	Not recommended for use in children but has been used when benefits believed to outweigh risks. Seek advice from medical microbiologist or infectious diseases specialist	p.o.: 1.5 g i.v.: 400–600 mg	NB: Use with caution in epileptics and in patients with previous central nervous system disorders.

Other miscellaneous antibiotics

Chloramphenicol is a broad-spectrum antimicrobial agent with activity against both Gram-positive and Gram-negative bacteria, but not *Pseudomonas aeruginosa*, and some of the more unusual microorganisms, including rickettsiae. Its major side-effects include those on the haematological system, including bone marrow suppression, both idiosyncratic, irreversible, leading to aplastic anaemia, and a reversible dose-related type. It may cause 'grey syndrome' in neonates and levels should be monitored in neonates and young children.

Fusidate sodium/fusidic acid is a narrow-spectrum antimicrobial agent mainly used for staphylococcal infections, usually with another antibiotic to avoid the development of resistance. Gastrointestinal and hepatic side-effects, including jaundice, are amongst those described.

Metronidazole is a nitroimidazole antibiotic with activity against anaerobic bacteria, including *Clostridium difficile*, and some protozoa. Gastrointestinal, including a metallic taste, and neurological side-effects are among the adverse reactions described.

Nitrofurantoin is used in the treatment of urinary tract infections. It has a wide variety of side-effects, some of which can be life-threatening. It should not be used in patients with renal impairment or in neonates.

Rifampicin is mainly used for the treatment of tuberculosis and prophylaxis against invasive disease caused by *Haemophilus influenzae* type b and *Neisseria meningitidis*, but is also used in combination with other antibiotics in selected infections. Rifampicin has a number of different side-effects, including discoloration of urine, tears and other body secretions. Hepatic enzymes are induced, affecting the metabolism of many other drugs, therefore drug interactions must be checked before rifampicin is prescribed.

Sulphonamides have activity against both Gram-positive and Gram-negative aerobic bacteria. Side-effects affect many systems, including allergic skin and systemic reactions and haematological changes. They should not be used in newborns. Trimethoprim has mainly anti-Gram-negative activity. Side-effects of trimethoprim include skin reactions, haematological changes and gastrointestinal disturbances and it should also be avoided in neonates.

Vancomycin is a glycopeptide antibiotic with a spectrum of activity that is almost exclusively against Gram-positive bacteria, aerobic and anaerobic, including MRSA. Among its side-effects are nephrotoxicity and ototoxicity, and rapid intravenous infusion is associated with a range of adverse events, including erythroderma ('red man syndrome'), severe hypotension, even cardiac arrest. Serum/plasma levels should be monitored. Some strains of enterococci are now resistant to vancomycin.

Antimicrobial	Route	Usual dose (mild to moderate infection)	Maximal dose (severe infection)	Usual daily maximal adult dose	Comments
Chloramphenicol	p.o., i.v.	Not appropriate	50–100 mg/kg per day divided into four doses	2–4 g	NB: (1) If using 100 mg/kg per day dosage consider possibility of reducing dose when clinically indicated. NB: (2) Consider performing serum/plasma concentrations to modify dose to avoid toxicity.
Fusidate sodium	p.o, i.v.	Usually not appropriate	20–50 mg/kg per day according to particular preparation composition and age, divided into three doses. See product information for each formulation	1.5 g	NB: There are different dosage recommendations for formulations as sodium fusidate compared with formulations as fusidic acid.
Metronidazole	p.o., i.v.	For anaerobic bacterial infections: 22.5 mg/kg per day in three divided doses. For giardiasis there are various regimens: 15 mg/kg per day p.o. divided into three doses for 5 days OR 30 mg/kg per day (maximum 1.2 g) as a single daily dose for 3 days	For anaerobic bacterial infections: 22.5 mg/kg per day in three divided doses	For anaerobic bacterial infections: 1–1.5 g	
Nitrofurantoin	p.o.	5–7 mg/kg per day divided into four doses	Not appropriate	200–400 mg	Some regimens suggest a lower dose of 3 mg/kg per day in four divided doses. NB: Contraindicated in neonates and in renal failure.
Rifampicin (rifampin)	p.o., i.v.	Not appropriate. Doses for prophylaxis: *Haemophilus influenzae* type b — 20 mg/kg (maximum dose 600 mg per day) once daily p.o. for 4 days, i.e. a total of four doses. For neonates less than 1 month of age the suggested dose is 10 mg/kg once daily for 4 days. *Neisseria meningitidis* — 10 mg/kg (maximum dose 600 mg) every 12 h p.o. for 2 days, i.e. a total of 4 doses. For neonates less than 1 month of age the suggested dose is 5 mg/kg every 12 h p.o. for 2 days	10–20 mg/kg usually once daily	600 mg	Also used for *Haemophilus influenzae* type 'b' and *Neisseria meningitidis* prophylaxis. NB: Higher dosage usually only used for tuberculous meningitis.

Antimicrobial	Route	Usual dose (mild to moderate infection)	Maximal dose (severe infection)	Usual daily maximal adult dose	Comments
Sulphonamides		Numerous	Numerous		NB: See local product information for availability and dosages.
Sulphamethoxazole–trimethoprim (co-trimoxazole)	p.o., i.v.	20–40 mg/kg per day sulphamethoxazole — 4–8 mg/kg per day trimethoprim divided into two doses	100 mg/kg per day sulphamethoxazole — 20 mg/kg per day trimethoprim divided into four doses for *Pneumocystis carinii* pneumonia	1600 mg sulphamethoxazole — 320 mg trimethoprim for mild to moderate infection (not *P. carinii*)	NB: Contraindicated in babies less than 2 months of age due to risk of kernicterus.
Trimethoprim	p.o.	6–10 mg/kg once daily OR as per product information	not appropriate	300 mg	
Vancomycin	p.o. (see Comments), i.v.	For p.o.: for *Clostridium difficile* only: 20–40 mg/kg per day divided into four doses p.o. For i.v: usually not appropriate	For i.v. only: 40 mg/kg per day divided into four doses. Some i.v. regimens recommend a loading dose of 15 mg/kg i.v. initially. Up to 60 mg/kg per day i.v. has been recommended for central nervous system infection	For *C. difficile* only 500 mg — 2 g p.o. For iv: 2 g	NB: (1) Oral dosage is for *C. difficile* treatment only. Conversely do not use i.v. administration for this indication. NB: (2) Monitoring of serum/plasma levels advised. NB: (3) Slow i.v. infusion.

ACKNOWLEDGEMENTS

I would like to thank Dr R. Pritchard for his help and comments in the preparation of this chapter.

BIBLIOGRAPHY

American Academy of Pediatrics. Antimicrobials and related therapy: Tables of antibacterial drug dosages. In: Peter G, ed. 1994 Red book: Report of the Committee on Infectious Diseases, 23rd edn. Elk Grove Village, IL: American Academy of Pediatrics, 1994.

Badewitz-Dodd L H (ed.). 1994 MIMS Annual, Australian edition, 18th edn. Crows Nest, Sydney: MIMS Australia (MediMedia Australia), 1994.

British Medical Association and the Royal Pharmaceutical Society of Great Britain. British National Formulary. Prasad A B, ed. Number 28. London: Pharmaceutical Press, September 1994.

Kilham H (ed.). The children's hospital handbook. Royal Alexandra Hospital for Children, Camperdown, New South Wales: Alken, 1993.

Sanford J P, Gilbert D N, Gerberding J L, Sande M A (eds). The Sanford guide to antimicrobial therapy 1994. Dallas: Antimicrobial Therapy, 1994.

Shann F, Duncan A, Butt W, Henning R, South M, Tibballs J. Drug doses, 8th edn. Parkville: Intensive Care Unit Royal Children's Hospital, Parkville, Victoria, 1994.

Shlaes D M, Binczewski B, Rice L B. Emerging antimicrobial resistance and the immunocompromised host. Clin Infect Dis 1993; 17 (Suppl 2): S527–S536.

Victorian Drug Usage Advisory Committee (Antibiotic Guidelines Sub-Committee, Mashford M L, chairman). Antibiotic guidelines 1994/1995, 8th edn. North Melbourne: Victorian Medical Postgraduate Foundation, 1994.

Index